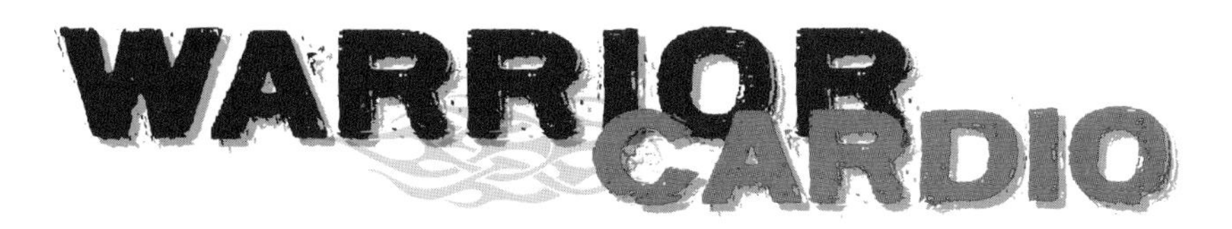
WARRIOR
CARDIO

THE REVOLUTIONARY METABOLIC TRAINING SYSTEM FOR BURNING FAT, BUILDING MUSCLE, AND GETTING FIT

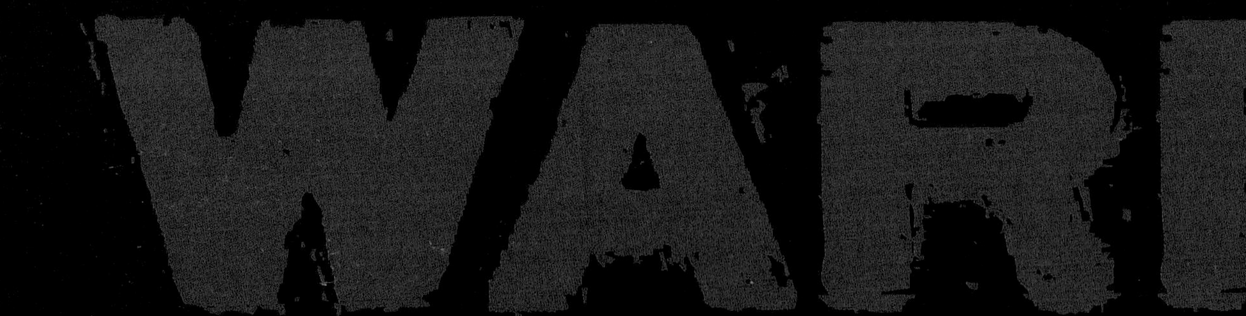

ALSO BY MARTIN ROONEY

Training for Warriors: The Ultimate Mixed Martial Arts Workout

Train to Win: 11 Principles of Athletic Success

Ultimate Warrior Workouts: Fitness Secrets of the Martial Arts

10R CARDIO

MARTIN ROONEY

wm

WILLIAM MORROW

An Imprint of HarperCollins*Publishers*

The information in this book has been carefully researched, and all efforts have been made to ensure accuracy. The author and the publisher assume no responsibility for any injuries suffered of damages or losses incurred during or as a result of following the exercise program or diet or supplement recommendations in this book. All of the procedures, poses, and postures should be carefully studied and clearly understood before attempting them at home. Always consult with your physician or qualified medical professional before beginning this or any diet and exercise program.

HarperCollins books may be purchased for educational, business, or sales promotional use. For information please write: Special Markets Department, HarperCollins Publishers, 10 East 53rd Street, New York, NY 10022.

FIRST EDITION

Designed by Renato Stanisic

Library of Congress Cataloging-in-Publication Data is available upon request.

ISBN 978-0-06-207428-7

12 13 14 15 16 OV/RRD 10 9 8 7 6 5 4 3 2 1

CONTENTS

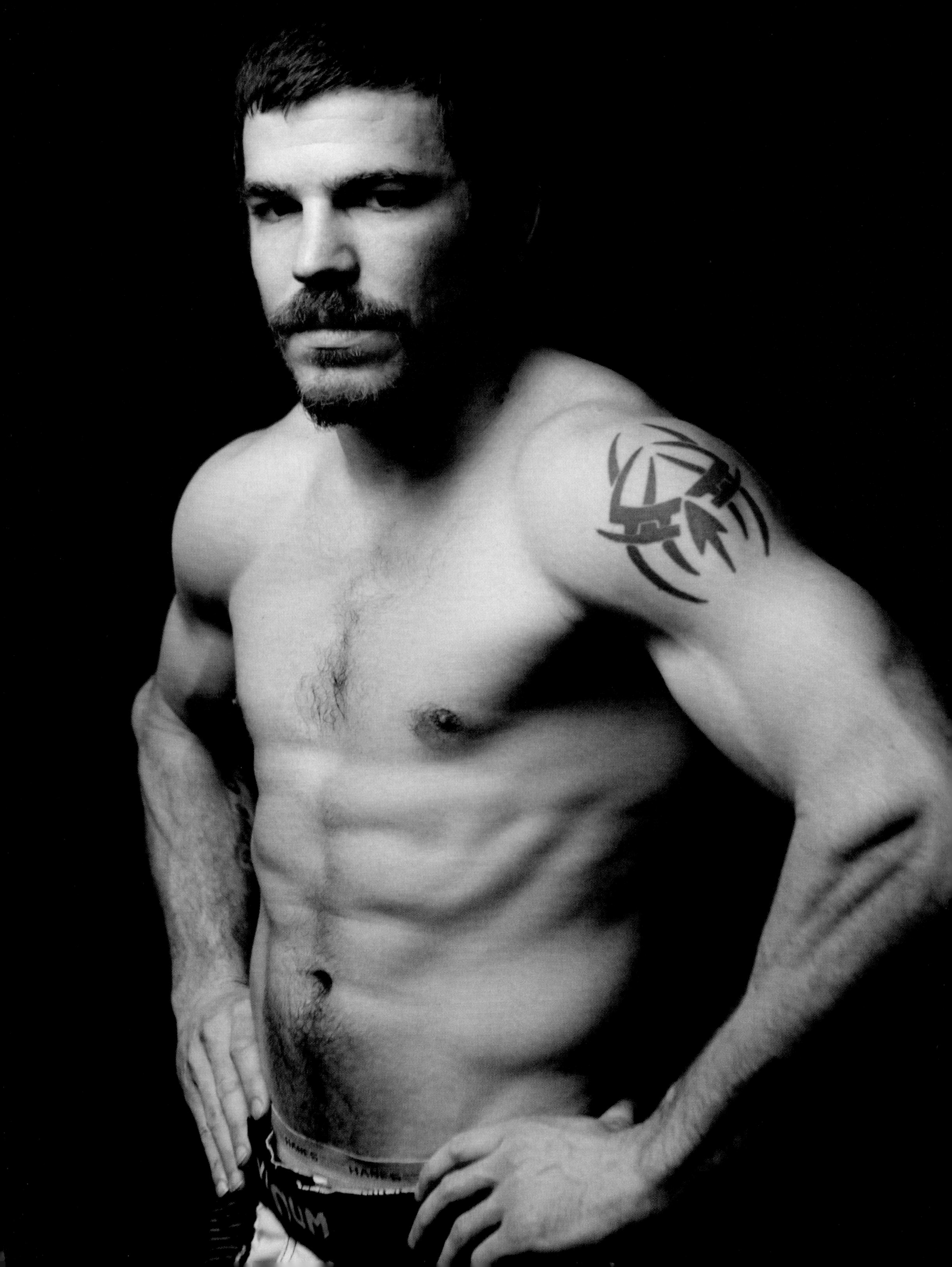

FOREWORD

The sport of Mixed Martial Arts has undergone a huge evolution since Royce Gracie won the first Ultimate Fighting Championships in 1993. To compete at the highest levels of MMA nowadays, a fighter must not only possess a high level of technical skill, but he must also be in top physical condition. He must place as much emphasis on becoming a world-class athlete as he does on perfecting his martial arts technique.

In April of 2008, I won a fight in the International Fight League that cemented me as a top local prospect on the brink of bigger fights against tougher opponents. At that time, Strength and Conditioning was the most neglected aspect of my training and I knew I would have to gain in size, strength, and endurance if I was to compete with the world's best lightweights. Backstage at that event, I met Martin Rooney and when he offered to train me and my brother Dan, we couldn't pass up the opportunity.

The initial sessions with Martin were not what I expected. I thought they were going to be the all-out, gut-busting sessions that I saw on TV with guys left half dead on the ground. I was actually disappointed when this was not what I received. My disappointment lessened as I started to get the one thing that I should have been more worried about: results. During the first year of our training with Martin, Dan and I made physical improvements, learned a lot about training, and fulfilled our dreams by being asked

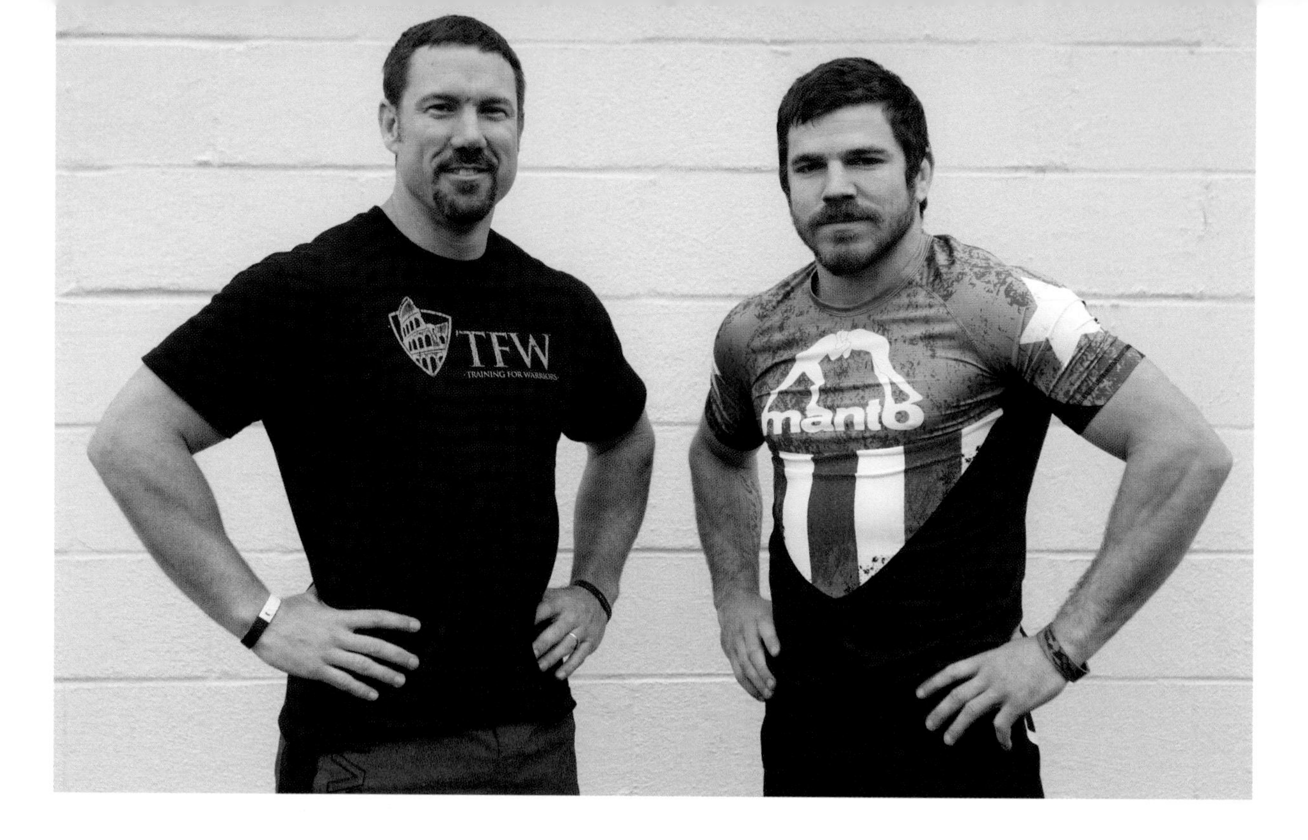

to fight in the UFC. As we signed our UFC contracts, we quit our construction jobs and went from hammering nails to pumping iron.

In the three years that I have been following the Training for Warriors system, I changed from that tough local-level fighter into a professional athlete. I have fought ten times for the UFC, going 9–1 over that span, and am currently ranked Top 10 in the world. I have not only been able to pack on 10 pounds of muscle and add hundreds of pounds to my lifts, but I have also stayed healthy. One secret to my success has been the design of Martin's training. I have taken Martin's philosophy and applied it to all other aspects of my fight preparation, from Brazilian Jiu Jitsu to Muay Thai to nutrition. We train hard, but we also train smart, which is an aspect that seems to be overlooked by many of my peers. MMA is becoming a worldwide sport, but it is surprising how few athletes really train like professionals. While the growing trend in MMA is fighters constantly getting hurt in training and pulling out of fights, I have become the fastest fighter to reach ten fights in UFC history.

The information in *Warrior Cardio* is professional training. As you will see in this book, the detailed warmups, speed training, strength training, endurance training, flexibility work, and nutrition are put together in a format that is easy to follow. *Warrior Cardio* will show you that Martin's approach to training is simple. If you train with him, Martin will help you get away from the current fads where everything has to be "extreme" and get back to the same movements that mankind has been doing for millennia. I have lived this training and reaped the benefits, and I have seen it consistently work with everyone else who has used it as well. Whether you are a fighter or not, I know you are going to benefit from the information contained in this book.

If you want to build strength, improve conditioning, lose fat, and/or gain muscle, *Warrior Cardio* will deliver results. I can say that with confidence because I know that it worked for me. Buy this book, live this system, and you will see results.

JIM MILLER
TOP RANKED UFC LIGHTWEIGHT
MAY 2011

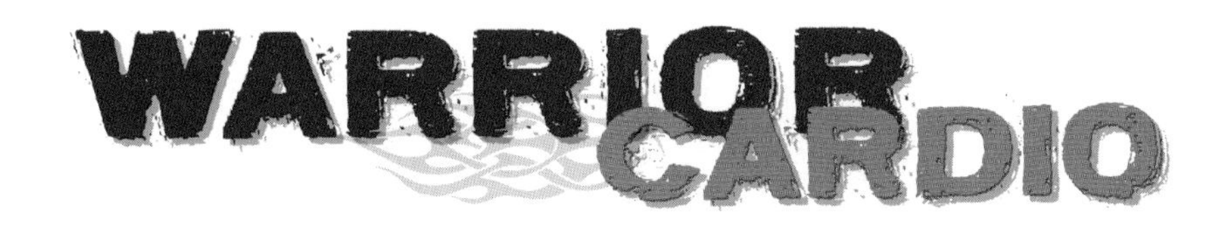
WARRIOR
CARDIO

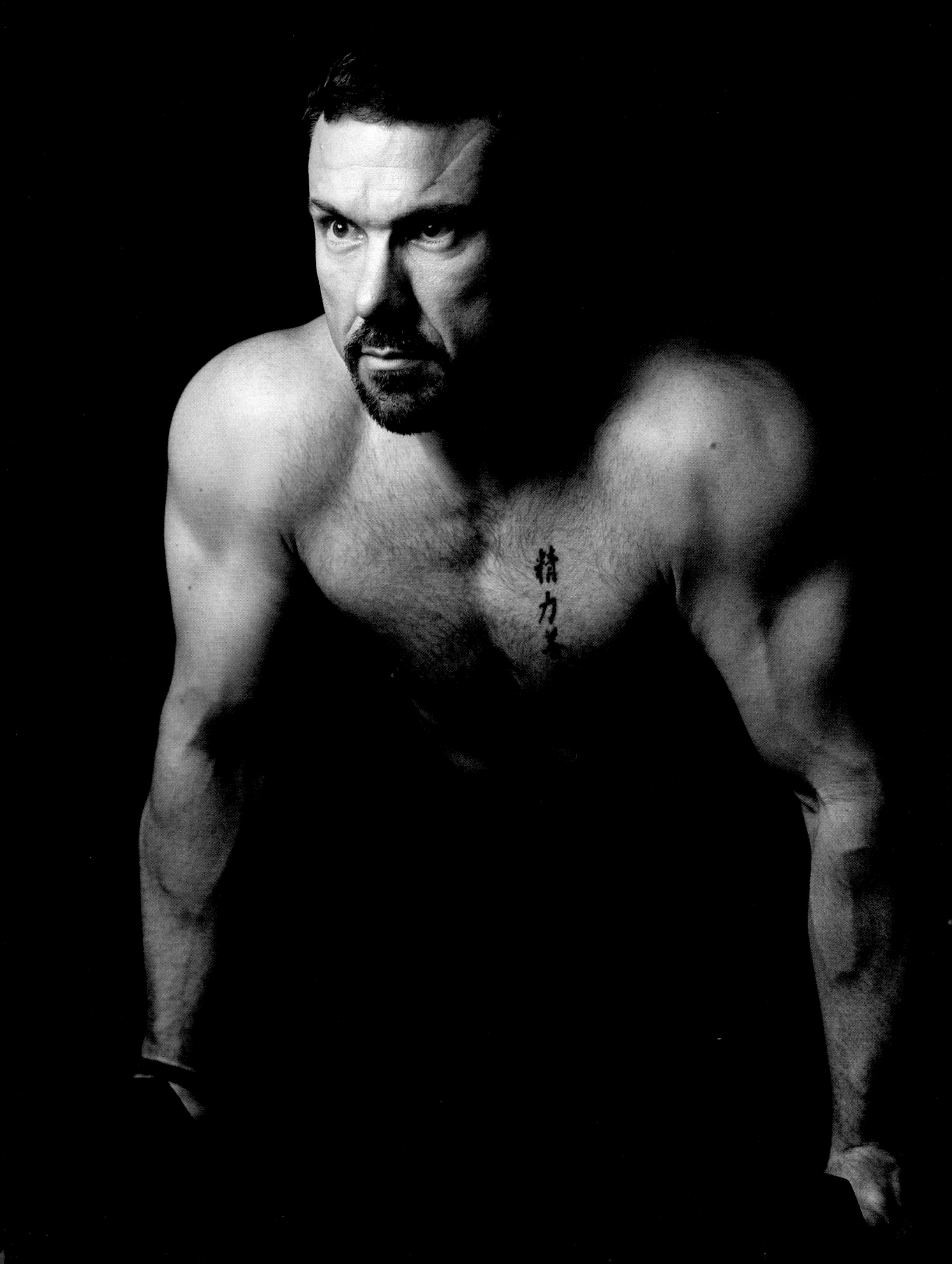

INTRODUCTION

From the dawn of man, we have recognized that an increase in energy expenditure leads to a faster heartbeat, an increase in body temperature, and a decrease in energy. Whether hunting for food, building a shelter, or covering some distance, our earliest ancestors had to be aware of the effects of this movement on their energy stores. As time has progressed and technology has improved, there has been an inverse relationship to the amount of energy expended for a given task. Today, we no longer have the daily mandatory physical demands that were once necessary for survival. As a result, energy expenditure has gone down, hard work has been experienced less often, and I believe that we have lost touch with the body's natural sense of response to exercise. Perhaps it could be said that we have lost touch with our "Warrior Within."

In the last 100 or so years, "fitness training" has become a necessity as a result of this decrease in workload. In the last 50 years especially, there has been a trend to replace the once mandatory physical demands with voluntary physical exercise to achieve the effects of caloric expenditure and health benefits that we know are essential to our health and longevity. In this same time period, there have been many interesting trends that have ultimately led to the current state of what is often referred to as "cardio" training. In the 1970s, Kenneth Cooper launched a concept of aerobics that got everyone doing something new: jogging. Following this movement, aerobics moved into the confined areas of gyms and fitness centers called "aerobics rooms." Since then, there has been an endless supply of gimmicks, gizmos, and gadgets designed to capture our imaginations just enough for us to ignore how contrived the exercises actually are. I say contrived because today, most "cardiovascular" activity is a far cry from the elementary movements and stressors for which the human body was designed. Most "cardio" training today is simply some kind of mildly interesting yet invented excuse to get someone to move around for about 30 minutes. Even today, complete sections of gyms are devoted to the glorified burning of calories on shiny treadmills and cycles designed more for look and feel than results. As the fitness trends moved from the gym to within the home, more and more contrived gadgets, topics, videos, and Internet programs were created to satisfy the never-ending need for modes of exercise. Since humans become quickly bored with every new contrived mode, there must be an endless supply of new gadgets, equipment, and ideas to keep pace.

Unfortunately, despite all of our shiny new equipment, statistics demonstrate that the world is not becoming more fit. Instead, we are getting increasingly obese and sedentary, even as the number one fitness request of most people is to lose fat. Why can't we get it right? I believe there are two reasons that are currently stopping us.

First, people and trainers select and prescribe exercises according to what I call the Illogical Four: Novelty, Coolness, Ability to Produce Soreness, and Ability to Produce Fatigue. What amazes me is that the veil of the Illogical Four has been pulled so strongly over our eyes that we no longer look for the reason why we started voluntary exercise in the first place: improvement in health and performance, a.k.a. results.

The first rule of the Training for Warriors system is that "We do not do something for nothing." Although it can be argued that many of the exercises contained in *Warrior Cardio* will satisfy the parameters of the Illogical Four, know that these are only a by-product in the pursuit of results. What makes this book different is that instead of just delivering the "how," I am also going to deliver the "why." By my outlining the exact science, readers can understand the purpose behind each exercise and avoid the haphazard approach that is currently plaguing physical training. My goal here is to, along with a team of the top professionals in the world, deliver the "new" science behind cardiovascular training and nutrition in a simple and condensed fashion. Once you are armed with the understanding of "why" this system produces results, you will be better engaged to apply the "how" to do it.

Secondly, I have noticed that a common excuse for people not to exercise or eat well is that they either don't know what to do or that things are too "complicated" for them to understand. Mastery is not about making something more complicated; it is about making complex things simple. The aim of this book is to give every warrior a simple format to follow. Once you have read *Warrior Cardio*, you can go to the gym and supermarket with a simple and quick list of things to execute that will give you the results you are looking for in the least amount of time. By the time you have finished this book, there will be no reason to doubt your level of competence for training again.

I will warn you: the training within this book is not easy. As I tell my fighters, nothing will ever replace hard work and practice. Warrior Cardio was created as I trained some of the greatest fighters on the planet.

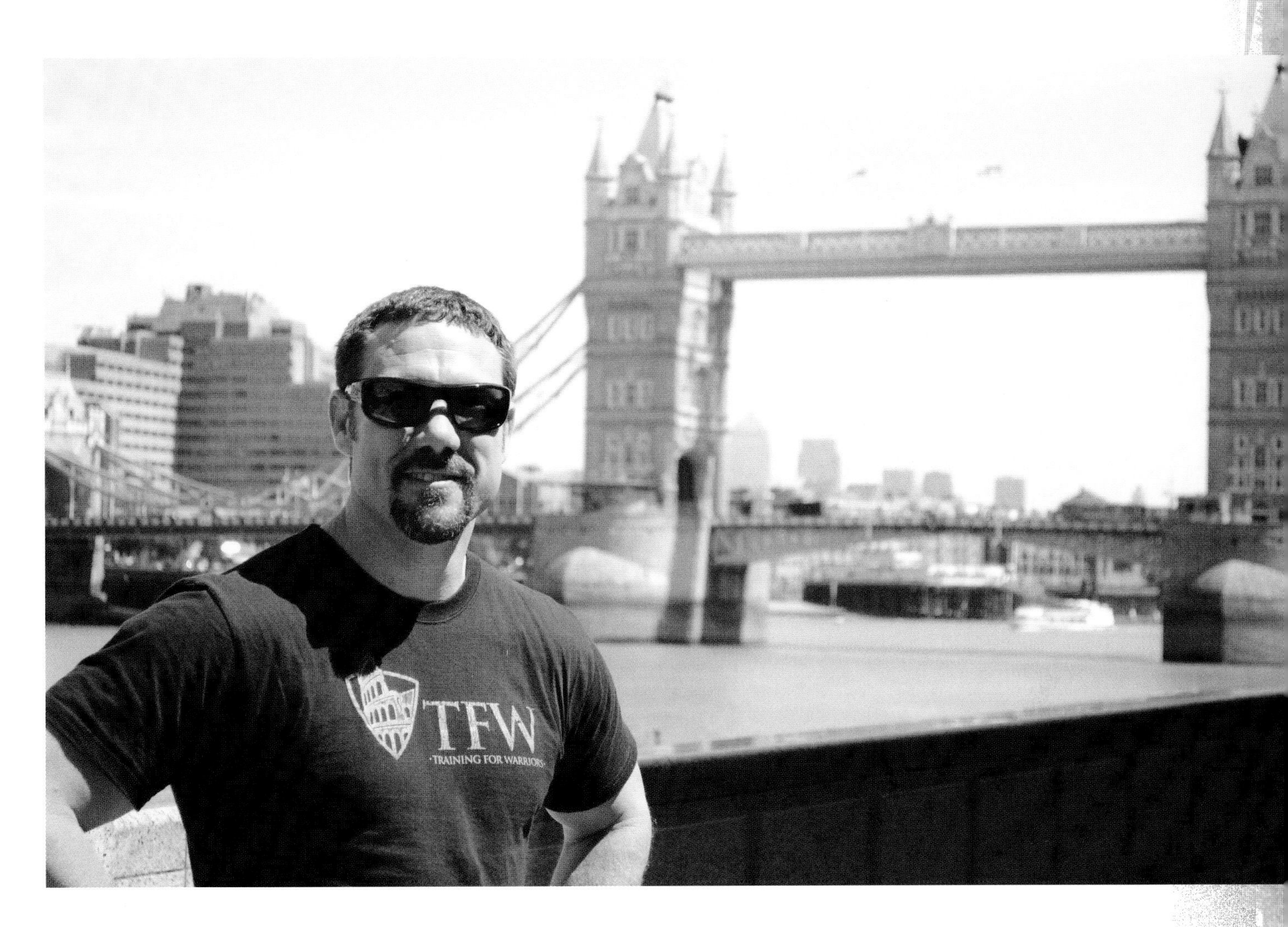

Although the original purpose was to best prepare my athletes for combat, I began to see that the fitness improvements, fat loss, and general well-being attained by my fighters was available to everyone. You do not have to be a fighter to train and look like one. Of course, I have also come to realize that we are, in some way, all warriors. Whether you need the energy to get through a stressful day of work, perform an athletic event, or play with your kids, we all face daily challenges to overcome.

When I polled people about what they wanted in this book, they asked for more science, more workouts, and more motivation. Within these pages, all of those requests are fulfilled. Using a vast amount of information and experience built with top athletes over the last 20 years, *Warrior Cardio* delivers a simple-to-follow program that can have anyone in the gym and working effectively. Everyone wants to build muscle and to burn fat. And nobody wants to waste time while trying to achieve these two goals. The world needs a solution. I believe that within this book, the solution can be found.

MARTIN ROONEY
THE QUEEN'S WALK
LONDON, ENGLAND
MAY 2011

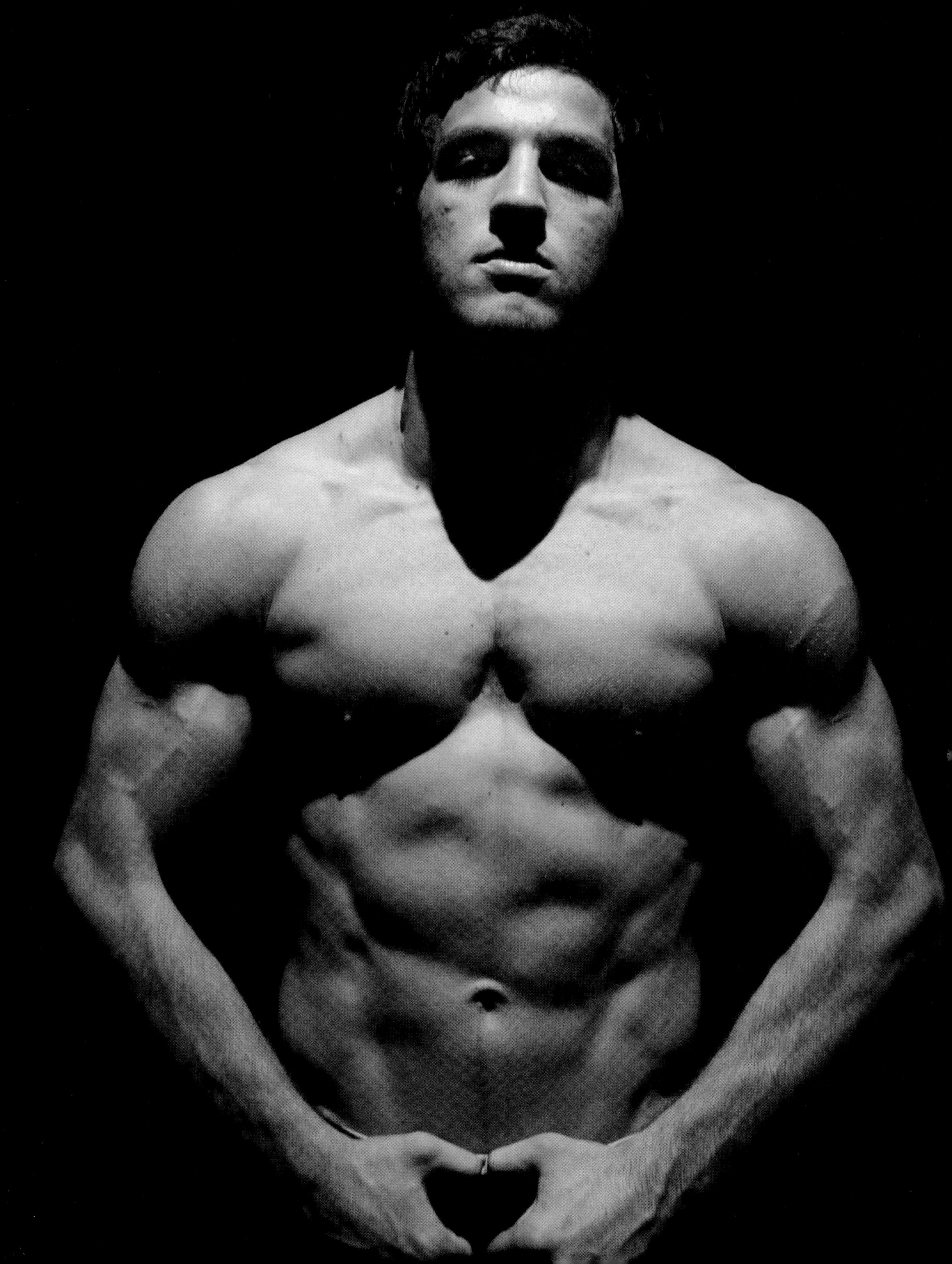

GETTING STARTED

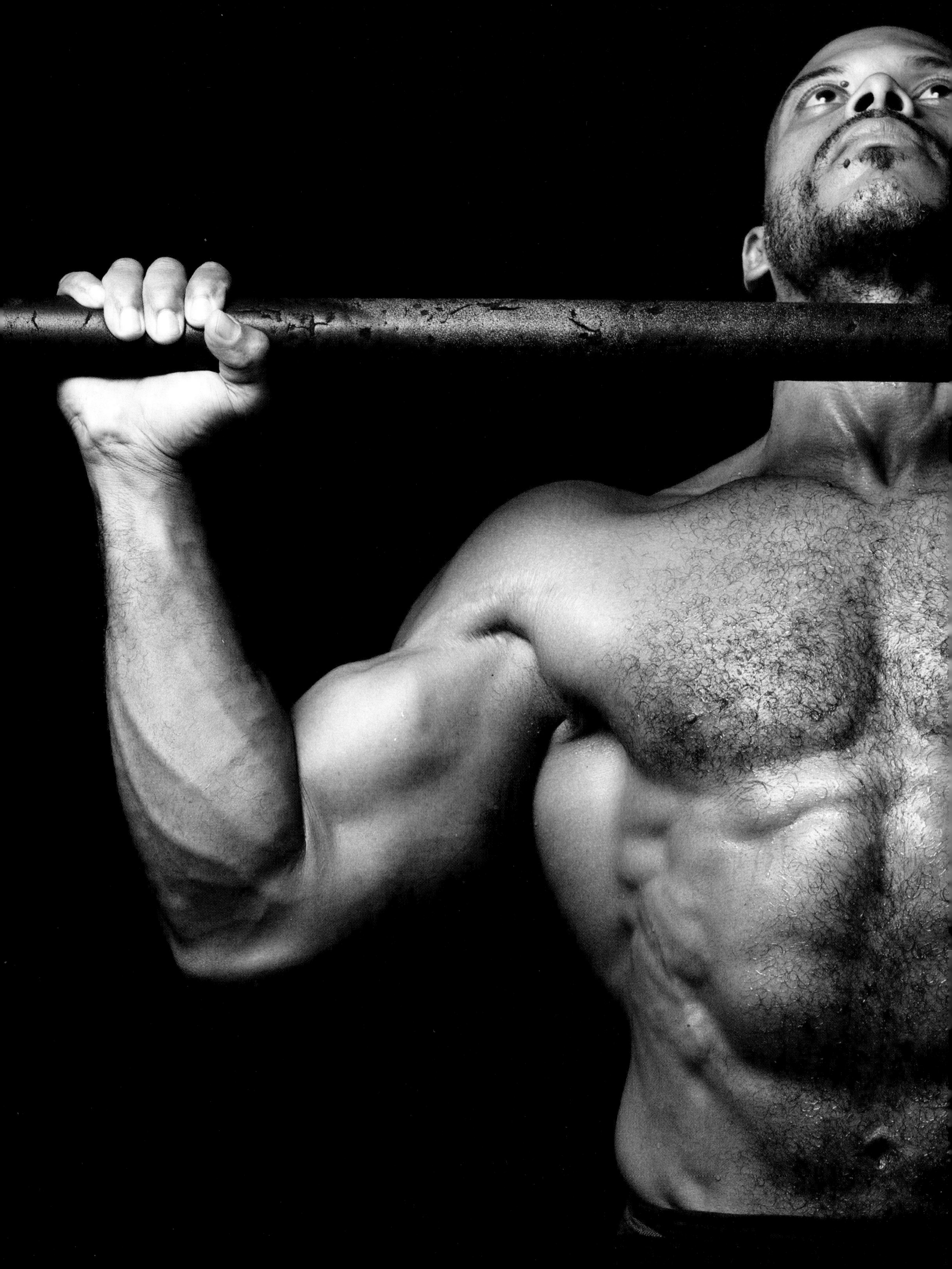

WHAT IS CARDIO ANYWAY?

"Cardio." It's a familiar word, especially if you're someone who exercises regularly. But do we all really understand what cardio is and how it works? Is it a 5-mile run or is it 30 minutes on the stationary bike? Can't cardio be improved by playing a game of pickup basketball or running some interval sprints, too? Once you start to realize that the concept of cardio is more nebulous than you might have originally imagined, it is easier to understand why people are having such a difficult time using this style of training to achieve results. Cardio, to answer the original question, is a term that refers to cardiovascular fitness, otherwise known as aerobic fitness. In the Training for Warriors system, Cardio is training focused on improving the capacity and efficiency of the cardiovascular system. Although you may think that training focused on cardiovascular benefits has been around for centuries, it actually only dates back to the onset of the 1970s fitness boom, which began with Dr. Kenneth Cooper's publication of a book entitled *Aerobics*. The fitness boom spawned many of today's biggest fitness-oriented corporations, including brands like Nike and Gatorade. Prior to that time, no one had ever heard of running shoes and sports drinks. You ran in your Converse Chuck Taylors or Red Ball Jets and drank water to rehydrate. Back then, the only time you ran was if you were trying to catch a bus or the coach made you do laps for being late to practice.

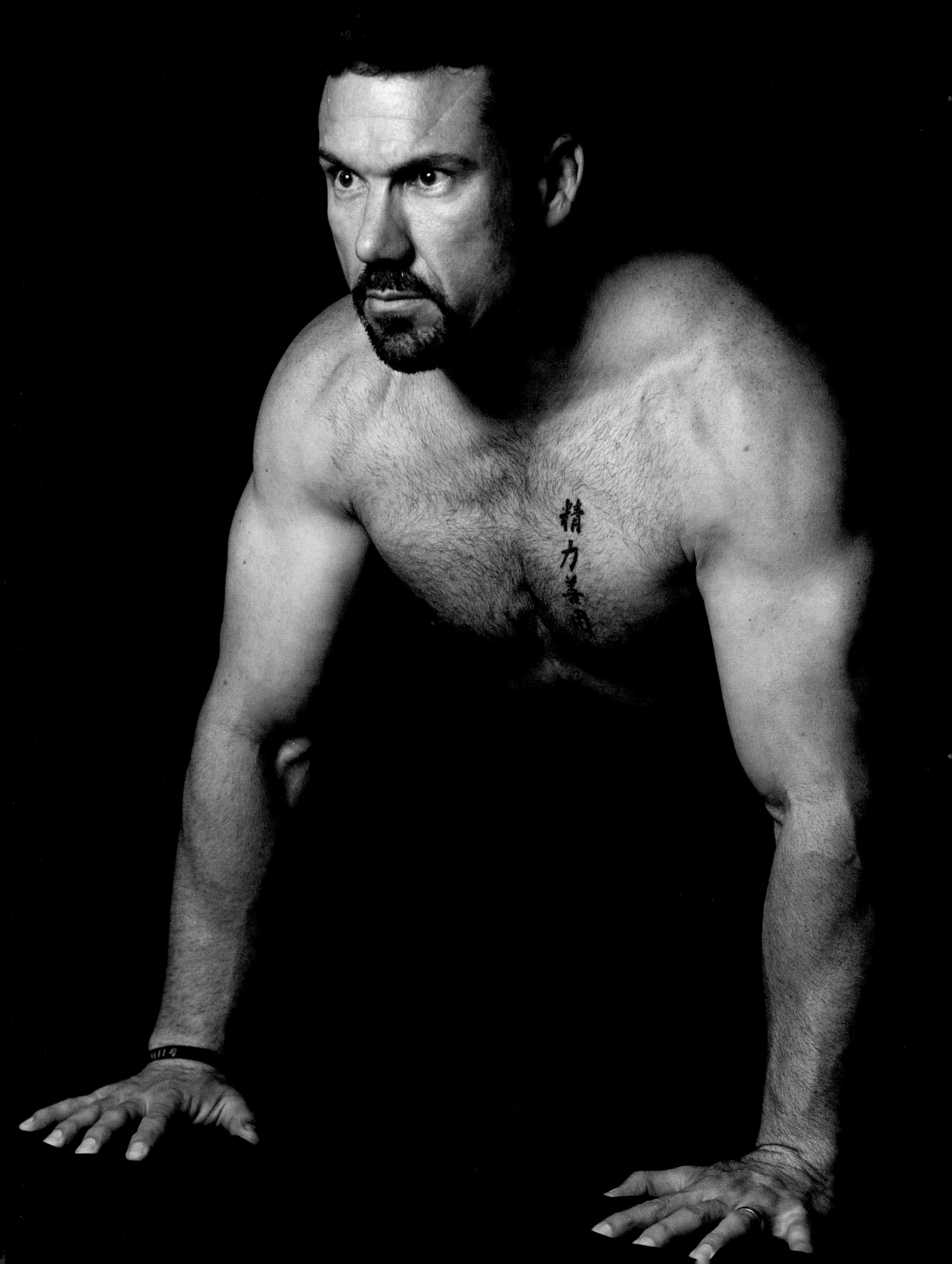
精力善用

Just as the running shoe and sports drink industries evolved, so has the concept of cardio fitness. Today we know that improving your cardio is not just a matter of getting out there and doing slow long distance runs. Modern sport science has revealed that conditioning for cardiovascular adaptations is no longer a one-size-fits-all proposition. Think about it this way: A man recovering from heart surgery will go through "phase I" cardiac rehabilitation. He will be monitored by a physical therapist while he walks very slowly in the hospital hallway. For him, this is cardio training. However, if I take a trained runner and have him do the same thing, there will be no training stimulus and no training adaptation.

If your ultimate goal is to improve your ability to run slowly over long distances, then the slow long-distance run approach may be okay, but it is also time-consuming and can place a lot of stress on body parts. Most people are unaware that there are better ways to achieve cardiovascular fitness. These styles can provide other benefits such as strength, power, muscle endurance, and flexibility. In addition, body composition can be improved—less fat and more lean body mass. This is the revolution in training behind the TFW system that will be presented in this book.

When I began this project, I realized that I did not have all the answers in terms of the science and methodology behind Cardio or Metabolic Training. In order to produce the level of book I wanted to create, I knew I had to present the science and research that backed up the training systems that would be used in this text. To do that, I needed to recruit and interview as many of the top people as I could. As I worked through this process, I recognized that my original professor and mentor, Dr. Tony Caterisano, has forgotten more than I will ever know about the science behind cardiovascular fitness. Dr. Caterisano, in addition to being one of my original training partners and a former javelin coach of mine, has been a Division 1 Head Wrestling Coach and powerlifting champion. Not only does he have an Exercise Physiology PhD behind his name, but more importantly, he's seen the real-world application of this style of training with thousands of athletes. Simply put, this guy has been a mentor to me over the last 20 years and he knows his stuff. That is why I could think of no one better to write the chapter on the science behind cardiovascular conditioning.

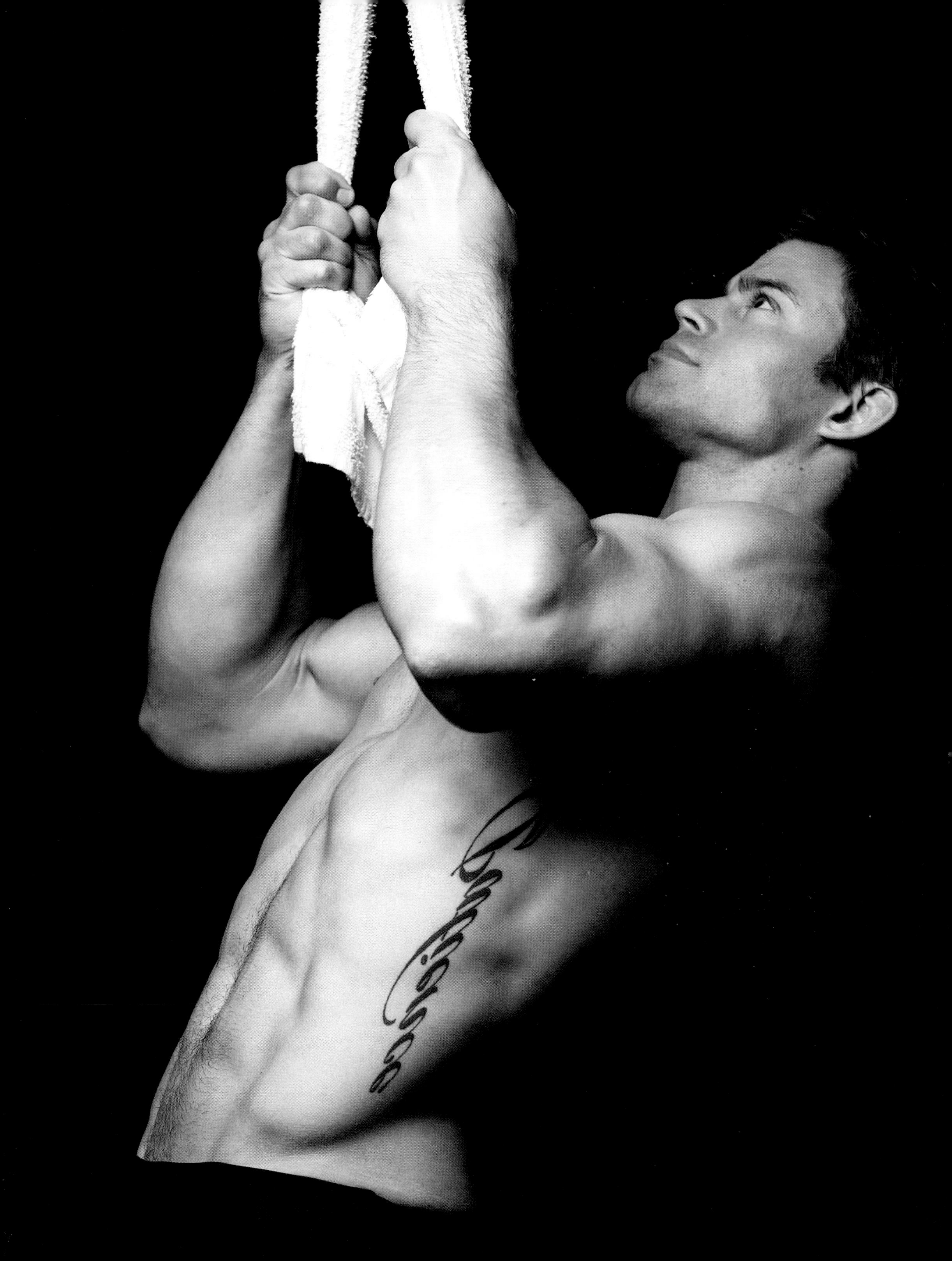

2

THE SCIENCE OF WARRIOR CARDIO

BY DR. TONY CATERISANO

In order to achieve the full results of this program, a working knowledge of the science of Metabolic Training is important. With a better understanding of how the body responds to this style of training and the correct application and long-term use of the training, you will be better armed to create and complete more effective workouts. We will begin with a review of the energy systems of the body, explain the science behind *Warrior Cardio*, deliver some examples of how to periodize the training, and finish with some concepts on program design.

HOW THE BODY TRANSFERS ENERGY

The human body was designed to do work—hard work. Our ancestors literally had to perform hard labor to get through a typical day. People didn't just hop in their cars if they had to go somewhere. Even the most affluent people had to walk or hitch up the old horse and buggy. Everything from farming to digging ditches to manufacturing goods had to be done manually.

In order to be able to do this and survive, our bodies had to learn to be adaptable.

Our bodies developed according to a "use it or lose it" principle that dictated which system got stronger and which got weaker. We maintain and develop the systems that we use most often.

Today, we have it too easy. We drive rather than walk. How many people have you watched as they circle the parking lot at the local supermarket or store just to get a parking space close to the front door? Labor-saving devices may save us time and effort, but we pay a big price by signaling to the body that our muscles and heart are not important systems to be maintained. We need to overload these systems every so often to keep them working at optimal levels, so that we have them when we need them. The goal of *Warrior Cardio* is to provide you with the information that will help you to properly understand and overload these systems. The first step toward this goal is to explain the different energy systems of the body and how they work.

ATP—THE RECHARGEABLE BATTERY OF THE MUSCLE

Energy is defined as the capacity to do work. The more energy we can *transfer and liberate* during a given activity, the harder we can train. You'll notice I didn't say "produce"; I said "transfer and liberate." This is because according to the first law of thermodynamics, energy can neither be created nor destroyed. Energy can only be transformed from one form to another (the electric light is a perfect example of electrical energy transforming to light energy), stored, and liberated to allow us to perform work.

Ask anyone where the energy we need for the human body comes from, and he or she will probably tell you "from food." If people really know their stuff, they may also correctly describe the "energy substrates," which consist of carbohydrates, fats, and proteins. The good thing about these energy substrates is that not only can we get them from dietary sources, but we also can store them in the body for use at a later time. But here is what some people don't realize: we don't use the energy from these sources directly. Instead, we transfer the energy into what we refer to as rechargeable batteries called adenosine-triphosphate, or ATP. In the same way that the battery in your cell phone draws energy from the charging unit plugged into your wall socket, the ATP molecule is able to take energy from food or stored sources such as body fat and "hold" it for future use. **This process of transferring energy from food to ATP can be either aerobic, which means "with oxygen," or anaerobic, which means "without oxygen."** As we will see later in this chapter, a combination of both aerobic and anaerobic systems are used in most forms of physical activity. ATP is often called "the currency of work" because just like with money, the more you have, the more you can expend.

ANAEROBIC ATP PRODUCTION

There are actually two systems that produce ATP without oxygen, or anaerobically. The first is often referred to as the ATP-CP system. Already charged ATP is stored right in the muscle, along with a substance called creatine phosphate (CP), from which additional energy can be quickly transferred. To use the currency analogy again, the stored ATP is like a wallet full of cash. The energy is immediately available to spend. The creatine phosphate also stores energy that can be quickly released, but this energy cannot be used directly by the muscle. Instead it must be transferred to recharge ATP. In this scenario, CP is like foreign currency. You can't spend it in the grocery store until you go to the bank and get it converted into dollars. The popular supplement creatine monohydrate is formulated to actually boost our levels of intramuscular creatine phosphate by three to four times normal levels, which is why it is so popular among weight lifters—it means that the reserve of energy available to recharge our ATP is greater.

The second anaerobic system is known as glycolysis. It involves the breakdown of the carbohydrate derivatives glucose and glycogen. Whenever we eat a carbohydrate, our stomach and small intestines digest and absorb most of it in a form called glucose. This causes a rise in our blood glucose level (what many people call their blood sugar), triggering a reaction from the pancreas to produce a hormone called insulin. Insulin opens up receptors on our muscle cells to allow glucose to enter those cells, where it can be used as fuel to make ATP or be stored as glycogen.

Glycolysis is a ten-step process where energy is "harvested" from the glucose and glycogen molecules to be transferred into ATP. It is not a greatly efficient process. In fact, only about 5% of the potential energy stored in glucose and glycogen is actually transferred to ATP. The remaining portion that is left, called pyruvic acid, has the potential to later become lactic acid, a substance that contributes to fatigue during prolonged exercise.

In fact you may have heard of the "anaerobic threshold," which is defined as the point at which the anaerobic system of ATP production results in high levels of lactic acid production. Some scientists define it as a certain level of lactic acid in the blood. It is also characterized by heavier breathing (increased ventilation) as your body tries to "buffer" that lactic acid, neutralizing it with bicarbonate to form carbon monoxide (CO_2). This CO_2 drives ventilation, giving us that out-of-breath feel during heavy exercise. We often use "rate of perceived exertion," or RPE, as a good indicator that a person has crossed his or her anaerobic threshold.

The two anaerobic systems for recharging ATP cannot sustain prolonged exercise because they are both very limited in terms of storage capacity and the amount of ATP that can actually be produced. They are good for short-term, high-intensity work where bursts of energy must be immediately available, but lack the staying power of the aerobic system that will be discussed next. These systems also have to be recharged once the high-intensity exercise is over, actually requiring the aerobic system to put the anaerobic systems back in order, ready for the next bout of hard work. This will be discussed later in more depth, as it is important for understanding how accessing the aerobic system produces results such as fat loss.

AEROBIC ATP PRODUCTION

The aerobic pathway is the great generator of ATP. It occurs in specialized organelles, which are tiny specialized structures called mitochondria inside the muscle cells. The mitochondria are often referred to as the "aerobic power plants" of the cell, since all aerobic chemical transformations take place here. Without getting into too much detail, the aerobic system takes carbohydrates, fats, and proteins and sends them through a series of chemical transformations inside the mitochondria. Think of it as a reverse assembly line in which large molecules are broken down into smaller components. At various intervals in this disassembly operation, energy is siphoned off and transformed into ATP. Given the relatively large number of chemical reactions that take place in the aerobic process, it takes several minutes before the system is up and running. This is why our anaerobic system is so important in providing energy immediately, especially during exercise that lasts only a few seconds.

Once the aerobic system is up and running

(often referred to as "steady state"), it is very efficient and generates lots of ATP, while generating only small amounts of lactic acid. **More importantly, this system is able to use fat as fuel—in fact it is the only energy pathway that can use fat.** As we will see later, this is most relevant to people who want to get rid of excess fat.

In his book *Aerobics*, Dr. Kenneth Cooper extols the value of aerobic exercise in preventing heart disease. This happens on many levels. The obvious one is that the cardiovascular system gets challenged (overloaded), which results in positive adaptations in the heart and circulation. Capillaries, the tiny blood vessels that supply our tissues with oxygen and nutrients, branch out and form tributaries, thus providing new routes for nourishment to vital organs, including the heart itself. Aerobic activity promotes the formation of high-density lipoproteins, commonly known as the "good cholesterol," which actually takes artery-clogging substances out of circulation. Additionally, it promotes fat burning, which helps prevent obesity. Since heart disease is the number one cause of death in America, it is no wonder that this book made a significant impact when it first came out in 1968. Dr. Cooper's approach was simple: keep the intensity low and increase the duration and frequency while staying within a "training zone" of moderately elevated heart rate.

As important as *Aerobics* was in starting the fitness boom, however, the "one size fits all" approach to aerobic conditioning outlined in the book has evolved into a more varied approach. For some, the low-intensity, long-duration program is fine, but for many people who aspire to higher levels of fitness, it may not be best. The goal of this chapter is to provide the knowledge to start taking cardiovascular training to a more advanced level.

THE AEROBIC SYSTEM AND EPOC

The aerobic system is stimulated in two ways. During low-intensity physical activity, the aerobic system can meet the demand for energy. So, if a walk or bike ride is kept slow, the aerobic system can supply energy and the exercise can last a long time without discomfort. As the intensity of the exercise increases (e.g., you progress from a slow jog to a fast run), the aerobic system uses more oxygen and energy substrates to meet the demand for ATP. The system has limits, and eventually it will become maxed out. The body's capacity to deliver and use oxygen at the cellular level is referred to as one's maximum oxygen consumption, or max VO_2.

The second way in which the aerobic system is stimulated is during recovery from high-intensity exercise, which depends primarily on the anaerobic pathway of ATP production. For example, sprinting as fast as possible requires high amounts of ATP and can only be maintained for seconds at a time. The high demand coupled with inadequate time for the aerobic system to meet the demand creates the need to "borrow" ATP from the anaerobic system. This ATP must be paid back during recovery, which is why we continue to breathe heavily for many minutes after a hard sprint. Our body will work hard to bring the energy stores, heart rate, and body temperature back to normal. The aerobic system requires energy in order to accomplish this return to normalcy, and that is why you can burn fat effectively with this style of training.

This phenomenon of recovery after high-intensity work used to be called "oxygen debt," but today goes by the acronym EPOC, which stands for excess post-exercise oxygen consumption. EPOC involves stimulating the aerobic system to produce the large amounts of ATP needed to restore the two anaerobic energy systems. EPOC is typically based on two factors: the fitness level of the person and the intensity of the exercise. The lower the fitness levels of the person and the higher the intensity of the exercise, the higher the EPOC. **During EPOC we burn more calories than we would at rest, and with very high-intensity exercise followed by active recovery, the caloric expenditure can approximate the same level as the amount burned on a long run.** This concept is essential to understand since it is a major explanation why you can not only build muscle, but also burn fat during the Warrior Cardio workouts contained in this book. So even though these workouts are brief, due to the nature of their demands on the body's energy stores, the body has to use additional energy to recharge. This increase in the caloric burn burns fat.

THE END OF THE SLOW LONG-DISTANCE RUN

For some, running slow long distances is fine, as long as they don't overdo it and are satisfied with focusing on modest goals. This type of exercise is good for burning fat, but because it is long and slow, it takes a relatively long time to get gains, and its repetitive nature leaves the door open to overuse injuries. Also, many athletes cannot get sufficient carry-over (sometimes referred to as "transfer specificity") to the conditioning needed in their particular sport by doing slow long distance.

Take jogging as an example—the motion is repetitive on every stride. The knee, ankle, and hip joints move with the same motion thousands of times in a moderately distanced jog. The joints must absorb the shock of a person's bodyweight landing on each leg with each foot strike. This downward acceleration can equal a force of two to three times a person's bodyweight depending on terrain, which means a 150-pound person must absorb 300 to 450 pounds of force on each leg. Of course, the human body is designed to run and handle most of the trauma (this is probably how our ancestors traveled prior to the use of horses and other beasts of burden), but consider that our physical environment has drastically changed. Today our bodies must deal with hard pavement, poorly designed shoes, and urban environments. We set higher standards of performance in competition, continually pushing the envelope on what our bodies can achieve in sport performance. Jogging and running just cannot provide sufficient training stimulus for many athletes unless they train at such a high level of volume and intensity that they end up injured. There is a need today for a new style of training.

THE WARRIOR CARDIO APPROACH

By purchasing this book, you have identified yourself as someone who wants to go beyond the mundane approach to cardiovascular fitness and find a better way to meet your training goals. Athletes in the fighting arts are arguably the best-conditioned athletes out of pure necessity—in the fighting arts, letting up for even one second can lead to defeat, and I mean this literally. You can't "take a play off" the way you can in some sports. Instead, the action is continuous and often the intensity of your effort is not controlled by you, but rather controlled by what your opponent is trying to do (which many times is all about hurting you). Now, we are not advocating that everyone who reads this book go to the ring, cage, or wrestling mat to compete, but wouldn't it be great to be in the type of physical condition where you could? Wouldn't it also be great if we could acquire a high level of conditioning and at the same time develop strength, power, speed, and agility? This is what Warrior Cardio is all about.

INTERVAL TRAINING AS A WAY TO STIMULATE THE AEROBIC SYSTEM

Whether you call it interval training, circuit training, metabolic training, or high-intensity training (HIT), at TFW we want you to understand the basic premise is the same: **using high-energy-requiring work bouts and short rest intervals to stimulate the aerobic energy pathway.** Unlike the aforementioned traditional aerobic training model in which you stay in a prescribed "heart rate training zone," the idea here is to temporarily exceed the normal training zone and reach heart rates that approach one's age-predicted maximum. This only can be maintained for relatively shorts bursts of physical activity, and must be immediately followed by low-level "active rest" to allow the heart rate to come down and prepare the athlete for the next high-intensity bout of activity. Although the bar complexes, Hurricanes, and circuits accomplish this, probably the simplest example to understand the concept of this style of training would be running intervals on a track. One could sprint 200 meters (half of a lap around most standard tracks) and then walk 400 meters to allow the heart rate to come down and the body to recover. Then there would be another 200-meter run, again followed by the recovery. This increase in heart rate followed by active rest is where all the results come from. To properly affect the intensity of the workouts contained in this book, however, there is one element that needs to be correctly applied: the work-to-rest ratio.

THE WORK-TO-REST RATIO

We describe the relationship between the actual high-intensity activity and the active rest as the "work-to-rest ratio" (work/rest ratio) in designing interval workouts. **The work-to-rest ratio is one of the keys of this style of training because it will ultimately regulate the volume and intensity of workouts.** Often we use time to determine the work/rest ratio. For example, in a 1–3 ratio, if it takes 30 seconds to run 200 meters, the rest interval would be 90 seconds, or 3 times the work interval. To transition into a higher-intensity workload, one could change to a 1–2 ratio or even a 1–1 ratio, meaning that the 30-second work bout would be followed by a 60-second or a 30-second recovery, respectively.

Another variation on the work-to-rest ratio is to use recovery heart rate in determining the rest interval. During the Category 1 Hurricane, for example, you might run a 20-second sprint on the treadmill and get your heart rate up to 185 beats per minute. You could then wait until your heart rate gets down to 120 beats/minute before starting the next sprint. **The beauty of this Training for Warriors approach is that it makes the interval correspond to the fitness level of the participant.** A more aerobically fit person will recover faster than a less fit individual and can therefore handle a shorter recovery interval.

As you will see in *Warrior Cardio*, you are not limited to running as your only cardio exercise. In the TFW system there are other high-intensity exercises that involve large muscle groups to achieve the work portion, such as resistance exercises, plyometrics, speed and agility training, and sport-specific exercises. The fact that the TFW system uses a variety of training methods allows for "training multitasking," in which more than just cardiovascular conditioning can be gained within a particular workout routine. You can develop strength, hypertrophy, power speed, and agility in an economical way that provides a better carry-over to the type of real-life stamina that one needs to compete.

THE SCIENCE OF INTERVAL TRAINING

According to the TFW philosophy, a Metabolic Training circuit is created by putting several intervals of work and recovery together, manipulating the intensity by selecting specific exercises for the work portion and varying the precise rest intervals. Most people are able to throw a circuit together. The goal for this section is to explain the science behind why this style of training works and the best ways to put your circuits together.

As mentioned earlier in the chapter, high-intensity activity requires large amounts of ATP to be available as quickly as possible. The aerobic system, with its high number of chemical reactions, cannot immediately provide this massive amount of ATP, so it must be "borrowed" from the anaerobic sources (the phosphagen system and anaerobic glycolysis). Just as when you borrow money from a close friend, that money has to be paid back in a timely manner (or you lose a close friend), this is precisely what happens during the rest interval. We earlier identified this as EPOC. So, it is during this rest interval and the recovery after a workout where EPOC occurs and where the aerobic system is required to regenerate ATP to pay the anaerobic system back.

What many exercise scientists are now learning is that the type and intensity of the exercises selected can have a great impact on the metabolic demand and EPOC, thus affecting how well one adapts to the training. For example, Dr. Peter Lemon recently published a commentary in the *American College of Sports Medicine (ACSM) Sports Medicine Bulletin* regarding research into "sprint interval training (SIT)," in which he reviewed several research studies on the subject. These studies compared SIT, which is a specific form of high-intensity training involving running, to more "traditional" running programs and found that in each study cited, SIT training produced as good aerobic training effects as traditional long-distance running, if not better, but "with a fraction of the time commitment" (Macpherson et al. 2010). Research from his lab also found larger fat loss among the SIT-trained subjects compared to the more traditionally trained subjects. Previous to Dr. Lemon's work, other studies by Mazzetti et al. (2007), Gibala (2009), and Trapp et al. (2008) found similar results when comparing high-intensity training to slower, long distance running. Across the board, the high-intensity subjects burned more body fat with less of a time commitment.

In our lab at Furman University, we wanted to see just how much extra energy was expended during circuit weight training, both between sets and during a 45-minute recovery period following the circuit. We also wanted to see if the amount of resistance used made a difference in the way the body recovered. We recruited experienced male weight lifters and had them perform one of two different weight circuits on separate days while measuring energy expenditure using a portable metabolic system that subjects could wear during weight lifting. The circuits included the same exercises, except that one was performed at 70% of each subject's one-repetition maximum (1RM), while the other was performed at 85% of the 1RM. The number of sets and reps was adjusted so that in each trial the subjects lifted the same volume of weight. So, for example, they lifted the lighter weight for more repetitions and the heavier weight for fewer repetitions so that the total pounds lifted were exactly the same. The results showed that lifting the heavier weight for fewer repetitions actually elicited greater energy expenditure than the lighter weight, even though the absolute volume of work was the same. This suggests that the heavier weight, which involved more muscle mass, needed more energy to restore the system, hence a higher EPOC. These results were published in *Medicine and Science in Sports and Exercise*, the official journal of the ACSM (Caterisano et al. 2007, Mazzetti et al. 2007, Caterisano et al. 2008).

The bottom line here is that the scientific studies support the idea that the adaptations achieved with interval training are similar to—if not superior to—more traditional forms of aerobic training such as distance running and low-intensity exercise on various cardio machines. In addition, intervals take less of a time commitment and can provide the opportunity for other fitness parameters, such as power and strength, to be trained at the same time.

PERIODIZATION OF TRAINING

Martin has a funny saying in which he believes that "the two most dangerous P-words in training are periodization and plyometrics." It's true, and the danger does not come from awareness, but from application. Many people can get confused by the concept of periodization. As a result of this, people are often paralyzed about what to do with training and then don't do anything at all. To put it simply, in order to accomplish anything, you need to have a plan. **Periodization is a training concept that plans and organizes workouts according to two important training variables—training and rest. The training loads are typically manipulated using two inversely related variables—intensity and volume.** It is a concept that was imported from the old Soviet training models that used training cycles of varying lengths with different training loads during different phases. Although there are thousands of pages written on the topic, the following two models should give you a working understanding of how periodization is commonly applied both in a competitive setting and for people looking to improve overall fitness.

THE LINEAR MODEL

In the classic or linear periodization model, training is broken down into different cycles that systematically manipulate the intensity and volume of work. Usually this style of periodization is used when an exact date of competition is known and an athlete has months of time in preparation for that event. The different cycles have different names. The smallest cycles, which often last one week, are referred to as minicycles. The collective term for a group of four minicycles might be called a mesocycle, and a group of four mesocycles a macrocycle, depending on how often it is repeated.

The common application would be that each mesocycle has a different focus leading up to an event. The first mesocycle, commonly known as the "preparation phase," would use low-intensity and high-volume training loads. In weight training, the intensity might be based on the amount of weight lifted or the speed at which a resistance exercise is performed. The volume could be based on the number of repetitions, the number of sets performed, the number of lifts per workout, and the number of workouts per week. For example, in cycle 1, an athlete might perform five sets of 10 to 12 repetitions with a relatively low resistance. The second mesocycle, often referred to as the "first transition phase," is characterized by an increase in the intensity and a decrease in the training volume. In this example, the athlete might increase the resistance and cut the volume to five sets of four to six repetitions in cycle 2. The third mesocycle, also known as the "competition phase," further increases the intensity while decreasing the volume. Continuing with our example, it may involve pushing the intensity to a high percent of the 1RM while dropping the volume to five sets of two to three repetitions. The last of the four mesocycles, sometimes referred to as the "second transition phase," can be either a tapering phase in preparation for competition or an active rest phase to provide recovery before entering the next macrocycle. This last phase may last only a week or two, and involves relatively low-intensity as well as low-volume training, often referred to as "unload cycles." Keep in mind that this classic periodization model is not the only form of periodization available, but it may be best for a competitive athlete attempting to reach high levels of performance just before a championship contest.

THE UNDULATING MODEL

A second form of periodization, called "nonlinear periodization" or "undulating periodization," is more suitable for those who are more interested in maintaining fitness over a long period of time. In this model, the training loads are changed more often, even from workout to workout. If you aren't a competitive athlete but still want a systematic way to add variety and recovery cycles into your workouts, this approach is best. Rather than 3-to-5-week cycles, in undulating periodization, the training loads and types of exercises are changed week to week or even day to day. You may have heard among some popular workout routines the term "muscle confusion" as the "secret" to which its promoters attribute their program's success. This is just another way of applying the concept of undulating periodization. By changing the training stimulus, you are exposing the body to new overloads. This keeps the workouts psychologically fresh and helps prevent the mental staleness of doing the same workouts week in and week out. In addition, it prevents the physical staleness the Soviets used to term "accommodation," in which adaptations to training render the training stimulus less effective.

The simplest way to design an undulating periodization program is to designate that some days in your weekly routine will be "heavy" days and some will be "light." In terms of weight training, a heavy day might mean lifting high percentages of the 1RM, and light would mean lifting smaller percentages of the 1RM. With interval training, a heavy day might be where the work-to-rest ratio is one-to-one, while a light day would be one-to-three.

In a Training for Warriors four-day-per-week workout program, with two resistance days and two metabolic conditioning days, the heavy lifting day might be Monday and the light lifting day would be Friday. The light conditioning day would be Tuesday and the heavy conditioning day would be Thursday. Of course, with the Warrior Cardio program, we are training strength, power, speed, and agility every workout—it is just that on each of these days certain exercises will be priorities. Wednesdays, Saturdays, and Sundays will be rest days.

Understanding how to use undulating periodization is essential for training an MMA fighter. Since a fighter may have matches pop up throughout a year, he has no specific season, trains year round, and has to be close to top condition at all times. With the undulating periodization model of the TFW system, the fighter can make progress in areas of strength and speed while still allowing for recovery. As an example of how a fighter using the TFW system would apply the training, his Monday workout might involve weight training for strength with no conditioning because he will have a wrestling or martial arts session later that day. He may do light conditioning circuits on Tuesday to supplement his fighting workouts, a light fighting technique workout on Wednesday, and a heavier conditioning session such as Hurricane training on Thursday. On Friday he may hit a higher-volume weight-training workout with fighting sessions later that day. Saturday and Sunday may be rest days or involve sparring work one of the two days. Much would depend on how close his next match is, if that information is known. **But the overall approach is to manage the energy expended throughout the week and make sure that recovery is taking place to make adaptation.** As the actual competition got nearer, more rest cycles would be included. The key here is not to overlook the fact that he has other training sessions besides what he does in the weight room.

The TFW philosophy states that if you are not a competitive athlete getting ready for a specific date, you are always "in season." Understanding this and undulating periodization, you need to pick the times to push yourself to the limit, but you shouldn't try to do this every day. You should interject lighter, low-intensity days along with complete days off. **Remember, just because something is hard doesn't mean it is an effective approach to optimal training results.** If that were the case, this chapter would be one sentence: Push yourself to your physical limits every workout. Unfortunately this is what some athletes, coaches, and personal trainers believe.

You can get more creative with undulating periodization, varying the training loads every workout, but just remember that if you are going to push the limit, when you rest, you must truly rest. The rest part also includes adequate sleep and good nutritional practices, which will be outlined later in this book. Your workouts can be perfect, but if you don't give your body enough raw materials to rebuild and adapt through proper nutrition and allow it the chance to go through normal sleep cycles, you won't make the best gains possible.

WHY PERIODIZE YOUR TRAINING?

The simple answer is to prevent overtraining. The work ethic for success in sport or any other endeavor has been deeply engrained in our minds from an early age. We are told that the road to victory is to outwork our opponent, and that we can make up for lack of natural talent with hard work. Now, this is true up to a point. If a talented athlete doesn't work hard, he may be defeated by a harder-working opponent. But the human body has a finite capacity to recover from hard workouts. Anyone can design a circuit interval that would make even the most well-conditioned athlete lose his lunch. But that doesn't mean that it is the most effective way to train. **Remember, it is the adaptation from the training, not the training itself, that pays off in results.** If you don't allow for the proper amount of recovery, overtraining can occur.

Some early symptoms of overtraining are:

- Decreases in strength, power, and speed despite adherence to workouts (especially the inability to reach previously attained personal bests).
- An increase in mental errors and loss of

skills. It can even manifest itself as loss of concentration in school, at work, and during other mental tasks.

- Psychological problems such as depression or loss of interest in competing or training.
- Increased susceptibility to illnesses such as colds and other infections that indicate that the autoimmune system is weakened.
- Insomnia or inability to get a good night's sleep. Also, waking up tired after eight or more hours of sleep.
- Loss of appetite, unexplained weight loss, and unusual muscle soreness.

These symptoms indicate that the body is under too much stress and headed for exhaustion. Many people believe that overtraining can be corrected by just taking a couple of days off, but studies show that it can take a month or more to recover from overtraining. By periodizing the training cycles you take the best approach to dealing with overtraining—you prevent it.

CONCLUSION

The goal of this chapter was to not only get you excited about the practice of *how* to get into "fighting shape" (whether literal or figurative), but also to present the theory that substantiates *why* you should follow this form of training. You should understand how the energy systems work and why interval training is the most time-efficient and effective way to stimulate cardiovascular adaptations, while at the same time gaining strength, power, and agility. You should also have a concept of how to apply the training to optimize the results you seek. The scientific research and proven results have also been presented to show that the TFW system works. Now it is up to you to take this information and allow it to strengthen your training approach and your fitness level.

REFERENCES

Caterisano, A., B.T. Patrick, J.M. Grossnickle, and R.F. Moss, "The effect of varying intensity on total energy expenditure during circuit weight training with equal volume," *Medicine and Science in Sports and Exercise*, vol. 40, no. 5, pg. S257, May 2008.

Caterisano, A., B.T. Patrick, R.F. Moss, and J.M. Grossnickle, "Variable training intensities with equivalent training volume affects EPOC in circuit weight-training," *Medicine and Science in Sports and Exercise*, vol. 39, no. 5, pg. S481, May 2007.

Gibala, M., "Molecular responses to high-intensity interval exercise," *Appl. Physiol. Nutr. Metab.*, vol. 34, no. 3, pg. 428–32, 2009.

Macpherson, R.E., T.J. Hazel, T.D. Oliver, D.H. Paterson, and P.W. Lemon, "Run sprint interval training improves aerobic performance but not max cardiac output," *Medicine and Science in Sports and Exercise*, vol. 42, no. 5, May 2010.

Mazzetti, S., M. Douglass, A. Yocum, and M. Harber, "Effect of explosive verses slow contractions and exercise intensity on energy expenditure," *Medicine and Science in Sports and Exercise*, vol. 39, no. 8, pg. 1291–301, Aug. 2007.

Trapp, E.G., D.J. Chisholm, J. Freund, and S.H. Boutcher, "The effects of high-intensity intermittent exercise training on fat loss and fasting insulin levels of young women," *International Journal of Obesity*, vol. 32, no. 4, pg. 684–91, Apr. 2008.

Tremblay, A., J.A. Simoneau, and C. Bouchard, "Impact of exercise intensity on body fatness and skeletal muscle metabolism," *Metabolism*, vol. 43, no. 7, pg. 814–18, July 1994.

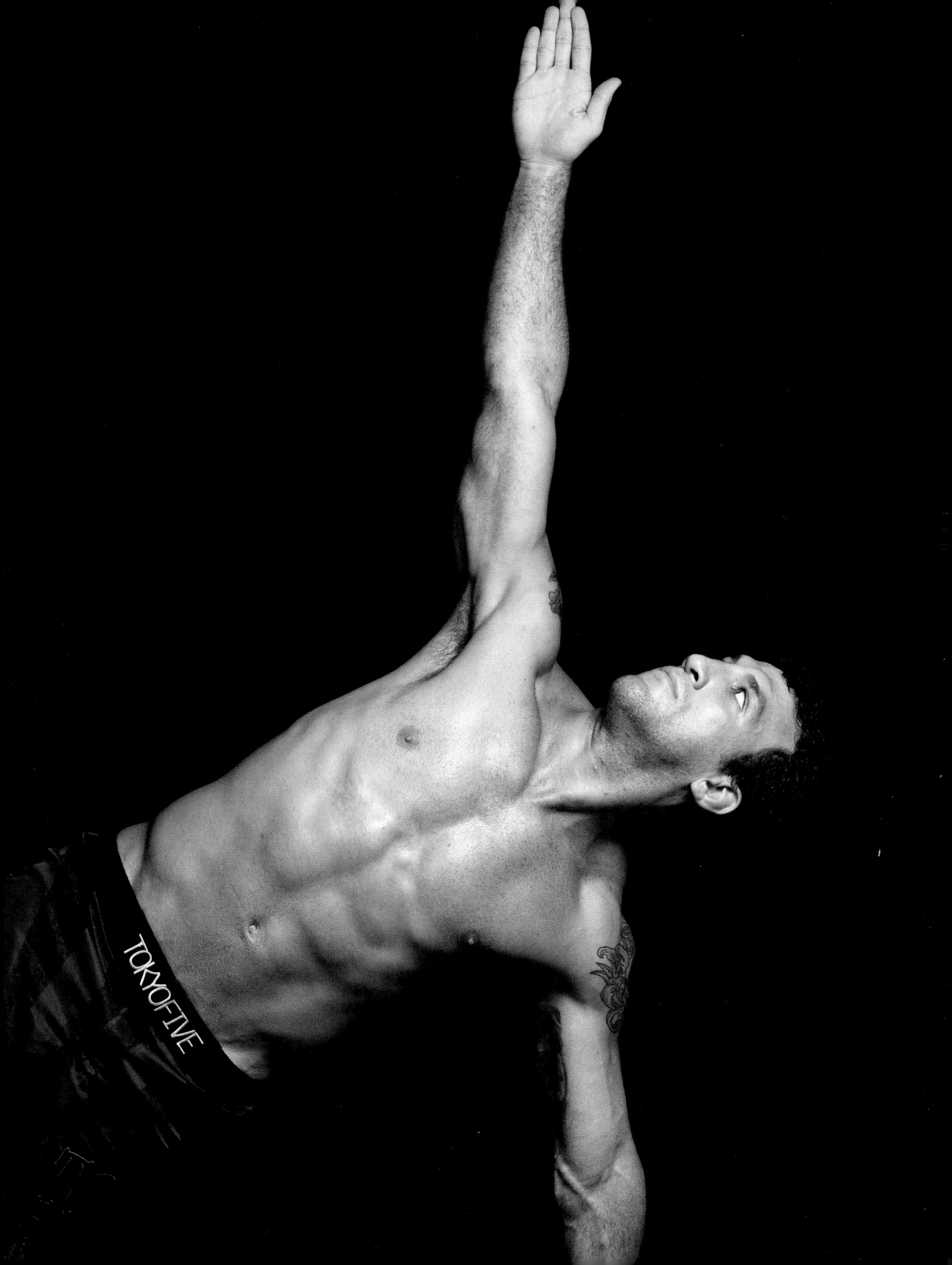
TOKYOFIVE

3

MENTAL CARDIO

CONTROL YOUR BREATHING, CONTROL YOUR MIND.
CONTROL YOUR MIND, CONTROL YOUR THOUGHTS.
CONTROL YOUR THOUGHTS, CONTROL YOUR ACTIONS.
CONTROL YOUR ACTIONS, CONTROL THE SITUATION.

In order to achieve the maximum benefit from the workouts in *Warrior Cardio*, you will have to work harder than you ever have before. These workouts are going to require your muscles and heart to become more conditioned, but those are not the only areas you will need to train. You will need to train your mind as well. When you train at this level or with this style, you must have a different way of thinking. Your mind has to be stronger.

Warrior Cardio is not just about developing physical stamina, but mental stamina as well. After years of training, I have found each one relies on the other. The only way for you to reach your goals of muscle gain and fat loss will be to develop both. The reason most people do not reach these goals is not because they lack the physical ability, but due to the absence of mental stamina. Because of the importance of stamina for the mind, I had to dedicate a section of this book to developing this rare form of fortitude. I refer to the active development of this fortitude as Mental Cardio.

THE LINK

In a way, the methods for developing Mental Cardio and Warrior Cardio are the same: a number of exercises are used in a circuit format to create a disruption that leads to adaptation and improvement. The physical training circuits in this book use a number of exercises linked as a circuit in order to create physical disruption, which will then result in gains in muscular strength and cardiovascular capacity once a response to that disruption takes place. The circuits of Mental Cardio use an examination of a number of concepts to create a disruption by challenging the way that you currently think so that your mindset and mental approach to training are stronger once a response takes place.

In both cases, the work you perform should show you where you are limited. In the physical circuit, if there are areas of weakness, you are forced to recognize them and work at them to improve. I am asking you to do the exact same thing with the areas of weakness you may find during the two Mental Cardio Circuits provided below. You need to recognize the areas in which you may be deficient and then work on them to improve. With improvement, I promise more rapid increases in both physical development and mental fortitude.

To train properly, you must have not only a physical training program, but also a mental approach to the training. This approach eventually becomes your training philosophy, built of the principles you most value and by which you live in accordance. These principles in both training and in life become your compass. If there are things that you stand for and that give you direction in your actions, you will not fall for the distractions that may hold you back or allow you to quit. Each workout in this book will force you to draw on your principles to push through and overcome the pain and fatigue that may come with these workouts. These should be seen as not an obstacle, but an opportunity for you to reach another level both physically and mentally. As you go through the workouts in the book, you should not just be looking at the physical limitations that are holding back your training, but at your mental limitations as well. By monitoring these concepts, only then can you manage them.

THE CIRCUITS OF MENTAL CARDIO

The following two circuits contain mental concepts that will be critical for the execution of the book. Every one of these principles can be developed and improved upon.

1. RESPONDER CIRCUIT

To perform this circuit, sit down with a piece of paper and write down the five mental concepts listed below. Spend 3 to 5 minutes writing down your thoughts on each concept in terms of whether you have any limitations in that area that can be improved upon and how you feel you respond to that concept. As you go through the workouts in this book, perform this circuit one time per week to analyze improvement and ongoing needs.

Conflict

Training often leads to a state of conflict. When people think of conflict, however, they often see themselves in a struggle against someone else. In the case of hard training, the struggle is with oneself. Learning to better deal with the internal conflict that occurs with hard training will allow you to better deal with other conflicts that you face in life. That is the power behind Warrior Cardio. The better you learn to manage internal conflict with hard training, the more mentally powerful you can become.

People often view conflict as something negative. You should begin to view the internal conflict you experience as a result of hard training as a positive experience that can be valuable. When you do this, you use internal conflict not as a reason to hold back or give up, but as an opportunity to build yourself up by increasing mental fortitude.

Conflict will appear all the time in this program. How you deal with this conflict will ultimately determine the results you achieve. For instance, there will be times you will not want to work out. There will be other times you will begin but want to give up. There will be part of you that wants to fight and part of you that wants to flee. This conflict, or inner battle, must be faced head on.

Overcoming conflict is about both being honest with yourself and holding yourself responsible. Being honest with yourself is one of the hardest things to do. Many find it difficult to state things as they really are. To blame one's circumstances on outside forces is much easier than holding oneself responsible.

For 3 to 5 minutes, ask yourself how you respond to conflict. Do you fight or flee? Can you be better in future workouts at facing your internal conflict?

Challenge

Most of us dream of hitting the lottery, getting more money to do less, or that our lives were easier in some way. Without the challenges, obstacles, troubles, failures, mistakes, problems, dilemmas, and even catastrophes, our lives would be less, not more. To achieve anything worthwhile in life, there has to be struggle. A challenge is not about what it is you want to achieve, but more about the struggle that it will require to surmount the obstacles to achieving it. A challenge is what you can use to test the limits of your physical skills and mental willpower. The result of a challenge will tell you what you are made of.

When using the workouts in this book, I want you to challenge the way that you think about the expectations you have for yourself. Simply put, if you have a low expectation for yourself, the challenge is weak and you will not go far. By constantly setting that ceiling higher and higher and increasing the challenge, you will move toward your goals.

My advice is to get most excited when things get most difficult. Welcome the challenge. A warrior gets fired up for the greatest obstacles because he knows they are his opportunity to find his greatness. The warrior that comes upon a roadblock should not see it as a stopping point, but an obstacle that can, must, and will be overcome to reach a higher level.

For 3 to 5 minutes, ask yourself how you respond to challenge. Do you welcome and look for better ways to challenge yourself? Can you do a better job of setting new and exciting challenges for yourself?

Change

Most people are afraid of change. But change in life is inevitable. It is not the changes in life that decide our destiny, but how we respond to those changes. All too often it is easier to just stay where we are. If you want to get to another level, you have to give up your old ways and dare to do something new. The same old exercises may no longer stimulate the warrior within, physically or mentally. That means it is either time to try something new or to make the old something more difficult.

There are a number of new ideas in this book. New ideas are agents of change, but many people are not receptive to them. All too often, a lack of mental flexibility leads to a lack of growth. When approached by new ideas, people first think up the reasons why something cannot work instead of why it can. My advice is to get excited by that fact that there is going to be more that you don't know than that you do know.

For 3 to 5 minutes, ask yourself how you respond to change. Do you welcome change or are you resistant? Can you improve your ability to recognize when it may be time to change and make the move away from something holding you back?

Choice

As human beings, our ultimate freedom is in our ability to choose. When people ask me about how to become more successful in any aspect of life, I simply instruct them to make better choices. Only you have the ability to choose your actions. No one can make you miss class, eat the wrong food, or turn on the TV. To be successful, you need to start making the choices that you know are best. In life, there are very few choices that can be considered "neutral." This means that a choice is either helping you or hurting you in terms of achieving your goals. Every breath you take, thought you think, decision you make, and piece of food you eat counts. It is your choice whether they move you forward or stand in your way.

Where you are right now in terms of fitness is a result of the choices you either did or did not make. Once you accept this responsibility, you will learn that your success or lack thereof will only be up to you. Once you realize this and hold yourself to a higher standard, you are primed to make instant improvement both physically and mentally.

I am not going to lie to you. Making the right choices all the time is going to be difficult. If it were easy, all people would have the fitness level and body that they desire. Just make sure not to confuse "difficult" with "impossible."

For 3 to 5 minutes, ask yourself how you respond to choice. Is it easy or difficult to make good choices? Do you recognize any areas in which better choices would greatly improve your success?

Comfort

Our bodies are always seeking out a feeling of comfort. Whether it's digesting a stomach full of food, healing an injury, or recovering from a tough Warrior Cardio workout, our body naturally attempts to remove discomfort from our personal experience. Even though discomfort is not something that many people regularly seek, being out of your comfort zone is often the key to personal development in both the physical and mental realms. Understanding this, you have to recognize that the more discomfort you can learn to tolerate, the greater an advantage you'll have over your competition.

In short, if you want to get the most from this book, you have to learn to be more comfortable being uncomfortable. These workouts will teach you how to do this. As you get used to the difficult nature of the training, you will develop the ability to tolerate harder and harder workouts. This mental skill will be critical to your success in other areas of your life. Once you begin to really train hard without fear of discomfort, other aspects of your life will also seem much easier.

For 3 to 5 minutes, ask yourself how you respond to discomfort. Do you seek out discomfort in order to improve yourself? What areas of your life would improve if you had a better ability to tolerate discomfort?

2. RECKONING CIRCUIT

To perform this circuit, sit down with a piece of paper and write down the six mental concepts listed below. Spend 3 to 5 minutes writing your thoughts on each, focusing on whether you have any limitations in that area that can be improved upon and your current level of development. As you go through the workouts in this book, perform this circuit one time per week to analyze improvement and ongoing needs.

Courage

If there is one principle that must be strongly developed in the warrior, it is courage. Courage can be described as the one principle that will guarantee the existence of all the other principles you adopt. Contrary to what many people think, courage is not fearlessness, but actually action taken in spite of fear. To start a new training program and follow a new philosophy requires courage. As with jumping out of an airplane, you have to recognize that the first step is the hardest. These workouts are not easy. You will need the courage to attack them and to overcome the fatigue they can produce. You will also have to develop the courage to stay committed to your goals despite opportunities to do otherwise. The possibilities to skip a workout or eat poorly will often present themselves. You must develop the courage to boldly say "no." Once you begin to see that there is nothing to fear, other aspects of your life will seem much less frightening as well.

For 3 to 5 minutes, assess your overall level of courage. Would people call you a courageous person? In what areas of your life would some added courage be of great benefit?

Concentration

Concentration can be described as making the most important thing the most important thing. The areas of your life in which you demonstrate the most concentration will also be the areas that deliver the greatest accomplishment. If you do not concentrate on your workouts or diet, it will be difficult to get the results you seek. When you concentrate, you must also be sure to concentrate on the right thing. During a workout, you should not concentrate on the pain or fatigue; you need to stay focused on the outcome. Concentrate your focus on the fat loss and increased muscle mass, not the pain.

By focusing your energy on what you want in the long term, you will insure that you do the necessary things in the short term. Concentration like this will no longer allow you to give up what you want most for what you want right now.

For 3 to 5 minutes, assess your ability to concentrate. Would people call you a person of great focus? In what areas of your life would some added concentration be of great benefit?

Competitiveness

Competition not only shows you where you rank in the world, but also offers feedback about your strengths or areas that need further development. Only by putting yourself "to the test" can you develop a true sense of your level of ability. Instead of solely thinking about external competition like yourself against an opponent, I want you to also address your "inner competitor" and drive to succeed. The workouts contained in this book demand your best effort. So, the ultimate goal of each workout is that you engage in competition against yourself.

By developing a higher level of competitiveness, you will be armed with the added energy to complete more difficult workouts and avoid opportunities to eat poorly. When you improve your ability to compete, you will recognize that the Path of Least Resistance does not intersect with the Road to Success.

For 3 to 5 minutes, assess your overall competitiveness level. Would people call you a competitive person? In what areas of your life would some added competitiveness be of great benefit?

Control

You must first accept responsibility that you are the only one in control of your destiny. A mentally strong person has the ability to control him- or herself under any situation. I believe that this is not an inherent ability, but an attribute that can be developed. The workouts in this book offer the opportunity to control yourself under difficult circumstances. There will be chances to skip workouts and stray from your diet. The key will be to exert self-control.

These workouts are going to push you to your limits. During the training, you are going to be in a fatigued state and experience pain. You will have to learn to control yourself and your emotions under duress. Once you learn to do this, you will have developed a useful ability that can be applied to areas outside of the training as well. Your ability to control yourself both physically and mentally under high stress will be the skill that eventually separates you from the competition.

For 3 to 5 minutes, assess your level of self-control. Would people describe you as someone with high levels of control? In what areas of your life would some added self-control be of great benefit?

Consistency

Consistency can be described as doing what you are supposed to do, when you are supposed to do it, all the time. Consistency is the best-kept secret behind why some people succeed and others fail. When you are consistent over time, small gains will eventually equal large ones. Your ability to be consistent will depend on two other important characteristics: discipline and perseverance. With these attributes, you cannot be stopped from achievement. Without them, you will never reach any goal you have set for yourself.

A classic training myth is that you can whip yourself into shape in a few weeks. To properly develop your physical and mental endurance, training needs to be all year long. If you are not prepared to train throughout the year, you do not really want to be a champion. I have found that the achievers do always what the mediocre do occasionally. If you just do a hard workout once in a while, this will not produce optimal results. Get consistent in your actions, and a little on top of a little will eventually become a lot.

For 3 to 5 minutes, assess your ability to stay consistent. Would people describe you as a consistent person? In what areas of your life would some added consistency be of great benefit?

Commitment

Commitment can be described as a pledge or promise to achieve something by a certain time under any circumstances. With firm commitment, you can stay the course even under the most trying situations. Most people, however, rarely commit to something even when they are actually doing it. They show up for workouts, but never go all out. Those people will never be satisfied, because deep down they know that they never gave their best. You should do the most with what you have been given. Unfortunately, most people go to their grave with their best works left inside of them. Most people never give their all and leave a little bit too much talent, skill, and possibility on the proverbial table of life.

To be successful in life, you must commit. You must go and put everything behind your commitment. There is no halfway in anything you do. When there is commitment, there is no doubt that you will achieve what you have set course to do.

For 3 to 5 minutes, assess your ability to commit to tasks. Would people describe you as a person of strong commitment? In what areas of your life would some added commitment be of great benefit?

Although you may see quick and steady progress in your physical performance, the development of a strong constitution takes more time. This is often a reason why people skip right to the physical exercise sections of this book. If you are willing to learn an exercise or circuit, you should be just as open to accepting new ways of thinking that can assist in leading you to faster results of losing fat and building muscle.

Your brain, just like any muscle of the body, grows in strength with proper use. Before you can build your body, I believe that you must first build your mind. I believe that perhaps the most important piece of anatomy to work with this book is not the heart or biceps, but the mind. And for the training in this book to work, your mind must be open. If your mind is not open to new ideas, these results will have a much harder time occurring.

The workout circuits contained in the book work to develop your physical armor. The two circuits of Mental Cardio should be used to strengthen your mental armor. If you choose not to perform them, that is okay, but know that you are only half the warrior you could be. The mental warrior eventually realizes the essence of training is not just the experience of the training, but what he learns about himself as a result.

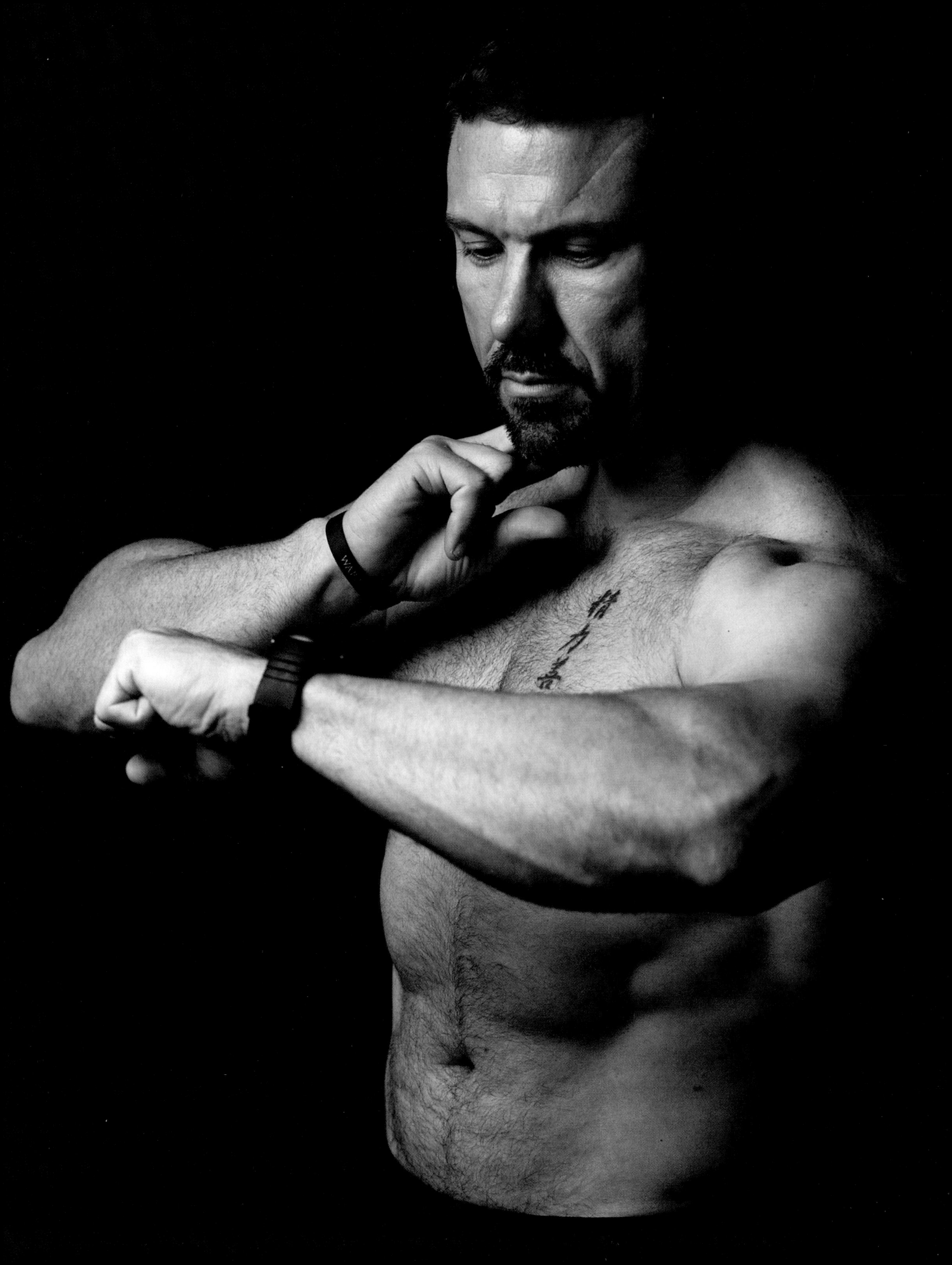

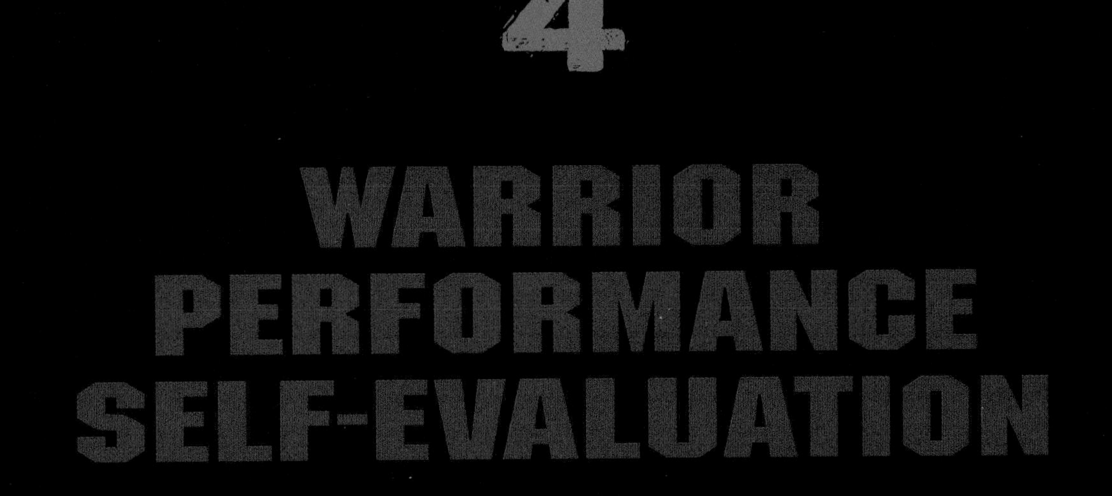

4 WARRIOR PERFORMANCE SELF-EVALUATION

We all know we have limitations, but rarely do we come across situations that force us to identify or examine them and then actually document them. This evaluation's purpose is to force you to find strengths, weaknesses, and areas of asymmetry in your body. By knowing these, you are then forced to make weaknesses into strengths and add symmetry to your physique and movement. If there are glaring issues found in your performance, this will also be the impetus to finally address and overcome them so you can be back to making progress.

An important note: If you find real issues that you think you can't address, then you may need to see a professional therapist who specializes in the particular issue.

All too often, fighters think that being injured is "part of the game" and fail to address the physical ailments that either start to creep up or are brought upon them. In each case, these issues need to be identified and addressed. You are not being "tough" by going through or around pain. You are being stupid.

Before you can help yourself, you must first know yourself. This evaluation will help you to do that from a physical performance standpoint. I am often amazed when I evaluate athletes who, although they are top players in their particular sport, rarely are aware of their true performance level. My goal was to create an evaluation that gave readers the ability to assess and better understand themselves.

Your challenge with this list, just like with the Warrior 20 you will find later in this book, will not be in understanding it, but in consistent execution to make improvements. As I have found, we are not in want of knowledge, but in action on that knowledge.

All too often, people will jump right to the exercise section and the circuits and get going. If you are really serious about your health, the key will be to go through this exam, document the results, and address them before training starts.

I believe that the most important physical characteristic we can possess is Relative Body Strength. Simple translation: how strong you are for how much you weigh. If you are stronger for your weight, this means you have an opportunity to jump higher, move faster, and more efficiently use your most important piece of exercise equipment, your body. Over the last decade of training thousands of top athletes, I have developed a performance evaluation that not only assesses current levels of strength and endurance, but also identifies areas of weakness.

WARRIOR 7 PERFORMANCE EVALUATION:

Resting HR
30-Meter Sprint
Vertical Jump
Broad Jump
3-Minute Pushup Test
3-Minute Chin-up Test
150-Meter Test

RESTING HEART RATE TEST

Resting heart rate is a measure of the number of times your heart beats per minute at rest. This test is an excellent assessment for your current level of cardiovascular conditioning. People who are more cardiovascularly fit usually have a lower resting heart rate because the heart has an increased ability to deliver blood to the body. The average resting heart rate for most people is between 60 and 80 beats per minute. Resting values below 60 indicate an increased level of fitness.

Administration

The best time to find your resting heart rate is in the morning before you get out of bed, or in the evening right before you go to sleep. When you take your pulse, use your index and middle finger on your carotid artery on your neck. Make sure you have been resting for a few hours and have not eaten close to the time of recording your number. Starting at zero, count the total number of beats while watching a clock for one minute and record your score.

ASSESSMENT

	Excellent	Above Average	Average	Below Average	Poor
Adults:	<49-55	56-65	66-73	74-81	>82

SPEED AND POWER TESTS

There are a number of ways to assess speed and power, but in the TFW system, we utilize the 30-meter sprint, the vertical jump, and the broad jump. I believe that these are not only quick and easy tests to administer, but also assessment tools that offer an incredible amount of information. The following is how to perform each test and a rating scale for adult men and women to assess their current levels of performance.

THE 30-METER SPRINT TEST

Why sprints are a good assessment tool

A sprint is an excellent way to gain knowledge about an athlete. In order to be fast, an athlete must have good relative body strength, low body fat, good coordination, and an excellent power output. Since power will tell you about your overall strength level and ability to use that strength quickly, this is a great predictive test for athleticism.

Administration

Mark off 30 meters with a tape measure and have a friend time you with a stopwatch. Sprint the 30 meters from a standing stationary position. Have the timer start the clock when you start running and stop the clock when your chest crosses the finish. Record your best of three times in seconds.

ASSESSMENT

Below is a scale to assess your current level of ability in seconds

	Excellent	Above Average	Average	Below Average	Poor
Males:	<4.0	4.2	4.4	4.6	4.6>
Females:	<4.5	4.7	4.9	5.1	5.1>

THE VERTICAL AND BROAD JUMPS

Why jumps are a good assessment tool

The broad and vertical jumps are excellent assessments of fitness. These tests are great assessments for an athlete's ability to express power. Since power is a measure of how well your nervous system can express both strength and speed, both jumps tells you a lot about your current conditioning.

Administration

To assess the vertical jump, stand with your dominant side facing a wall and reach your hand as high as possible without going up on your toes. Mark the highest point of your fingers. Then, using chalk on the hand, jump as high as possible and touch the wall, leaving a chalk mark at the highest point. Using a tape measure, assess the difference between the two marks. This will be your vertical jump.

To assess a broad jump, stand with the tips of your toes behind a line marked on the ground with the feet slightly less than shoulder-width apart. Stretch out a tape measure to 11 feet from the line. From this position, you are allowed to swing your arms back and then forward to create momentum while jumping. You must take off and land with both feet. Your jump won't count if you land on one foot or fall backward during landing. To record your distance traveled, measure from the start line to the back of the closer heel.

ASSESSMENT

Vertical Jump

	Excellent	Above Average	Average	Below Average	Poor
Males:	30"	25"	22"	20"	18"
Females:	24"	20"	18"	16"	13"

Broad Jump

	Excellent	Above Average	Average	Below Average	Poor
Males:	9'6"	9'	8'	7'6"	6'6"
Females:	9'	8'	7'	6'6"	5'5"

ENDURANCE TESTS

There are a number of ways to assess endurance, but in the TFW system, we utilize the 3-Minute Pushup Test, the 3-Minute Chin-up Test, and the 150-Meter Test with every athlete. The following is how to perform each test and a rating scale for men and women to assess their current levels of performance. Note that for the 3-minute tests, there is only one score. This is because I believe that men and women can attain the same level of relative body strength and endurance and, therefore, should be measured on the same scale for these tests.

THE 3-MINUTE PUSHUP TEST

Why pushups are a good assessment tool

This pushup test is a fantastic challenge to test both upper body strength and endurance of your chest, arms, and core. Although this test initially sounds easy, many athletes are often surprised by the results.

To perform a good pushup

Begin in the pushup position with arms straight, the hands under the shoulders, and core held tight. The arms should be rotated so that the crease of the elbow faces forward. Keep the back straight and lower the torso to within 2 inches of the ground while keeping the elbows close to the body. Extend at the elbows to return to the original position.

Administration

Begin in the up position. Start the timer before the first rep. For a rep to count, you must go all the way down (chest 2 inches off the floor) and lock out the elbows at the top. You can rest however/whenever you want, but the clock must keep running. Poor reps in terms of body position or putting down a knee before a rep is completed do not count toward the total. Stop counting when 3 minutes have elapsed and record your score.

ASSESSMENT

Below Average: Under 54
Average: 55-74
Good: 75-99
Excellent: 100-110
Extraordinary: 111+

THE 3-MINUTE CHIN-UP TEST

Why chin-ups are a good assessment tool

The chin-up is not only a fantastic exercise to increase the size and strength of the muscles of the back and arms, but this posture-improving exercise can also predict a lot about your athletic potential. The chin-up works more upper-body muscle mass than most exercises and is one of the best tools to assess your Relative Body Strength.

To perform a good chin-up

Begin holding the bar with the elbows extended and the palms facing you (supinated grip). Lift the feet from the floor and then "pull" your body upward until the chin rises over the bar completely. While pulling upward, keep the "kipping," or using the legs to assist, at a minimum. Lower under control until the elbows are as close to extended as possible.

Administration

Begin in the hanging position with your feet off the floor. Start the timer before the first rep. For a rep to count, you must go all the way up (chin must rise over the bar) and come close to lock out the elbows at the bottom. You can rest however/whenever you want, but the clock must keep running. Poor reps in terms of jumping from the ground, chin below the bar, or not enough elbow extension do not count. Stop counting when 3 minutes have elapsed and record your score.

ASSESSMENT

Below Average: Under 19
Average: 20+
Good: 30+
Excellent: 40+
Extraordinary: 50+

THE 150-METER TEST

Why this test is a good assessment tool

This test gives you an excellent look at your energy production and efficiency. It evaluates speed, speed endurance, and how well you are able to use all three energy systems that are described in this text. This test, like the 3-minute tests, is also good for assessing mental toughness.

Administration

Mark off 37.5 meters with a tape measure. Sprint this distance four times, as fast as possible (total running distance is 150 meters).

The test consists of three total rounds of sprinting with 15 seconds of recovery time between rounds. Record the time after each round.

ASSESSMENT

EXCELLENT
Males time for round 1 = 23 s, round 2 = 26 s, round 3 = 31 s
Females time for round 1 = 26 s, round 2 = 29 s, round 3 = 34 s

AVERAGE
Males time for round 1 = 25 s, round 2 = 30 s, round 3 = 36 s
Females time for round 1 = 30 s, round 2 = 35 s, round 3 = 40 s

POOR
Males time for round 1 = 28 s, round 2 = 34 s, round 3 = 40 s
Females time for round 1 = 34 s, round 2 = 39 s, round 3 = 45 s

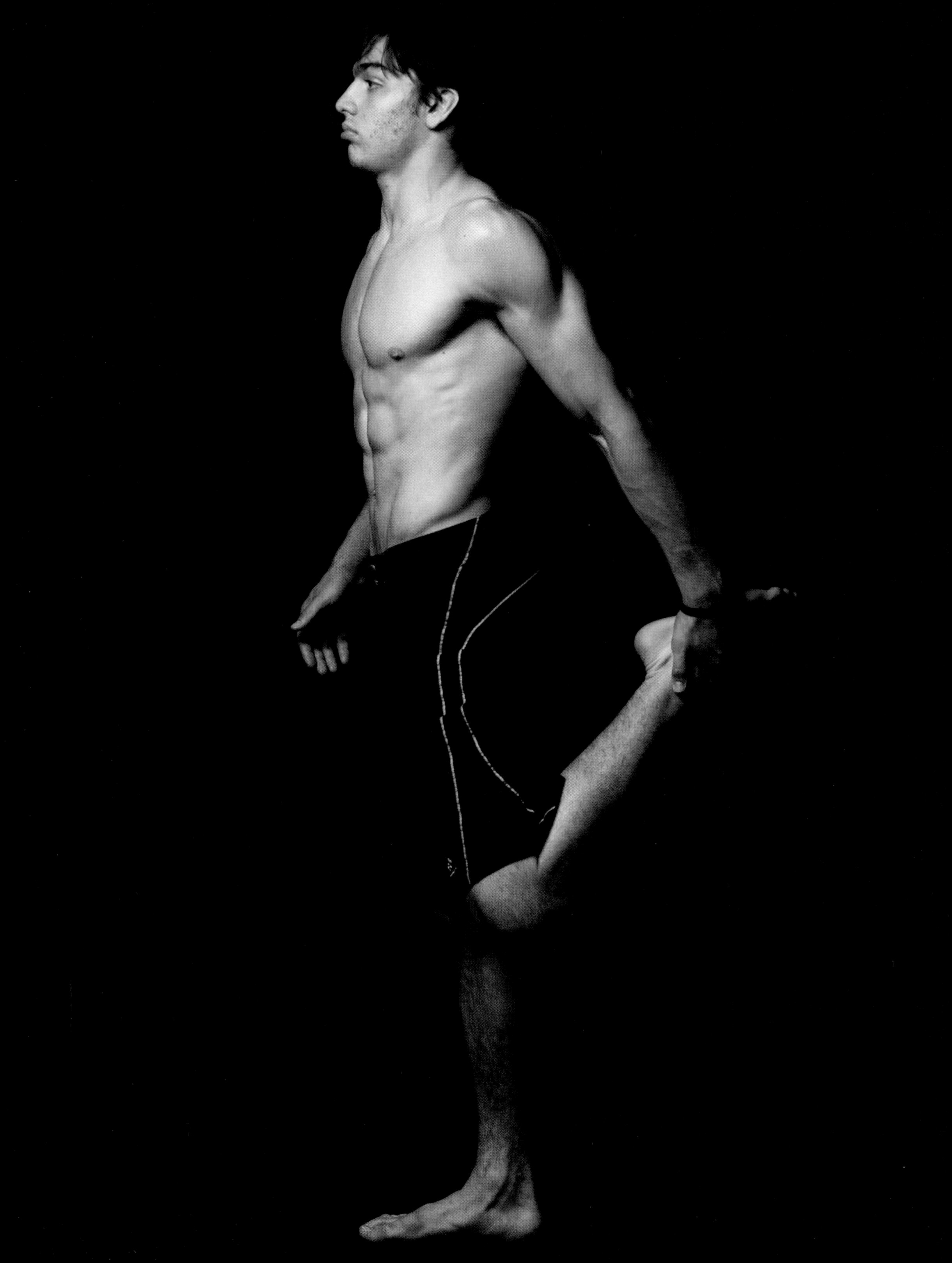

5

WARRIOR PREHAB 15

If you had a Ferrari and it got a deep scratch in the door, a flat tire, or an alignment issue, would you get it fixed? Of course. Yet when we have similar nicks and pings in our bodies, we rarely address them. Even less common is working to train the body so that these issues do not appear in the first place. This work is commonly known as prehabilitation.

I like to define prehab as "something people know they should do, but that nobody does!" Essentially, these are the exercises that you do so that you never need to do rehab. Whether you fight or sit in a chair all day, it can lead to tightness and weakness of the body. Doing the Warrior Prehab routine in this chapter will undo that. Although these may seem like simple and basic stretches, it is often the simple and basic stuff that people skip, wanting to jump right into some of the more difficult workout routines. But you cannot put on your tie before you put on your shirt. If you don't have the proper ranges of motion that these movements require, decreased performance or injury is a possible outcome. I like to tell my athletes that a little on top of a little eventually becomes a lot. If you spend a little time on these exercises, you will see pains disappear, ranges of motion increase, and numbers in the gym improve.

Once you have put yourself through the Warrior Prehab, I am sure that you will immediately be reminded of some areas of tightness that you need to work on, as well as alerted to areas of asymmetry that you may not have known about. In either case, the main purpose of the Warrior Prehab is to make you more aware of your body.

These exercises are to be performed before every TFW workout. They focus on every section of the body and address the most common areas of weakness and range-of-motion loss in most athletes today. By performing these exercises, you will be opening and closing the door hinges of your body so that they will never get rusty. You can use this routine before the warmup, and I also suggest that you spend extra time performing the exercises that address your greatest needs in the evenings throughout the week. You should be able to complete these exercises in about 15 minutes. The best investment people can make is an investment in themselves. Don't you owe it to yourself to invest in improved performance, decreased injury, and training longevity?

These exercises should not be performed to the point of pain. The key is to increase range of motion. With the photos of each exercise, there is a description of how the exercise is to be performed and for how long or how many repetitions.

For every stretch performed, pay particular attention to whether there is pain or asymmetry on either side. If you notice either of these things, you may want to visit a medical professional to investigate further.

1. BALL FOOT ROLL

Using a ball of the hardness of your choice, begin by placing your toes on the ball. Applying slight pressure, press the sole of your foot into the ball and roll it over the top of the ball until the ball is at the heel. Roll the ball back toward the toes and repeat for about 20 passes on each foot.

This exercise is used to improve the mobility of the foot. As you are performing the passes, you can roll the ball more under the outside and inside of the foot.

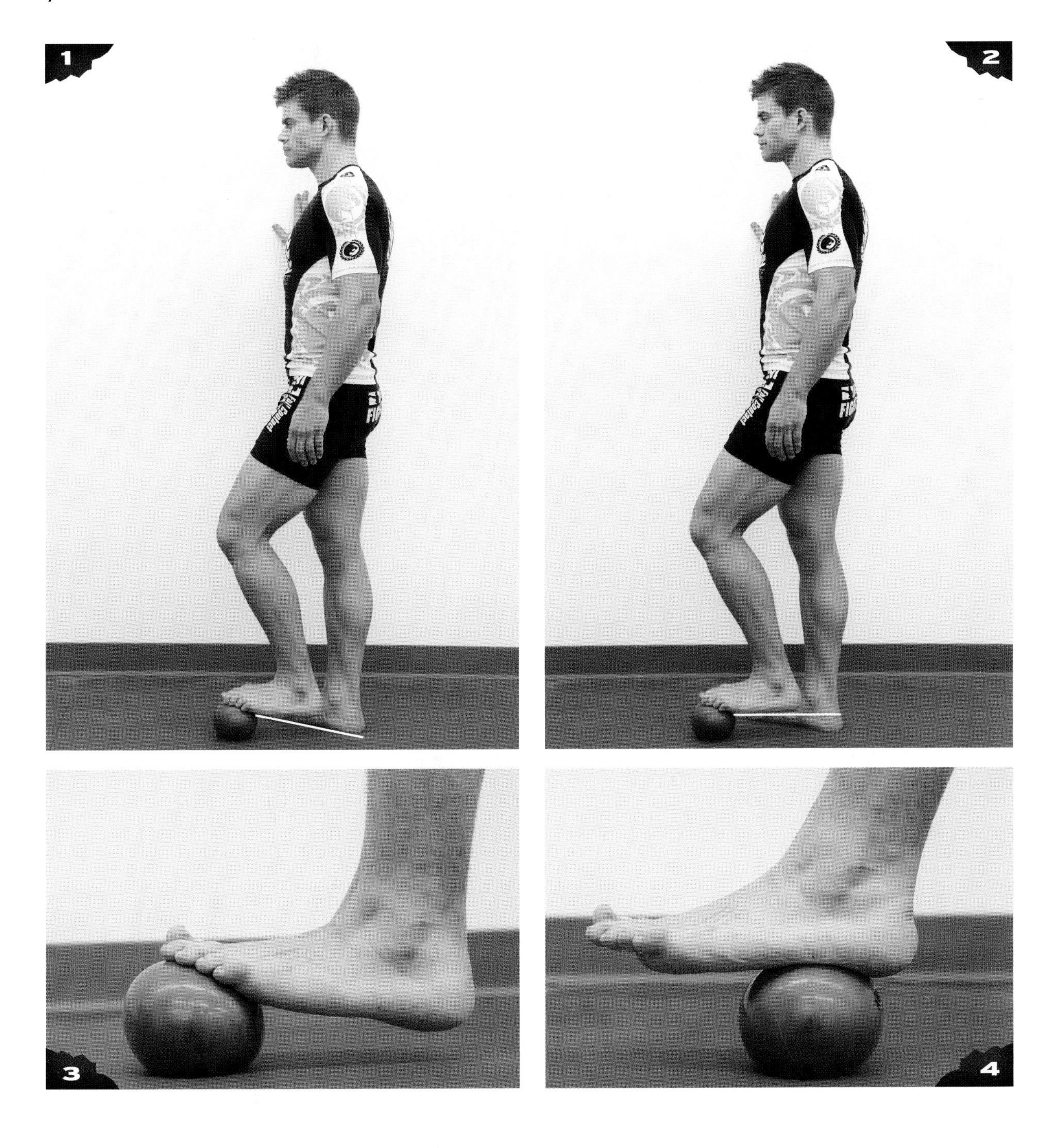

2. IT BAND FOAM ROLL

Lie on one side and place the foam roller under the IT band. This is the area along the outside of the thigh that starts at the top of the hip and runs down to the outside of the knee. Using your arm to balance, slowly roll the outside of the leg over the foam roller. If there is any area of increased soreness, stop and hold the pressure on that spot until the soreness is reduced. Work your way down the leg toward the knee. Repeat on the other side.

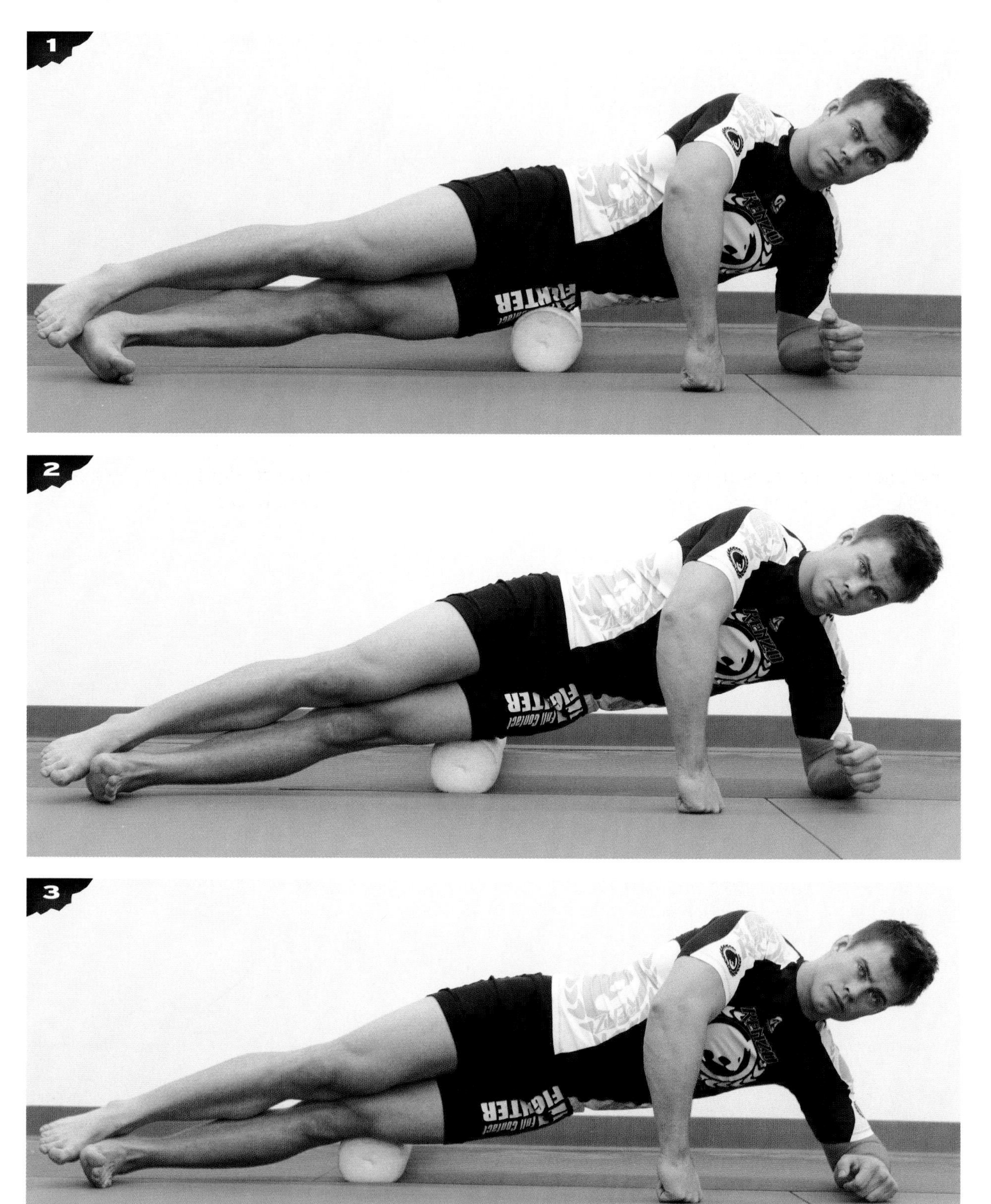

3. PIRIFORMIS FOAM ROLL

Begin by sitting one hip on the foam roll. Lift the foot on the side on which you are sitting and cross it over the other leg. While balancing on the opposite hand and foot, slowly roll the buttock over the foam roll in search of tender areas. Sit on any tender spots until the soreness reduces. Repeat this on the other hip.

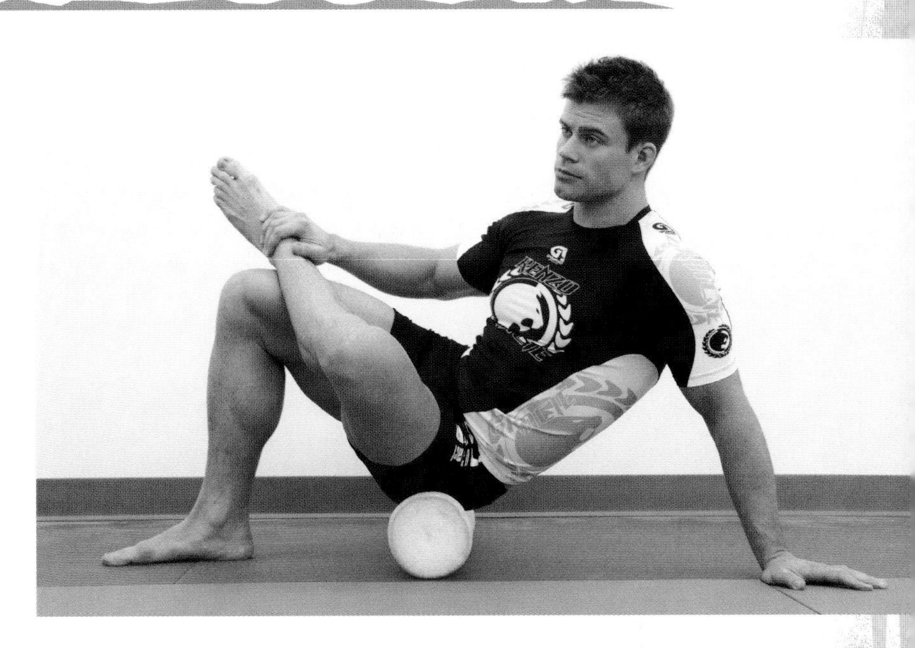

4. HIP INTERNAL AND EXTERNAL ROTATION STRETCH

Begin seated on the floor. Bring the sole of one foot to the inside of the opposite thigh while bringing the other foot to the buttocks. In this position, you can lean to either side and forward to increase the stretch on either or both of the hips. If this stretch is painful on the knees (in particular on the leg with the foot to the back), begin with that leg held straight out and ease the foot back over a number of workouts. Hold this stretch for 30 seconds on each side.

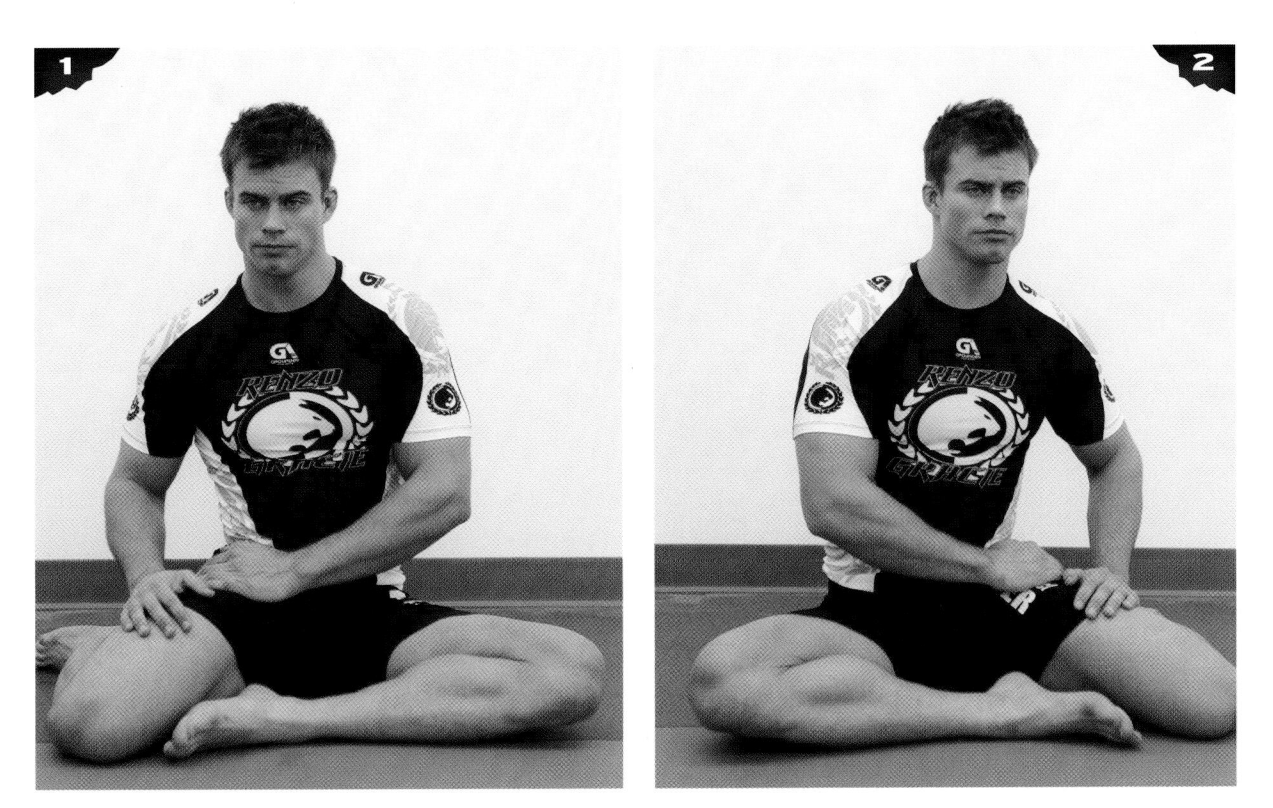

5. STANDING GASTROCNEMIUS STRETCH

Begin standing and support yourself with both hands on a wall. Bring one foot behind the body and keep the chest and back leg at about a 45-degree angle to the wall. While keeping the heel of the back foot flat to the ground, slowly move the hips toward the wall. Hold the stretch for 20 seconds and repeat for 2 reps on each leg.

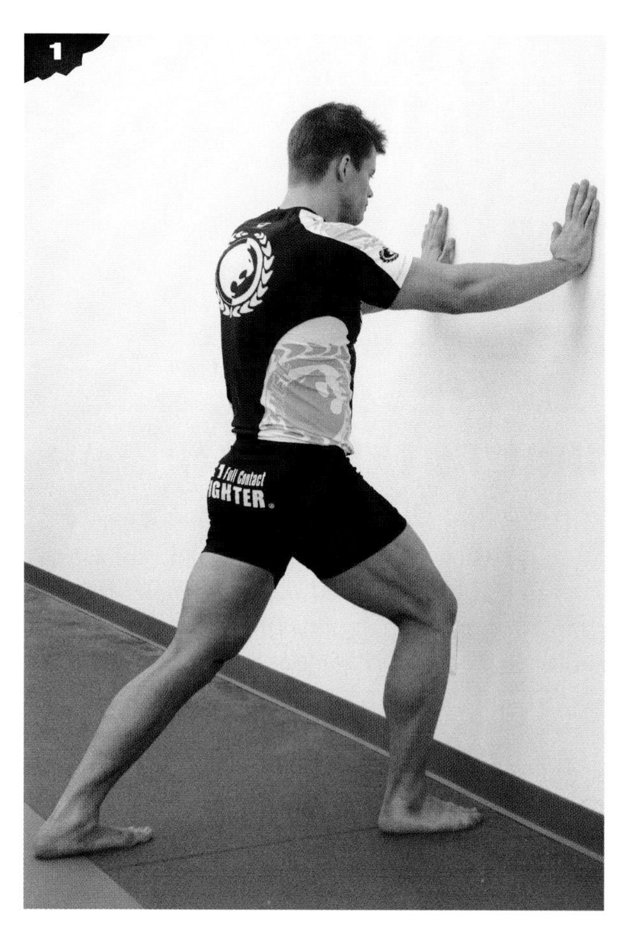

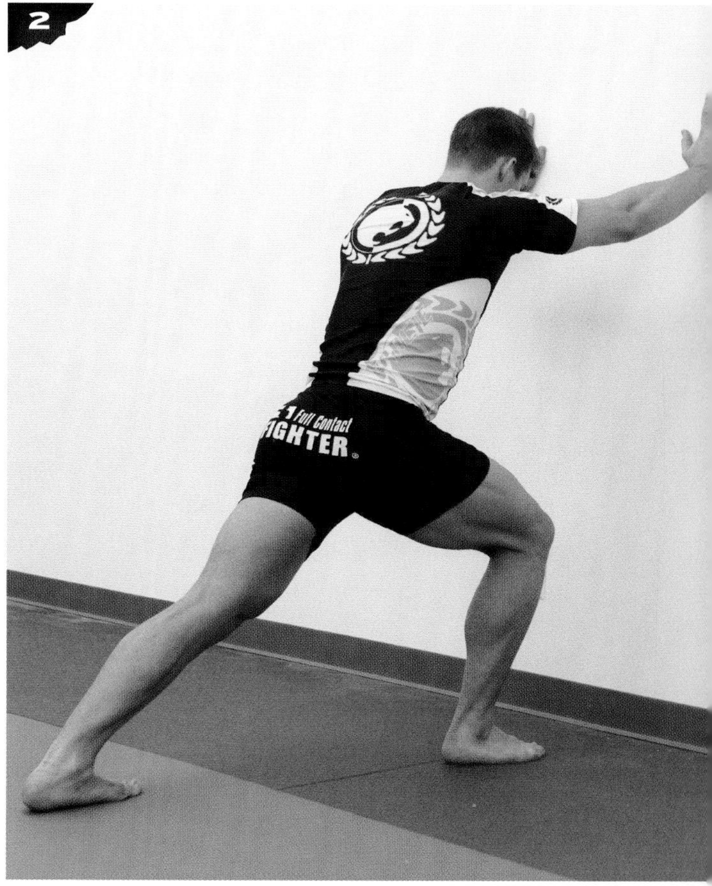

6. STANDING QUADRICEPS STRETCH

Begin standing and support yourself with one hand on a wall if necessary. While keeping the knee directly under the hip, bring the foot up behind the hip and grab onto the foot with the hand on the same side. Pull the foot up while making sure to maintain an upright position with the upper body. Hold for 20 seconds and repeat for 2 reps on each side.

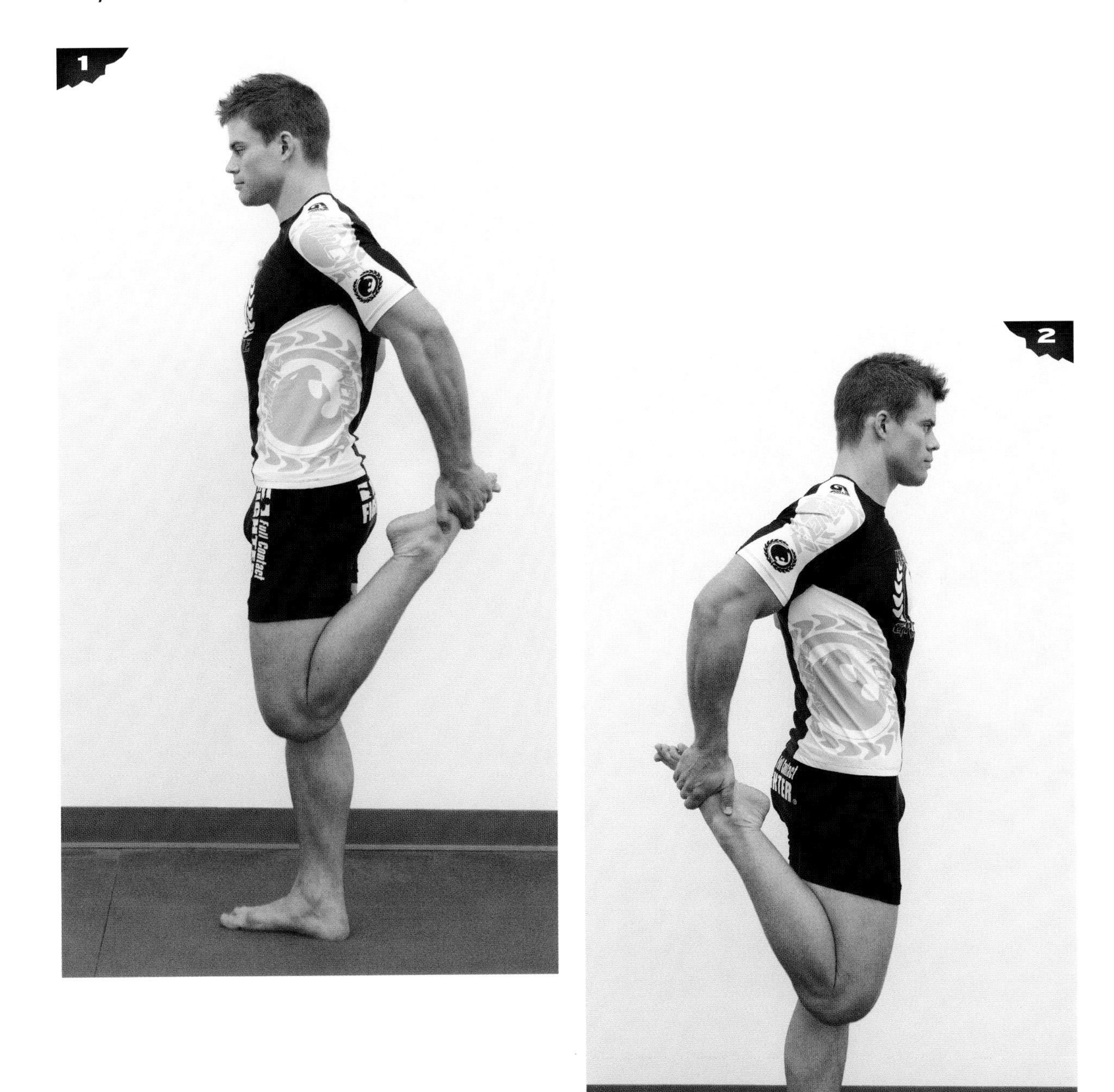

7. STANDING HAMSTRING STRETCH

Begin standing. Cross one foot over the other while making sure that neither foot is farther forward than the other. Bend forward as if to touch the toes. There will be a much greater stretch felt on the back leg. Hold for 20 seconds and repeat for 2 sets on both sides.

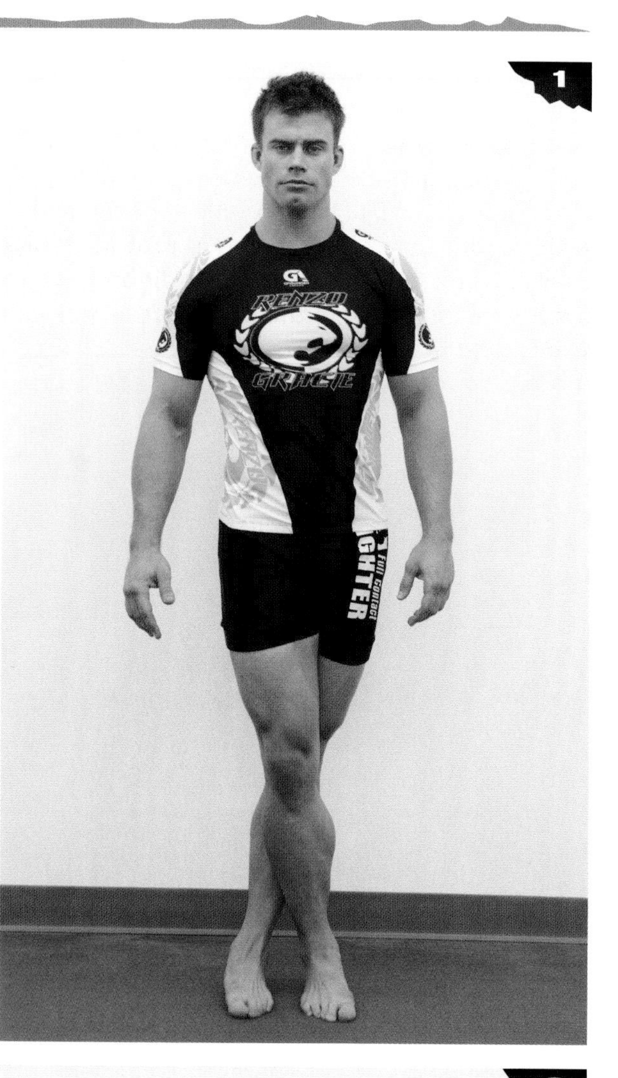

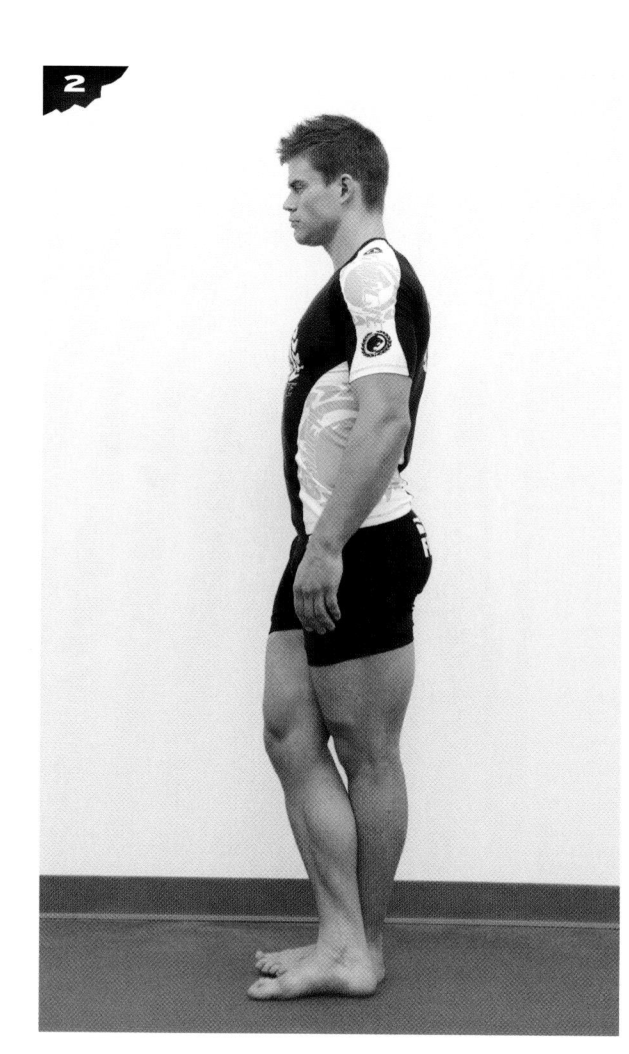

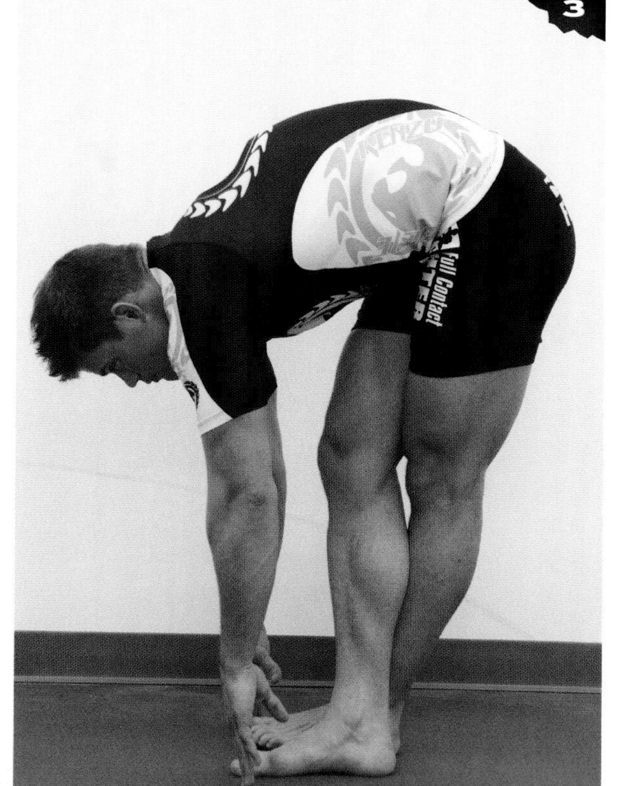

8. WALL SOLEUS/HIP FLEXOR STRETCH

Begin facing a wall on one knee, with the foot nearer to the wall only an inch or two away. In order to determine the correct distance to perform this stretch, lean forward at the hips to see if you can touch the knee to the wall while still keeping the heel of the front foot on the ground. If this is possible, move the front foot back slightly and continue to repeat the process until the heel can no longer be kept on the floor. Once this point is reached, slide the back knee backward slightly to also stretch the hip flexor on the back leg in addition to the soleus and ankle on the front. Hold for 20 seconds and repeat for 2 sets on both sides.

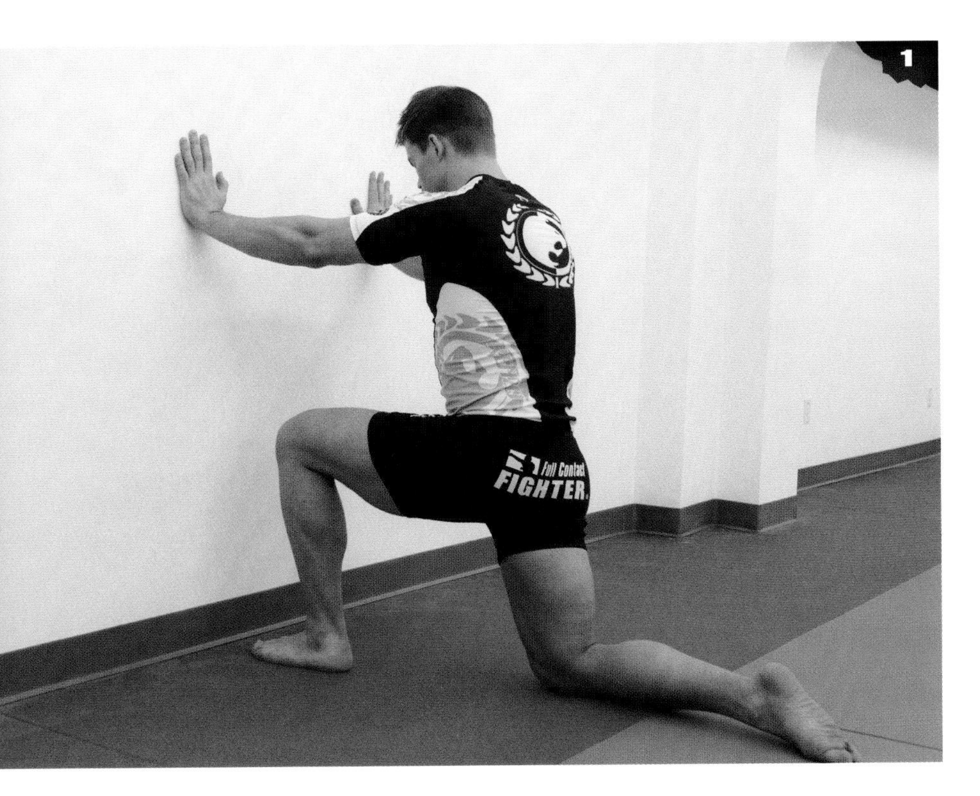

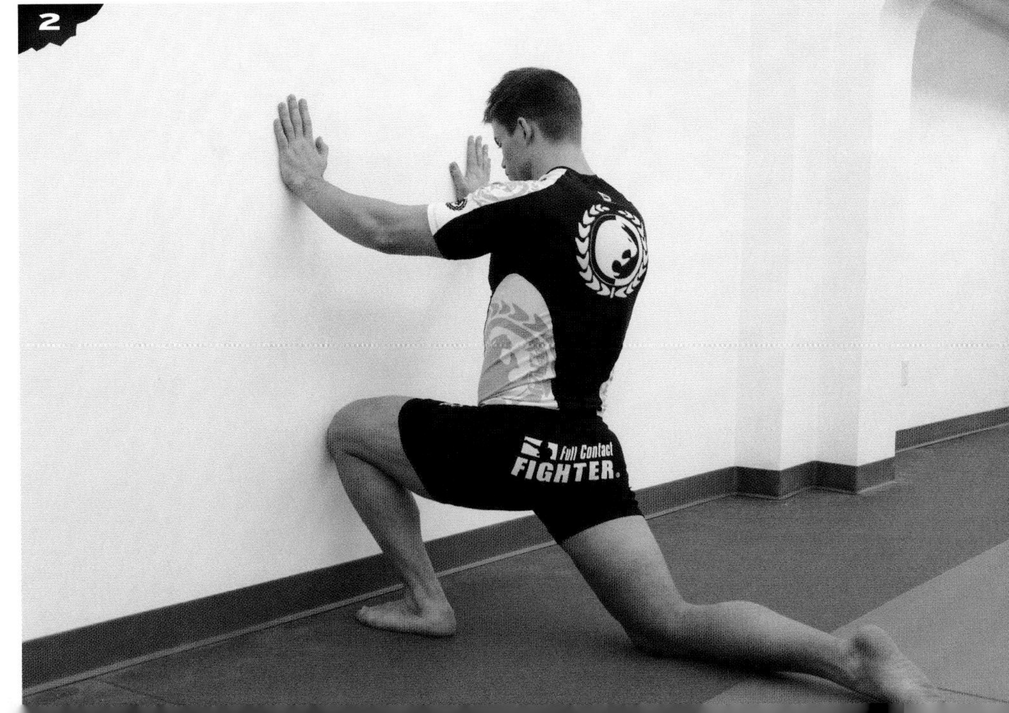

9. SEATED GLUTE, ANKLE, AND SHOULDER STRETCH

Begin sitting on the edge of a bench with one leg crossed over the other and the hands supporting the weight of the body. Move the hips slightly forward until you can drop them straight down. This movement will create a stretch on the hip of the top leg, the ankle of the bottom foot, and the shoulders and pectoral muscles. Bring the bottom foot back to create more stretch on the ankle if needed. Perform this stretch for 20 seconds and repeat for 2 sets on each side.

1

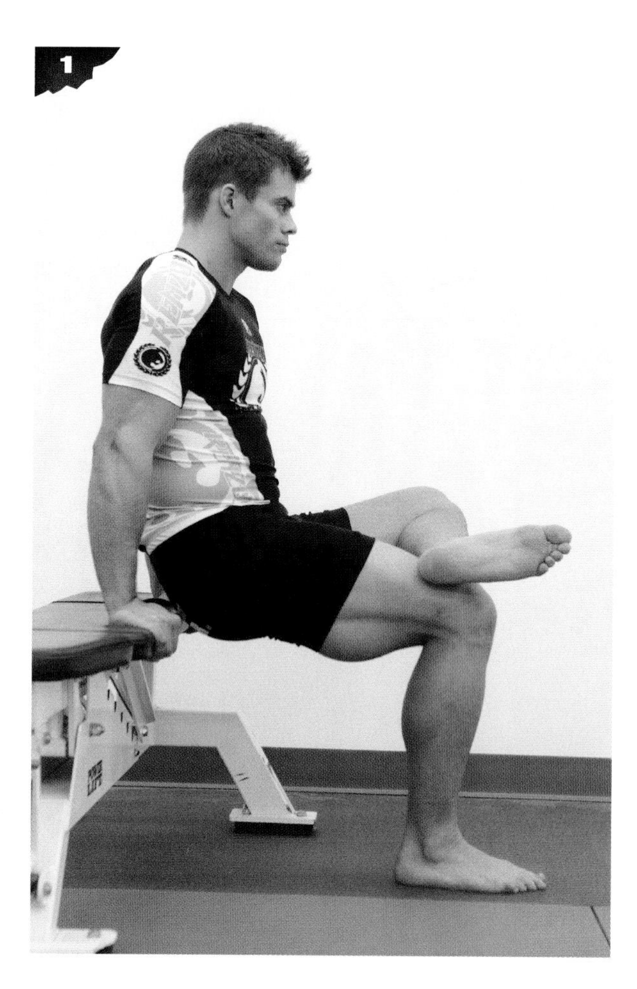

2

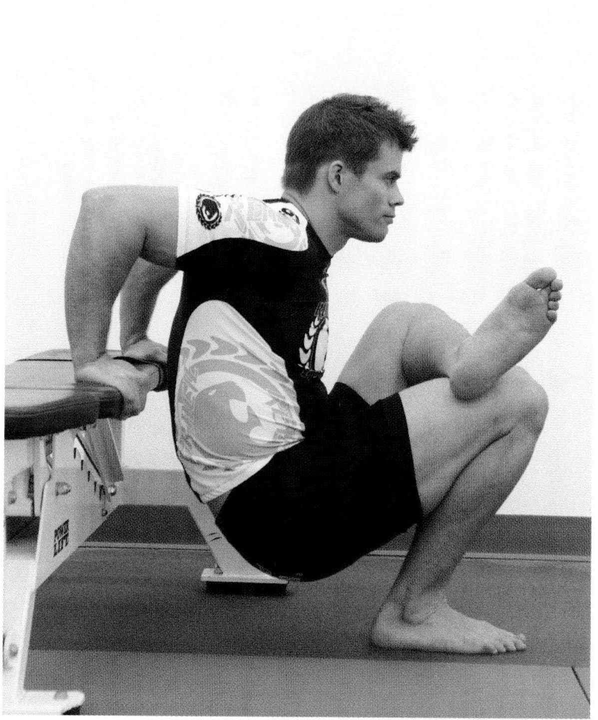

10. SUMO SQUAT

At this point in the Warrior Prehab 15 routine, the increased mobility of the ankles, hips, and hamstrings should allow you to perform a deeper squat.

Begin in the deep squat position while grabbing onto the toes with both hands. While maintaining a grip on both sets of toes, extend at the knees and hips in order to raise the hips as high as possible. Even if you are unable to attain straight legs, hold the top position for 20 seconds and repeat for 2 sets on both sides.

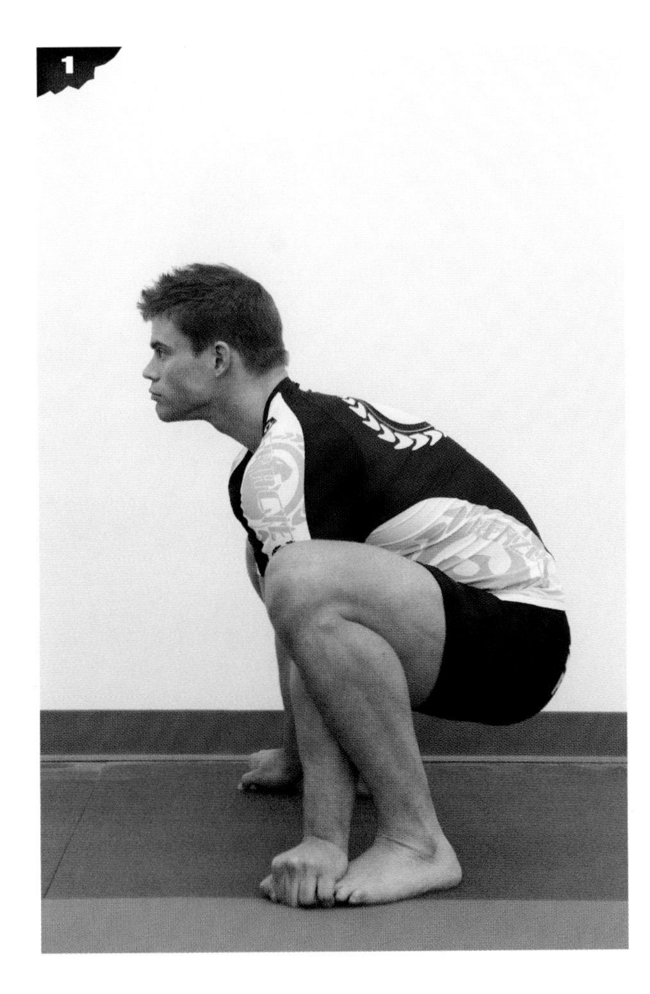

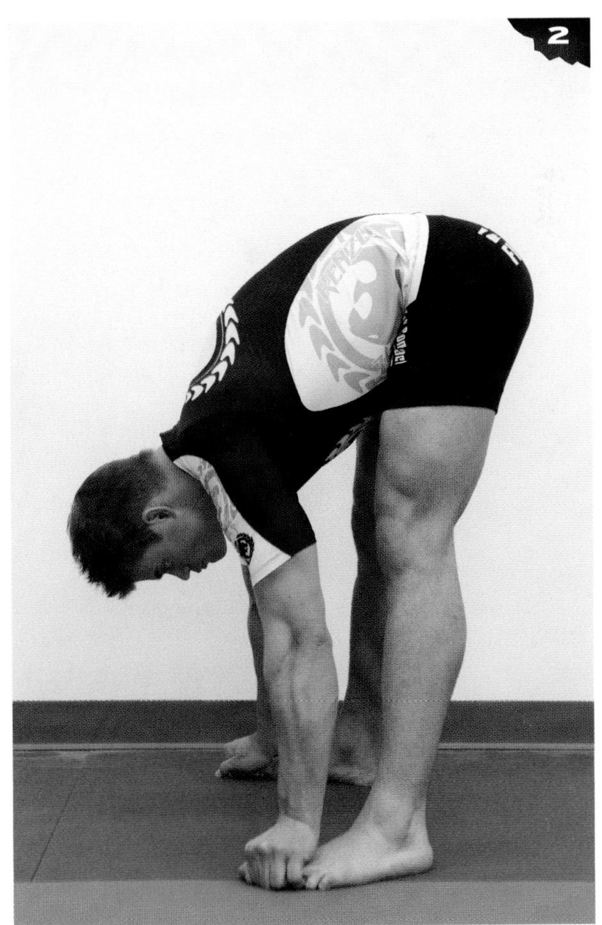

11. LATISSIMUS STRETCH

Begin kneeling and place the palms flat on the floor in front of you. While keeping the elbows extended, lower the head and chest to place a stretch on the lats. Hold this stretch for 20 seconds and then repeat for 3 repetitions.

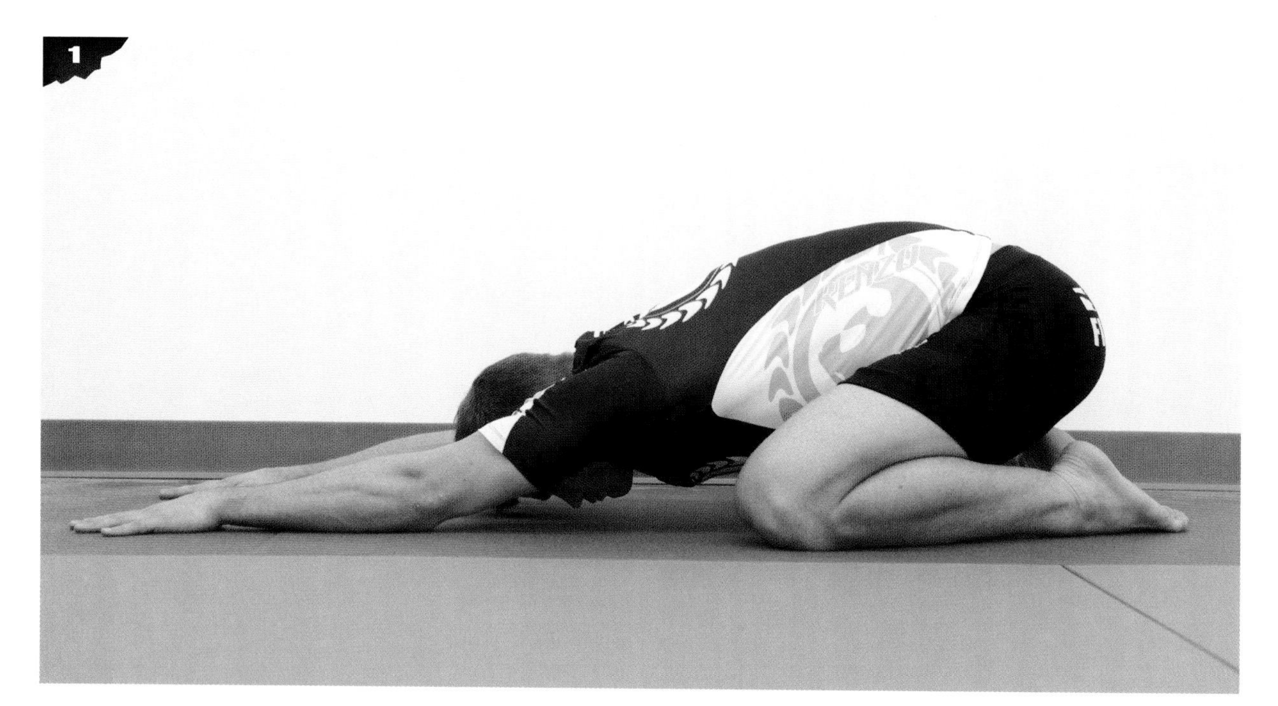

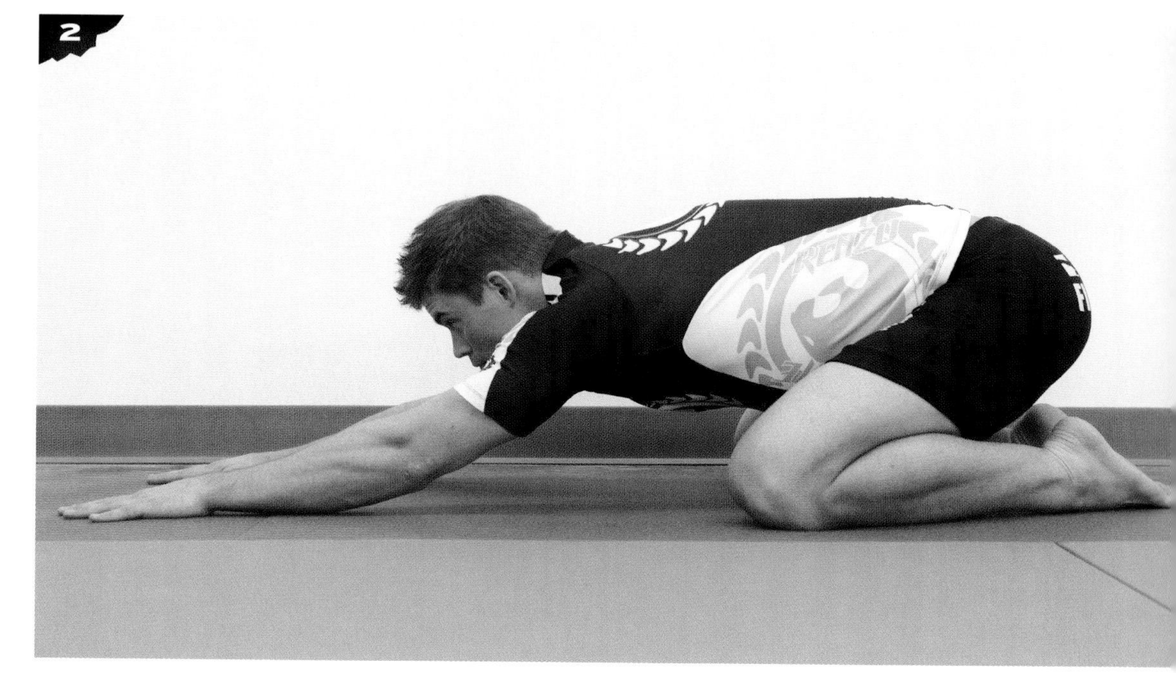

12. ABDOMINAL STRETCH

Begin lying facedown on the floor with the hands held at the sides at chest level. Press the hands into the ground to lift the upper body from the floor while keeping the hips and thighs down. Look upward with the head to increase the stretch on the neck. Hold the stretch for 20 seconds and repeat for 3 repetitions.

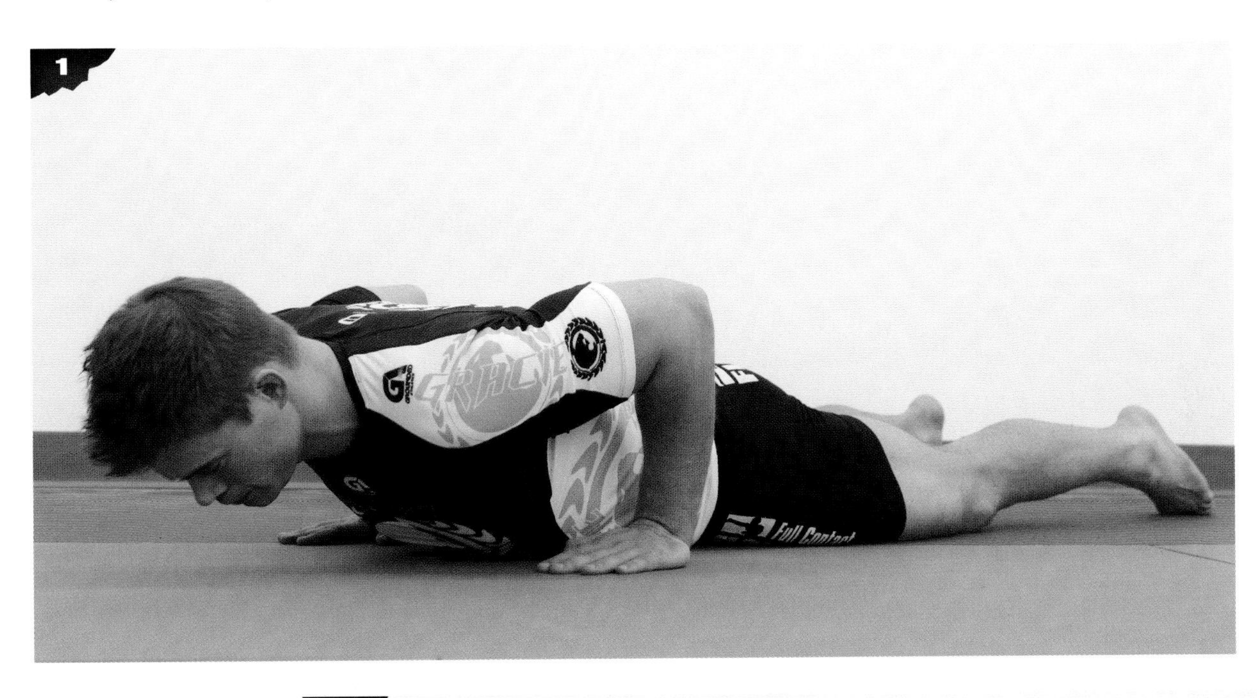

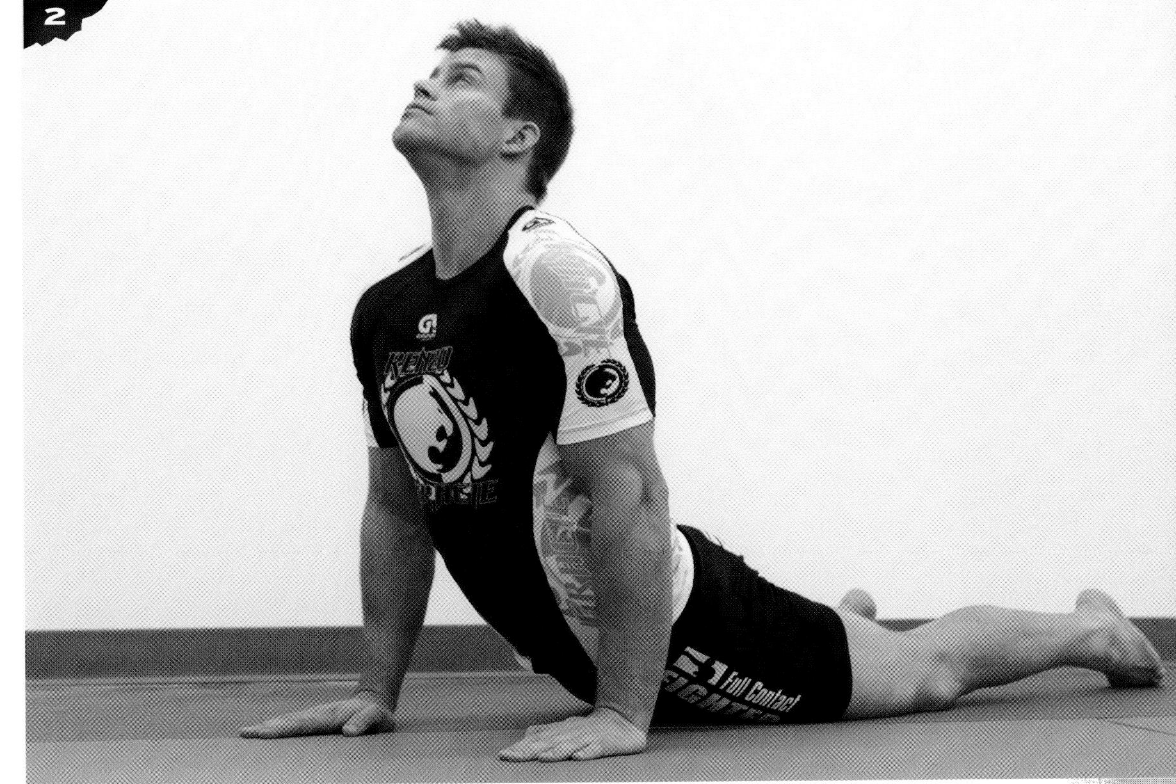

13. CORNER PECTORAL STRETCH

Begin standing facing into a corner with the hands held slightly above the head and the elbows at a 90-degree angle. Keeping the feet about two feet from the corner, slowly lean the chest forward, creating a greater stretch on the chest and shoulders. Hold the stretch for 20 seconds and repeat for 3 repetitions.

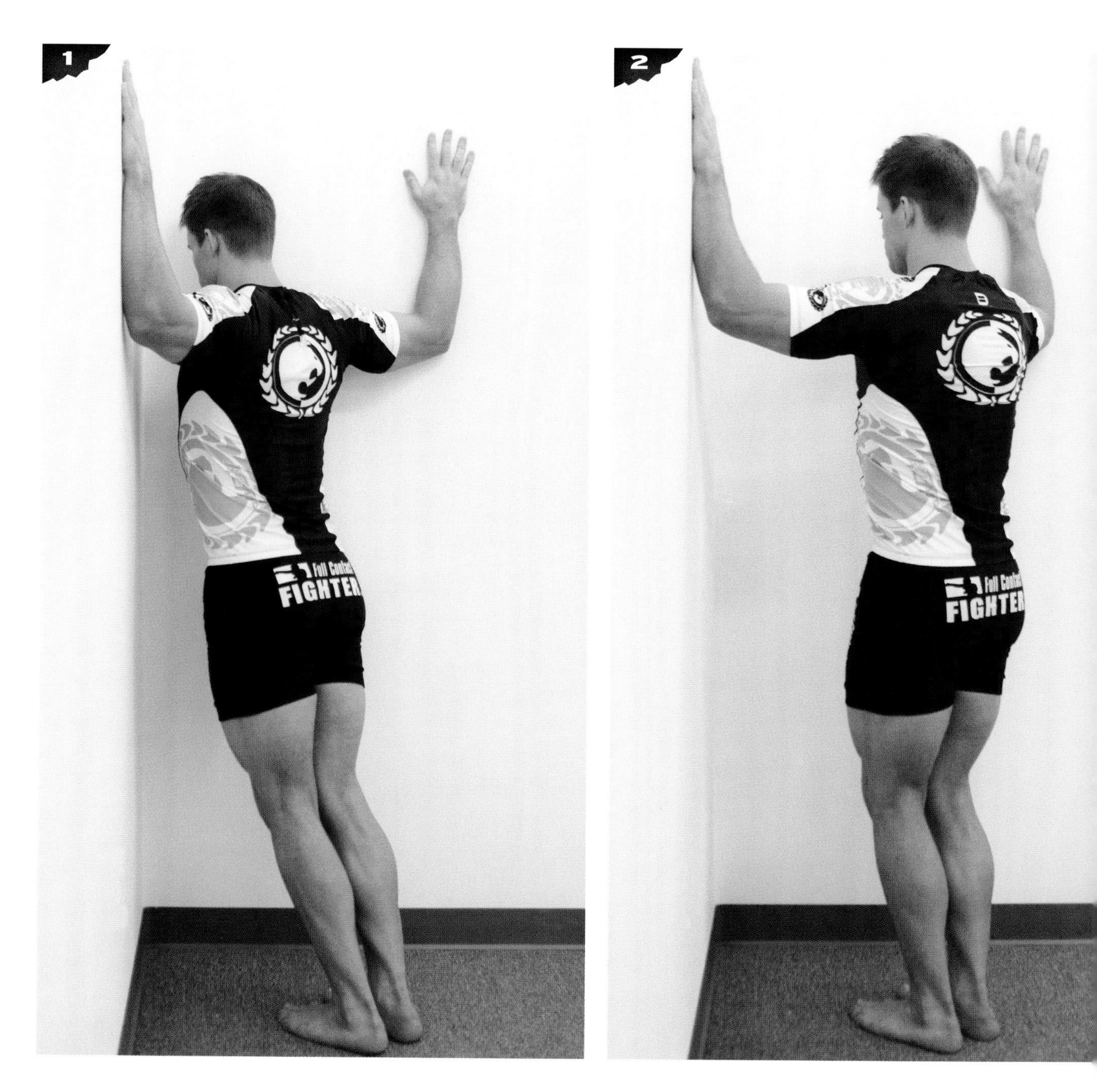

14. THORACIC STRETCH

Begin lying on a bench with hands held behind the head. The chest and head should be held off the bench so that the middle of the back is supported while the head is held up by the hands. To perform the stretch, open up the elbows and look upward so that the head drops as low as possible past the bench. Hold this stretch for 20 seconds and repeat for 3 repetitions.

1

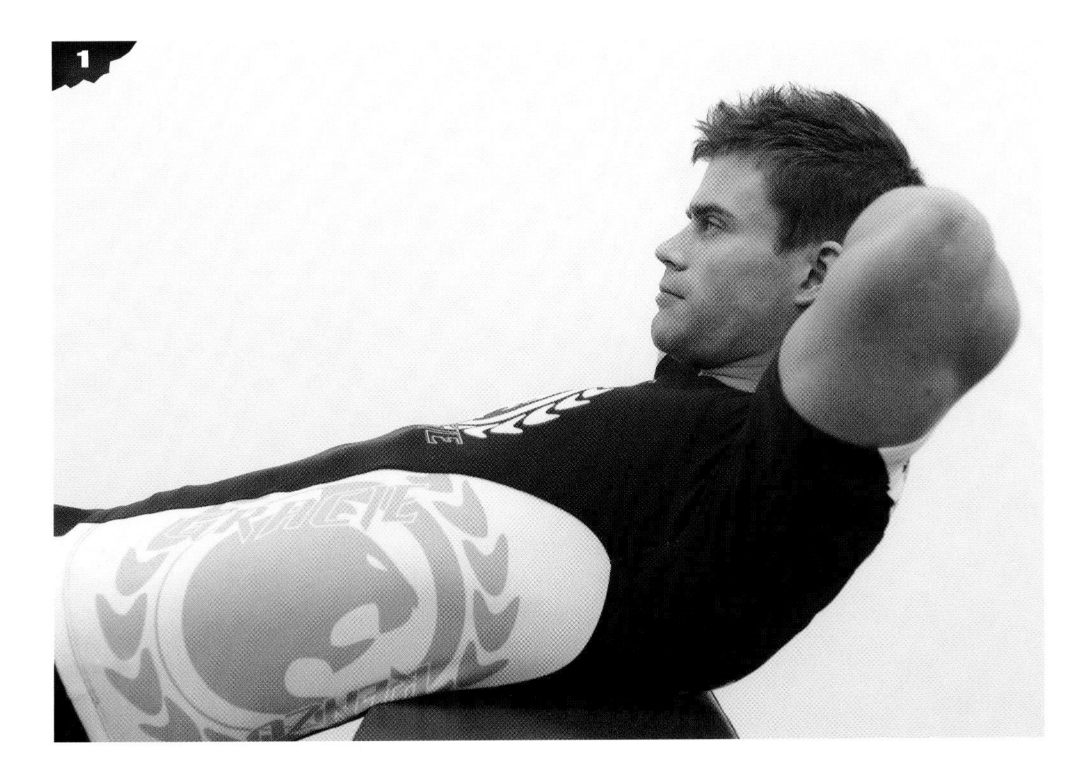

2

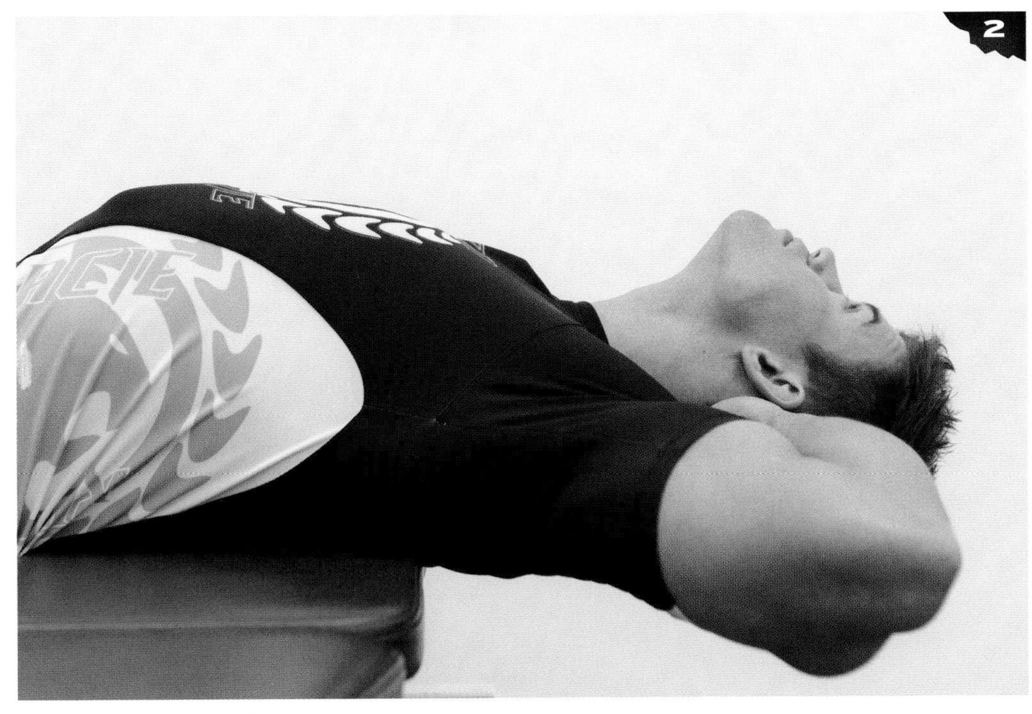

15. WALL SLIDE

Begin standing with the back against the wall and the hands held over the head so that the backs of the wrists and hands are also flat against the wall. Lower the hands so that the elbows come down toward the sides of the body. Keep the wrists, hands, and elbows as flat to the wall as possible while trying to maintain the same position of the torso. Take about 3 to 5 seconds to lower the arms and then repeat for 8 to 10 repetitions.

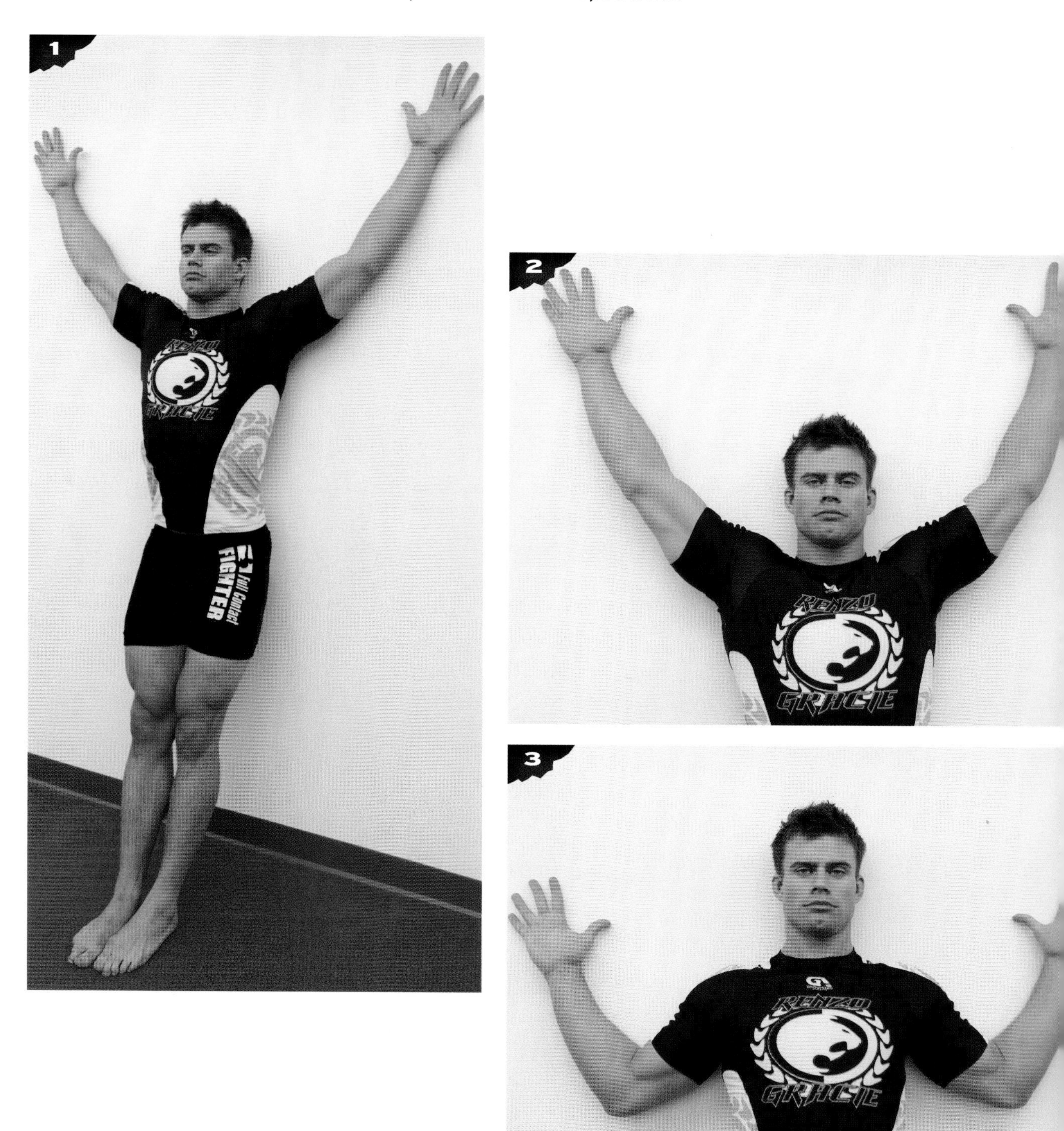

TFW PREHAB 15 CHEATSHEET

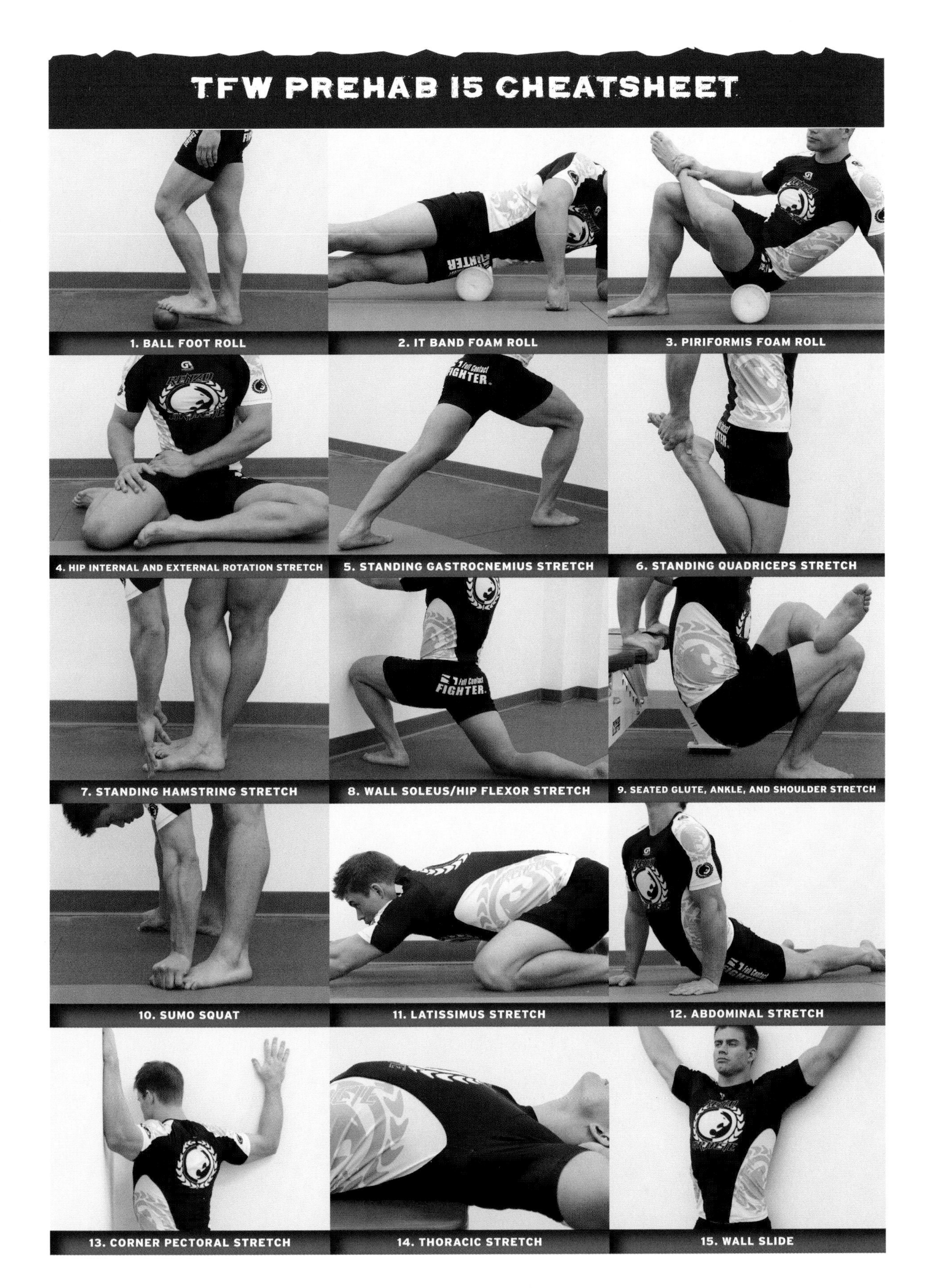

1. BALL FOOT ROLL
2. IT BAND FOAM ROLL
3. PIRIFORMIS FOAM ROLL
4. HIP INTERNAL AND EXTERNAL ROTATION STRETCH
5. STANDING GASTROCNEMIUS STRETCH
6. STANDING QUADRICEPS STRETCH
7. STANDING HAMSTRING STRETCH
8. WALL SOLEUS/HIP FLEXOR STRETCH
9. SEATED GLUTE, ANKLE, AND SHOULDER STRETCH
10. SUMO SQUAT
11. LATISSIMUS STRETCH
12. ABDOMINAL STRETCH
13. CORNER PECTORAL STRETCH
14. THORACIC STRETCH
15. WALL SLIDE

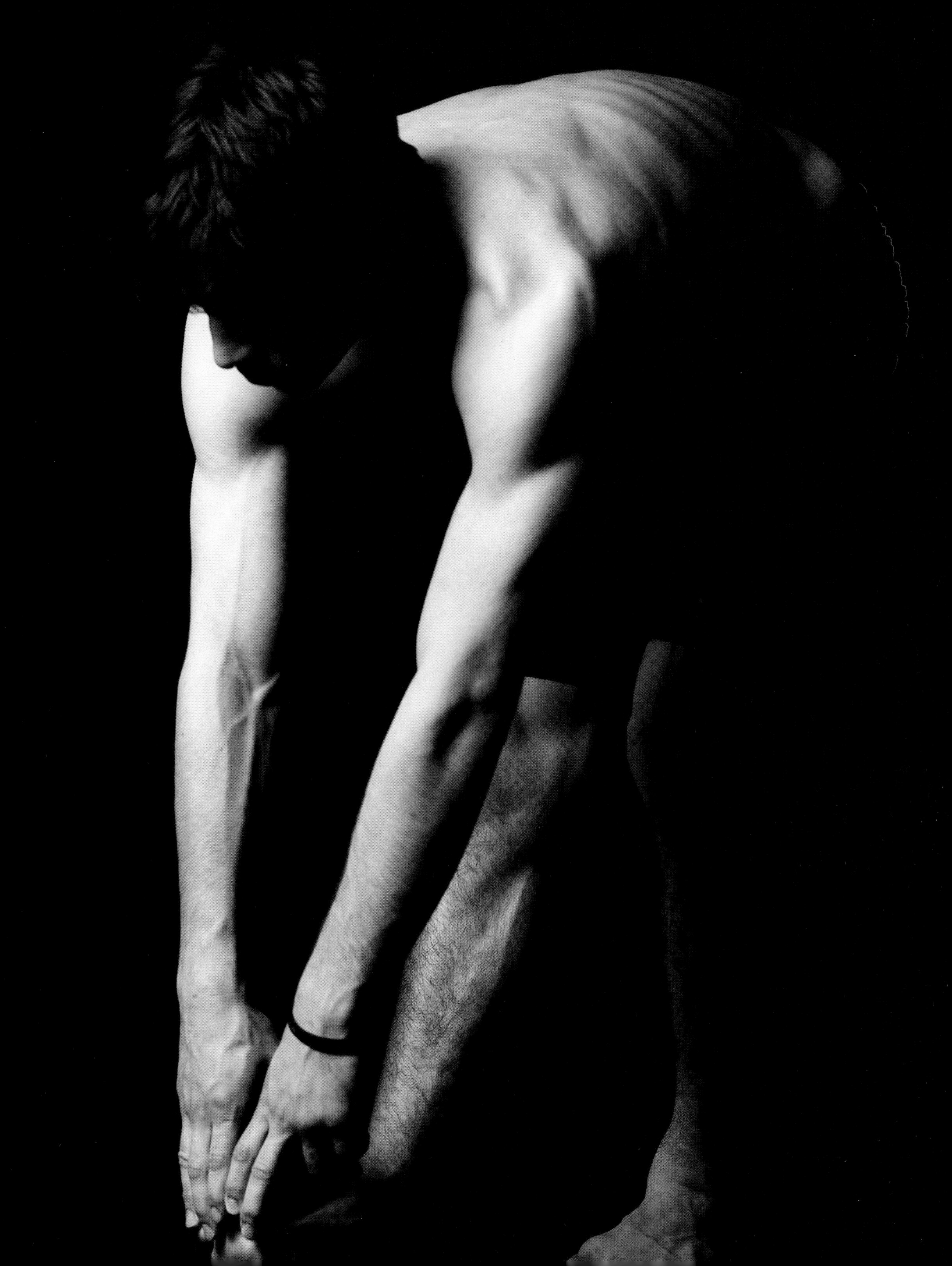

6

WARRIOR CARDIO WARMUP

The metabolic forms of training contained in this book are very demanding. A common mistake with this style of training is to use either an inadequate warmup or no warmup at all. Since a trainee often thinks that Metabolic Training sessions are great at getting the heart rate up and increasing core temperature, they often decide to jump head-first into the session. Don't do this.

The warmup is the cornerstone of TFW training. In most of the books out there, the warmup is quickly glazed over as if it were unimportant. This is definitely not the case here. In fact, this chapter is perhaps the most important.

Once you've performed the Prehab 15 exercises, you must still go through a 15-to-20-minute warmup to get both the body and mind prepared for what is to come. The entire process of prehab and warmup should take less than 30 to 40 minutes to complete. Since the Metabolic Training sessions contained in this book should not take more than 20 minutes to complete (and some take much less, leaving time for core work and flexibility), there is no excuse for you to skip the warmup.

There are a number of reasons that this Warrior Warmup must be employed before a Metabolic Training session:

1. A proper warmup is first and foremost about injury prevention. If you are injured, you cannot train. If you are injured because of an improper warmup, this is a training tragedy.
2. A proper warmup for metabolic sessions is necessary to burn off adrenaline and get the body to a steady state of oxygen consumption. This will make the training session more effective both in performance and in fat-burning capability.
3. A proper warmup can be used to increase heart rate and blood flow to the muscles and raise their temperature, which will lead to improved strength and power development.
4. A proper warmup can be used to increase speed of movement, balance, and neuromuscular stimulation, allowing you to turn muscles on and off faster.
5. A proper warmup can be used to increase flexibility and improve range of motion.
6. A proper warmup can also be used to build strength.
7. A proper warmup can be used to improve balance and coordination of movement.
8. A proper warmup gives you an opportunity to focus on the upcoming workout and set the tone for the session. The warmup is the buffer between your life in and outside of training.

To perform this warmup, all you need is one lane with 10 yards of space.

This warmup has four different portions: Mini Plyo Hops, Movement Drills, the Upper-Body Band Routine, and the Hip Circuit. The first two portions can be performed together and the last two portions can be performed whether you are doing an upper- or lower-body-focused session.

The Warrior Warmup contained in this book differs from the original warmup contained in *Training for Warriors: The Ultimate Mixed Martial Arts Workout*, but either variation can be utilized before a training session.

A. MINI PLYO HOPS AND MOVEMENT DRILLS

Mini Plyo Hops are used to increase heart rate and core temperature and to stimulate the nervous system for activity. If possible, these are to be performed in bare feet. For these drills, it's best to use or create an actual line on the floor, which forces you to use better form, but you can imagine the line if necessary.

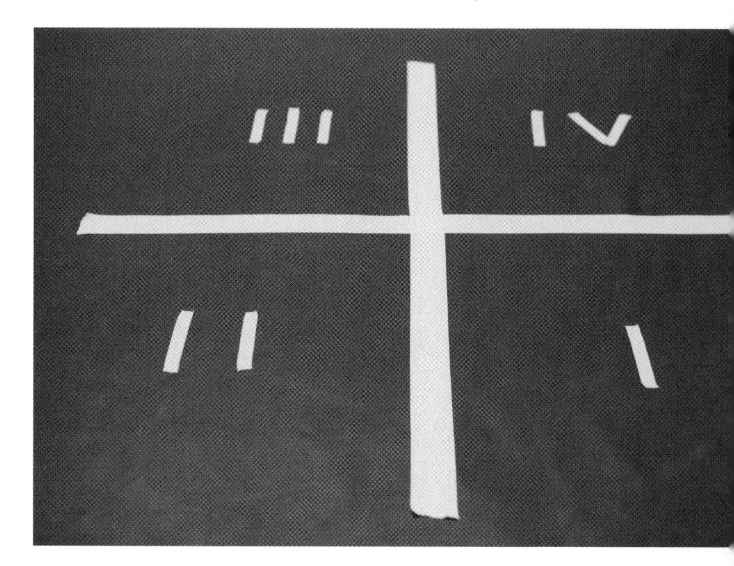

The hops are to be performed as quickly as possible. I like to describe the hops as having the shape of an upside-down tornado. Your feet should move to the described boxes, but you should keep your torso stable in one place over the line. This will force you to engage your core while the feet move under you to manage your balance.

There are sixteen different hopping variations. In between every two variations performed, you are to perform one walking drill for 10 yards down and back.

1. TFW CROSS JUMPS: 1—4

Begin standing in section 1 of the cross. Jump 20 times back and forth in between sections 4 and 1. Each hop counts as one jump.

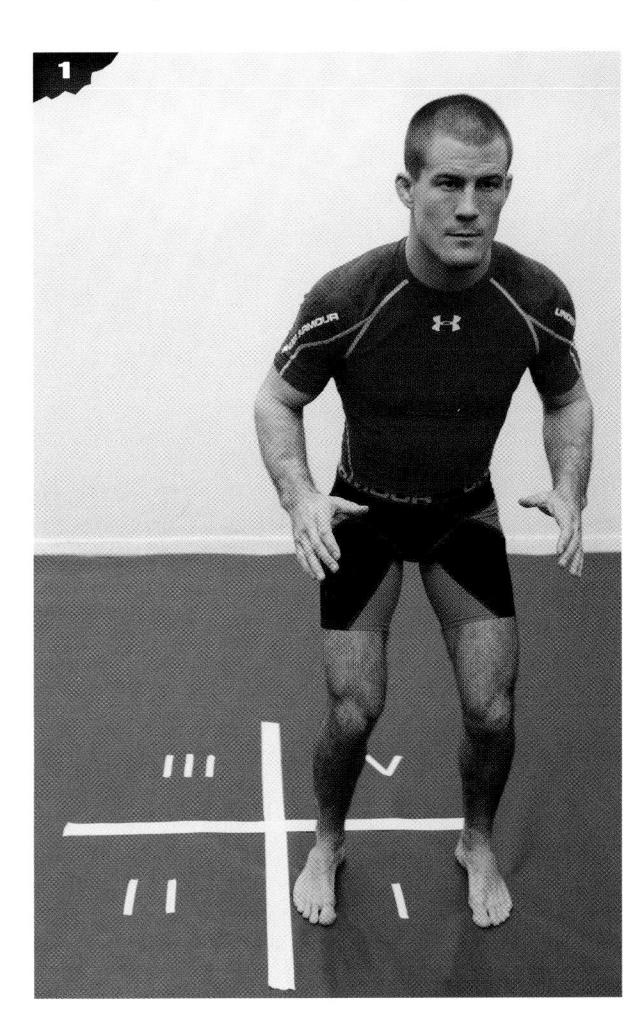

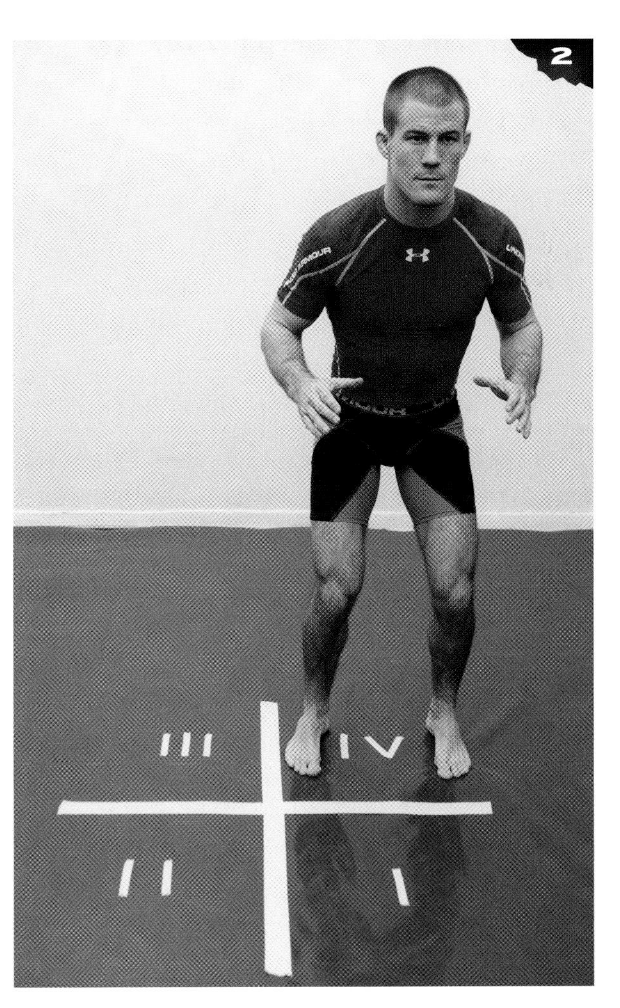

2. WALKING KNEE TO CHEST

Walk three steps and pull the right knee to the chest as high as possible. Hold for 1 second, walk three more steps, and pull the left knee to the chest as high as possible. Make sure to keep the back straight and rise up on the toes while pulling the knee up. Get 3 to 4 stretches on each leg.

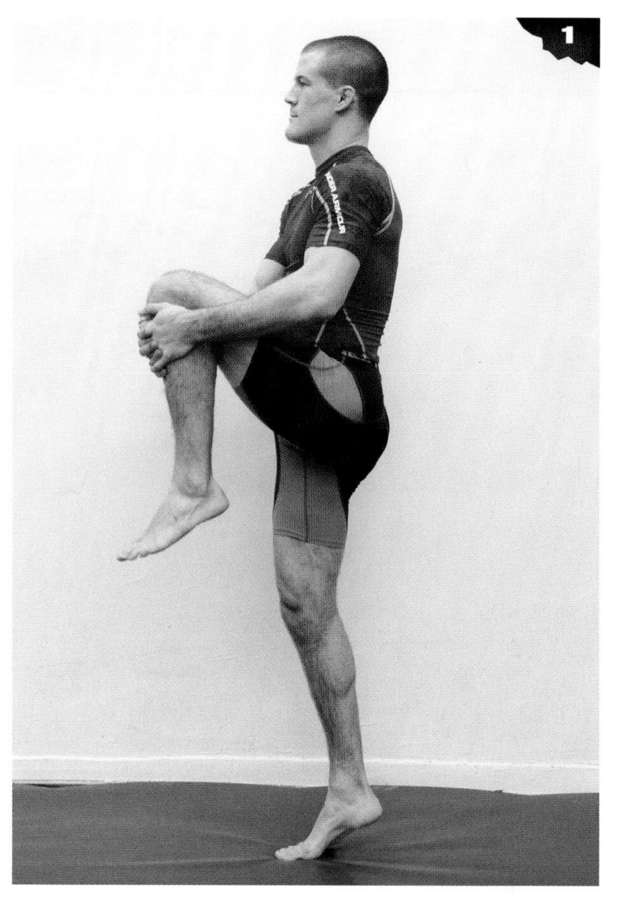

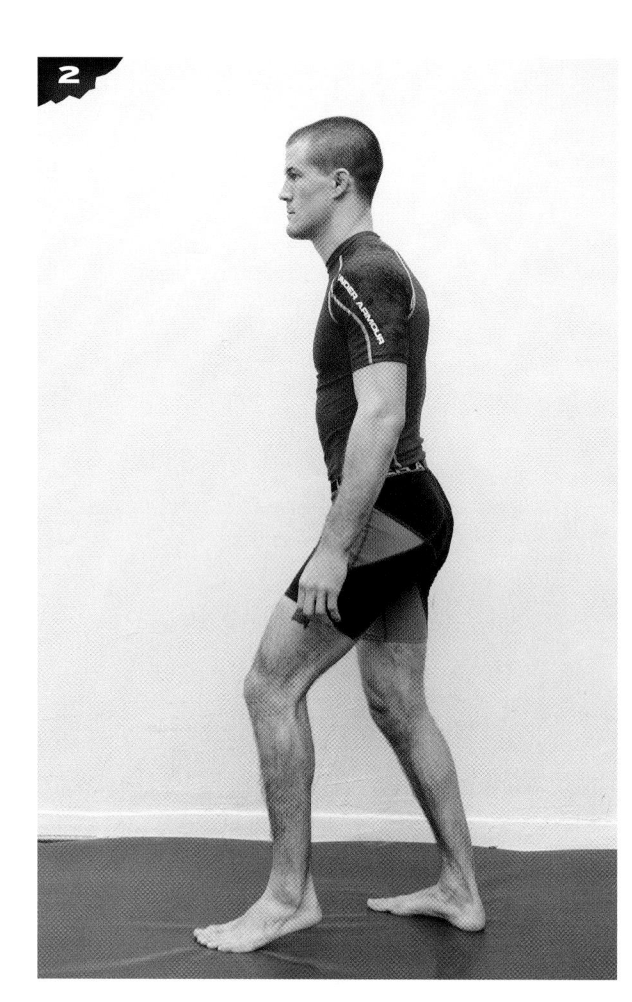

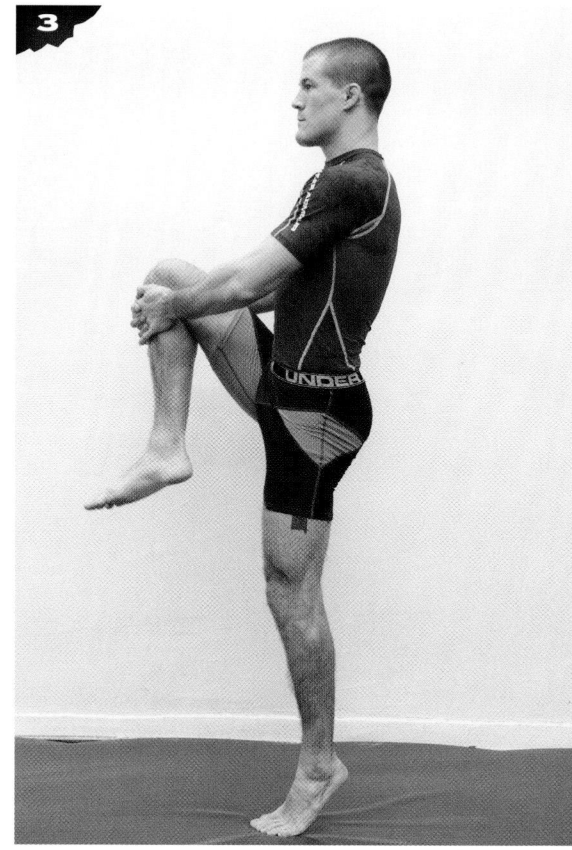

3. TFW CROSS JUMPS: 1–2

Begin standing in section 1 of the cross. Jump 20 times back and forth in between sections 2 and 1.

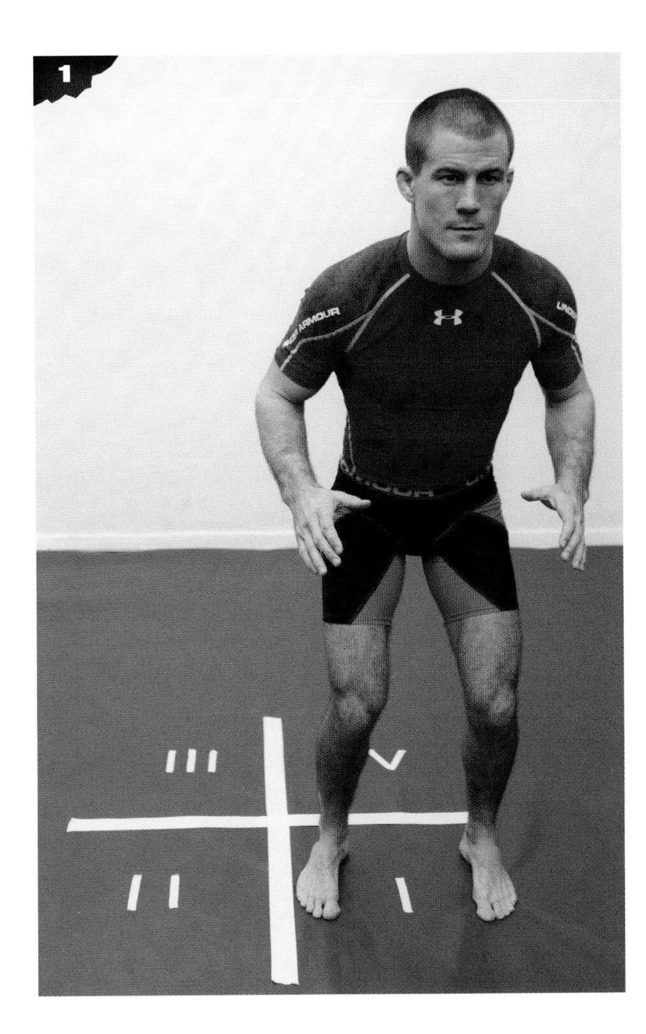

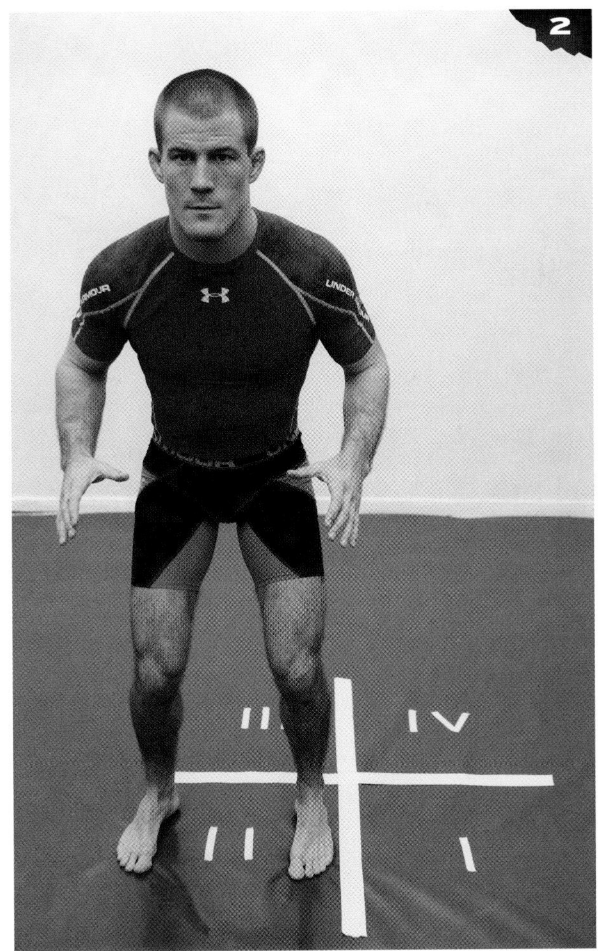

4. REPEAT THE WALKING KNEE TO CHEST.

5. TFW CROSS JUMPS: 1–3

Begin standing in section 1 of the cross. Jump 20 times back and forth between sections 3 and 1.

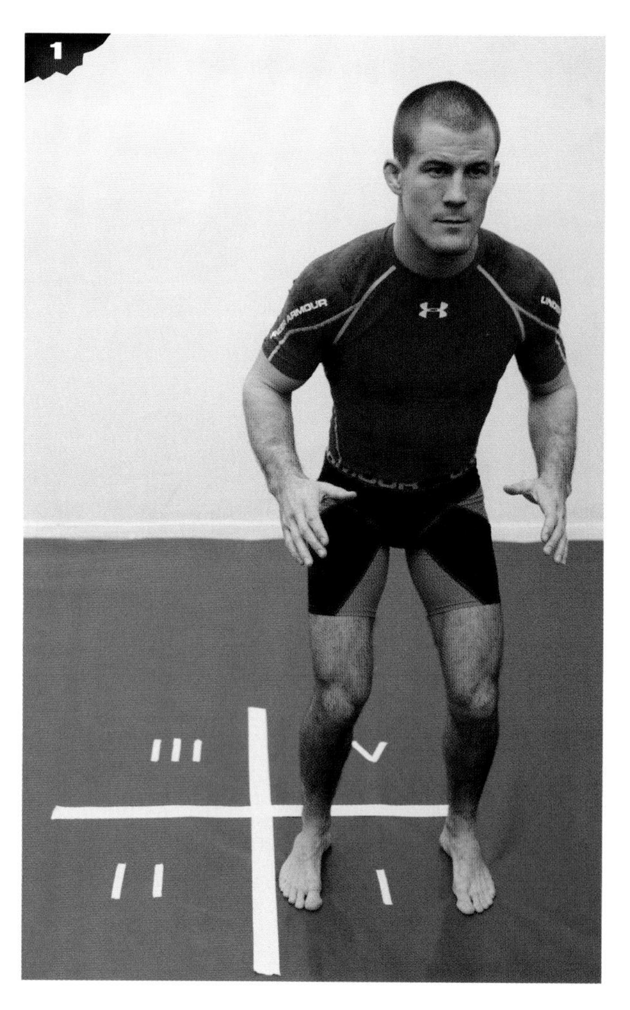

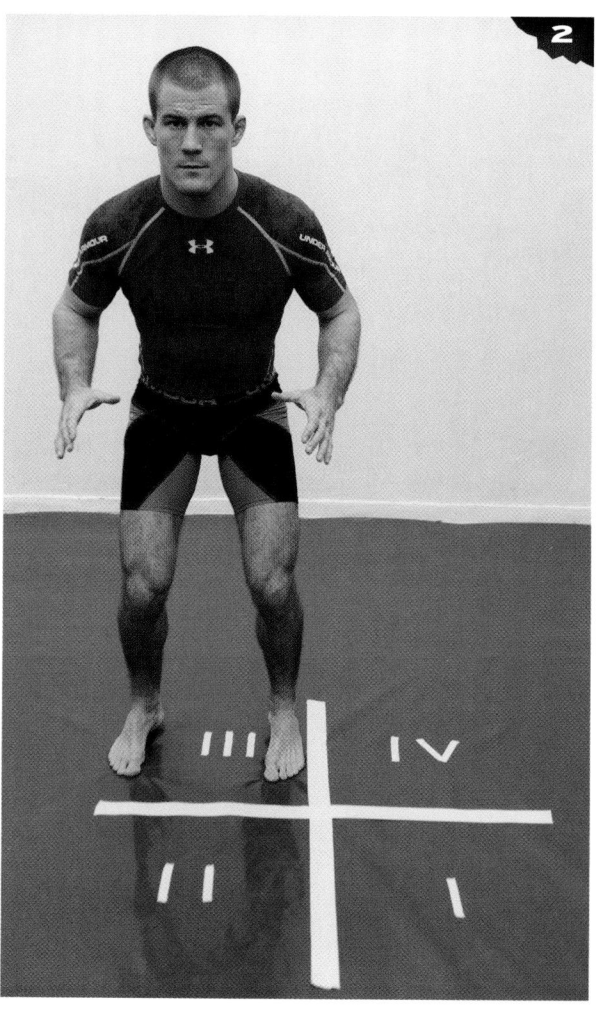

6. WALKING CRADLE STRETCH

Walk three steps and then grab one foot and under the knee on the same side. Pull both the foot and knee upward to create a stretch on the hip. Hold for 1 second, release, and then walk three more steps and pull up the opposite leg in the same fashion. Make sure to keep the back straight and rise up on the toes while pulling the knee up. Get 3 to 4 stretches on each leg.

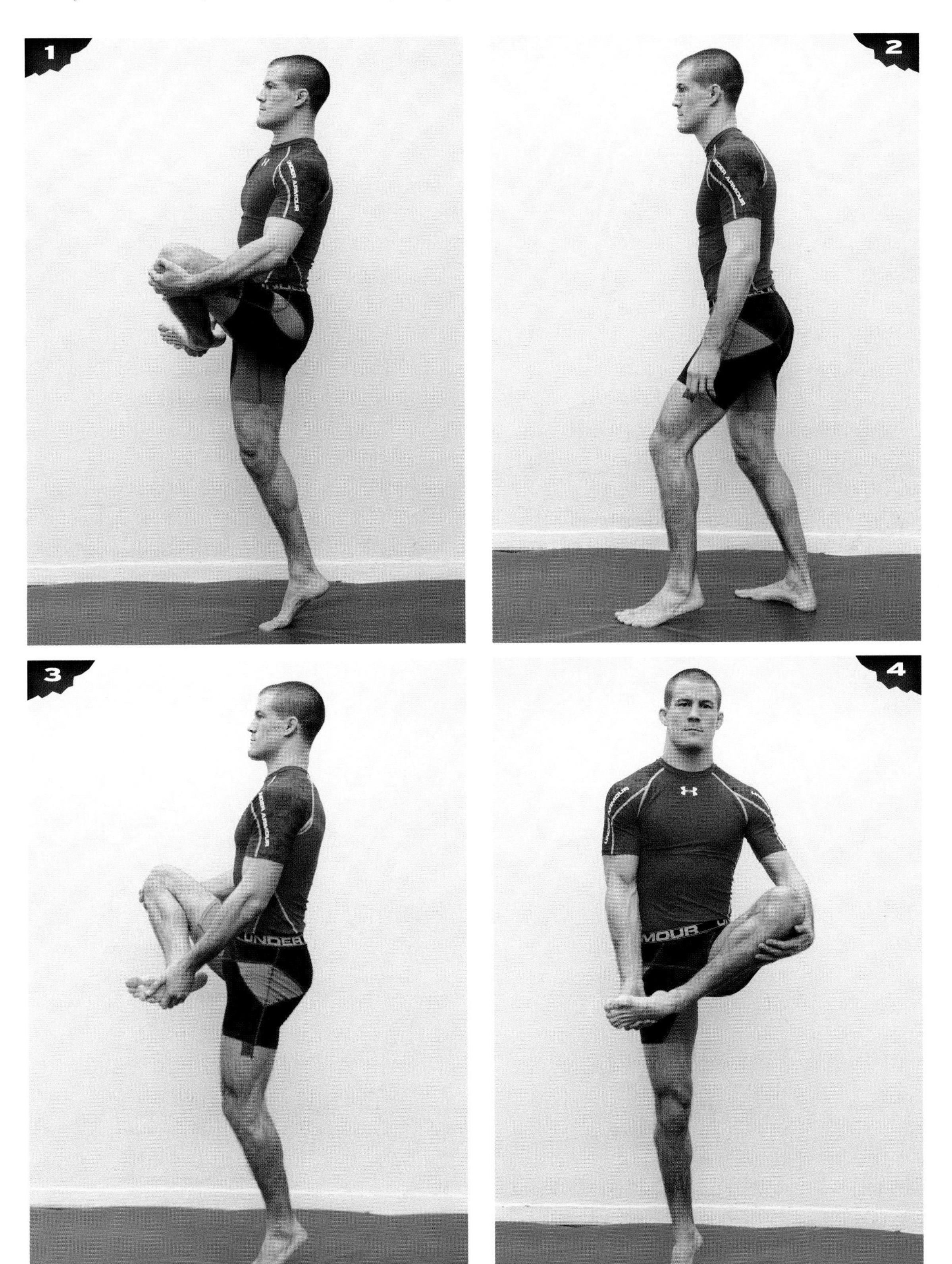

7. TFW CROSS JUMPS: 2—4

Begin standing in section 2 of the cross. Jump 20 times back and forth in between sections 4 and 2.

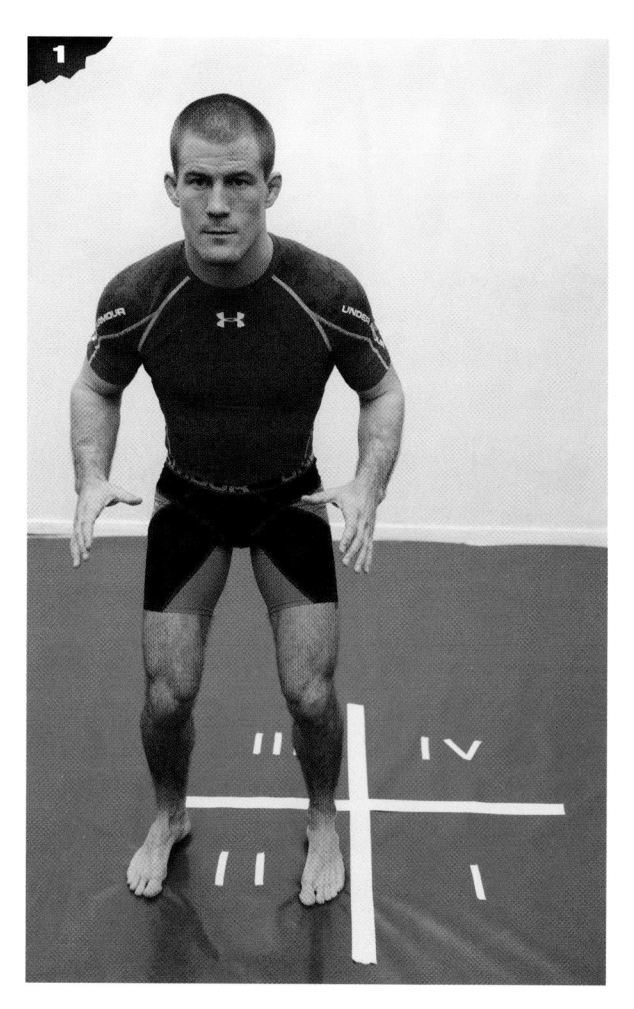

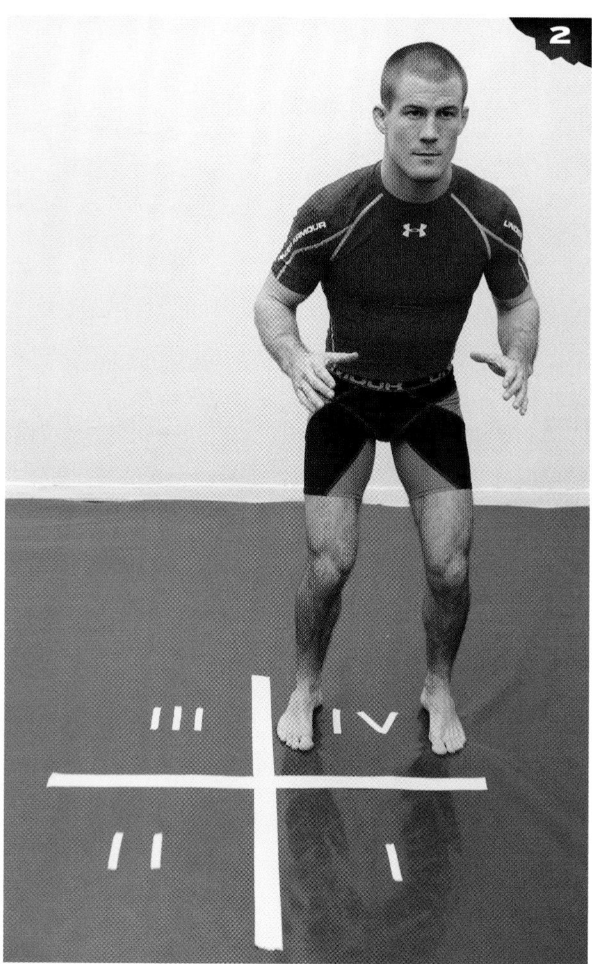

8. REPEAT THE WALKING CRADLE STRETCH.

9. TFW CROSS JUMPS: 1, 2, 3

Begin standing in section 1 of the cross. Jump in sections 2, 3, and 1. Complete 10 total revolutions.

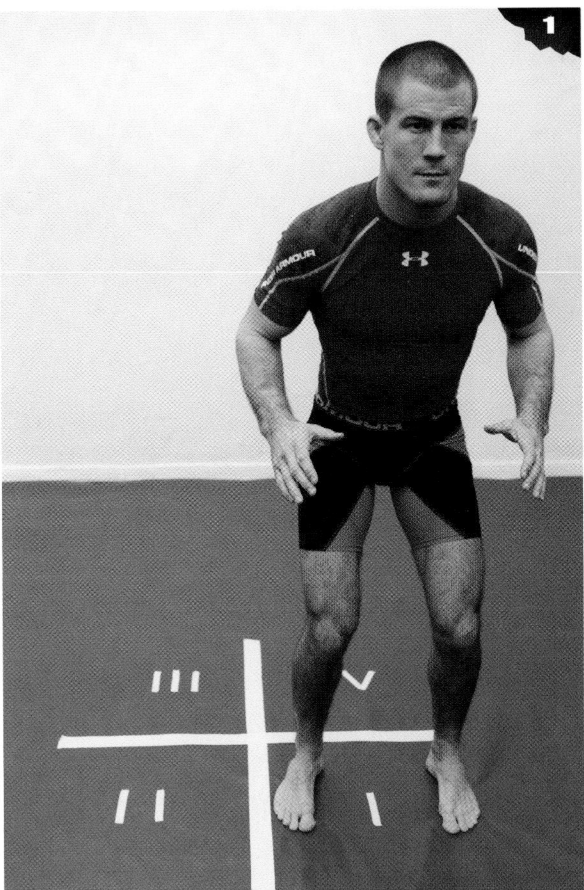

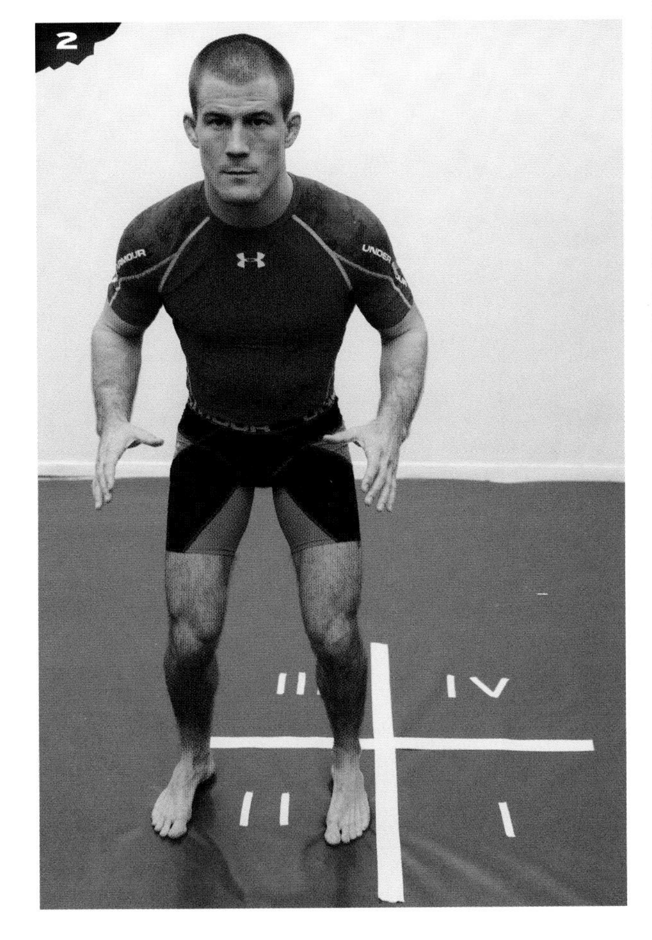

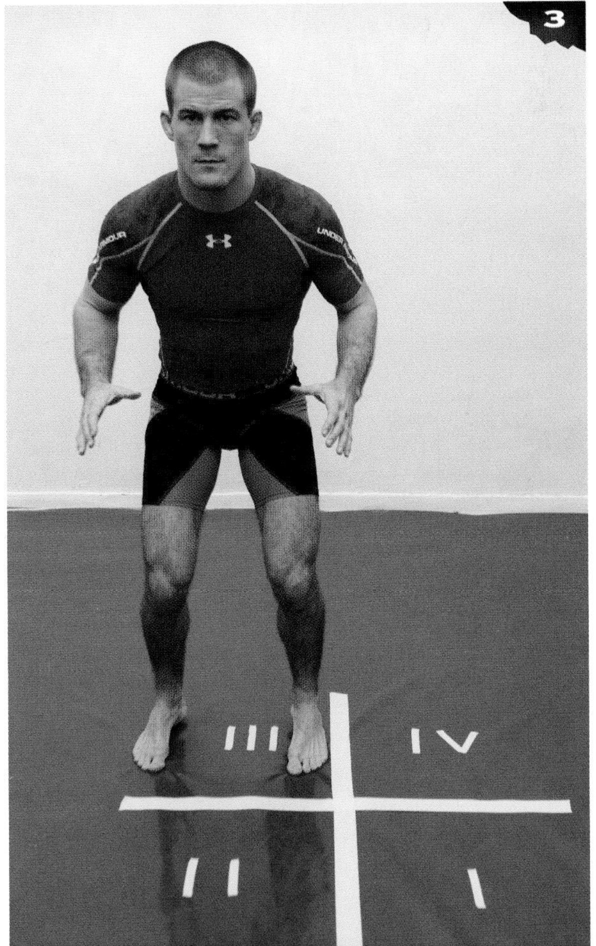

10. WALKING QUAD STRETCH

Walk three steps and then grab the ankle behind you while keeping the chest tall and both thighs parallel. From this position, lean forward as if to touch the toes while pointing the working thigh backward. Stand under control, walk three steps, and repeat on the opposite side. Get 3 to 4 stretches on each leg.

1

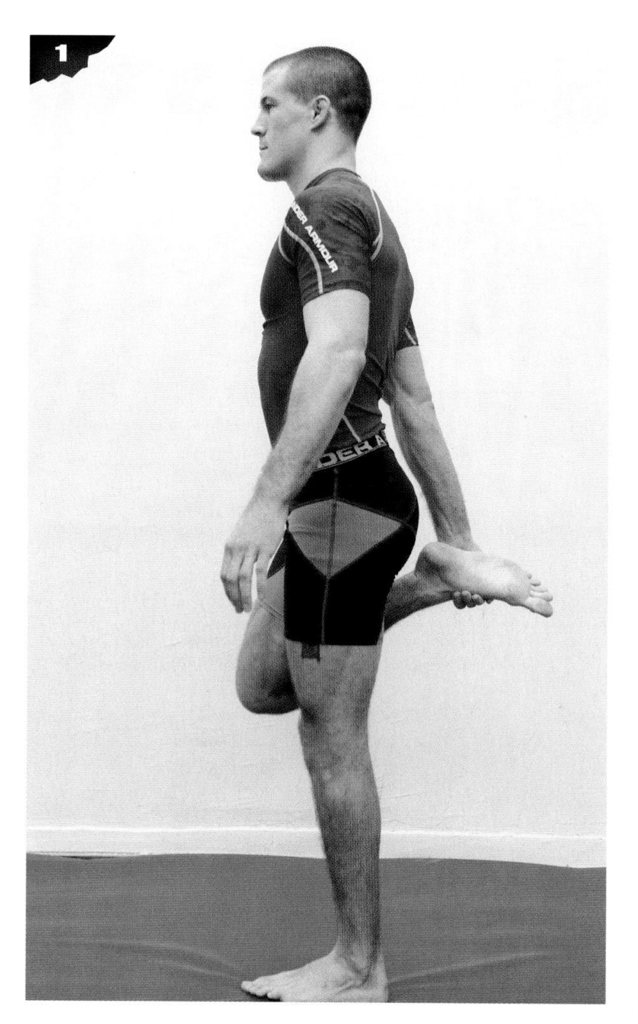

2

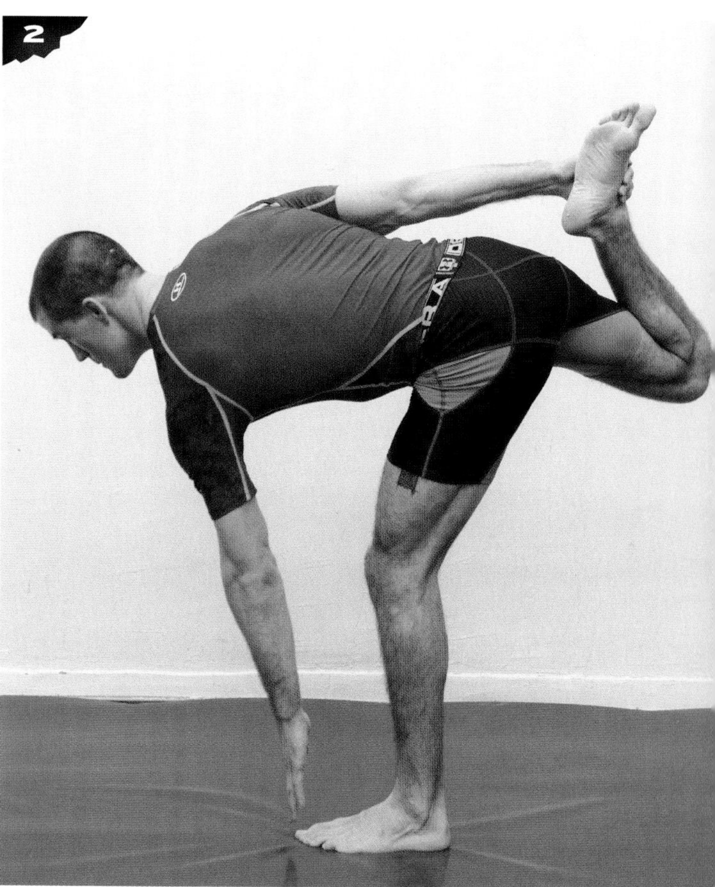

11. TFW CROSS JUMPS: 2, 1, 4

Begin standing in section 1 of the cross. Jump in sections 2, 4, and 1. Complete 10 total revolutions.

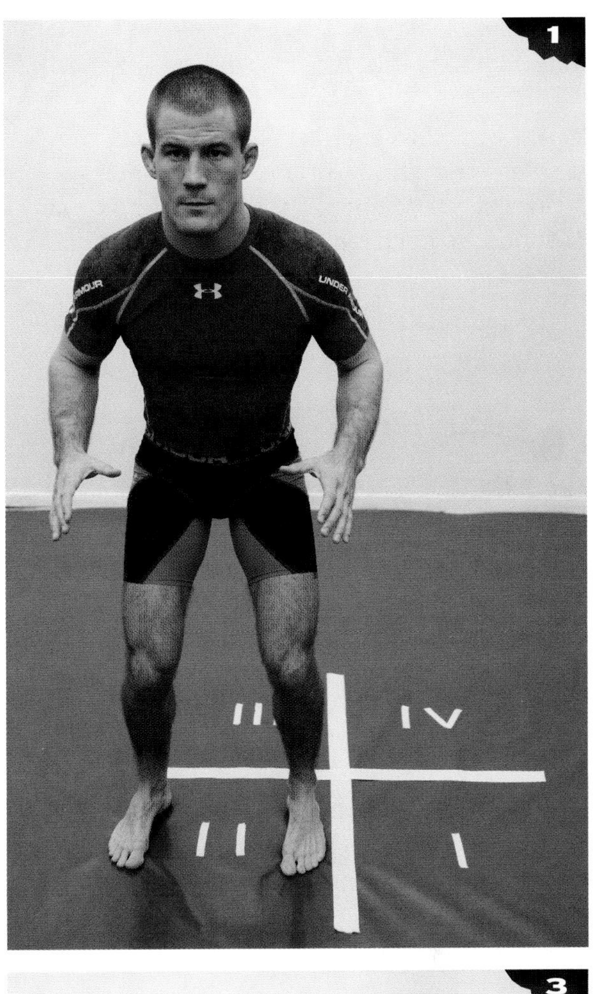

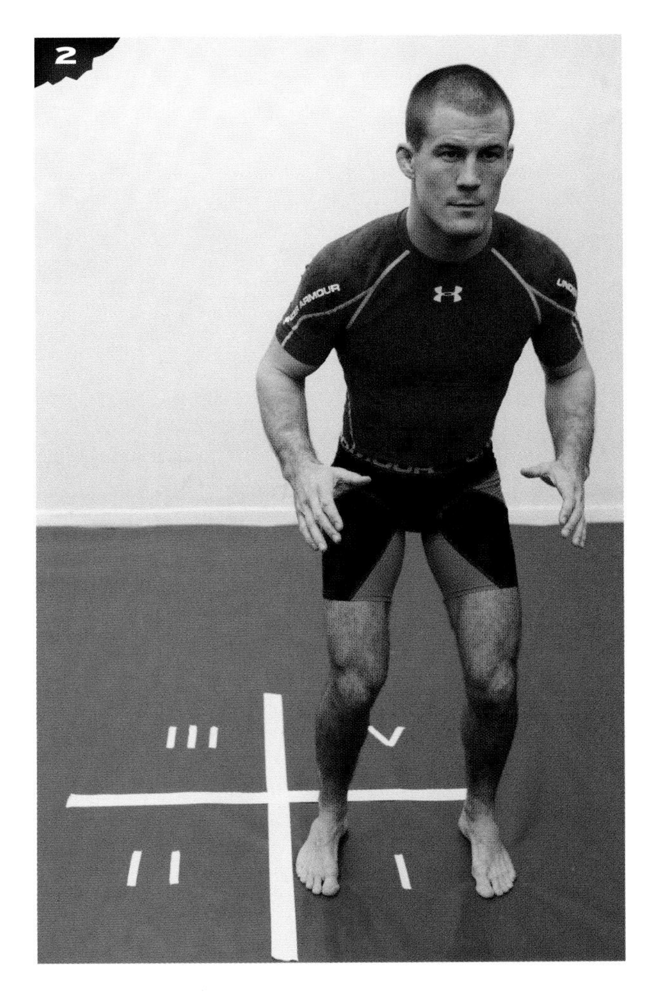

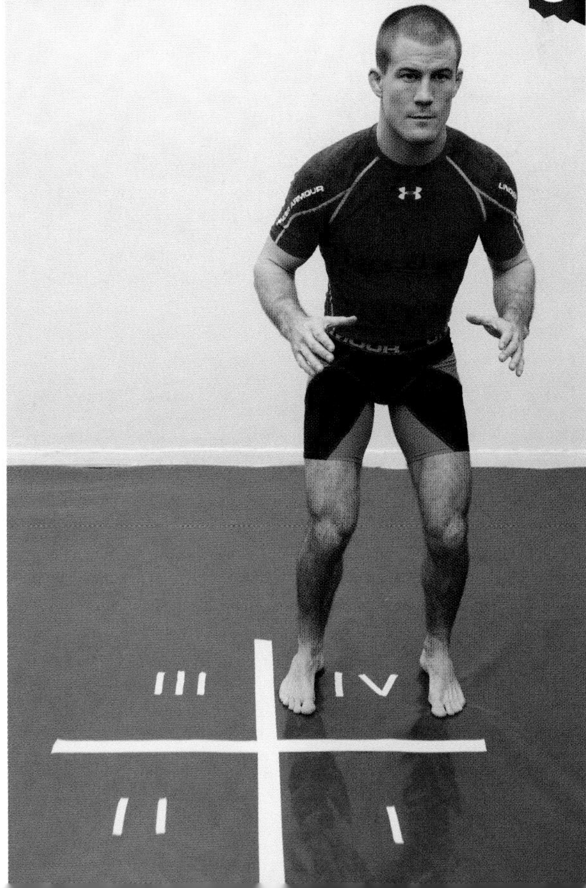

12. REPEAT THE WALKING QUAD STRETCH.

13. TFW CROSS JUMPS: STAR JUMPS

Begin standing with one foot in section 1 and one foot in section 2. Jump and bring both feet together on the intersection of the TFW cross and then jump the feet into sections 3 and 4. Jump back to the intersection and then the start position. This completes one repetition. Complete 10 total repetitions.

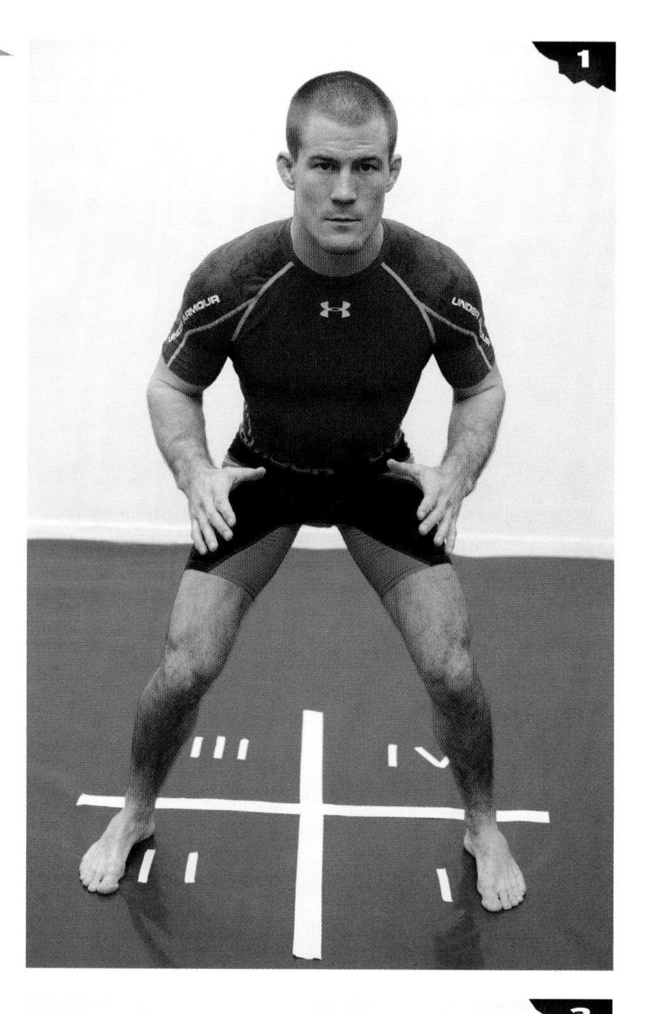

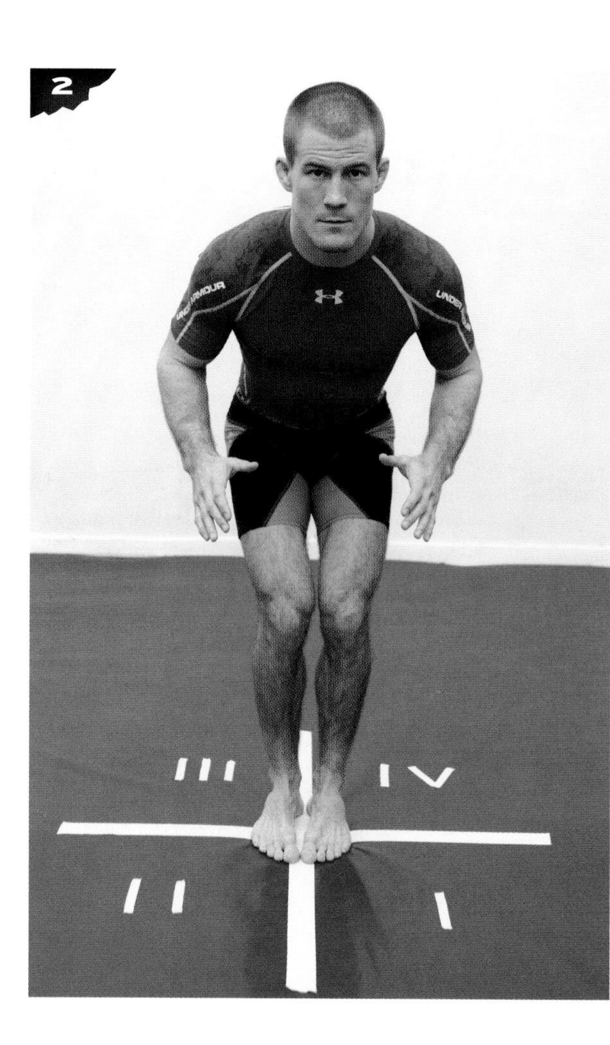

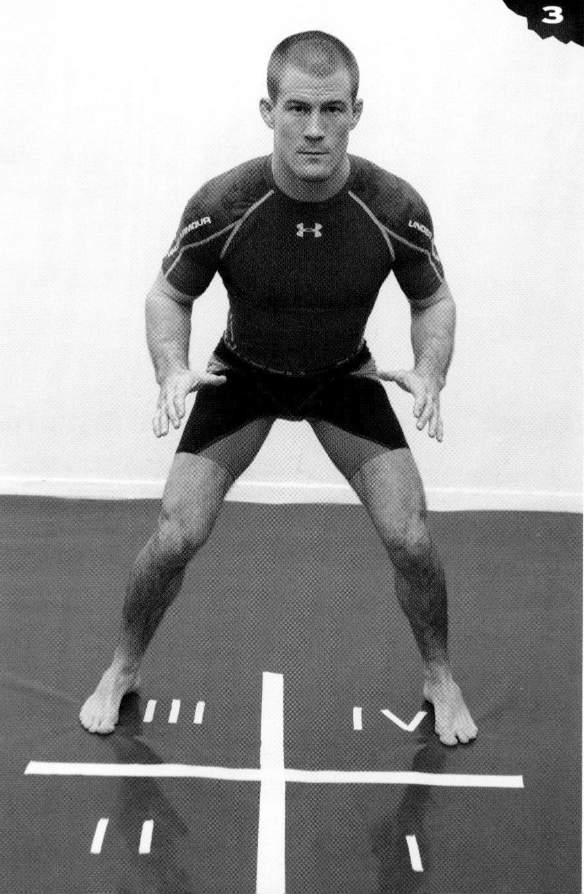

14. WALKING HAMSTRING KICKS

Walk three steps and kick up the right leg as high as possible. Keep the knee as extended as possible while touching the toe with the opposite hand. Walk three steps and repeat on the left side. Get three to four kicks on each leg.

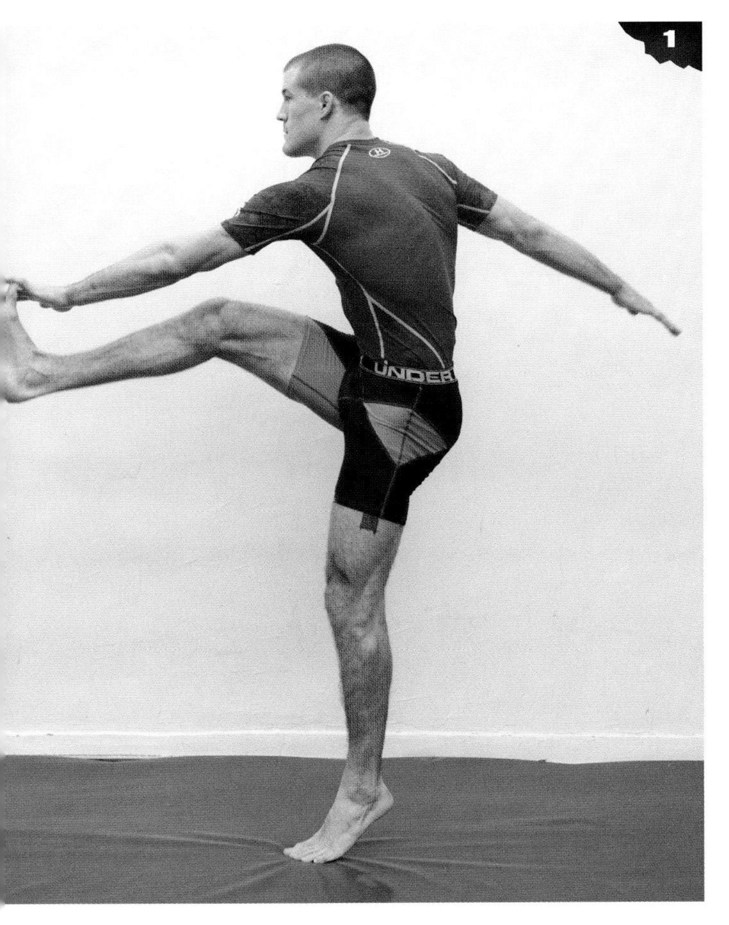

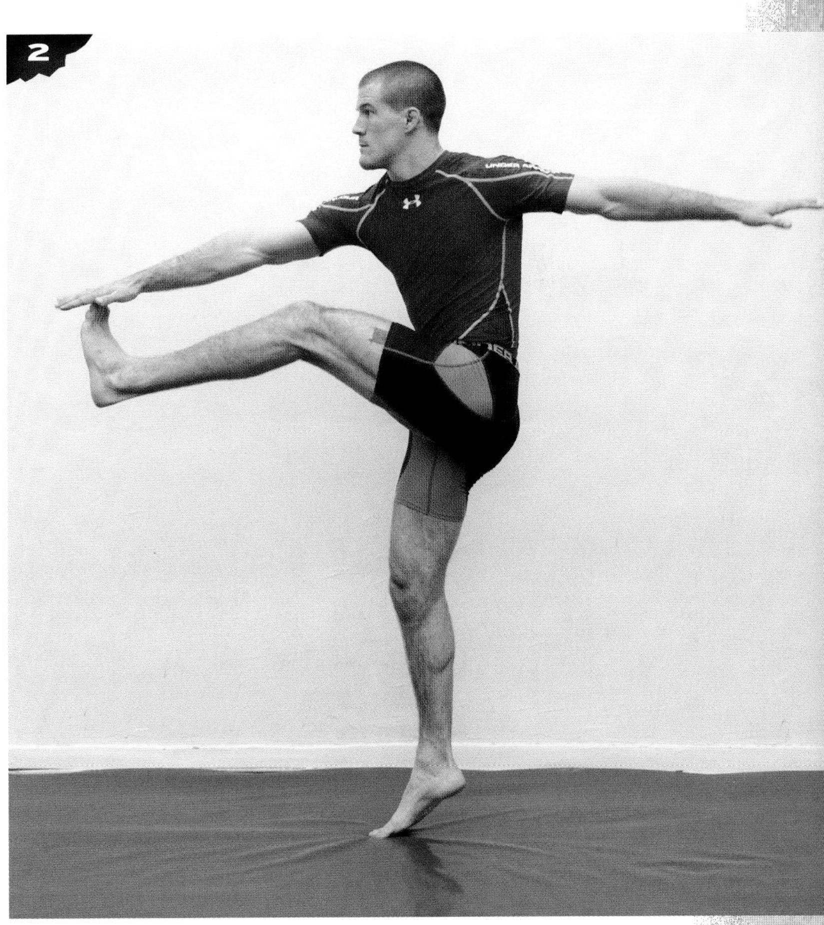

15. REPEAT THE STAR JUMPS.

16. REPEAT THE WALKING HAMSTRING KICKS.

17. TFW CROSS JUMPS: SINGLE LEG 1–4

Begin standing on one foot in section 1 of the cross. Jump 10 times back and forth in between sections 4 and 1. Repeat on the other foot for 10 jumps.

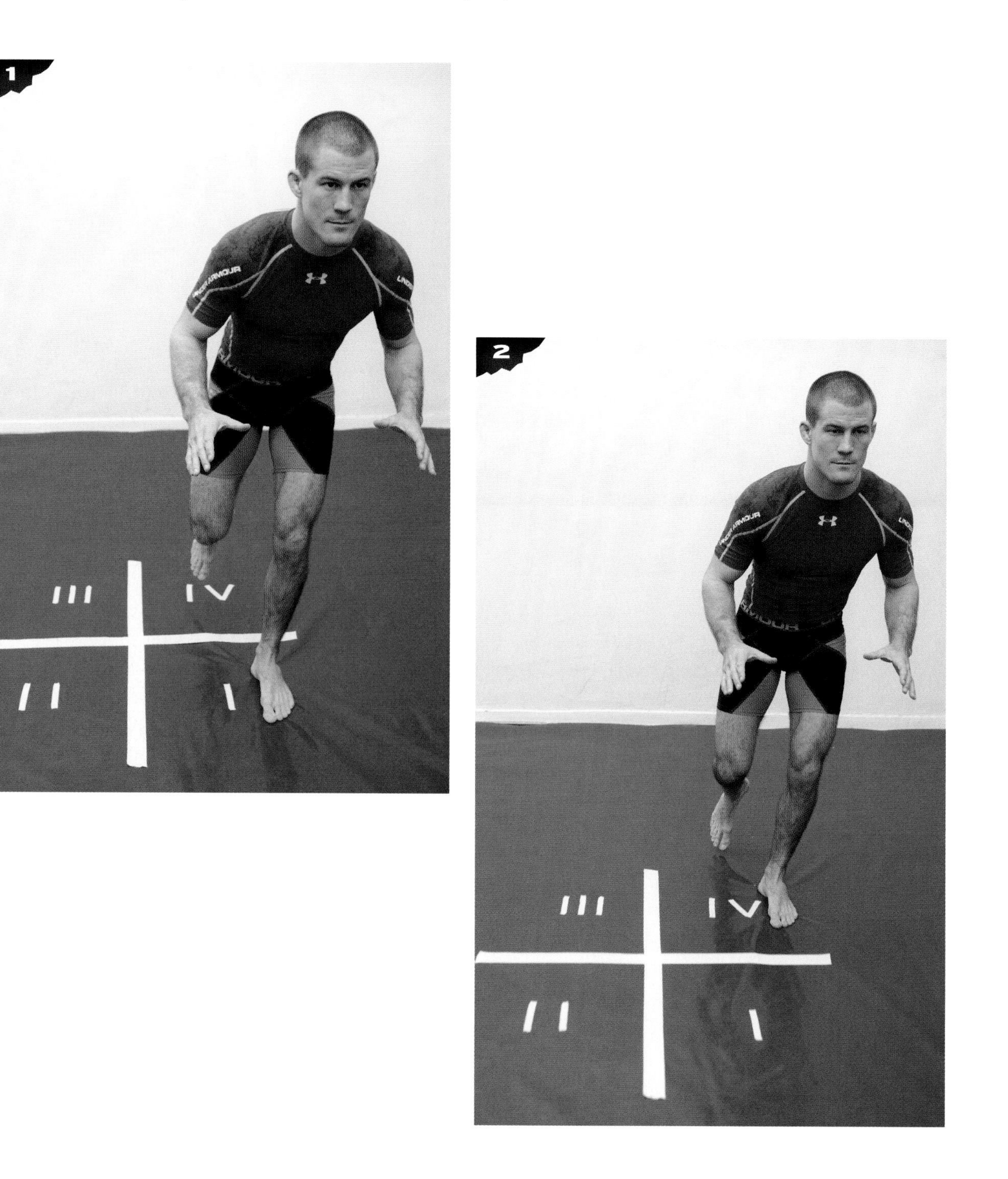

18. WALKING SIDE LUNGE

Begin standing, and lunge to the side and hold the stretch for 2 to 3 seconds. Stand back up to the original position. Side shuffle for three steps and then repeat the stretch. Get 5 to 6 stretches.

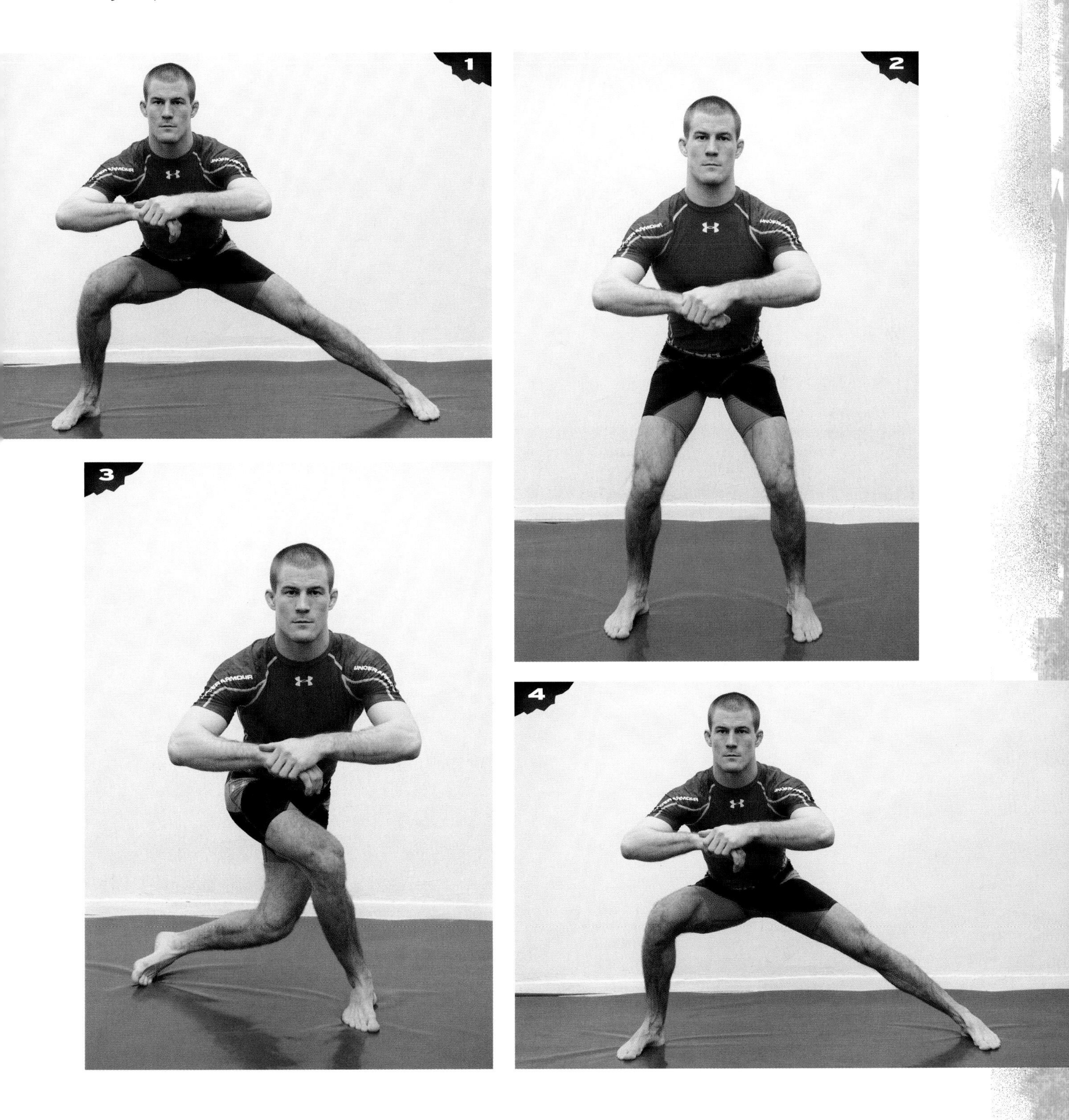

19. TFW CROSS JUMPS: SINGLE LEG 1–2

Begin standing on one foot in section 1 of the cross. Jump 10 times back and forth in between sections 2 and 1. Repeat on the other foot for 10 jumps.

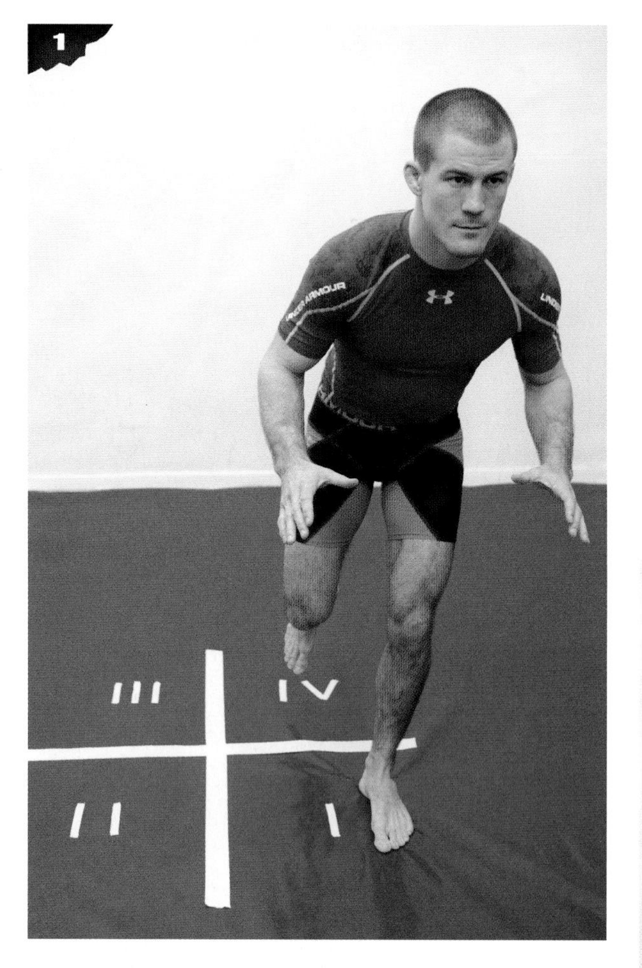

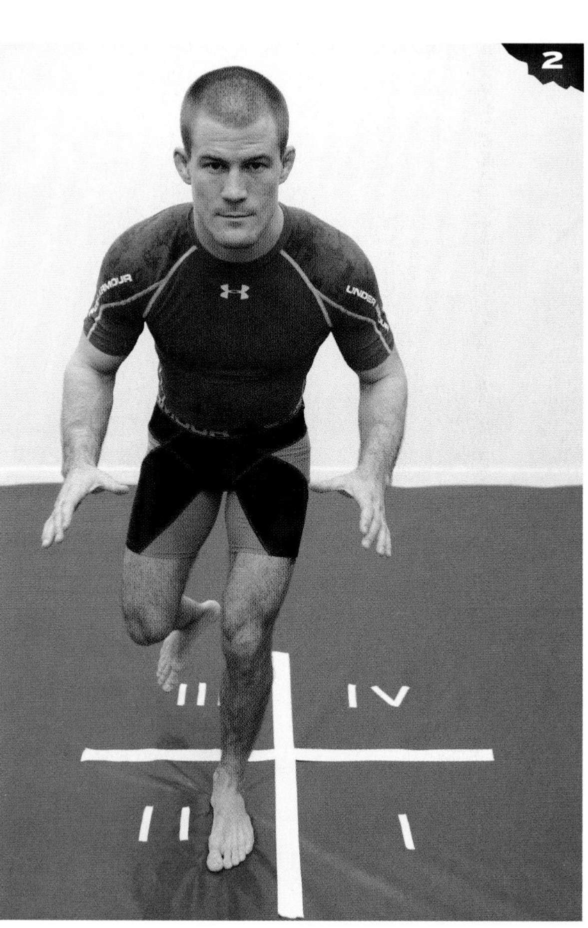

20. REPEAT THE WALKING SIDE LUNGE, BUT THIS TIME ON THE OTHER SIDE.

21. TFW CROSS JUMPS: SINGLE LEG 1–3

Begin standing on one foot in section 1 of the cross. Jump 10 times back and forth in between sections 3 and 1. Repeat on the other foot for 10 jumps.

1

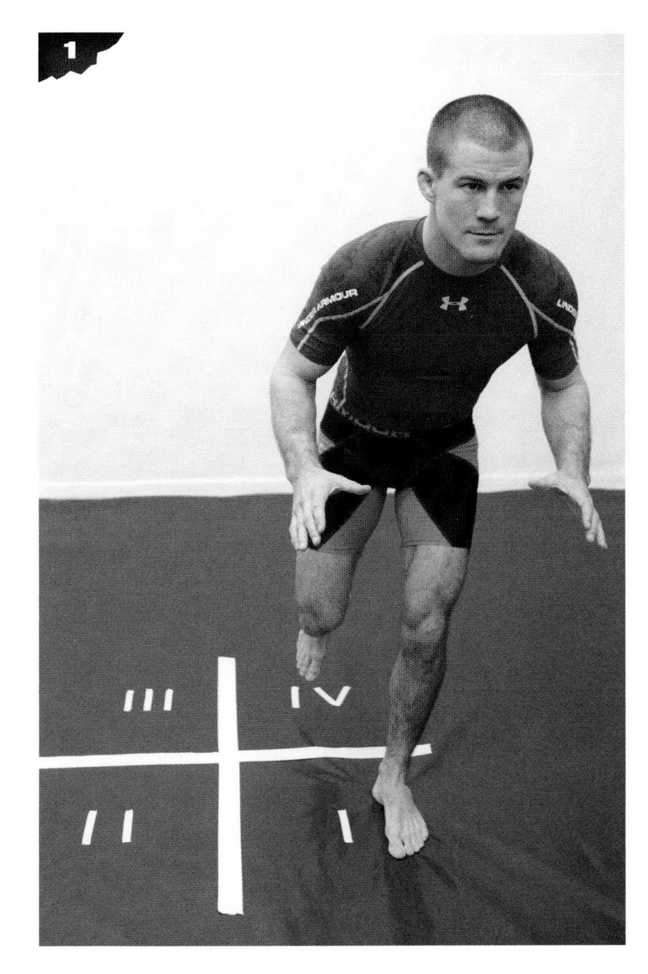

2

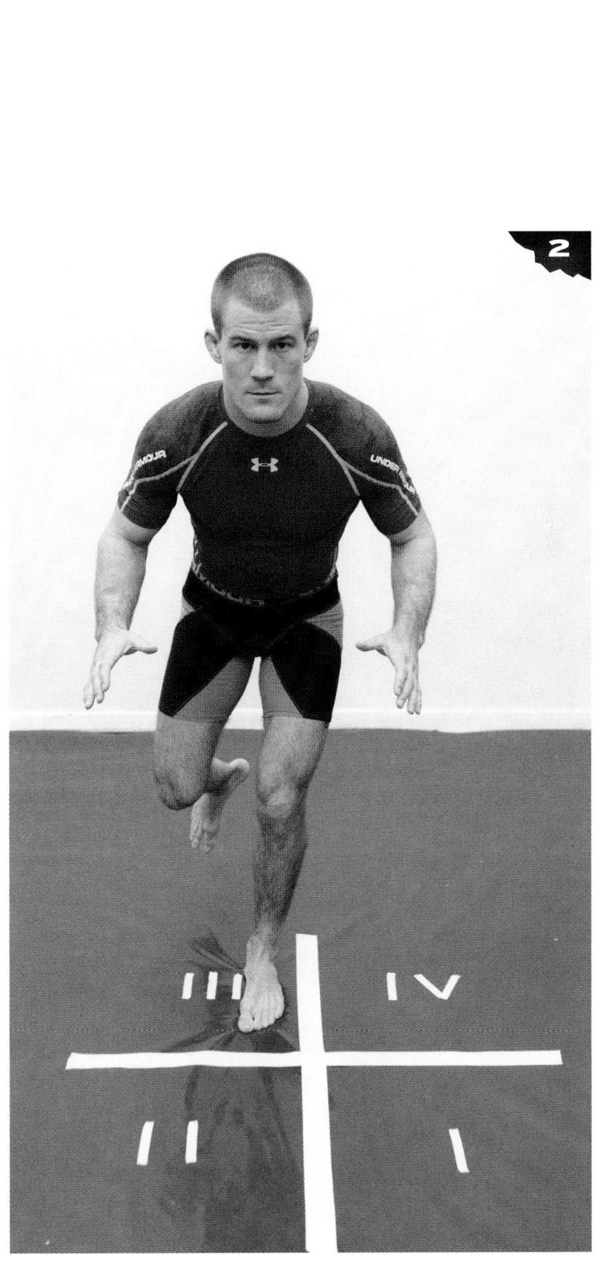

22. WALKING CROSS-LEGGED HAMSTRING

Walk three steps forward and cross one foot over the other so that the toes are at equal position forward. Reach down in order to touch the toes and hold the stretch for 2 to 3 seconds. Walk three more steps and cross the opposite foot over the top. Get 3 stretches on each side.

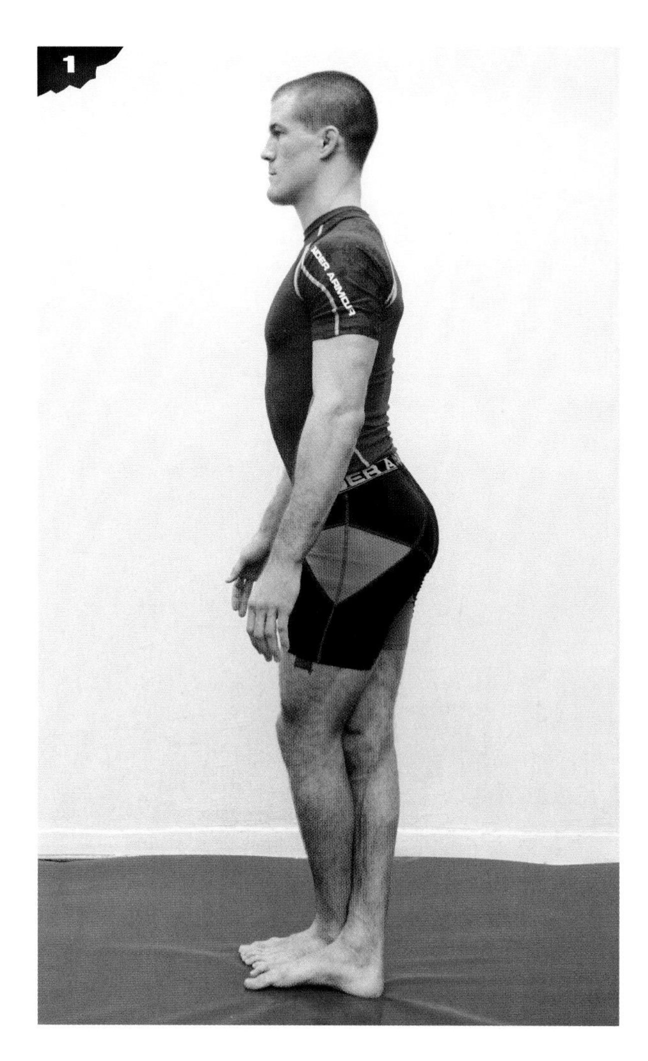

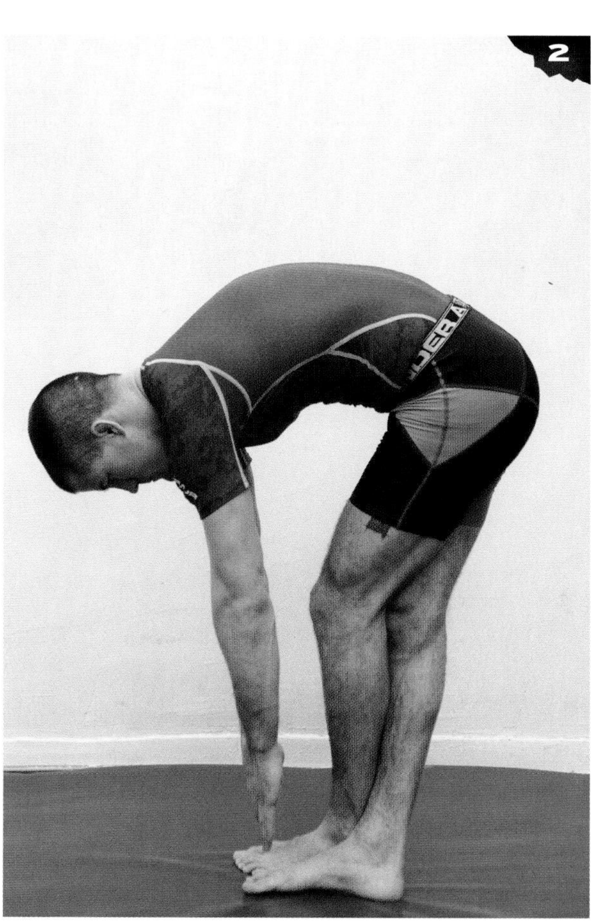

23. TFW CROSS JUMPS: SINGLE LEG 2–4

Begin standing on one foot in section 2 of the cross. Jump 10 times back and forth in between sections 4 and 2. Repeat on the other foot for 10 jumps.

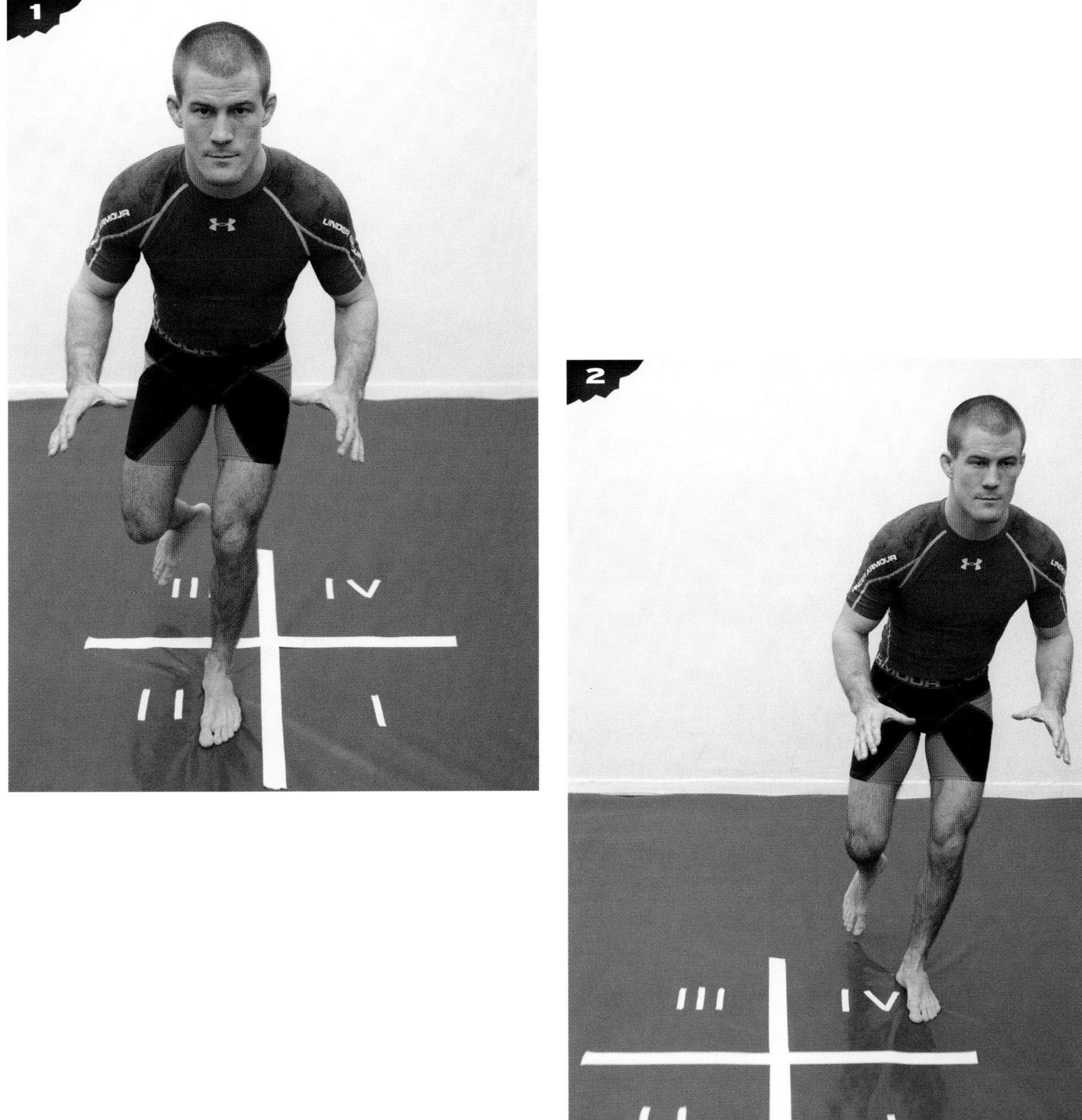

24. REPEAT WALKING CROSS-LEGGED HAMSTRING.

25. TFW CROSS JUMPS: 1-2-3-4 JUMPS

Begin standing in section 1 of the cross. Jump in sections 2, 3, 4, and 1. Complete 6 total revolutions.

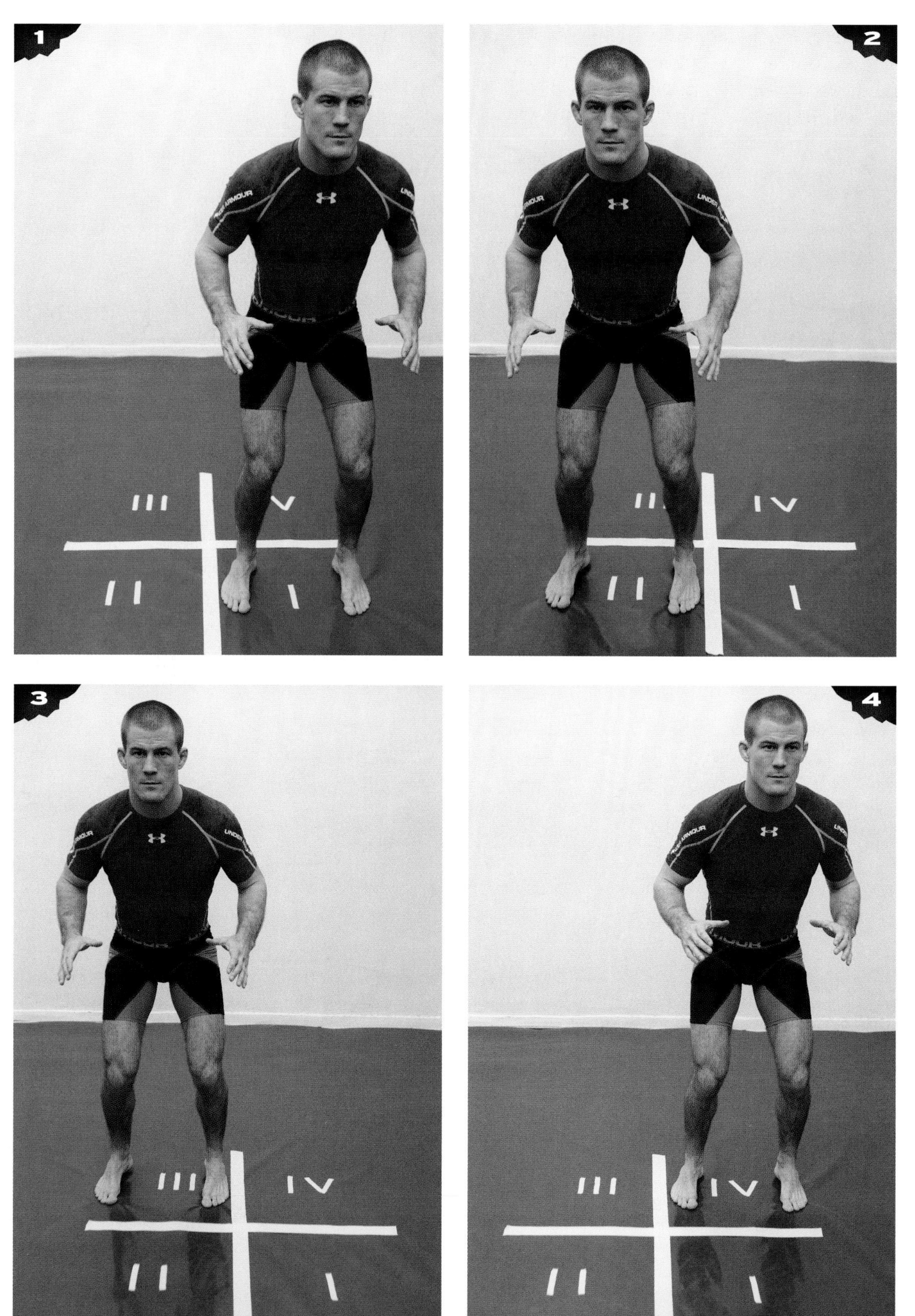

26. WALKING LUNGE AND TWIST

Begin standing with the arms out to the sides. Lunge forward on one leg so that the back knee almost touches the ground. Hold the position and twist the upper body into the direction of the front leg. Twist back, stand up, and repeat on the other side. Perform four twists to each side.

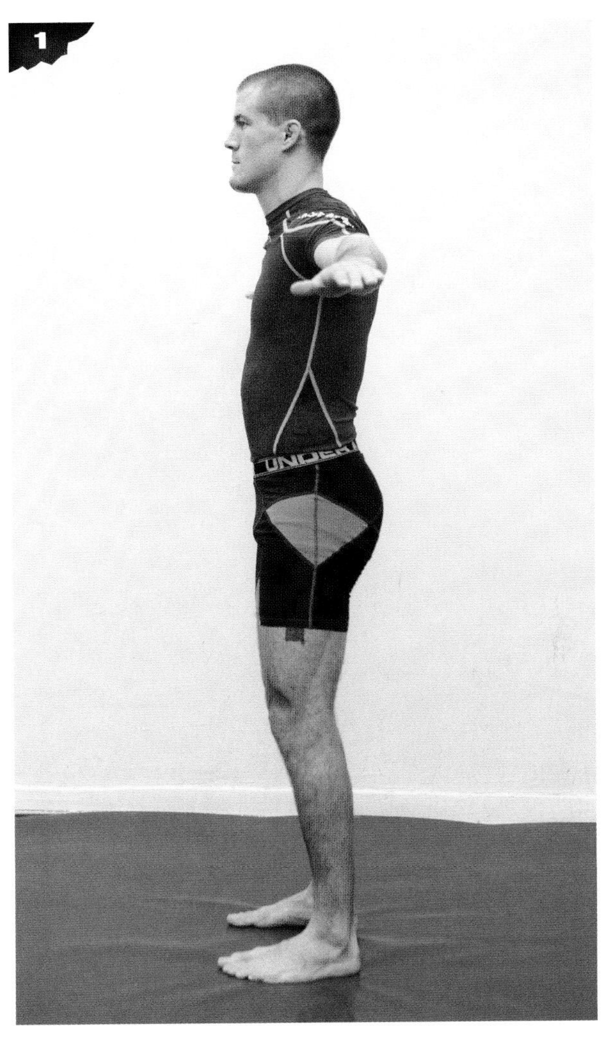

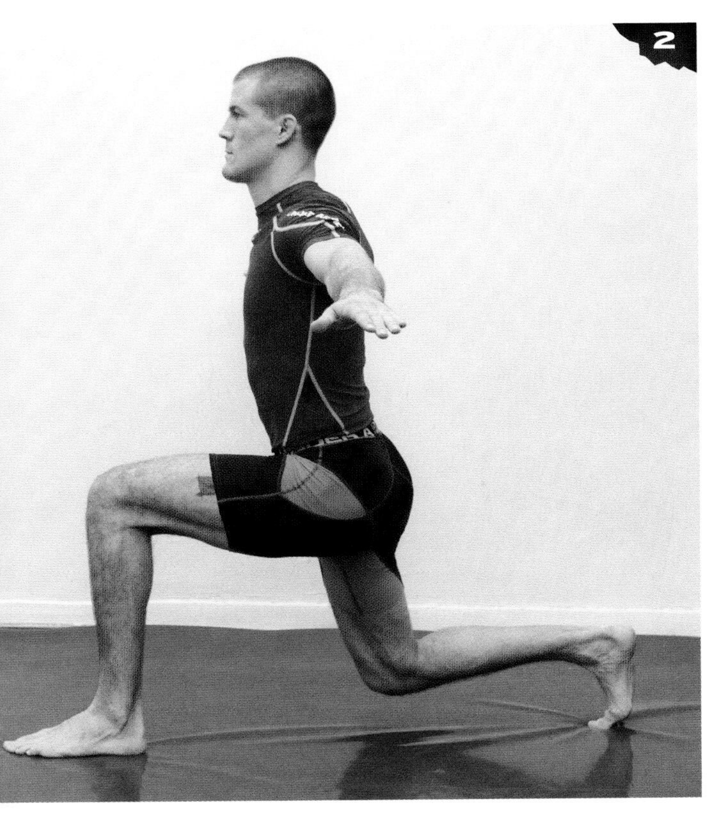

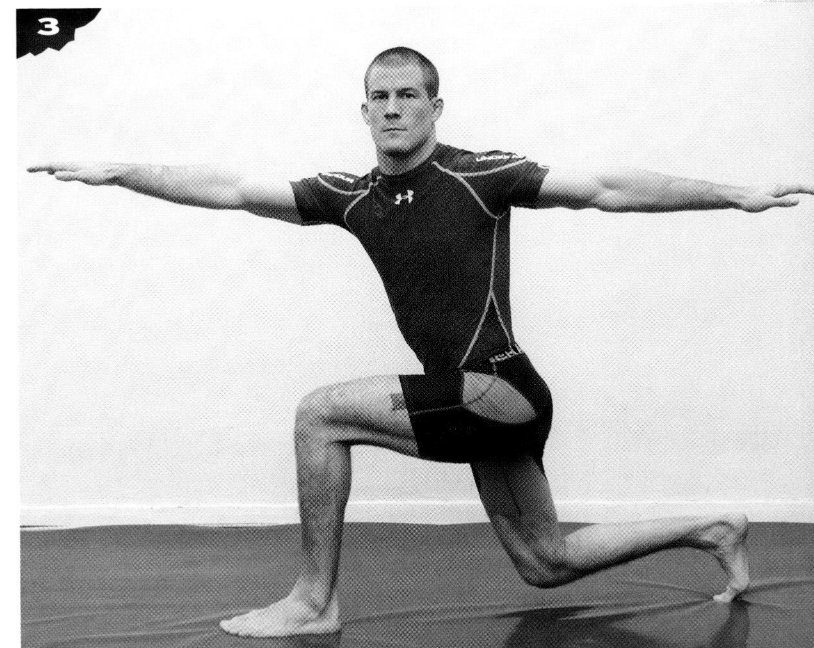

27. REPEAT THE TFW CROSS JUMPS: 1-2-3-4 JUMPS.

28. REPEAT THE WALKING LUNGE AND TWIST.

Following these you will perform two range-of-motion exercises for the upper body that will get you ready for the Upper-Body Band Routine.

29. L-STRETCH FOR THE SHOULDER

Begin standing with arms held out to the side and elbows at 90-degree angle. Lower one hand so that it is in the opposite position of the other. Hold the stretch for 2 seconds and then switch to the other side. Repeat for 10 total holds.

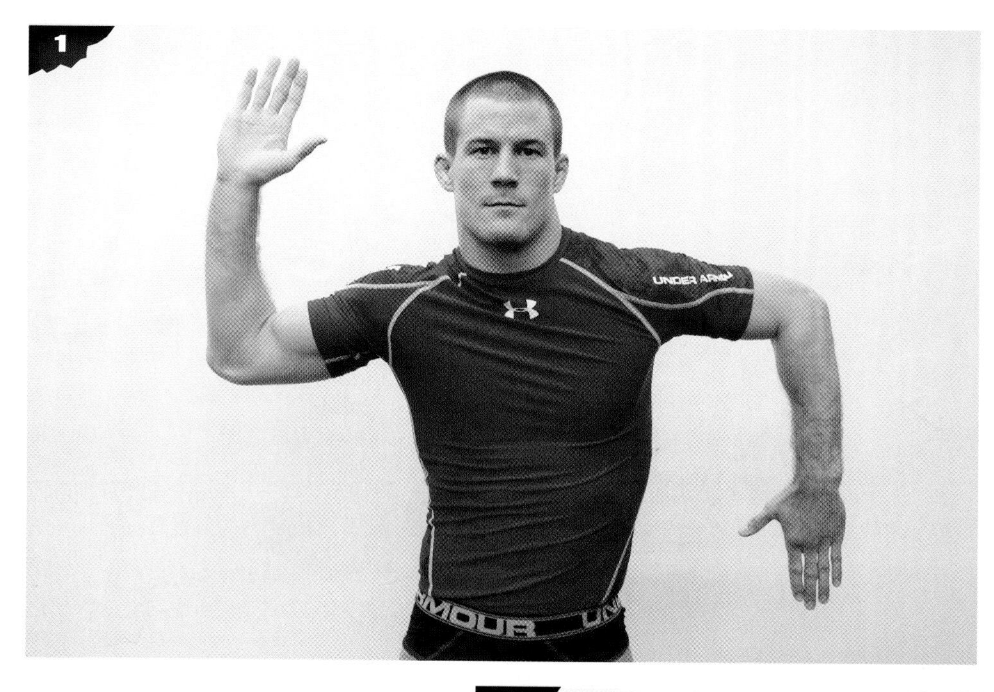

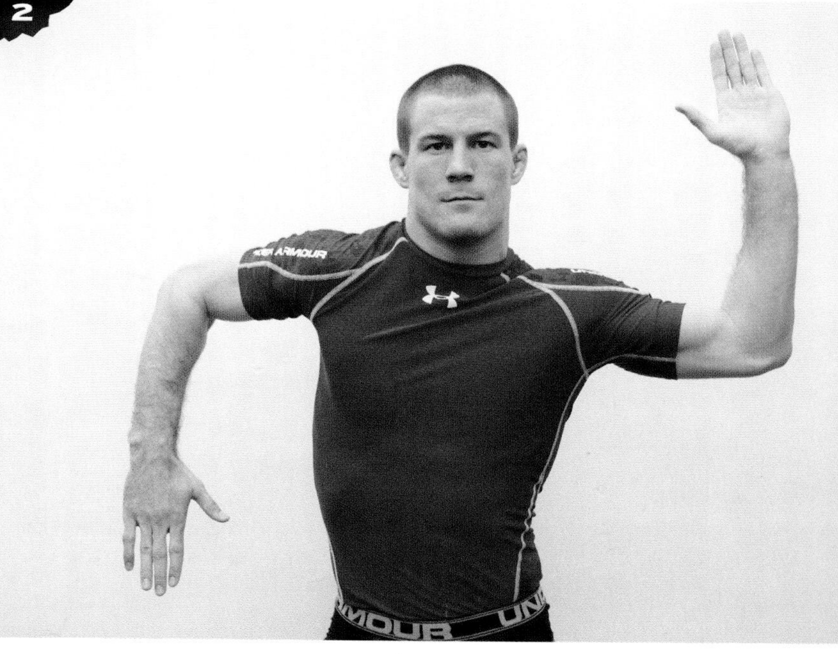

30. T-STRETCH FOR THE SHOULDER

Begin standing with the arms held out straight to the sides with one palm up to the ceiling and the other down. Turn the second hand until it also faces the ceiling. Hold for 2 seconds and then switch to the other side. Repeat for 10 total holds.

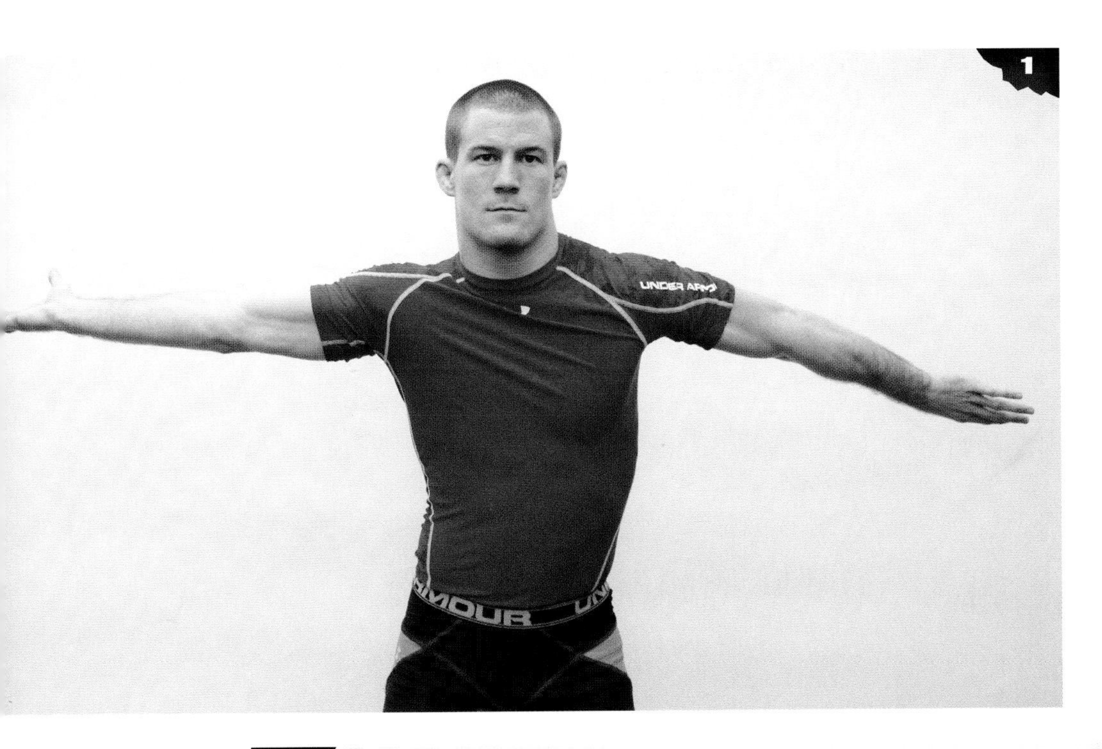

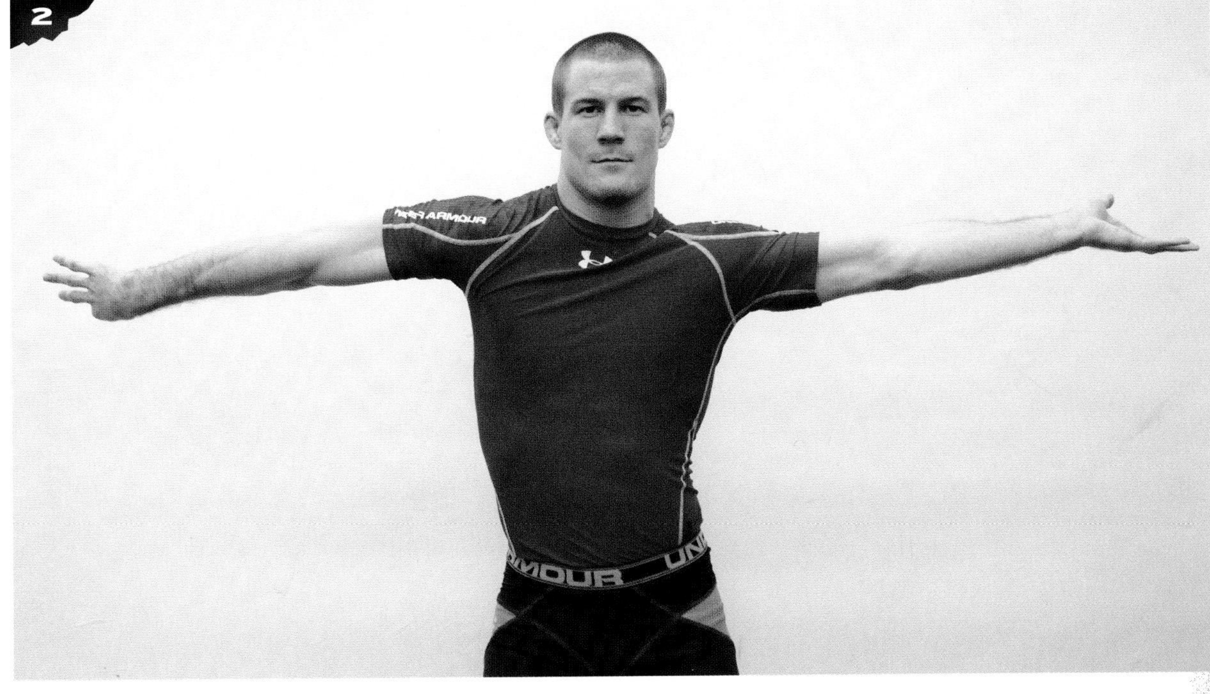

Once the Mini Plyo Hops and Movement Drills are performed, you are to perform the TFW Hip Circuit, which is then followed by the Upper-Body Band Routine.

The ten exercises of the TFW Hip Circuit are to be performed for 1 set of 6 repetitions on each leg. These exercises are to be performed in the order listed.

B. TFW HIP CIRCUIT

The key to these exercises is to make sure there is a 1-second hold at the contraction point of each exercise. During that second, the goal is to contract the muscles, which are working as hard as possible. These exercises are not to be performed quickly without any attention to the tempo. Over time, the 1-second hold will produce results.

1. BRIDGE

Begin lying on the back with knees bent and arms crossed over the chest. Drive both feet into the ground and lift the hips by squeezing the glutes and quads. Hold for 1 second and lower back down under control.

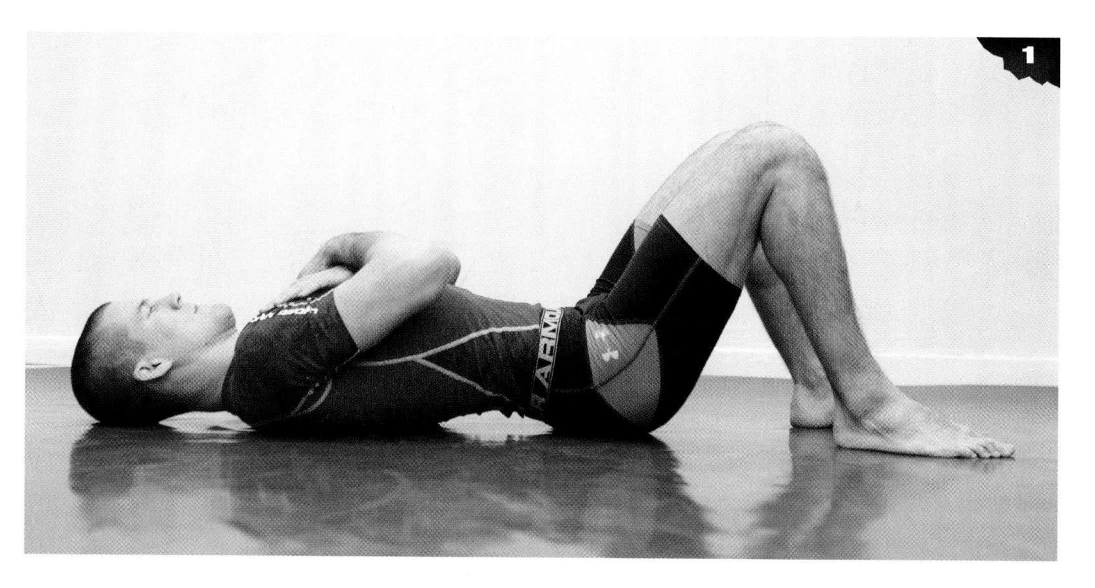

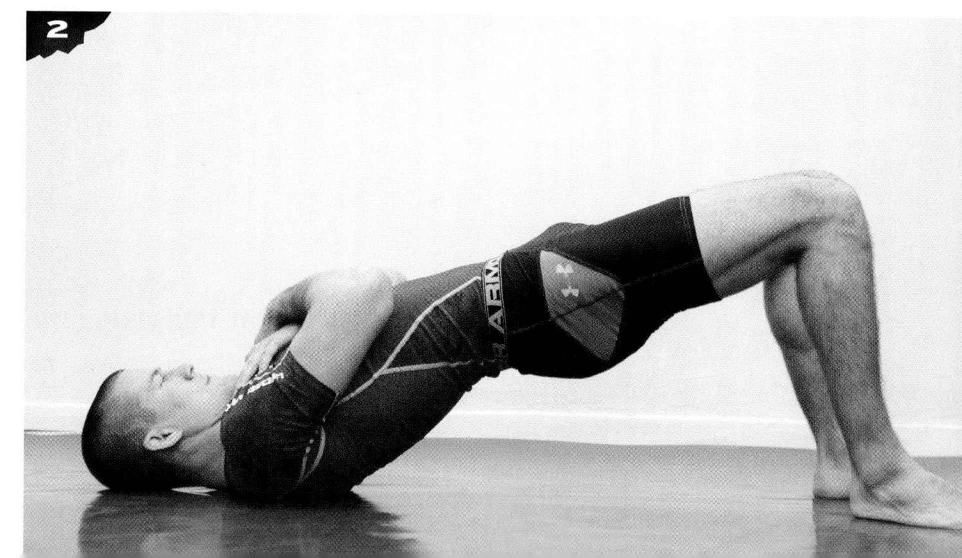

2. SINGLE LEG BRIDGE

Begin lying on the back with one knee held to the chest and the other foot on the ground. Drive the planted foot into the ground and lift the hips by squeezing the glutes and quads. Hold for 1 second and lower back down under control. Perform on both sides.

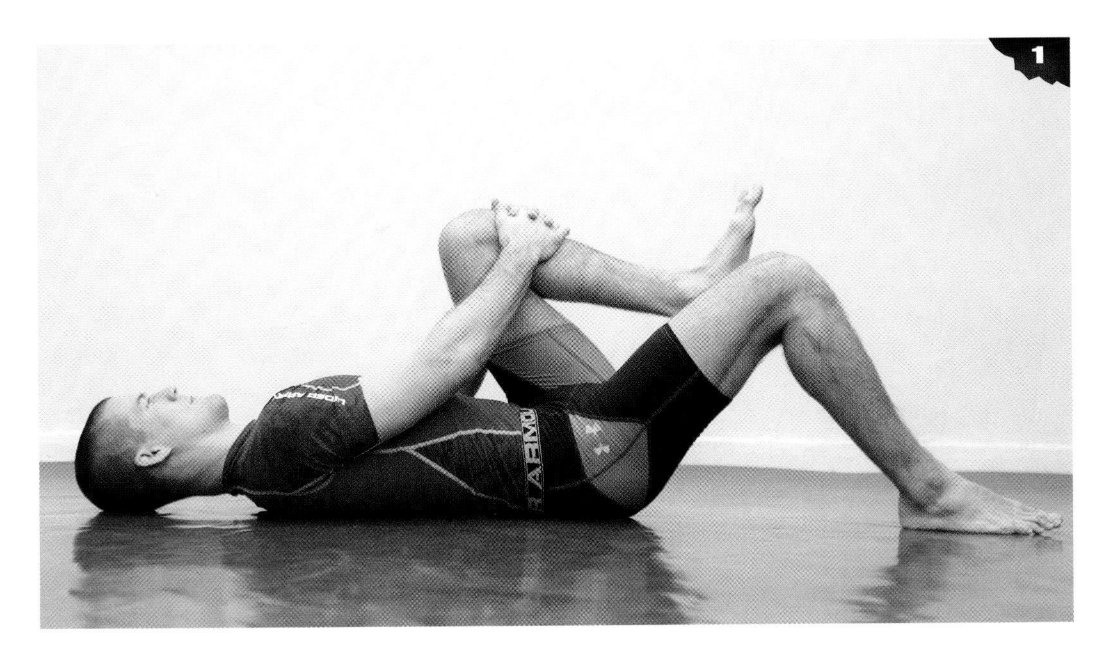

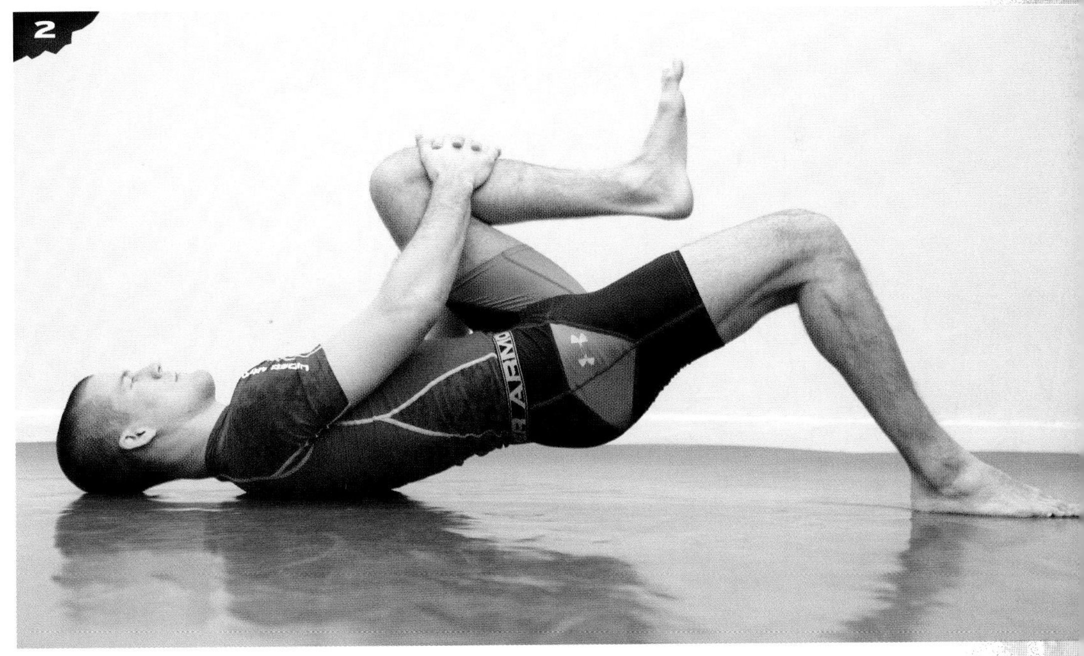

3. SINGLE LEG HIP POP-UP

Begin seated on the floor with the legs straight and the hands placed on the ground by the hips. Press with both hands and one foot into the ground and while keeping the knees locked straight, lift the hips as high as possible. Hold for 1 second and lower back down under control. Repeat on both sides.

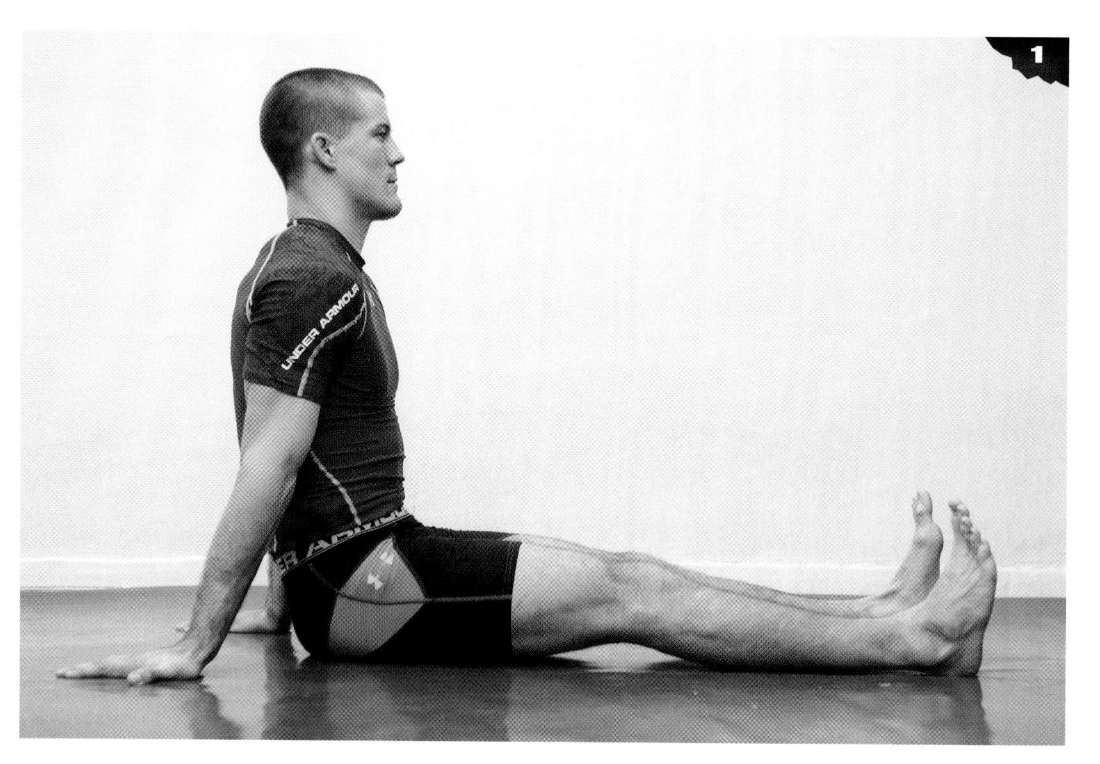

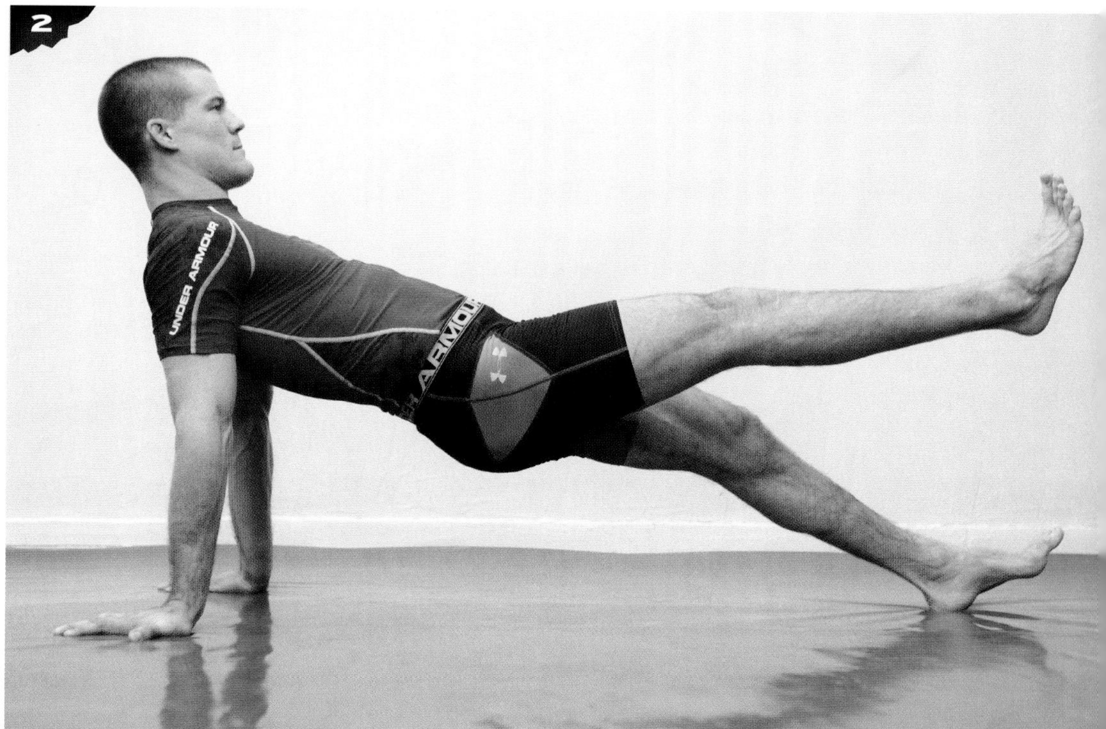

4. HURDLER HIP LIFT

Begin seated in the Hurdler position on the ground, with one leg extended out front and the other pulled behind the hip. While leaning slightly away from the back leg, lift the back foot toward the ceiling. Hold for 1 second and lower back down under control. Repeat on both sides.

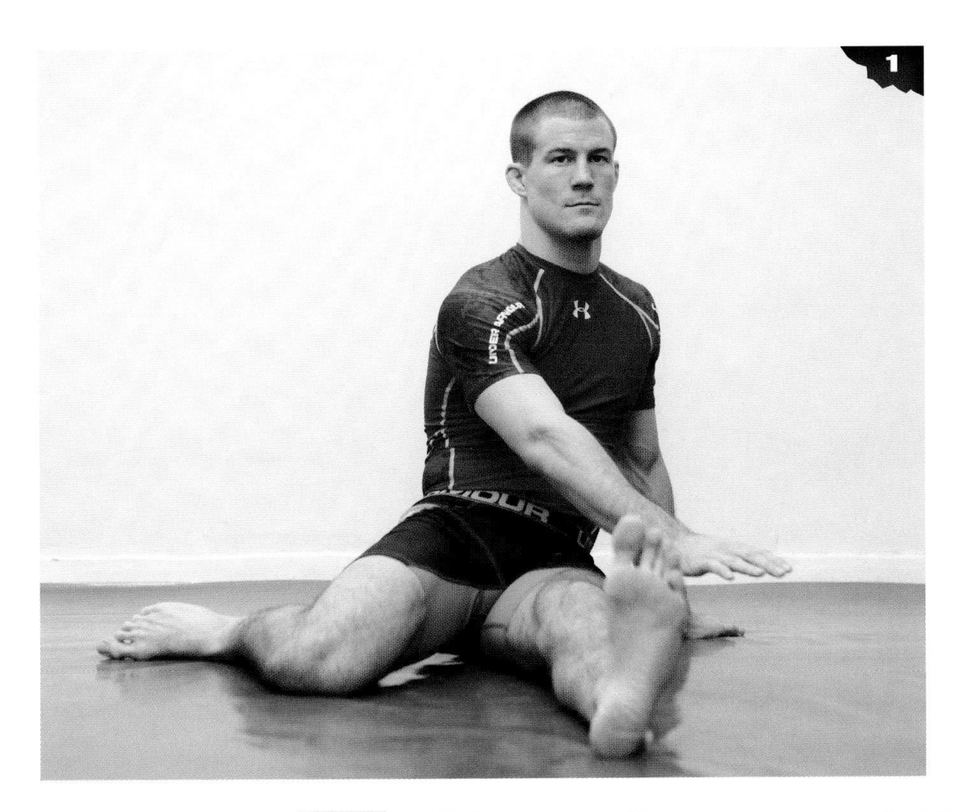

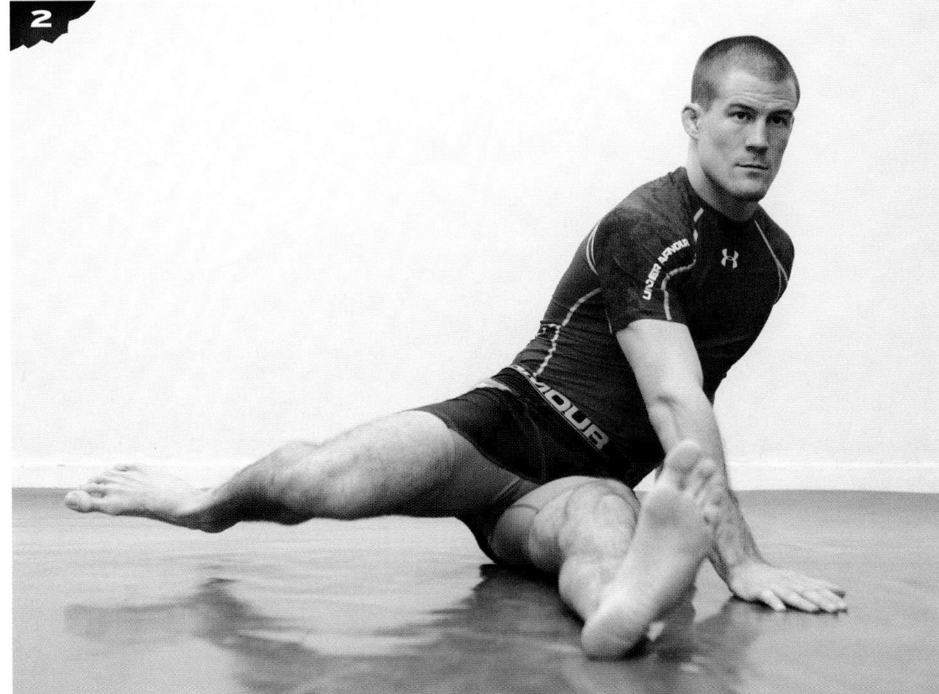

5. FIGURE-4 LIFT

Begin lying on the stomach with one leg crossed over the other, in the figure-4 position. While keeping the hips square with the floor, lift the bent knee out to the side as high as possible. Hold for 1 second and lower back down under control. Repeat on both sides.

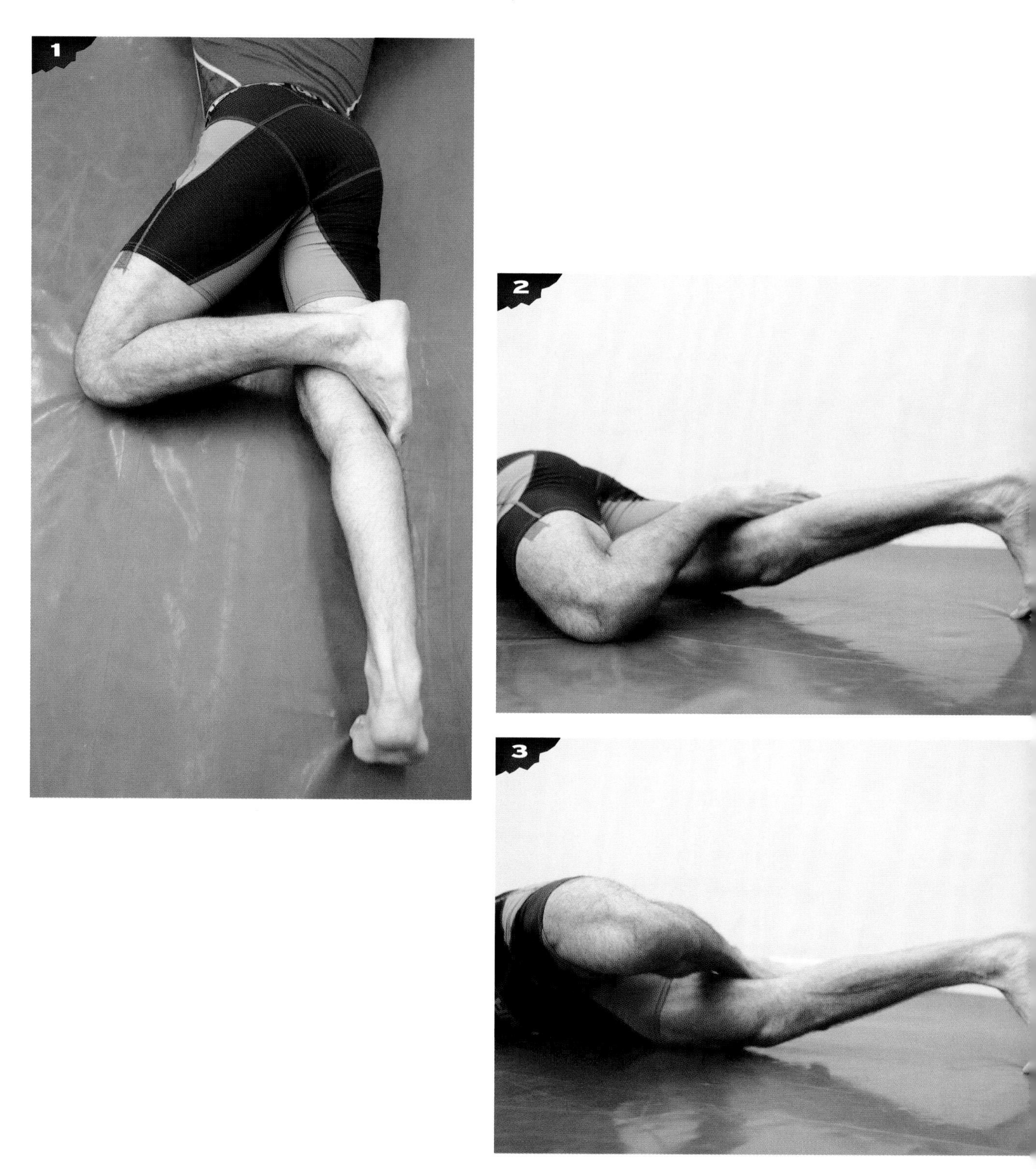

6. DONKEY KICK

Begin lying on the stomach with the chin on the hands and one leg bent at 90 degrees. Lift the sole of the foot toward the ceiling while maintaining the bend in the knee. Hold for 1 second and lower back down under control. Repeat on both sides.

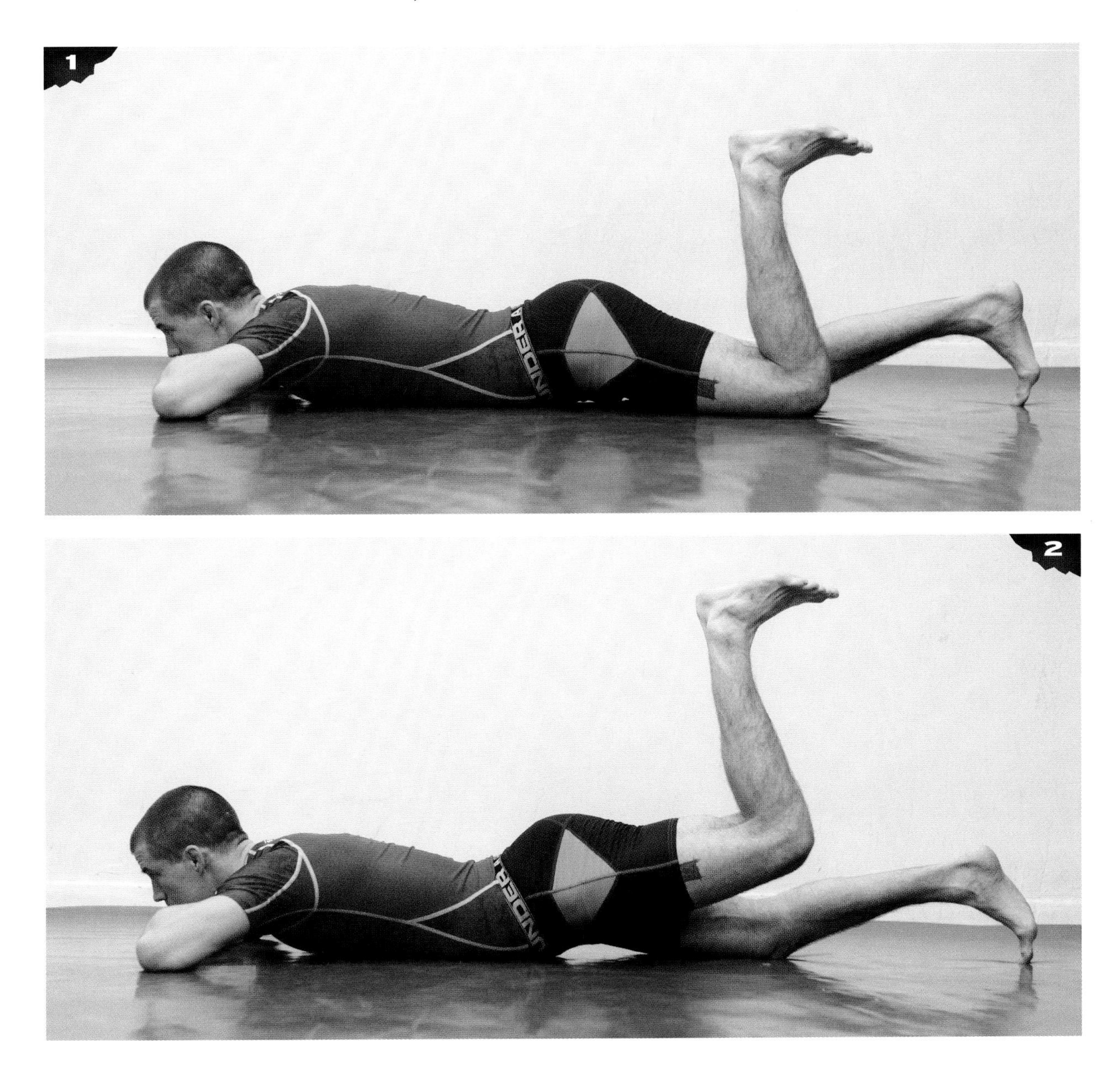

7. KNEE TO ELBOW

Begin lying on the stomach with the chin on the hands and both legs straight. Bring one knee up toward the elbow and hold for 1 second. Return to the start position and repeat on both sides.

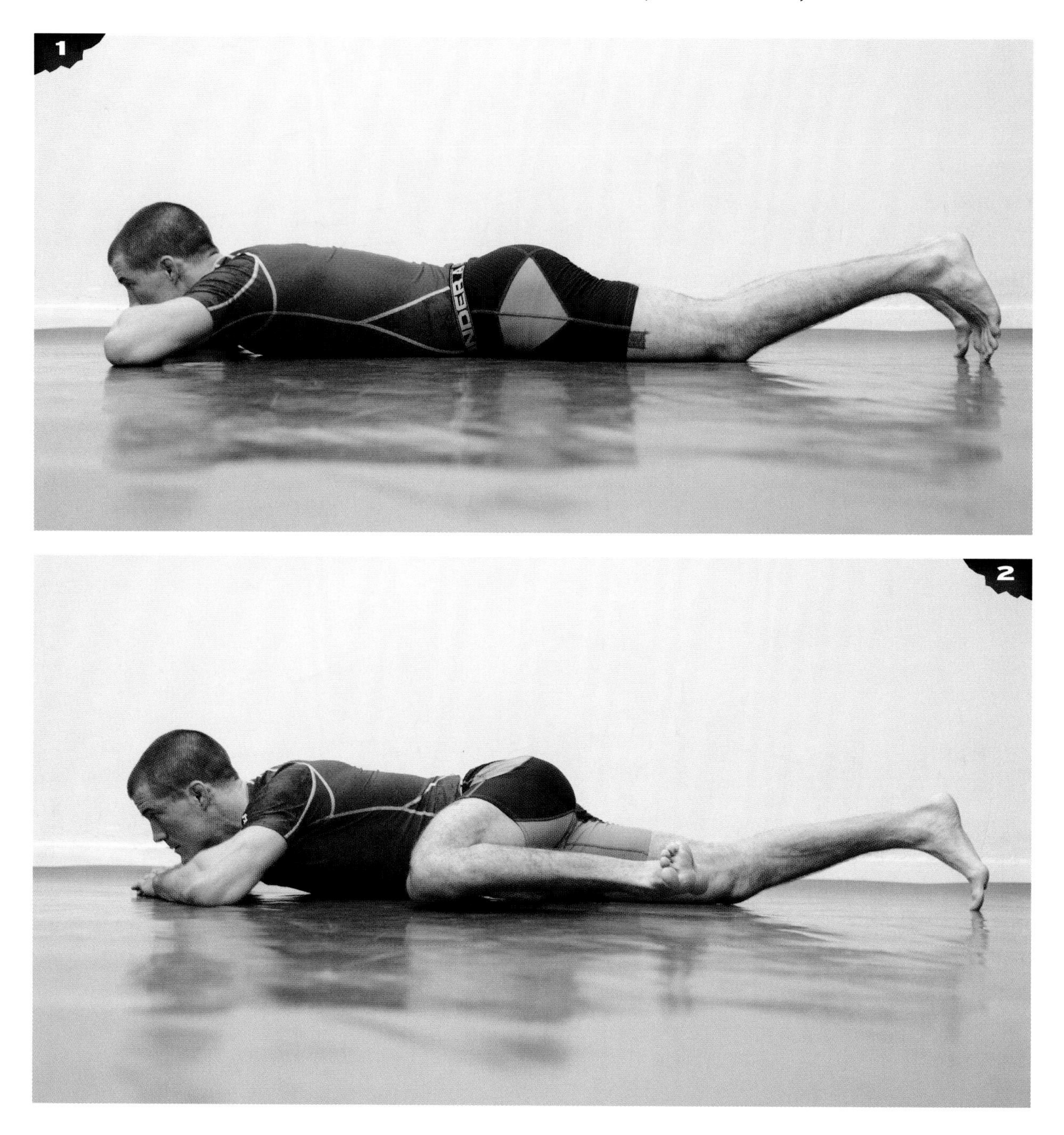

8. LATERAL SLIDE

Begin lying on the stomach with the chin on the hands and both legs straight. While keeping the toes pointed down, bring one leg out to the side and hold for 1 second. Return to the start position and repeat on both sides.

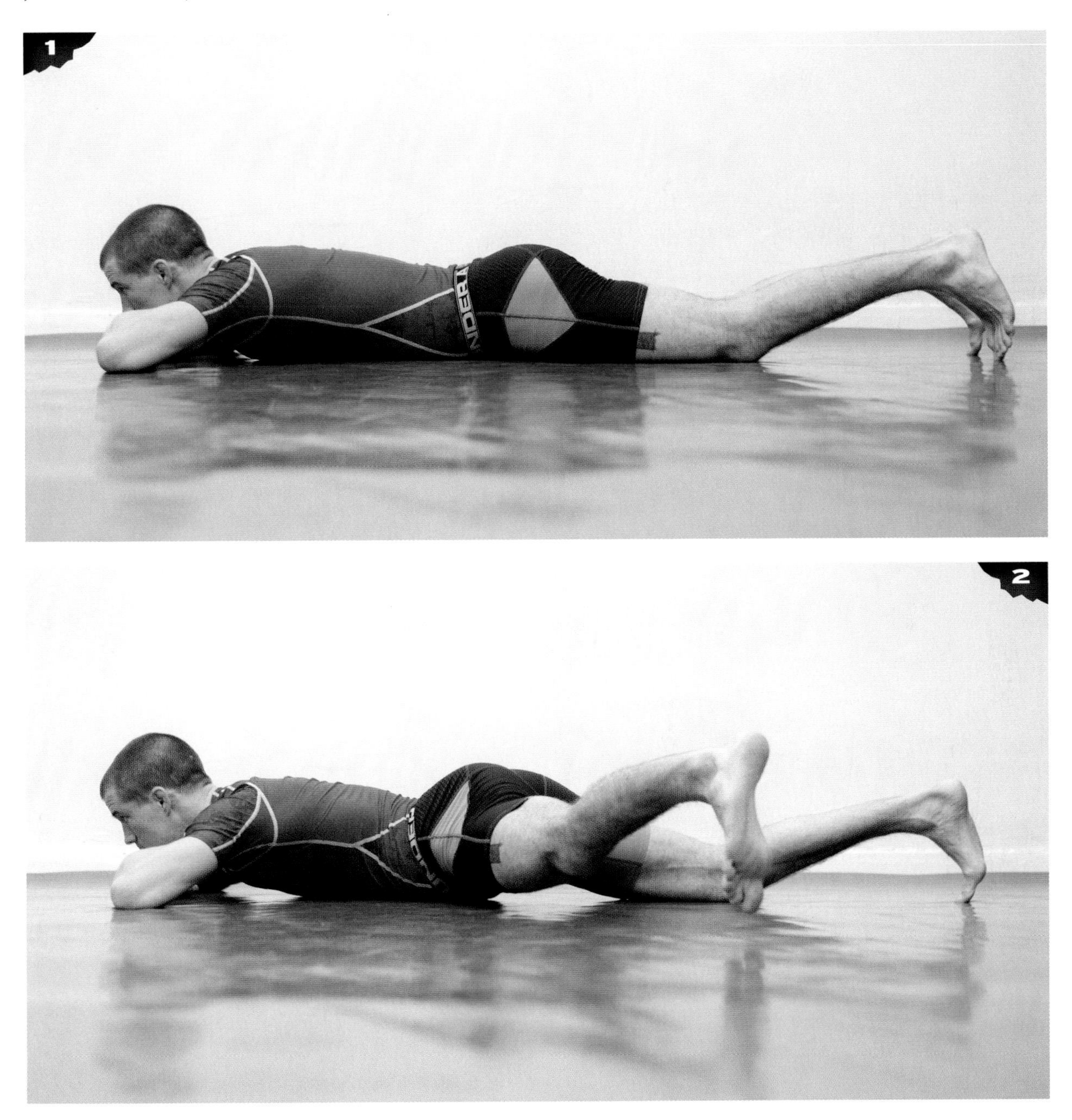

9. LATERAL RAISE

Begin on the hands and knees with the elbows locked, back flat, and one leg straight out to the side. Lift the outside foot as high as possible while keeping the elbows as straight as possible. Hold for 1 second and lower back down under control. Repeat on both sides.

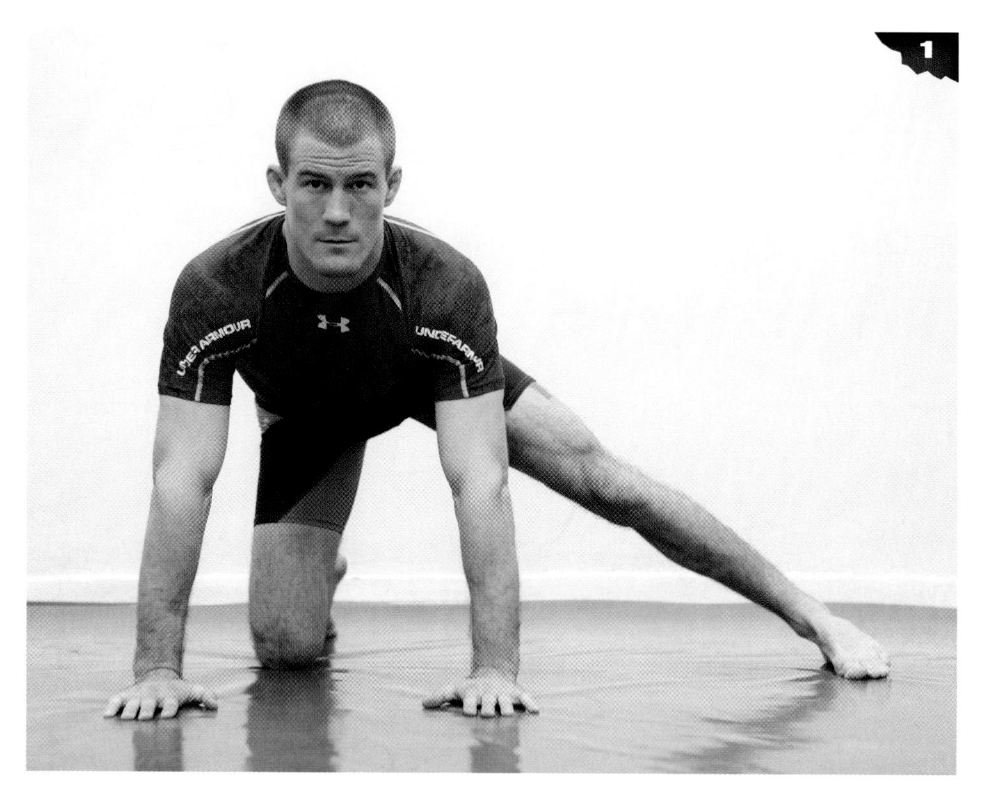

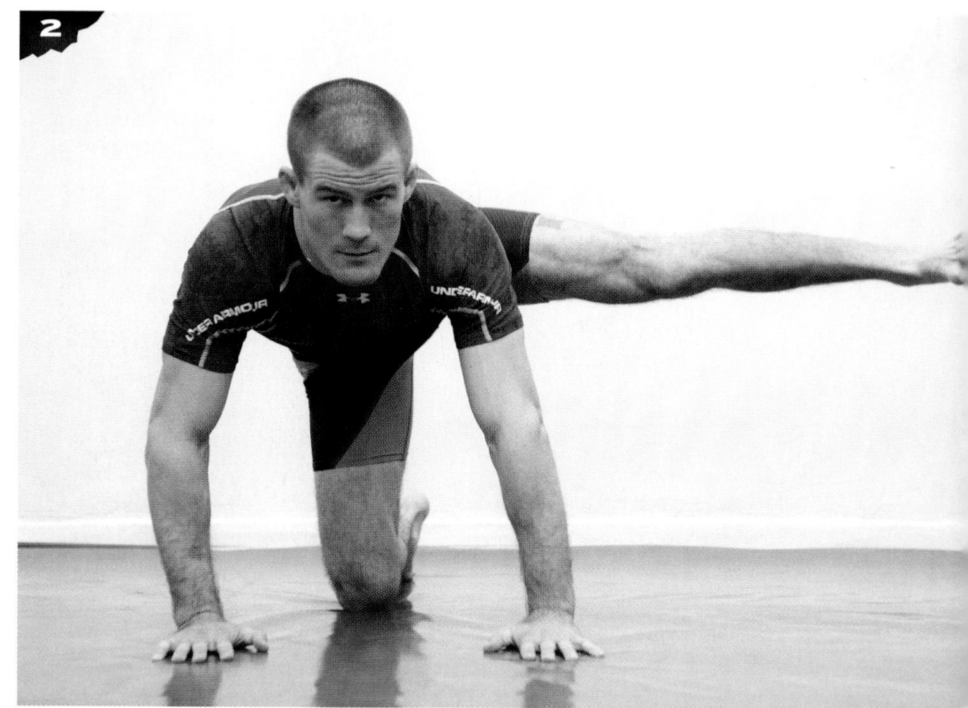

10. LATERAL KICK

Begin on the hands and knees with the elbows locked, back flat, and one leg straight out to the back. Lift the back foot to head height and then kick the foot out to the side while keeping the knee straight. Hold for 1 second and return the foot to the start position. Repeat on both sides.

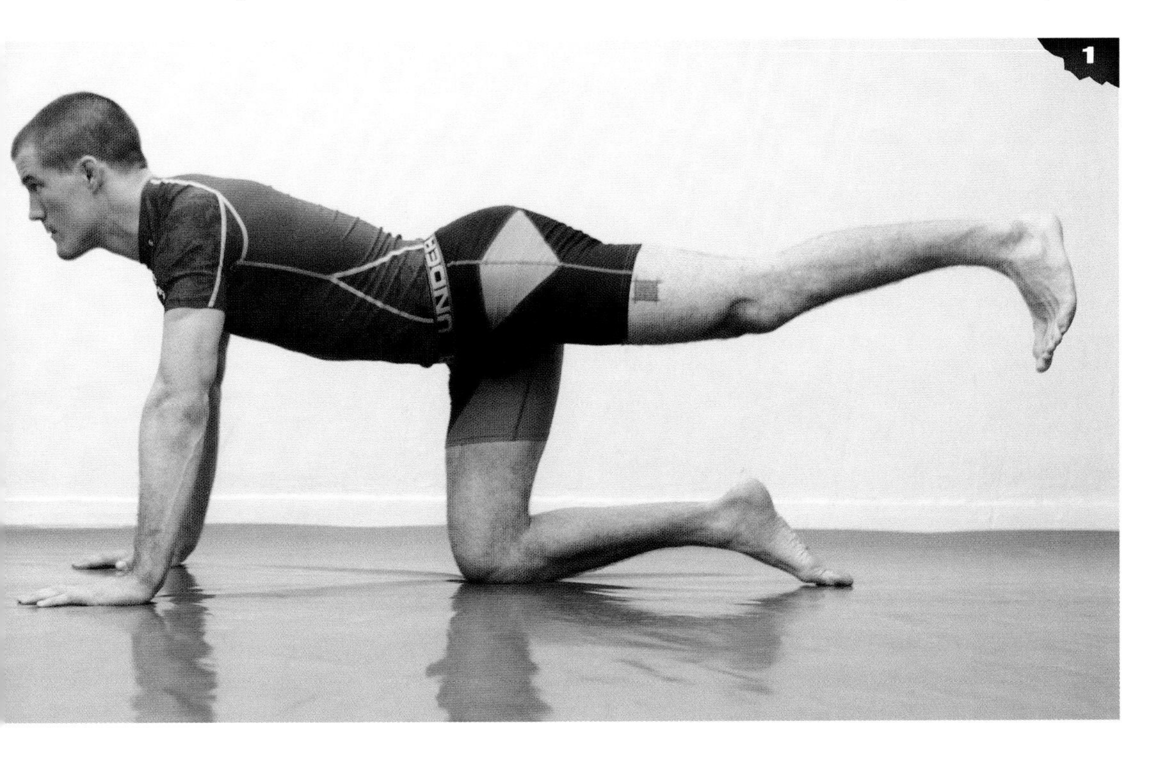

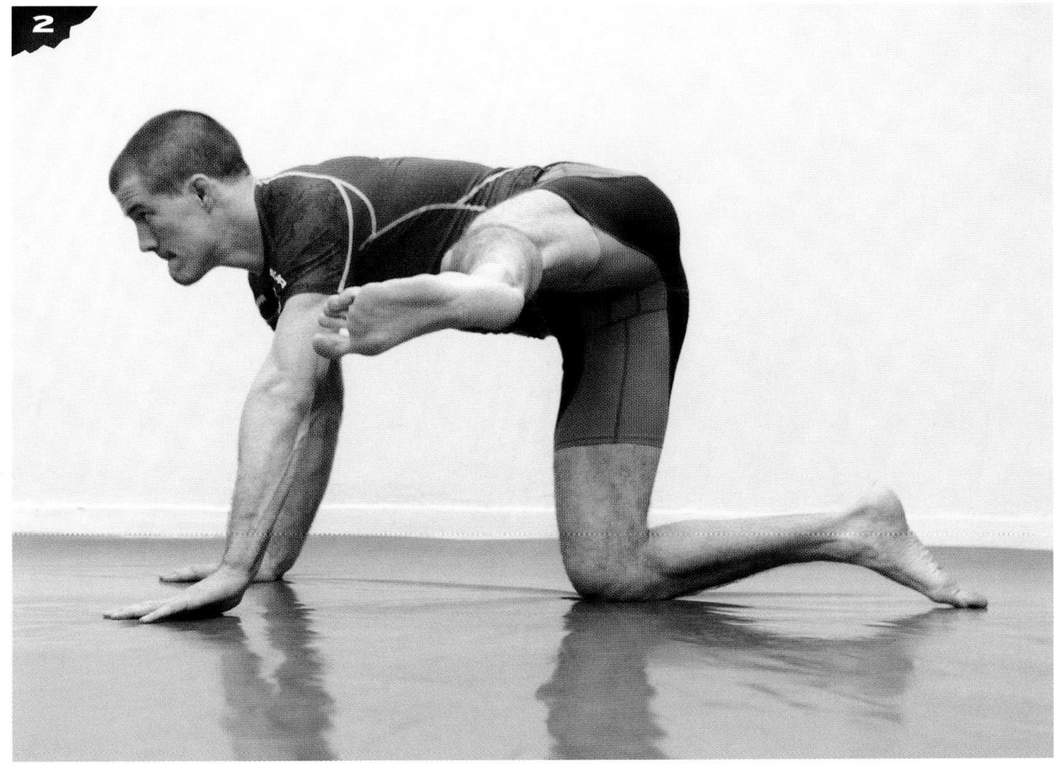

C. UPPER-BODY BAND ROUTINE

Following the TFW Hip Circuit, each of the six exercises of the Upper-Body Band Routine is performed for 2 sets of 8 repetitions. The band that is selected should be of moderate tension. This means that the 2 sets of 8 repetitions should lead to a good burn at the completion of each set, but not be overly difficult to perform. All drills are to be performed standing.

1. BAND FORWARD FLEXION

Start standing with one or both feet on the band or with the band hooked to something on the floor. Begin with the hands held at the hips and then raise the hands out in front of the body. Hold for 1 second and lower back down under control.

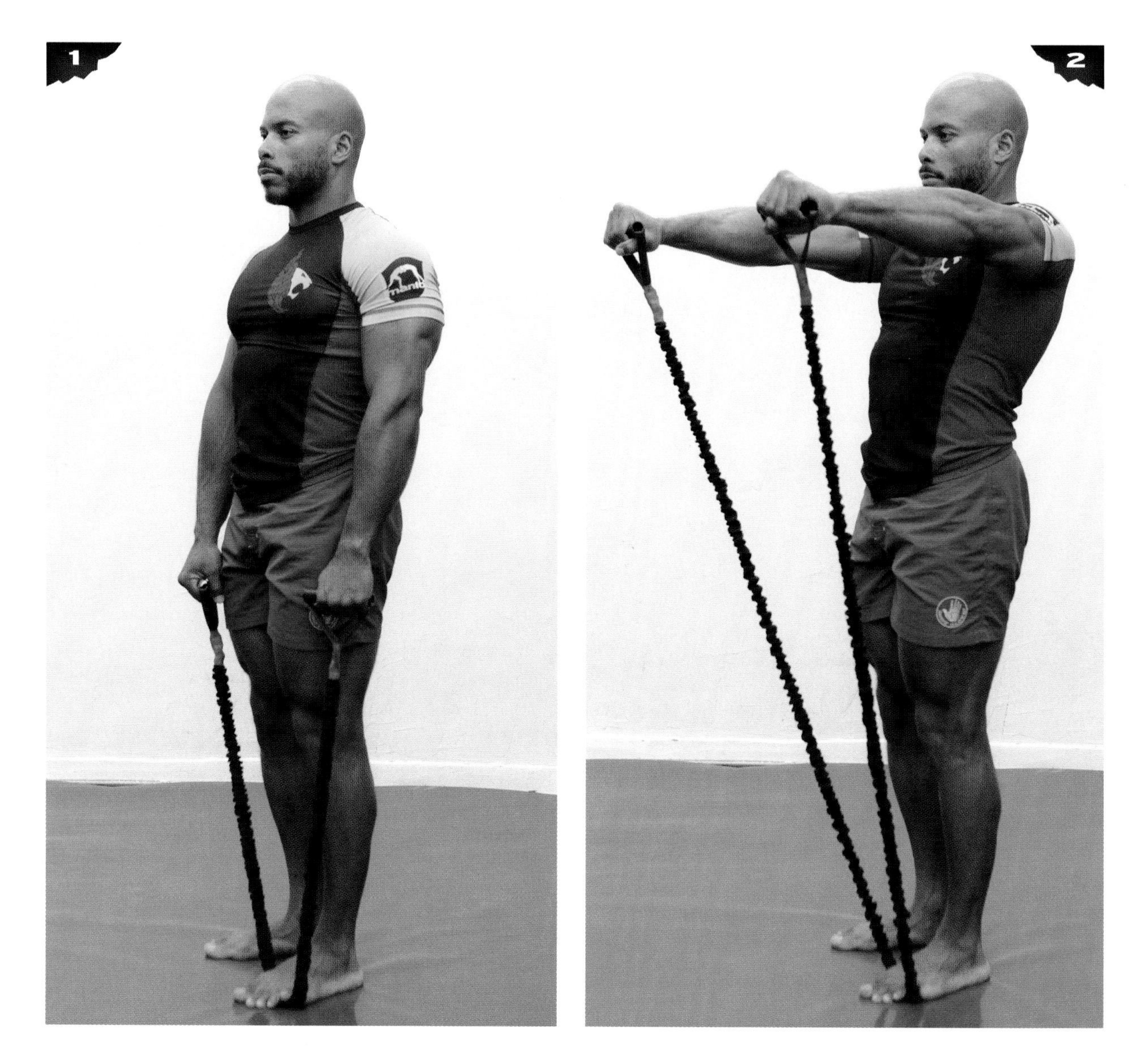

2. BAND HIGH PULL

Start standing with one or both feet on the band or with the band hooked to something on the floor. Begin with the hands held at the hips and then pull the elbows upward while bringing the thumbs close to the chin. Hold for 1 second and lower back down under control.

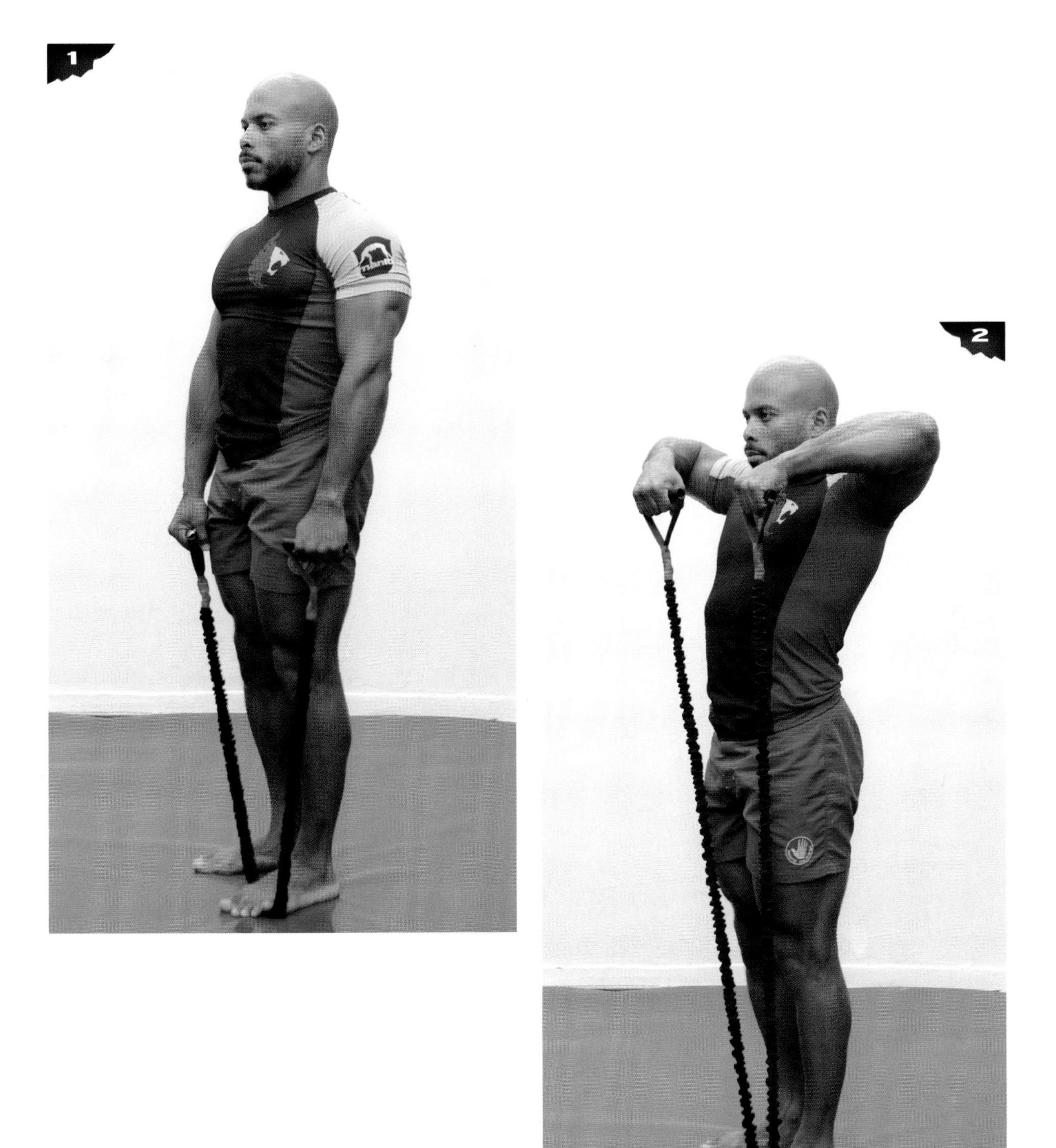

3. BAND LATERAL RAISE

Start standing with one or both feet on the band or with the band hooked to something on the floor. Begin with the hands held at the hips and then raise the hands up to the sides of the body at shoulder height. Hold for 1 second and lower back down under control.

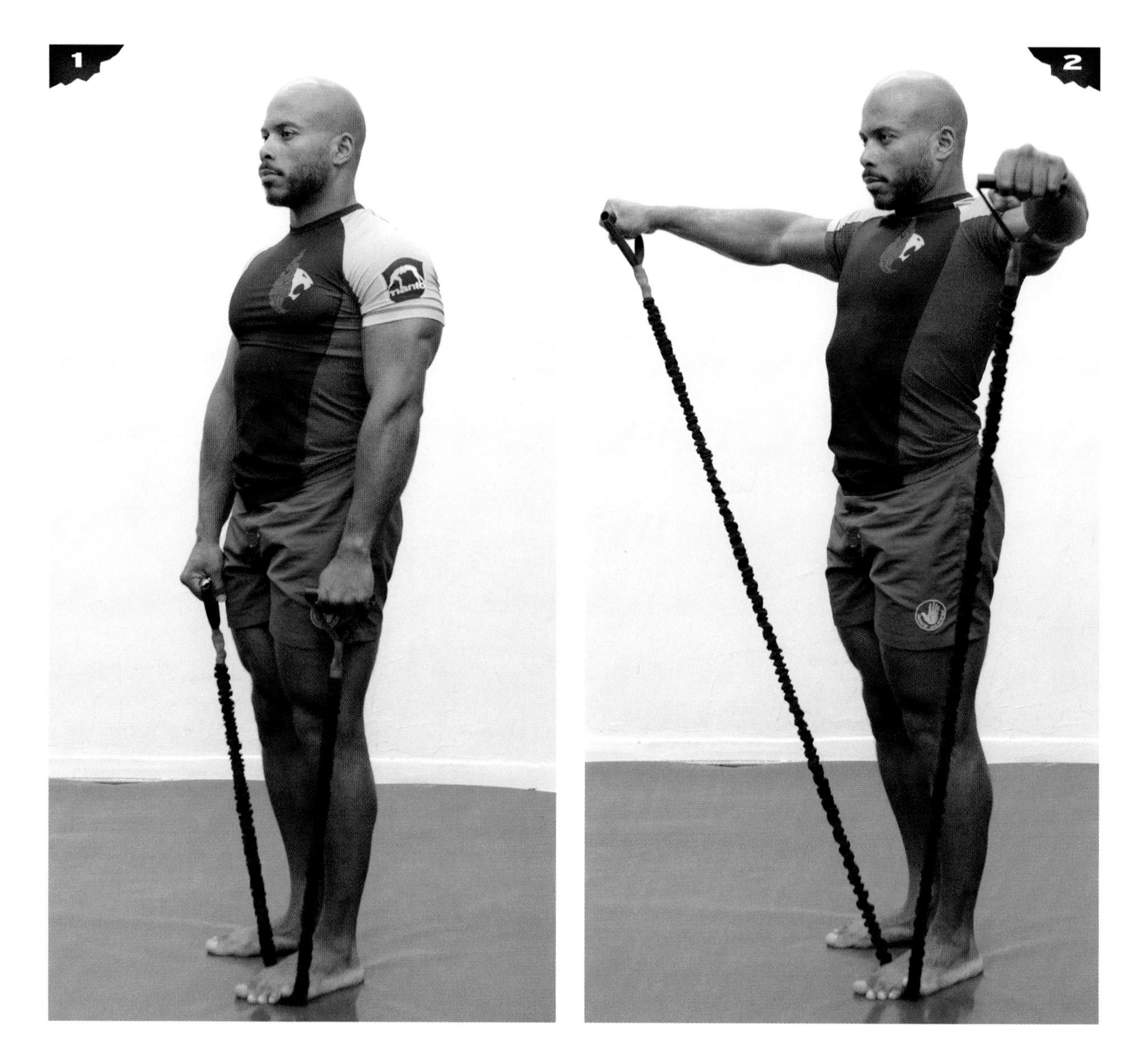

4. BAND ROW

Hook the band onto something at chest height. Begin with the elbows extended and the hands held together in the front of the body at shoulder height. Pull the hands to the armpits. Hold for 1 second and return to the start under control.

1

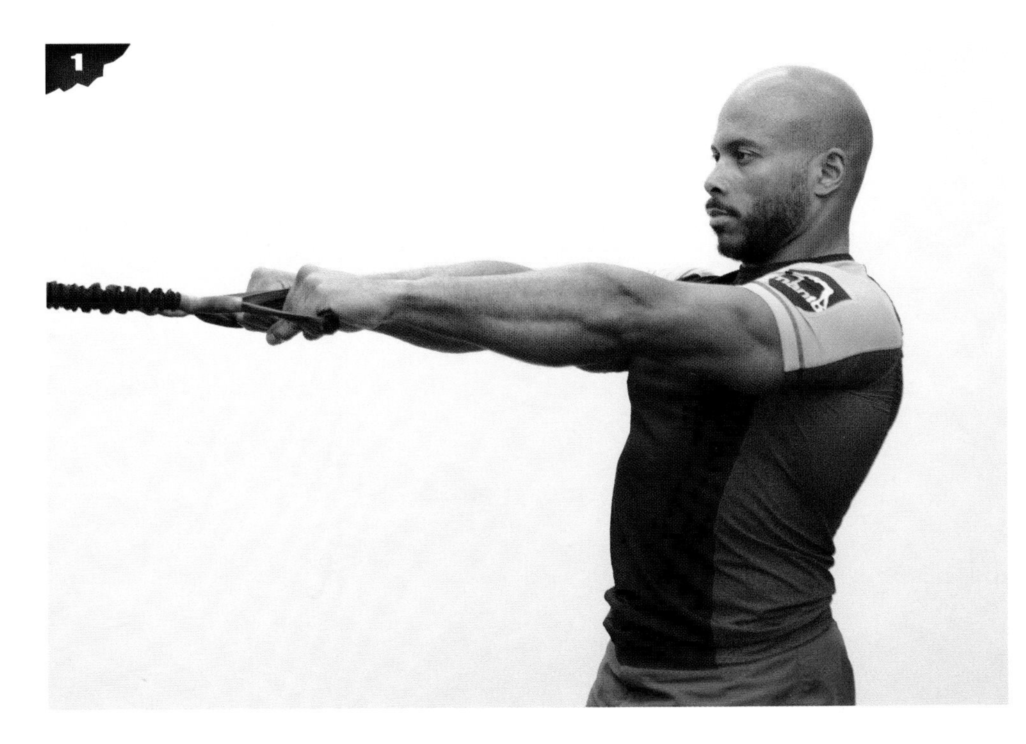

2

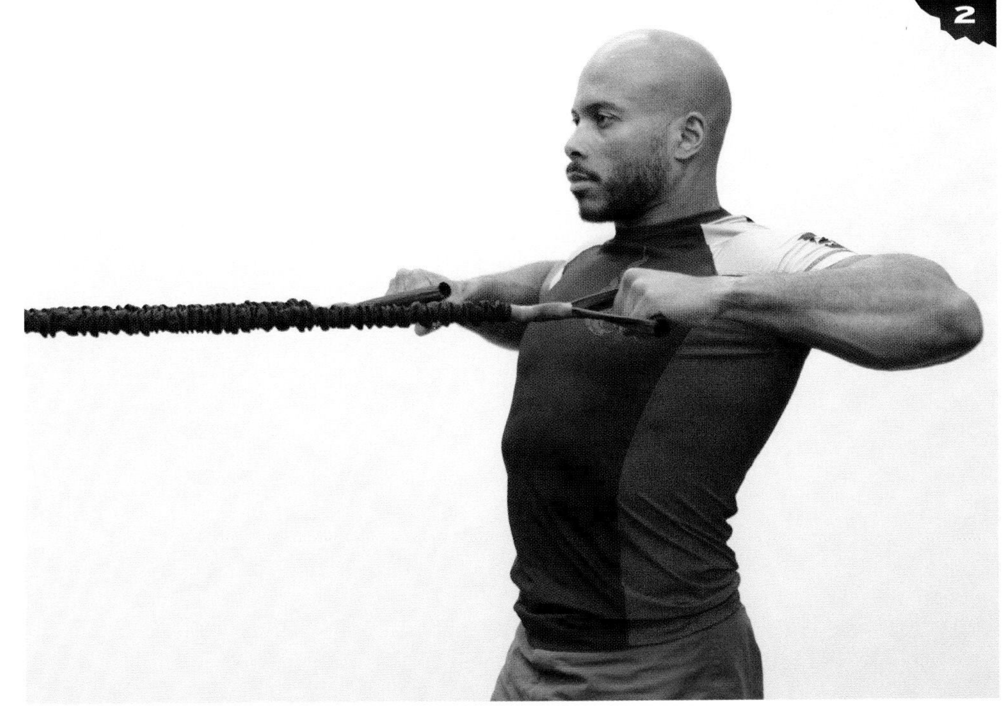

5. BAND EXTERNAL ROTATION

Hook the band onto something at chest height. Begin with the elbows extended and the hands held together in front of the body at shoulder height. Pull the elbows back and the hands up to the height of the top of the head. Hold for 1 second and return to the start under control.

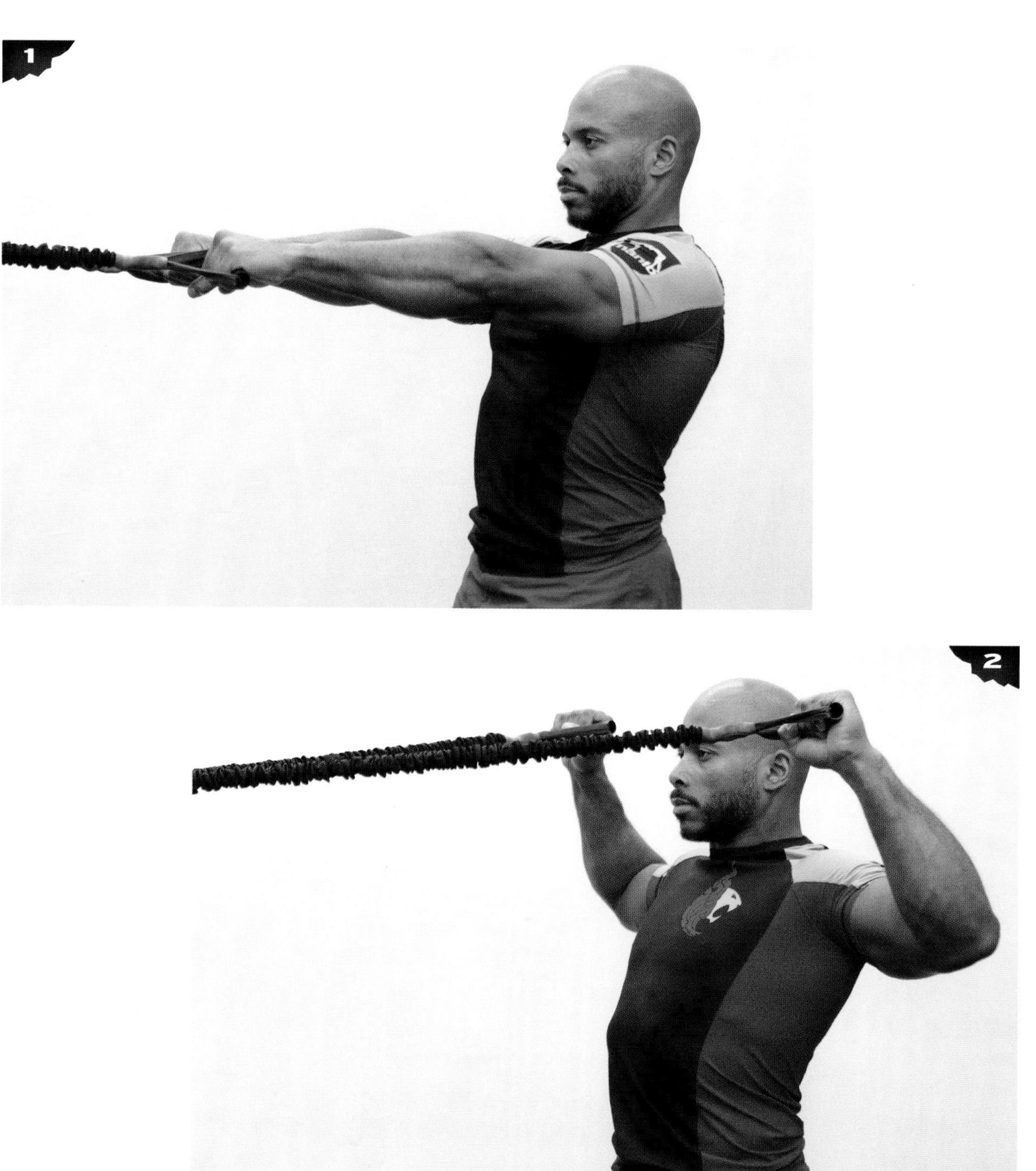

6. BAND EXTENSION

Hook the band onto something at chest height. Begin with the elbows extended and the hands held together in front of the body at shoulder height. Pull the hands down and behind the hips. Hold for 1 second and return to the start under control.

1

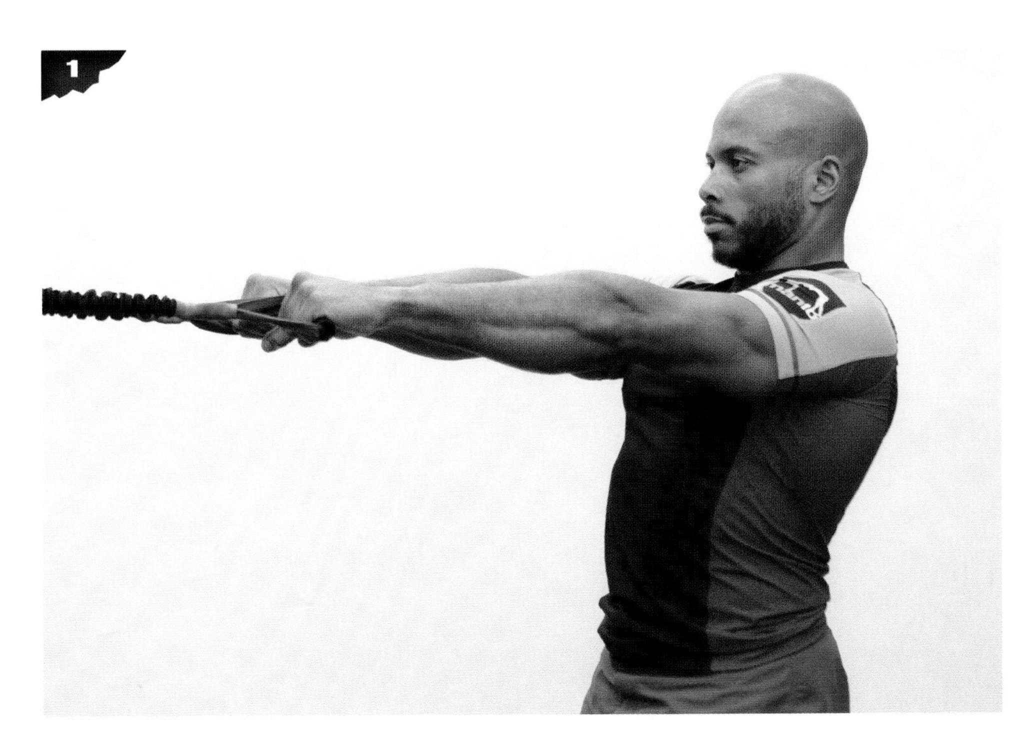

2

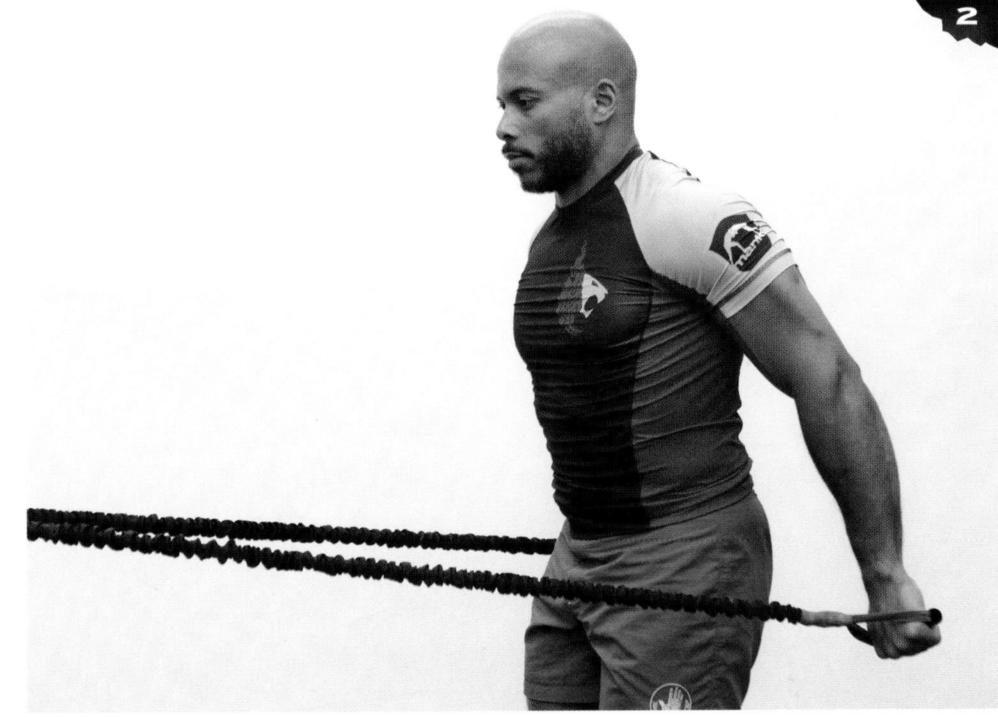

TFW WARMUP CHART CHEATSHEET

MINI PLYO HOPS AND MOVEMENT DRILLS

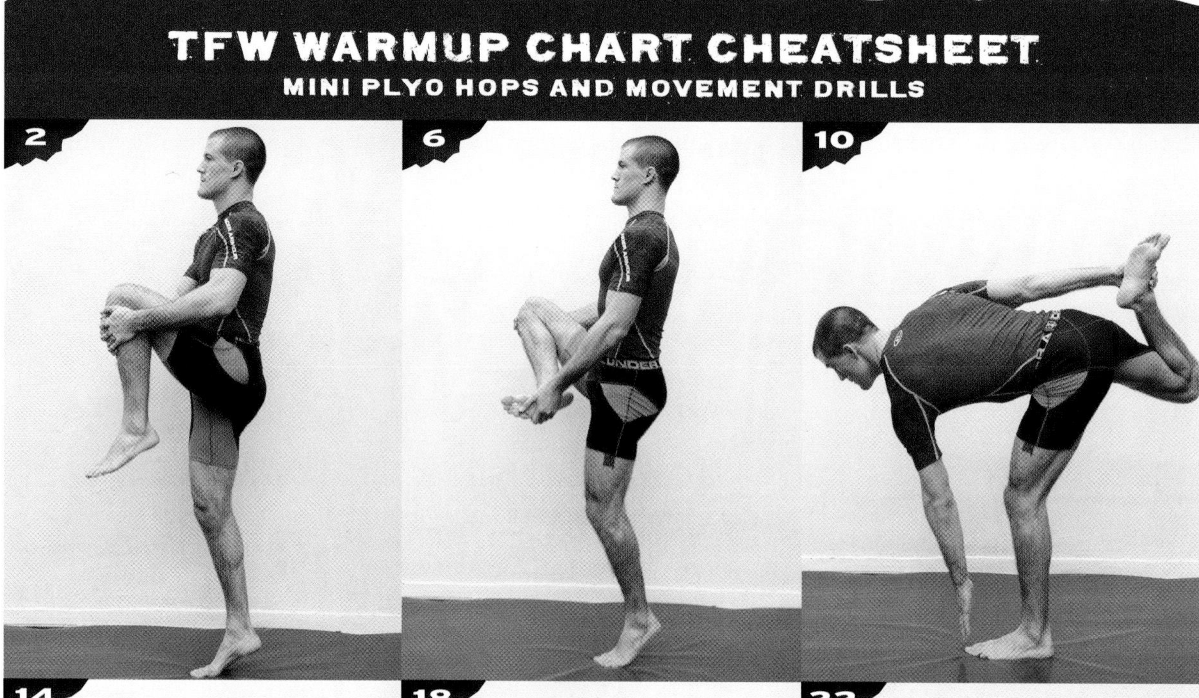

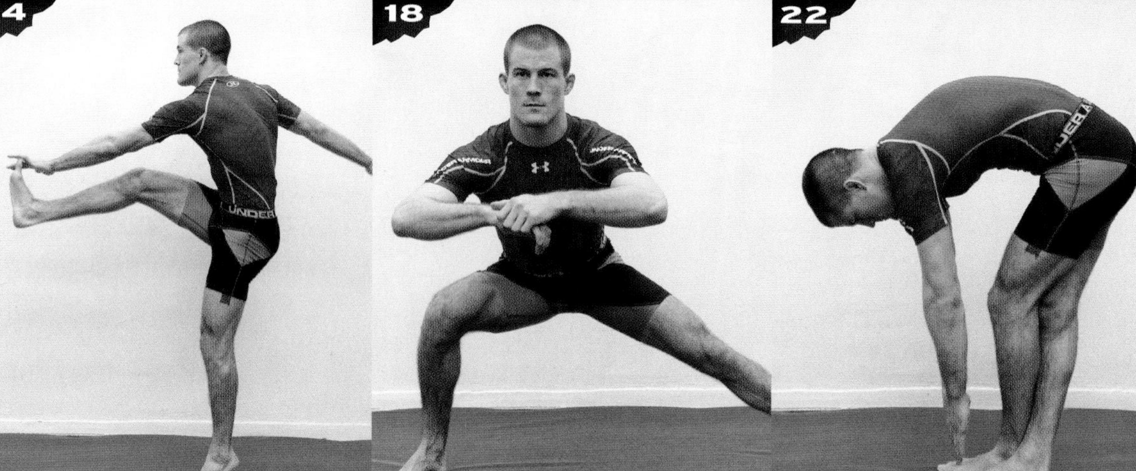

1. TFW CROSS JUMPS: 1-4
2. **WALKING KNEE TO CHEST**
3. TFW CROSS JUMPS: 1-2
4. REPEAT THE WALKING KNEE TO CHEST
5. TFW CROSS JUMPS: 1-3
6. **WALKING CRADLE STRETCH**
7. TFW CROSS JUMPS: 2-4
8. REPEAT THE WALKING CRADLE STRETCH
9. TFW CROSS JUMPS: 1, 2, 3
10. **WALKING QUAD STRETCH**
11. TFW CROSS JUMPS: 2, 1, 4
12. REPEAT THE WALKING QUAD STRETCH
13. TFW CROSS JUMPS: STAR JUMPS
14. **WALKING HAMSTRING KICKS**
15. REPEAT THE STAR JUMPS
16. REPEAT THE WALKING HAMSTRING KICKS
17. TFW CROSS JUMPS: SINGLE LEG 1-4
18. **WALKING SIDE LUNGE**
19. TFW CROSS JUMPS: SINGLE LEG 1-2
20. REPEAT THE WALKING SIDE LUNGE, BUT THIS TIME ON THE OTHER SIDE.
21. TFW CROSS JUMPS: SINGLE LEG 1-3
22. **WALKING CROSS-LEGGED HAMSTRING**
23. TFW CROSS JUMPS: SINGLE LEG 2-4
24. REPEAT WALKING CROSS-LEGGED HAMSTRING
25. TFW CROSS JUMPS: 1-2-3-4 JUMPS
26. WALKING LUNGE AND TWIST
27. REPEAT THE TFW CROSS JUMPS: 1-2-3-4 JUMPS
28. REPEAT THE WALKING LUNGE AND TWIST

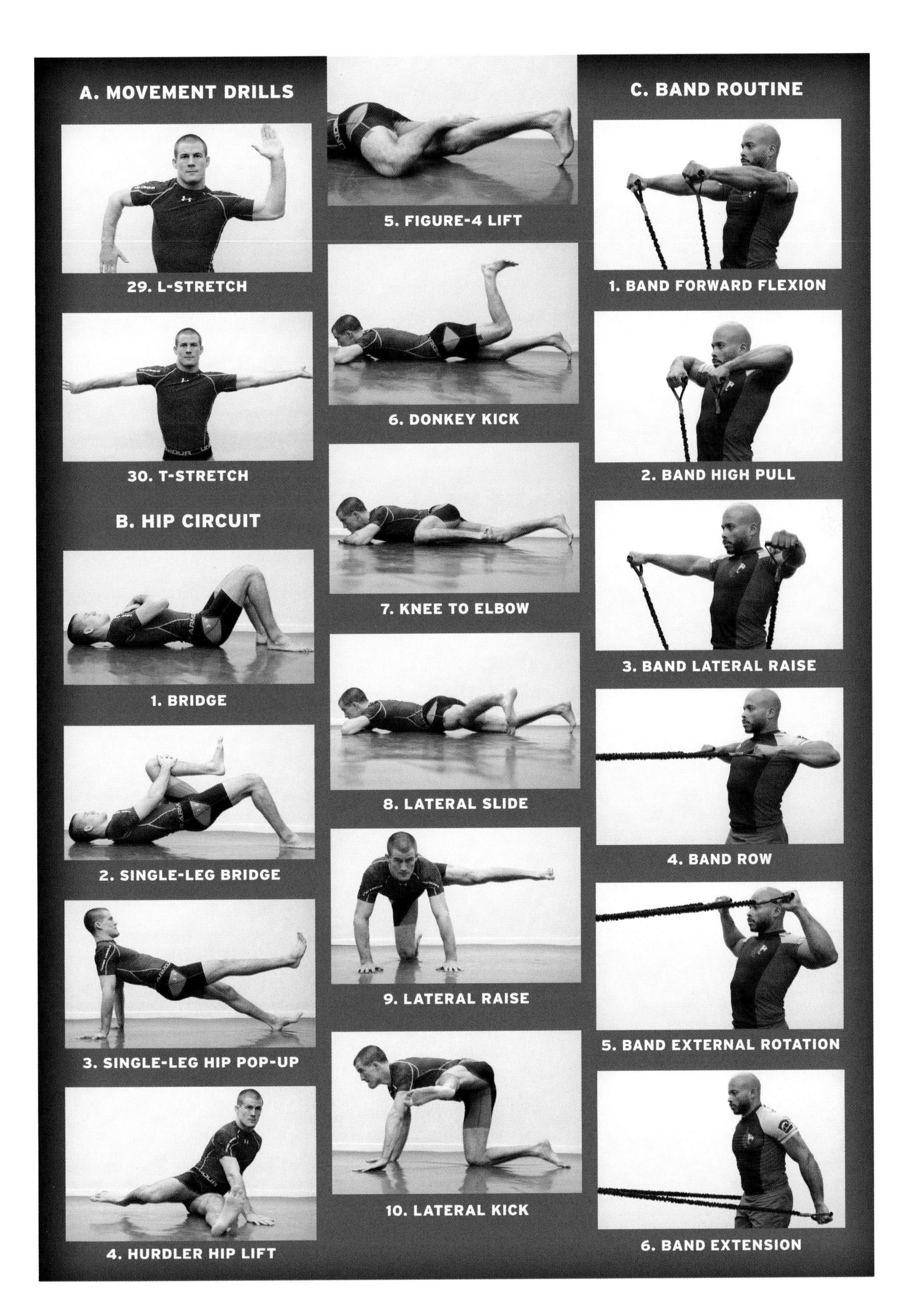
A. MOVEMENT DRILLS
29. L-STRETCH
30. T-STRETCH
B. HIP CIRCUIT
1. BRIDGE
2. SINGLE-LEG BRIDGE
3. SINGLE-LEG HIP POP-UP
4. HURDLER HIP LIFT
5. FIGURE-4 LIFT
6. DONKEY KICK
7. KNEE TO ELBOW
8. LATERAL SLIDE
9. LATERAL RAISE
10. LATERAL KICK
C. BAND ROUTINE
1. BAND FORWARD FLEXION
2. BAND HIGH PULL
3. BAND LATERAL RAISE
4. BAND ROW
5. BAND EXTERNAL ROTATION
6. BAND EXTENSION

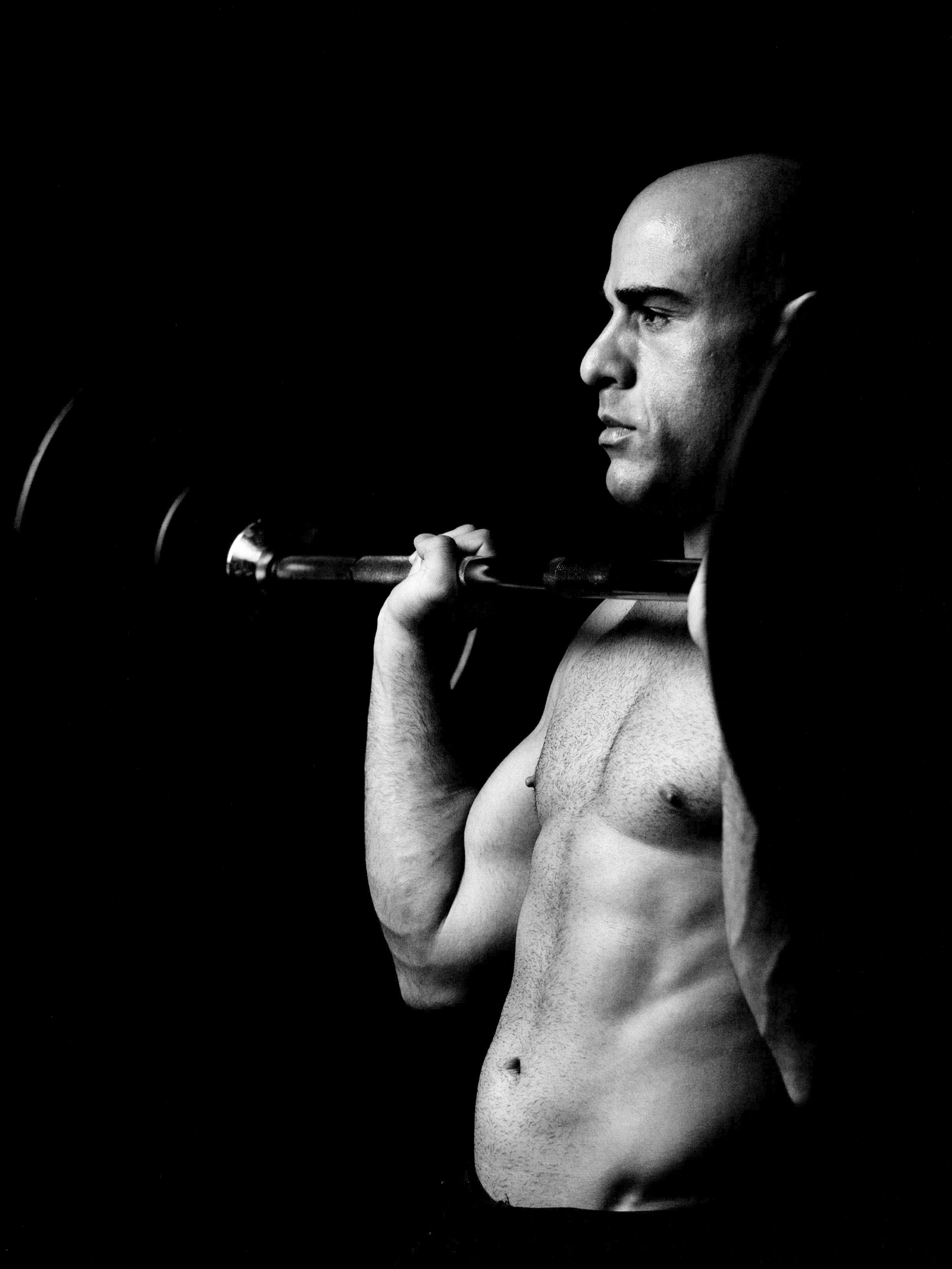

METABOLIC TRAINING

This part of the book will focus on the different forms of Metabolic Training that are commonly used in the Training for Warriors system. Although this list does not cover every form of Metabolic Training imaginable, that is not the purpose. The purpose is to deliver a number of different metabolic workouts that can be both monitored and measured.

Regardless of the name it is given, every form of Metabolic Training listed in this book is some form of a circuit, meaning a series of exercises performed in a row with periods of rest in between the individual exercises and the next series. This should make it easy to understand that regardless of the method you choose, every form of Metabolic Training has the ability to improve cardiac capacity, increase strength and muscle mass, and decrease fat. These results will depend entirely on the proper application of the form of training used.

Since we have identified that most people rarely perform these sessions with results in mind (remember the Illogical Four—Novelty, Coolness, Ability to Produce Soreness, and Ability to Produce Fatigue?), most people also do not pay attention to detail when performing this style of training. Just as you would not use weights without knowing the load, these sessions must also be graded and measured to be effective. This paradigm is what distinguishes the TFW system.

Speaking of application, you need to recognize that there are a number of ways in which the intensity of a circuit can be altered. Understanding these acute variables of training and how to adapt them during a workout will help you to design your program, prevent injury, and increase results.

10 FACTORS THAT AFFECT THE INTENSITY OF A METABOLIC SESSION

1. **Exercise Selection**

   If the circuit involves a number of complex movements with weight, the circuit will naturally be more intense to perform.

2. **Speed of Movement**

   If the circuit involves a number of movements that require great speed throughout the event, there will be an increased energy demand.

3. **Muscular Emphasis**

   If the circuit involves a number of movements that invoke smaller muscles (i.e., using ropes, medicine balls, etc.), there can be an increase in heart rate as a result.

4. **Duration of the Circuit**

   If the circuit increases in time, there is a chance that it will also increase in metabolic demand.

5. **Number of Exercises**

   With more exercises, usually there is a corresponding increase in time and, therefore, an increase in demand.

6. **Monitoring of Repetition Maximums**

   If there are an increasing number of repetitions within a set amount of time, there will always be an increased metabolic cost.

7. **Exercise Intensity (Weight)**

   The more difficult the exercises are to perform in terms of intensity, the larger the demand and subsequent oxygen debt.

8. **Total Number of Circuits**

   If there are more total circuits performed, there will be an obvious increase in demand.

9. **Rest Periods Between Exercises**

   Also known as the work-to-rest ratio, the shorter the amount of rest between exercises, the greater the demand of the circuit.

10. **Rest Periods Between Circuits**

    The length of rest periods between circuits will affect the overall intensity of the workout session.

The purpose of these chapters is not only to deliver a number of options when addressing the Metabolic Training days of the TFW system, but also to give you perspective on how to properly apply and monitor this style of training. All too often these forms of training are used solely to produce fatigue and soreness while looking new and cool. In the TFW system, these training tools are used to produce results. Metabolic Training is a powerful tool, but only when used correctly. With improper application, this style of training can also be damaging—the goal here is to show you how to apply it correctly.

During any Metabolic Training session, there are a number of rules that you must abide by. If you follow the TFW 10 Commandments of Metabolic Training, you will not only perform a more adequate circuit more safely, but you will also guarantee yourself a better opportunity to achieve results.

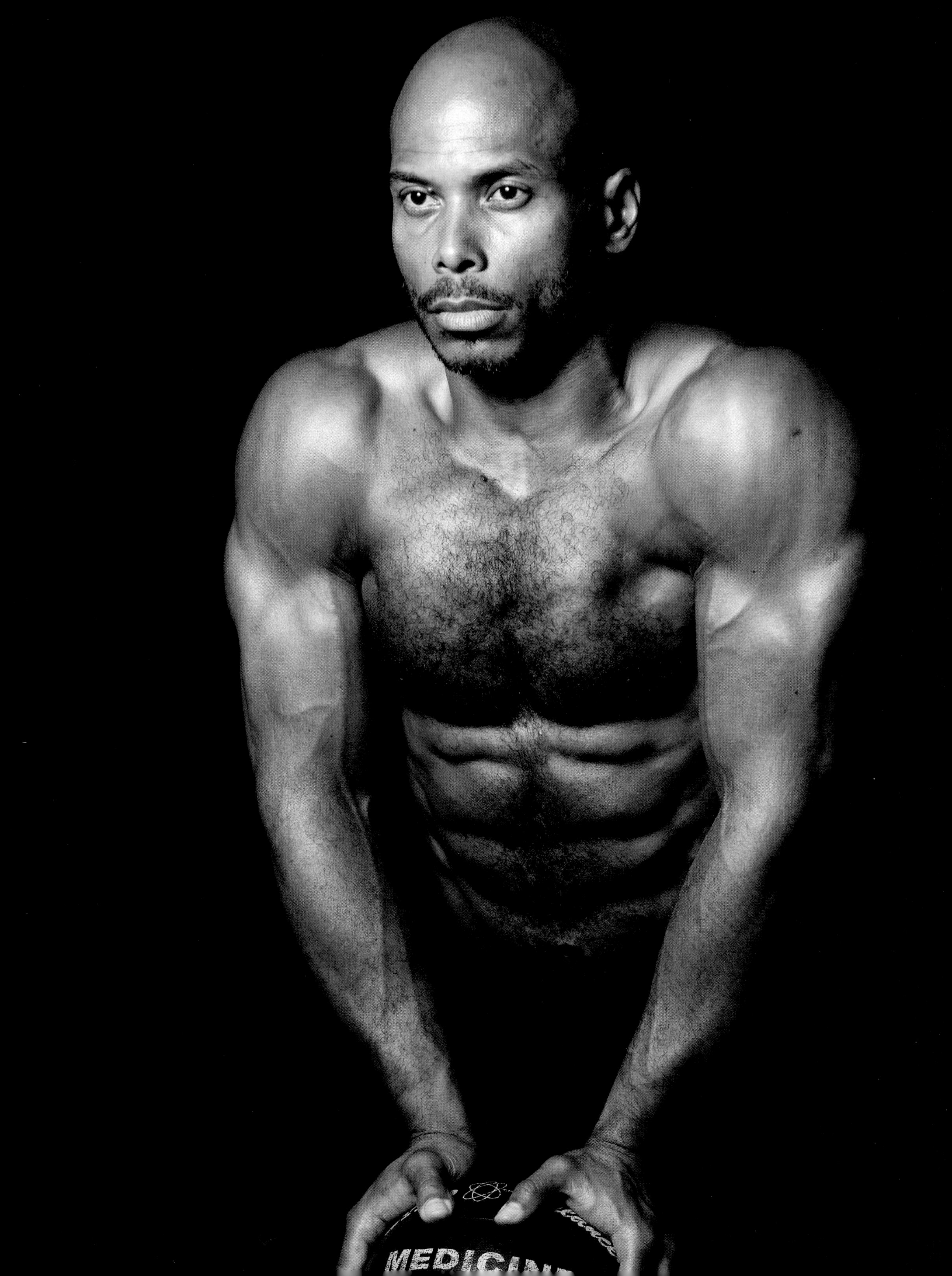
MEDICIN

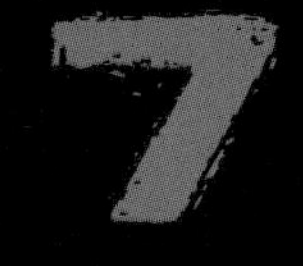

THE TRAINING FOR WARRIORS

10 COMMANDMENTS OF METABOLIC TRAINING

1. **Thou shalt not sacrifice technique for intensity.**
   Working hard or being fatigued is not an excuse to use terrible form. Although the workouts in this book ask for high intensity, you must also make sure that the exercises are performed well.

2. **Thou shalt not confuse fatigue or soreness with being productive.**
   The goal of the training is not complete exhaustion or the search of fatigue. Yes, these sessions may produce soreness and fatigue, but that is not the goal. The goal of the sessions is improvement.

3. **Thou shalt make sure that there is ample recovery between sessions.**
   In addition to monitoring the work/rest ratio, you must also make sure to recover in between sessions. Many of the workouts contained in this book are both physically and mentally demanding. Although they are fun, that is not an excuse to do them too often. Make sure you find the amount of recovery your body needs and stick to it.

4. **Thou shalt monitor and record heart rate and HRV during every metabolic session.**
A huge reason to do Metabolic Training is to affect the cardiovascular system. Why then would you not monitor that system during the workout? Your heart rate and its ability to recover (which is known as heart rate variability, or HRV) are critical to understanding the session's performance level and whether you are improving. Make sure to check it and record it for every session.

5. **Thou shalt become proficient in the exercises required before making them into a circuit.**
You should demand that before you throw a new exercise into a circuit, you are already very good at that exercise. Exercises added to a circuit should be ones you are the best at, not the worst.

6. **Thou shalt choose appropriate exercises (specificity and variety) and the correct weights (intensity) for these exercises.**
These sessions are tough, but adding too much weight or exercises you are not ready for is not making them tougher; it is being careless. Make sure that you select the correct exercises and weights. This will insure good, safe training.

7. **Thou shalt always monitor work-to-rest ratios.**
A main way to control the intensity of a session is through the work/rest ratio. To pay no attention to this variable throws caution to the wind. Each session should be planned and monitored according to this variable between both individual exercises and sets.

8. **Thou shalt follow appropriate progression of training.**
You cannot rush physiology. You must build up your body over time for these workouts. Although the most difficult sessions may be attractive, you have to wait until your body is ready. Following a proper progression will lead to training longevity.

9. **Thou shalt have a plan for what you are looking to achieve with the session.**
Failing to plan is planning to fail. Whether it is heart rate, number of repetitions, increased weight, a better time, or a new personal best, you must have a goal to make the session effective. A plan makes sure you are not just "in" the session, but "into" that session.

10. **Thou shalt utilize a proper warmup before the session.**
A warmup is critical to get the body to a steady state to prepare for demanding metabolic sessions. Without a proper warmup, there is an increased chance of injury.

Through understanding the factors that affect a metabolic session and following the TFW 10 Commandments of Metabolic Training, you should now be prepared to begin experimenting with the workouts contained in the following chapters. Remember, the training in this book can be a powerful tool when used wisely and a damaging form of training when abused. A tool is only as effective as the person wielding it.

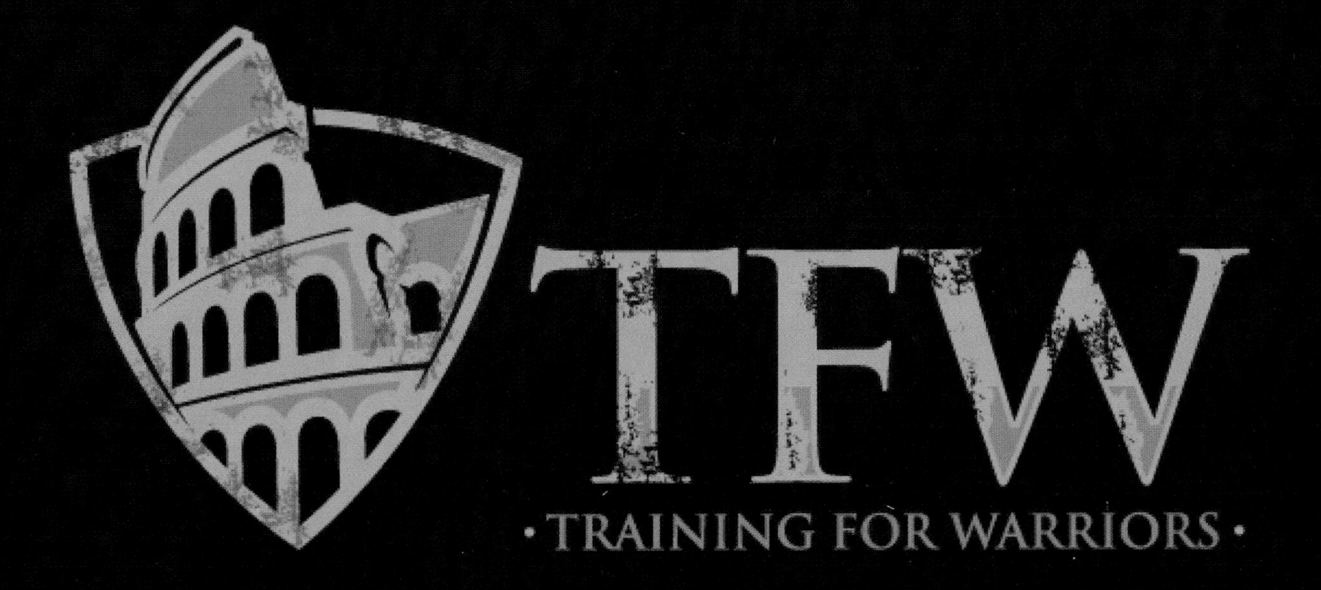
TFW
• TRAINING FOR WARRIORS •

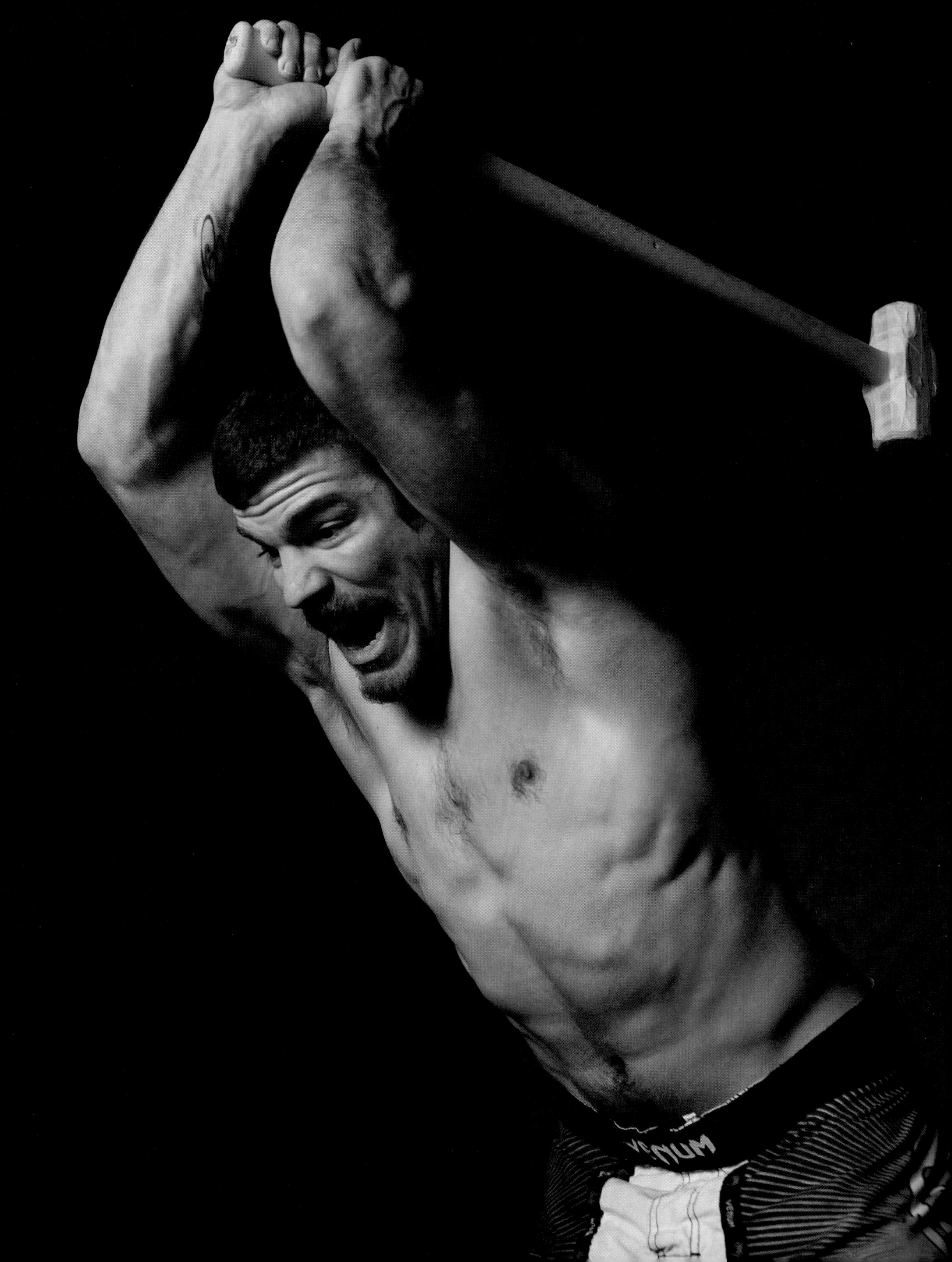
VENUM

8

ENERGY CIRCUITS

As a result of the recent explosion of circuits being used in commercial gyms, this is perhaps the most popular form of Metabolic Training today. Different forms of energy circuits have been used for decades in sport preparation, but now a number of forms are becoming commonplace in gyms around the world. During an energy circuit, a number of different exercises are performed back to back with little rest for a set time period. A circuit commonly uses anywhere from three to ten exercises. If there are multiple repetitions of that circuit, there is often the use of rest in between.

An energy circuit is an excellent opportunity to utilize a good bit of variety since almost any exercise can be thrown into the circuit. Whatever exercises you choose, it is important to make sure that you utilize good form on every exercise. Although variety is a good thing to stimulate both the mind and the heart, this is not an excuse to sacrifice technique for intensity. All too often practitioners use poor technique as a result of moving too quickly, increased fatigue, or improper motor patterns caused by inadequate practice. As I've mentioned, the goal is to create a cardiovascular stimulus, but quality of exercises should not suffer at the hand of intensity.

There are a number of ways that circuits can be performed. In the Training for Warriors system, the most common energy circuit we perform is one that mimics the specific time demands of an MMA fight, so each circuit "round" lasts 5 minutes. To keep the variety high, we perform five exercises during each round for 1 minute each. There can be a 10-to-15-second transition from one exercise to another, but the goal is to complete as much work as possible during each of the 1-minute intervals during the 5-minute round.

Once the round is completed, we traditionally use a 2-minute rest period in between energy circuits and rarely perform more than three total rounds. You can use shorter or longer work-to-rest ratios in between rounds, to either increase or decrease the intensity of the training session.

A. STRONGMAN CIRCUIT

1. FARMER'S WALK

Begin standing, holding a heavy dumbbell or implement in each hand with the elbows extended. Walk for 20 yards down and back as many times as possible in the time allotted.

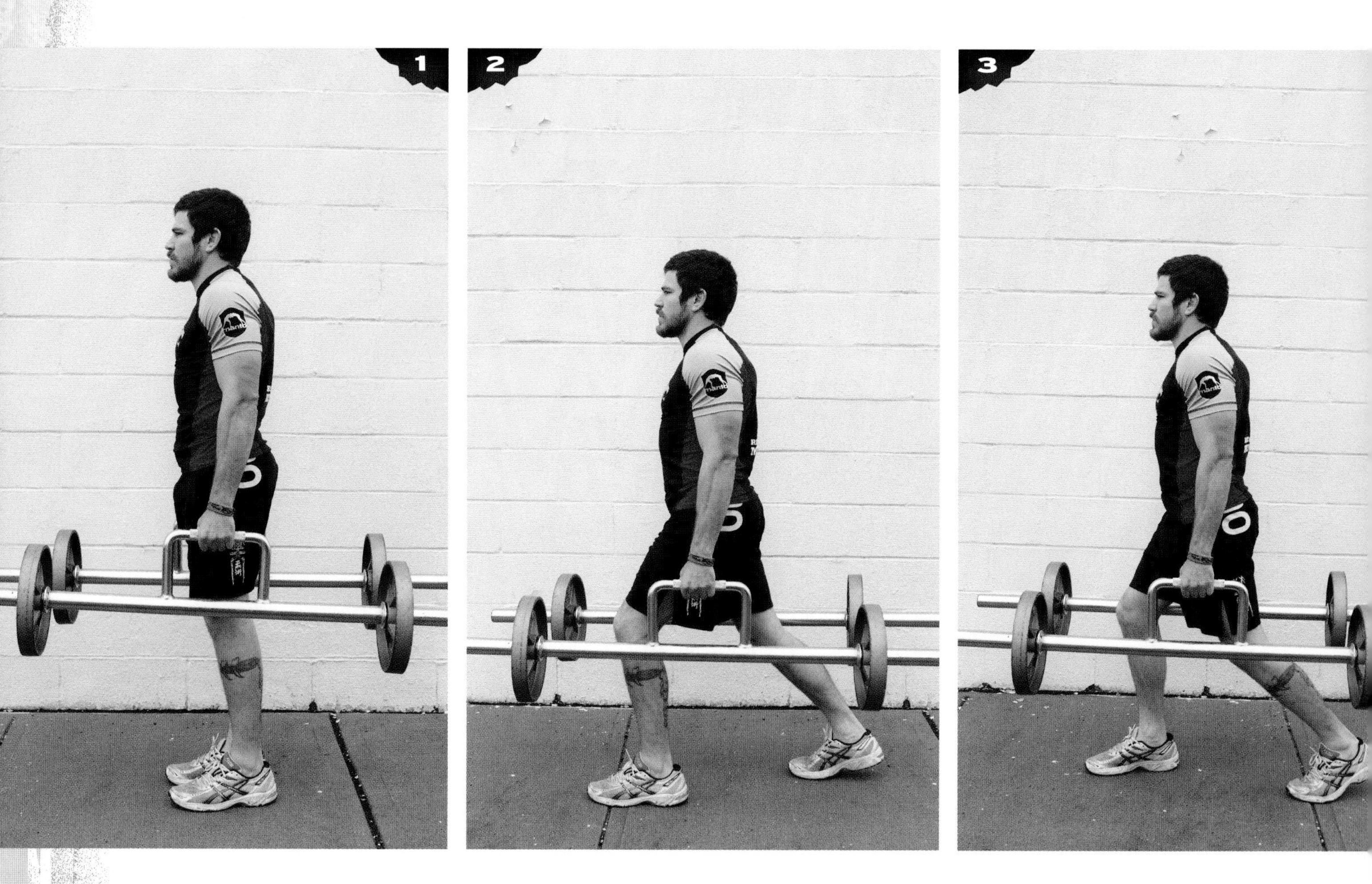

2. SANDBAG DRAG

Begin facing the sandbag while gripping the bag with both hands. Drag the bag backward for 20 yards, using a toe-heel foot contact. Repeat for the distance as many times as possible in the time allotted.

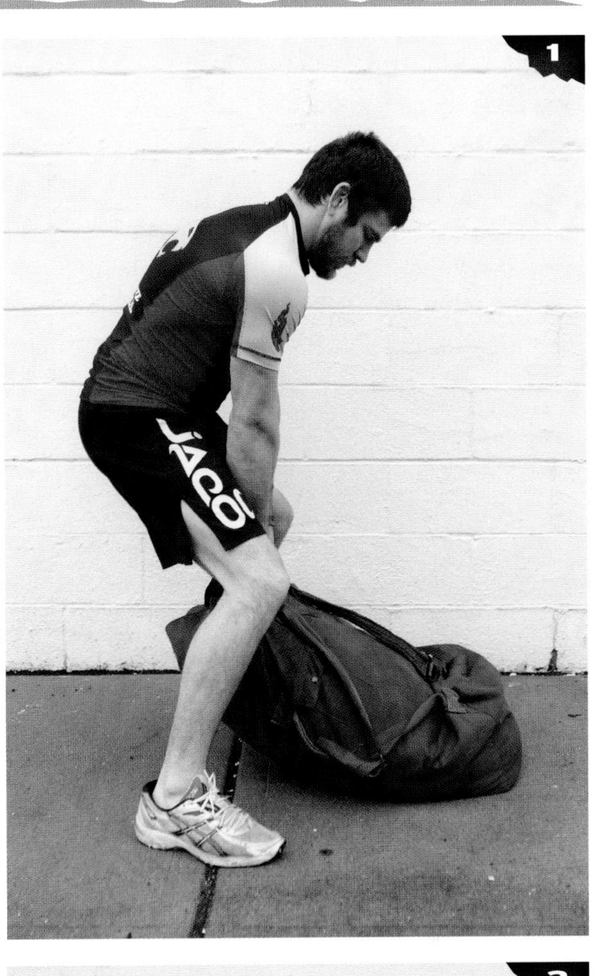

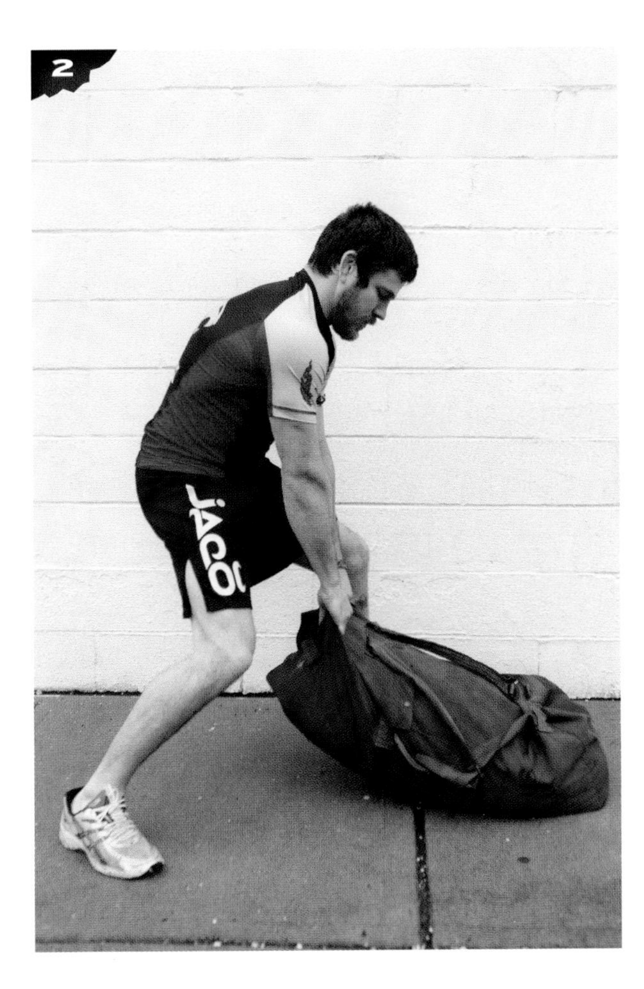

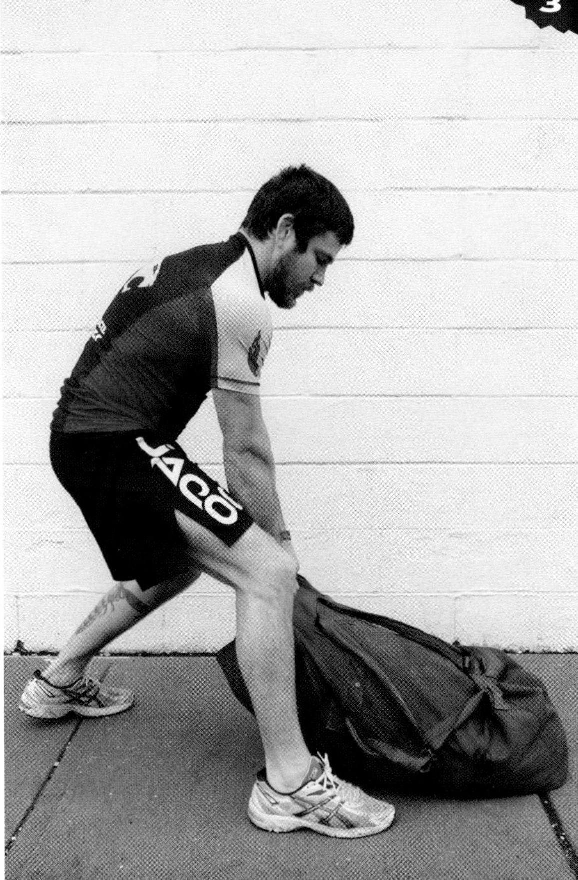

3. ARM-OVER-ARM ROPE PULL

Begin standing with the single rope in both hands. Pull the rope to the hip with the far hand and then grab farther down the rope with the opposite hand. Repeat for as many grips as possible in the allotted time.

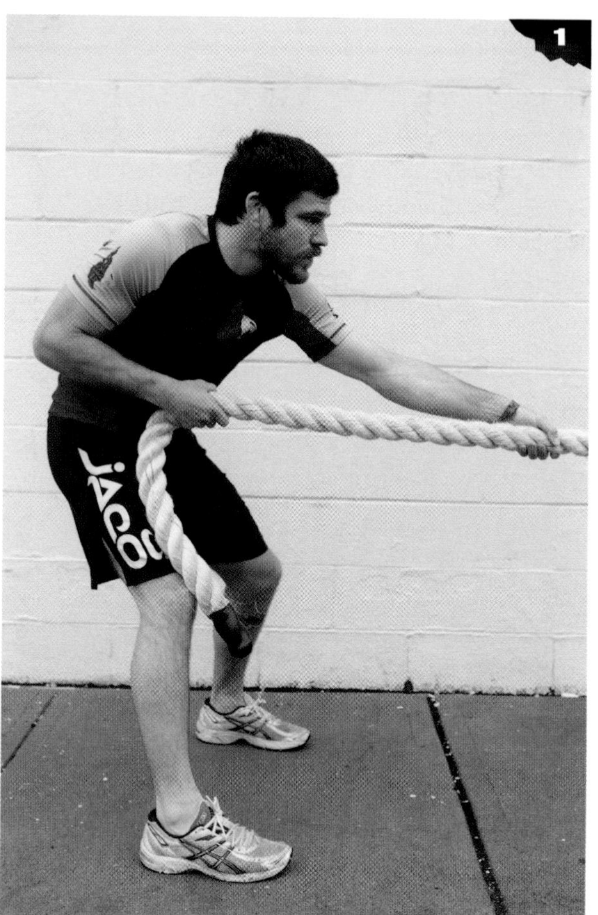

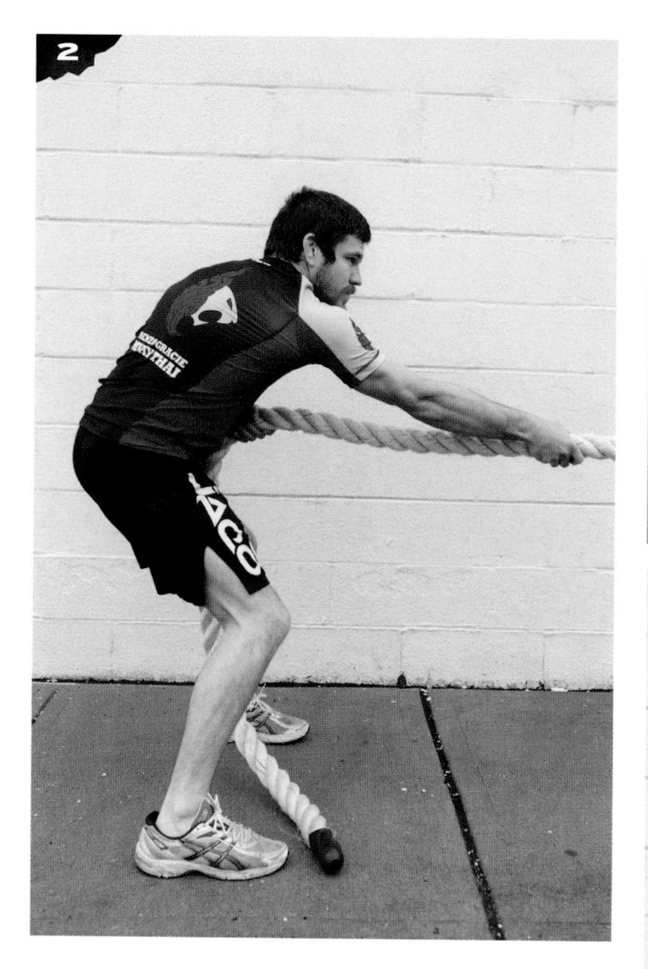

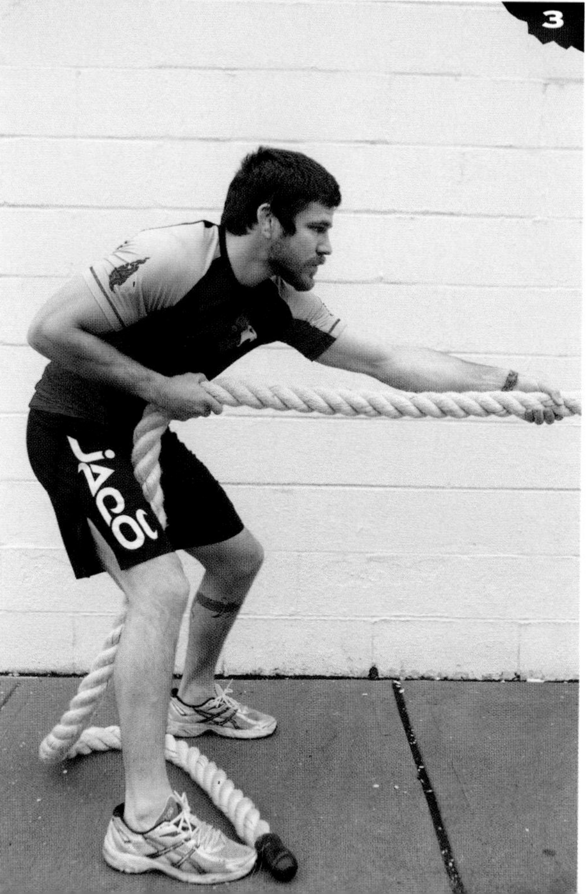

4. PROWLER PUSH

Begin using the high grip on the Prowler. Taking as big steps as possible, push the sled 20 yards. Run around to the other side of the sled and push it back using the low grip. Repeat for as much distance as possible in the allotted time.

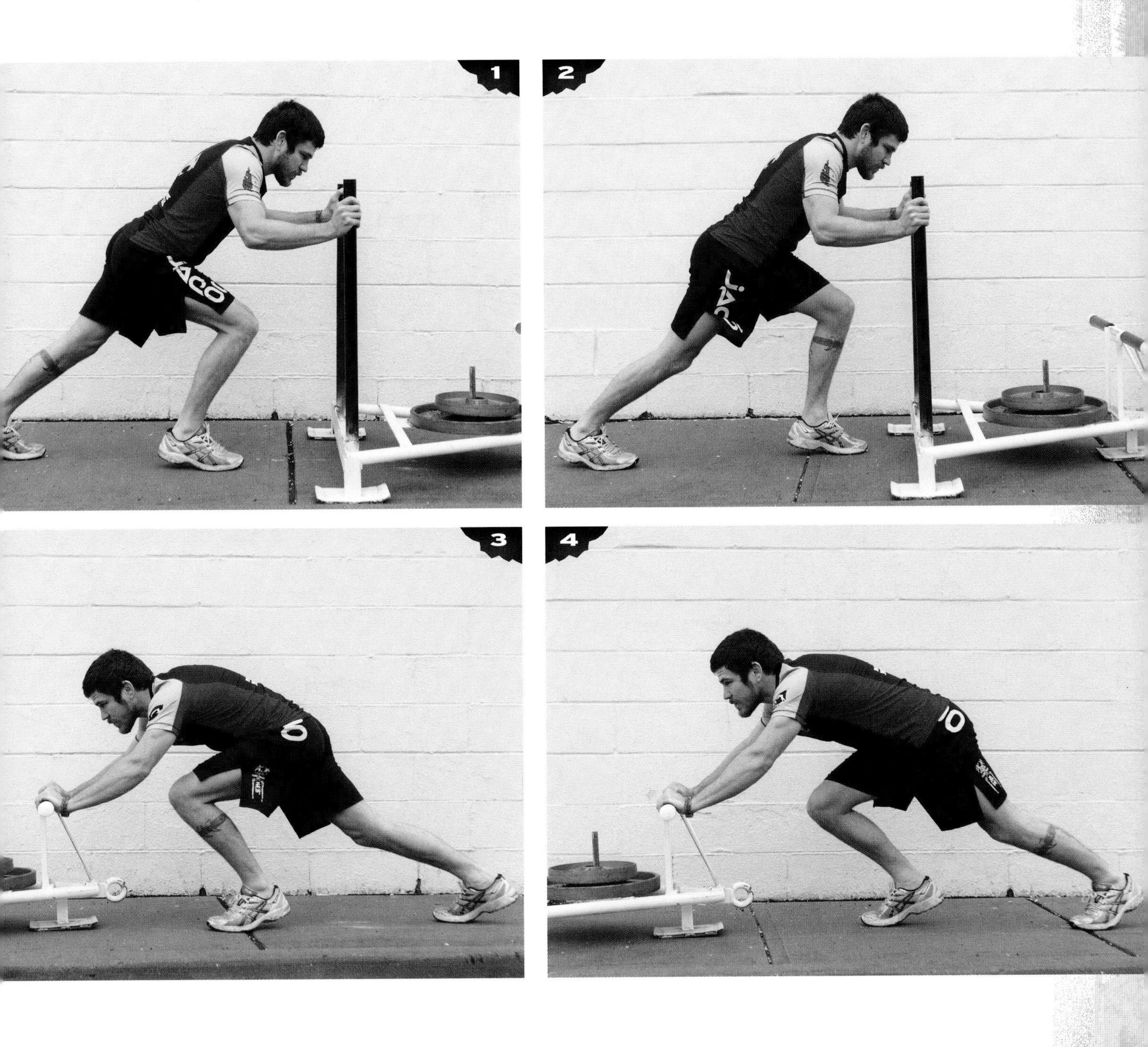

5. TIRE FLIP

Begin facing the tire. Bend down and grab both hands under the bottom rim. Using the legs, lift the tire onto one side while keeping the elbows extended. Turn the hands over and push the tire down as hard as possible. Run to the opposite side of the tire and flip it back to the other side. Repeat for as many reps as possible in the allotted time.

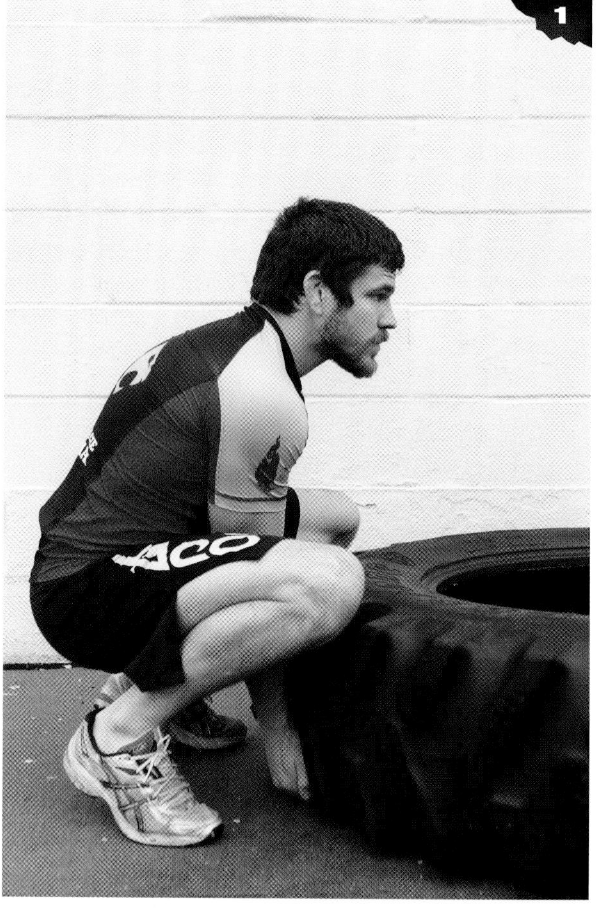

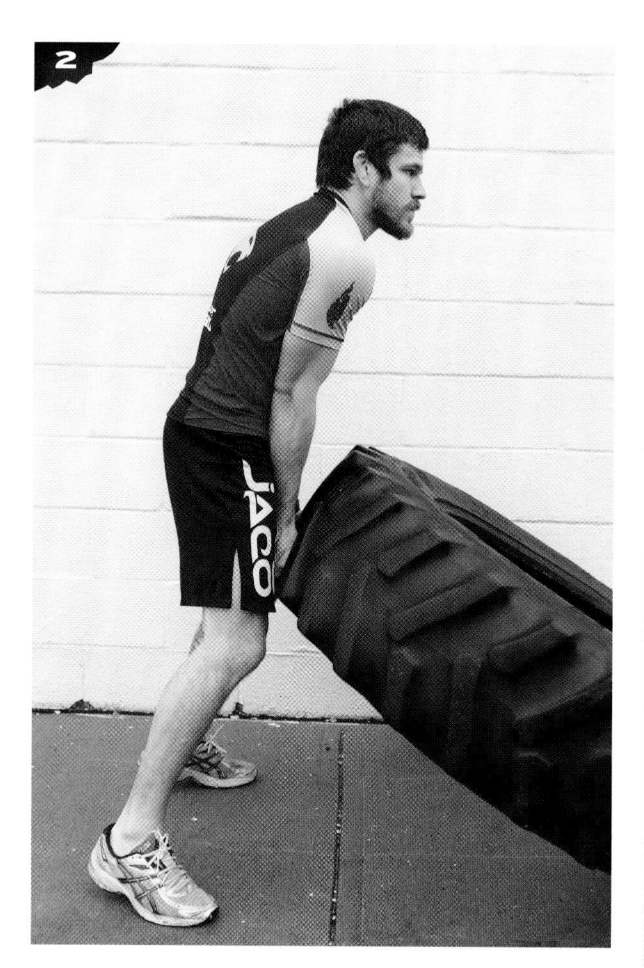

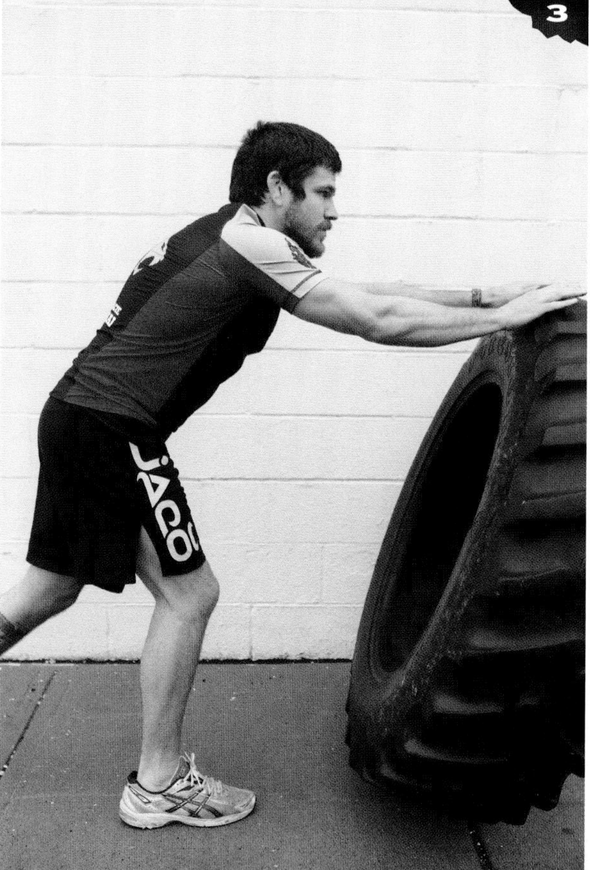

B. POWER CIRCUIT

1. ROPE

Begin standing, holding one end of the rope in each hand. Start by performing 10 double arm waves by bringing the arms up and down as violently as possible. Then perform 10 alternating waves by bringing each arm up and down one at a time. Then perform 10 outward circles by bringing each arm up and out to the sides and back down. Once all 30 reps are completed as fast as possible, start back at the beginning and repeat for the allotted time.

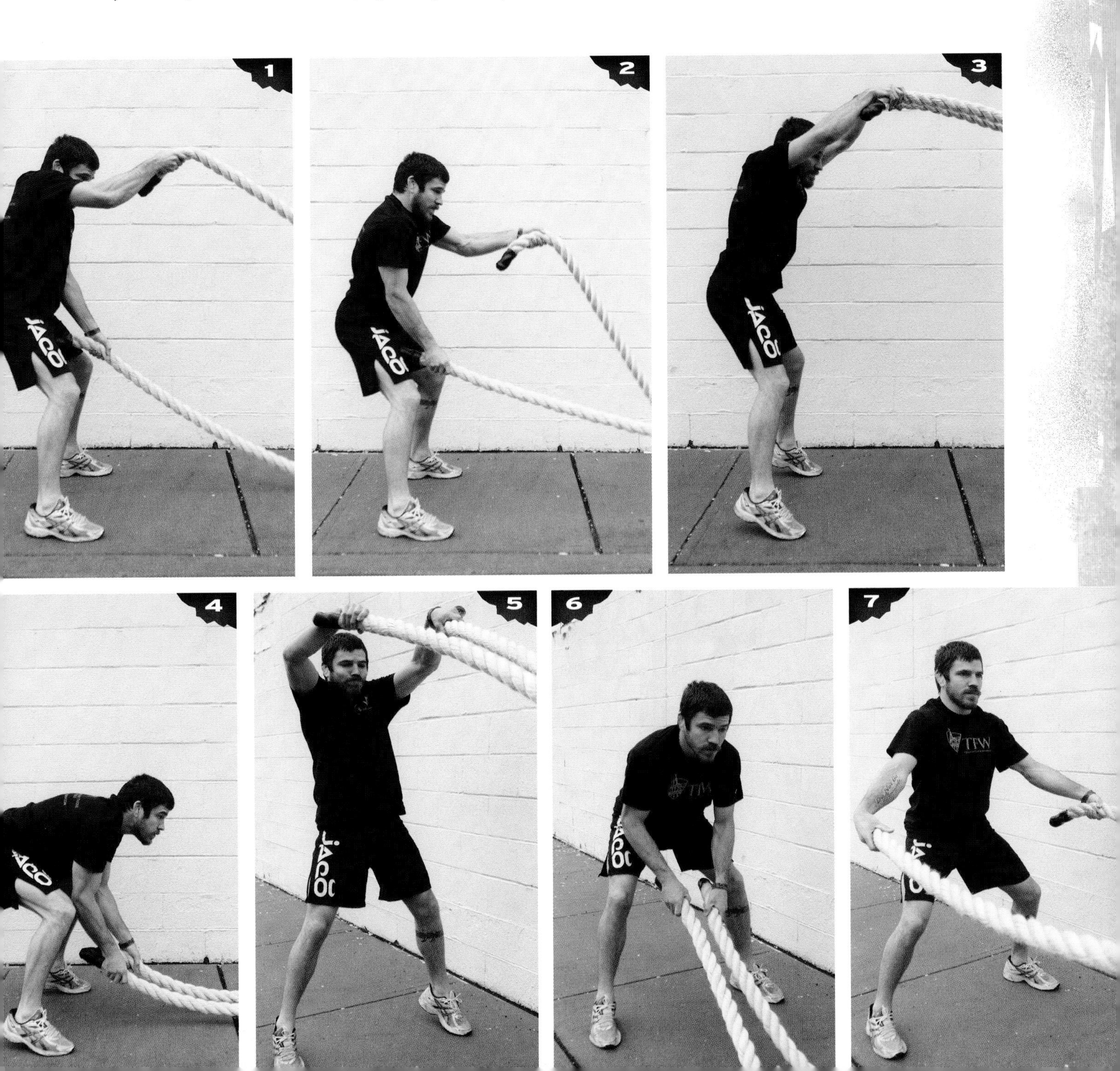

2. KETTLEBELL SWING

Begin standing with the kettlebell in both hands. Swing the bell between the legs while squatting down. Extend at the knees and hips and swing the bell forward to shoulder height. Repeat for 10 reps. Then perform 10 more reps using each arm single-handed. Once the 30 reps are completed, start back at the beginning for the allotted time.

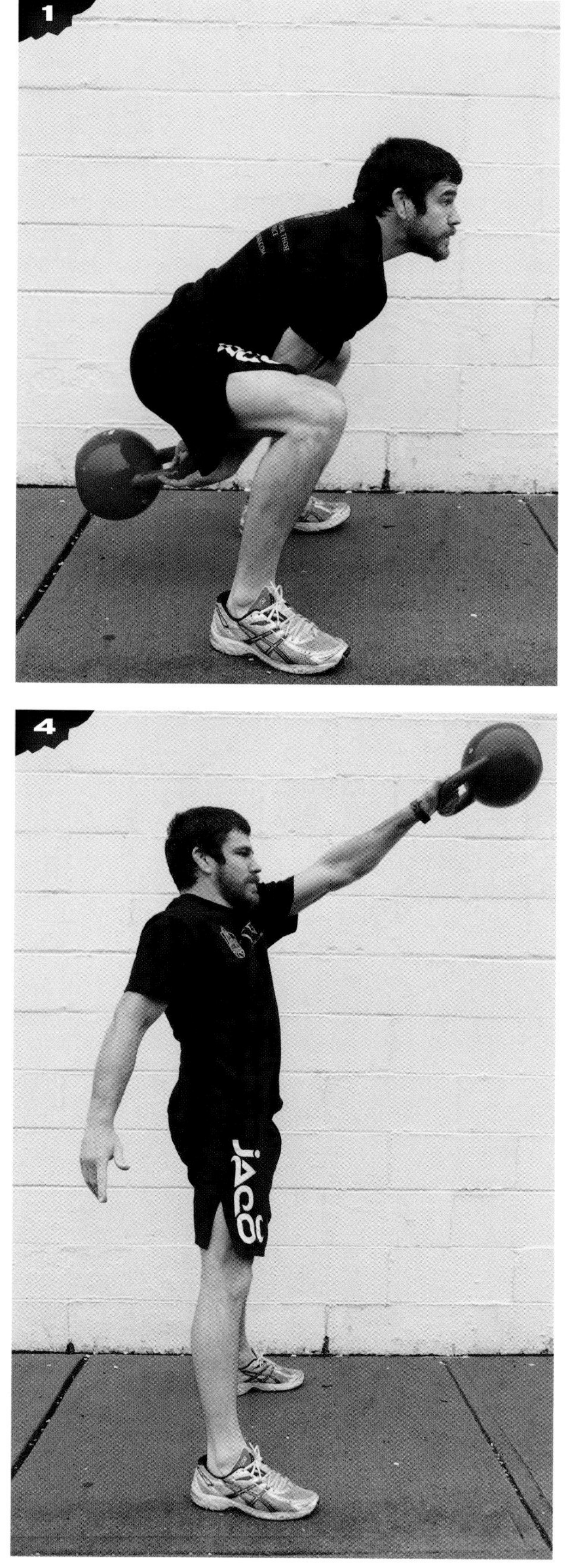

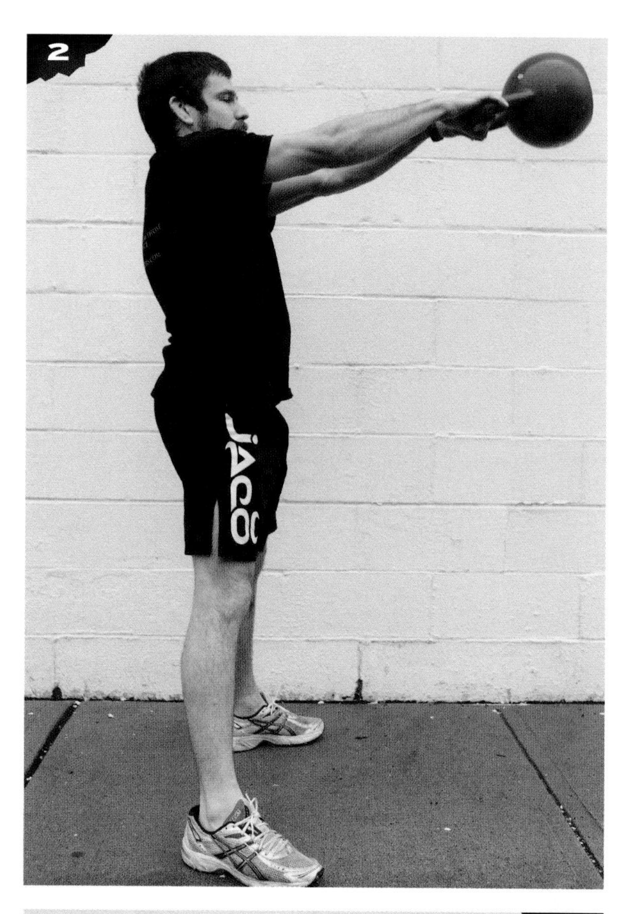

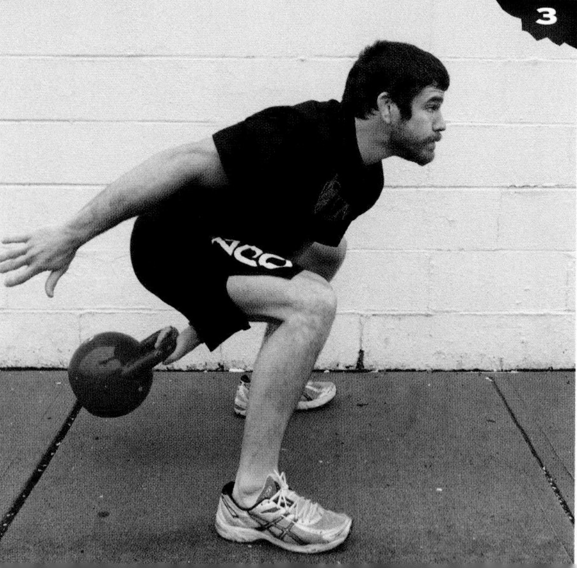

3. MED BALL SLAMS

Begin holding the medicine ball in both hands overhead. Fire the ball into the ground as hard as possible. Recover the ball and repeat for as many reps as possible in the allotted time.

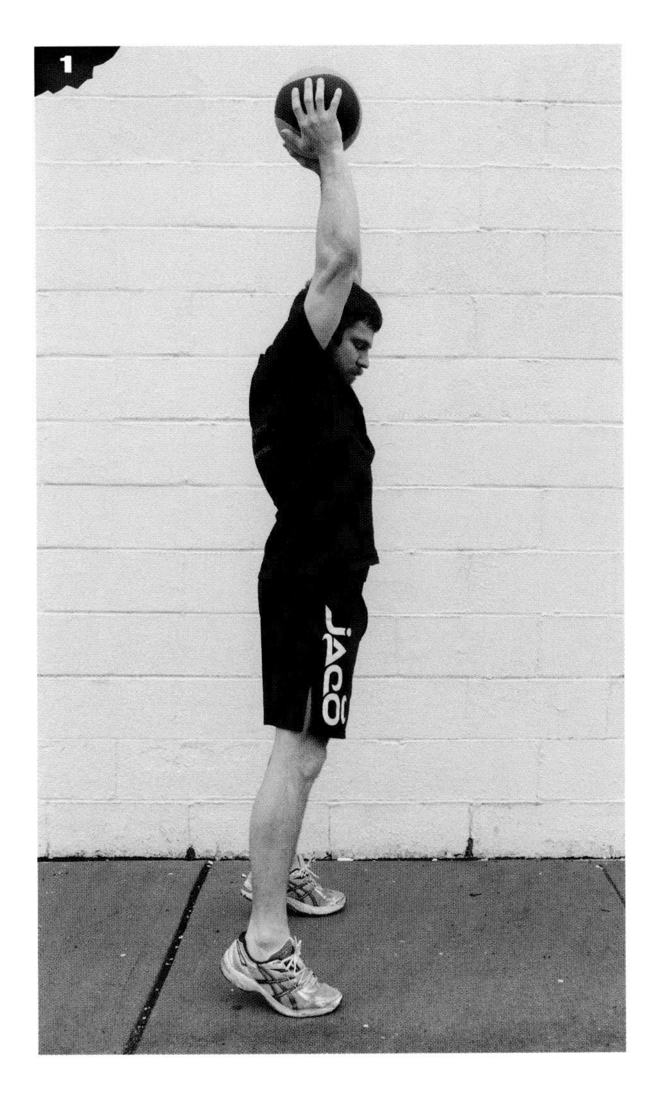

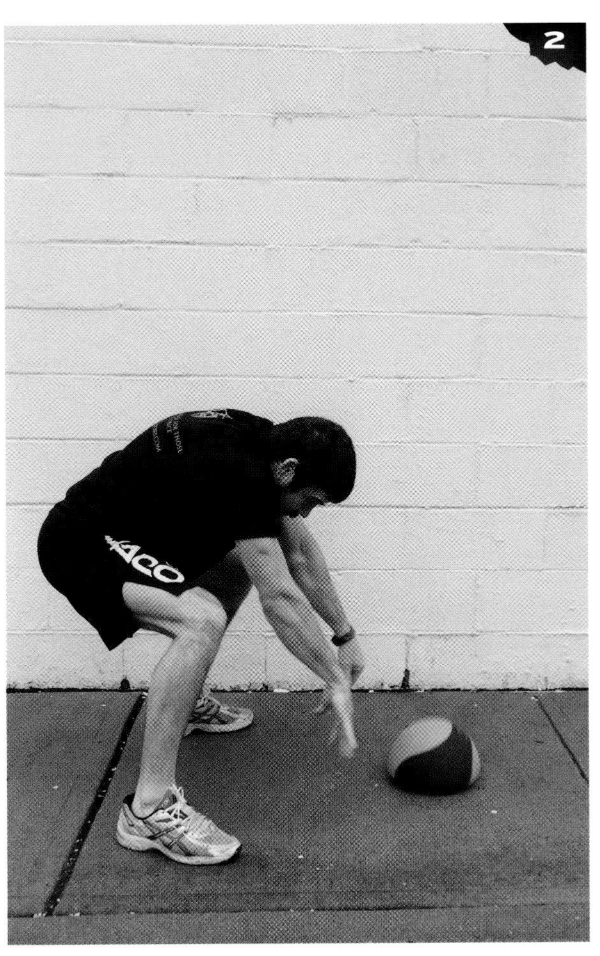

4. SLEDGEHAMMER SWINGS

Begin facing the tire with both feet forward, holding the hammer. Bring the hammer back and over one side of the body and hit the tire as hard as possible. Return the hammer over the other side of the body and repeat for as many reps as possible in the allotted time.

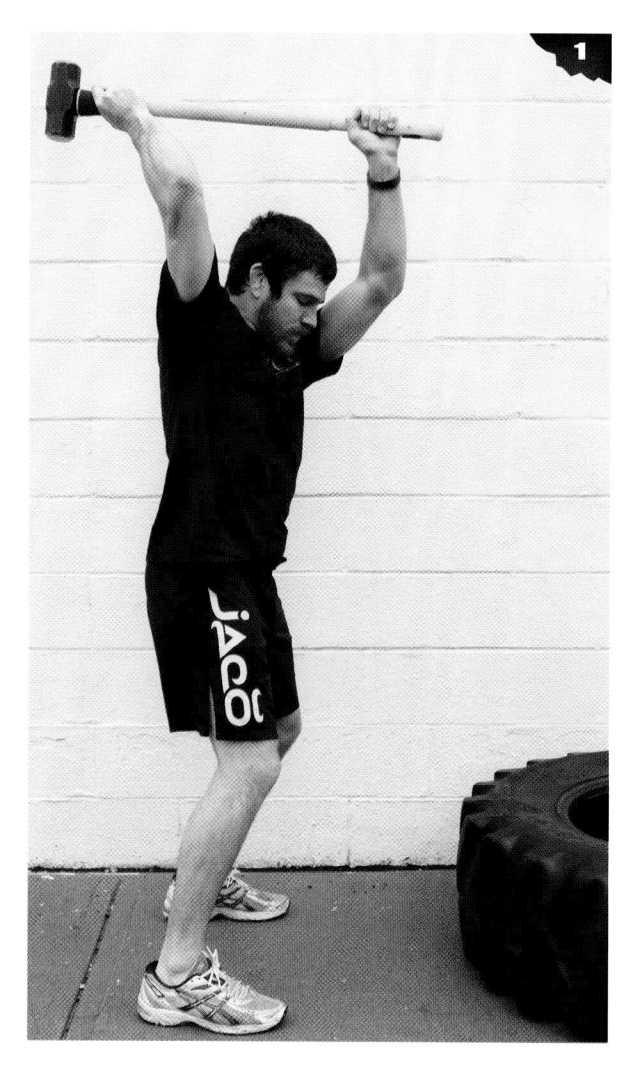

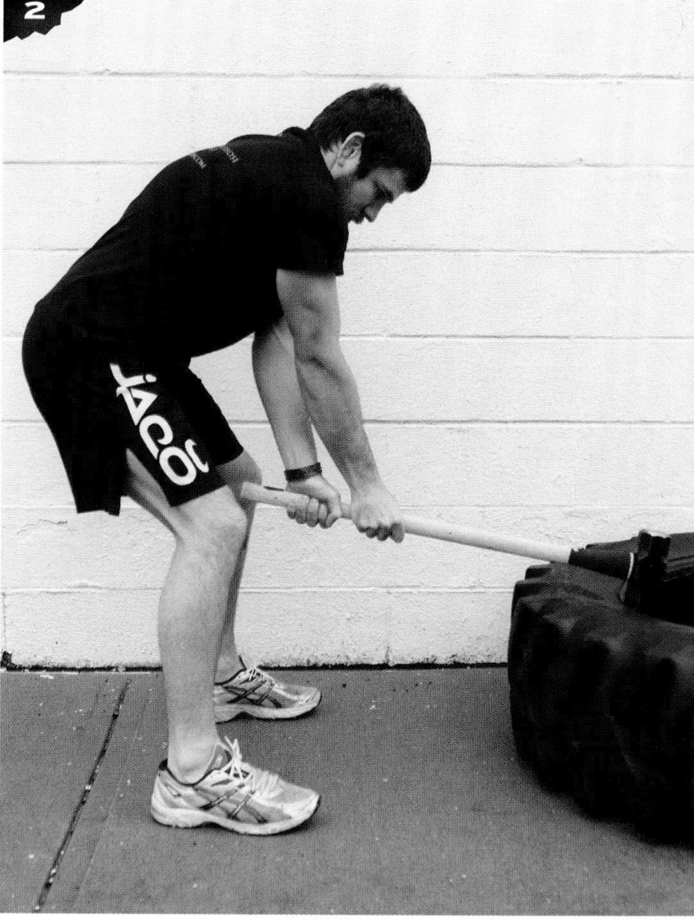

5. LADDER

Begin standing with both feet inside the ladder. Jump the feet outside and forward one box. Jump the feet back into the box and repeat for the length of the ladder and back. Once completed, begin running with high knees, using one foot in each box, down and back the length of the ladder. Once this second set is finished, perform side steps through the ladder using two feet in each box down and back up the ladder. Once the third set is completed, start at the beginning and complete as many reps as possible in the allotted time.

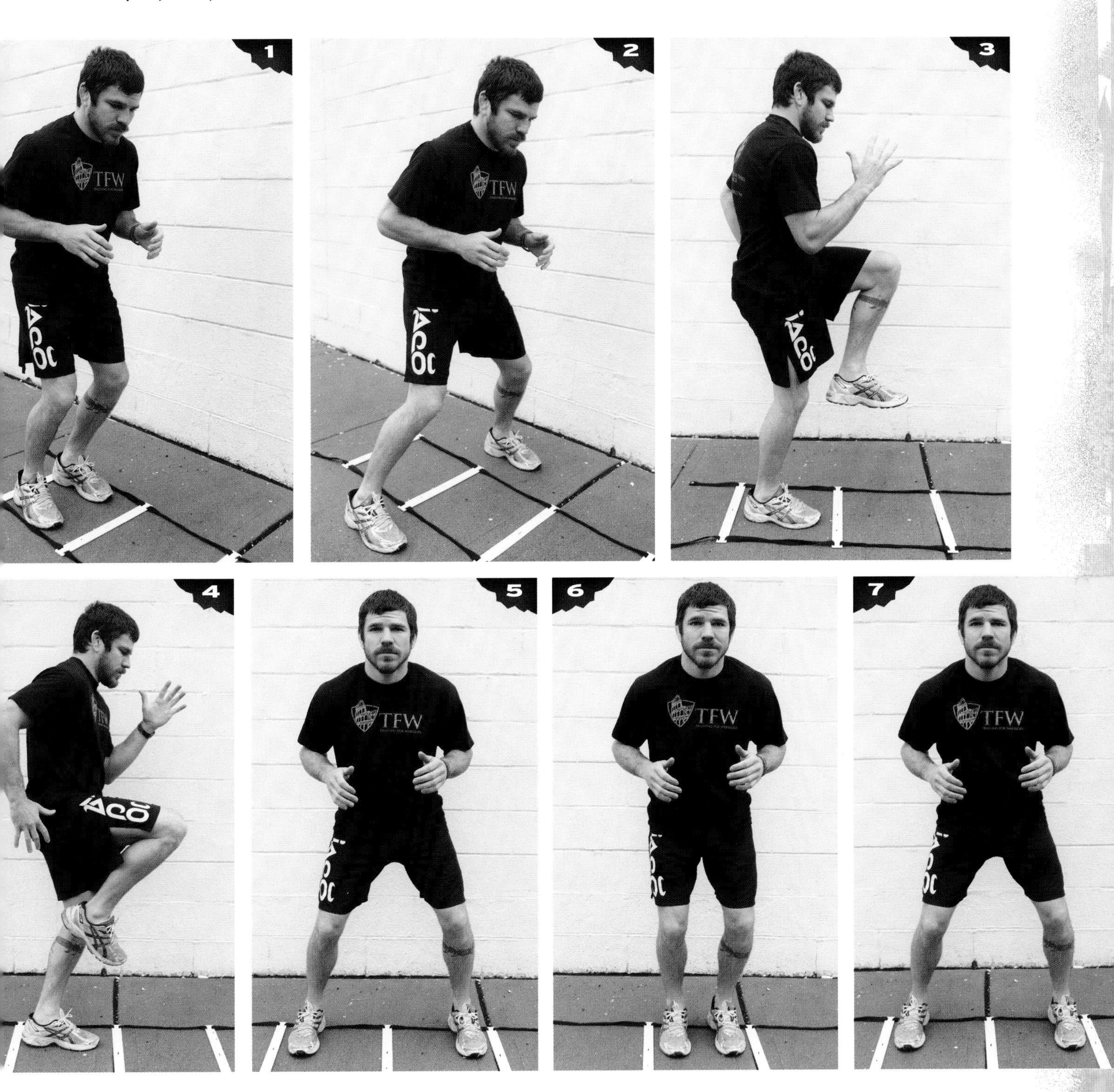

C. FIGHTER CIRCUIT

1. HEAVY BAG PUNCHES

Begin facing the heavy bag at an arm's length away. Perform as many alternating punches with each hand against the bag as possible for the required time. Keep the hands high and at the chin when not punching.

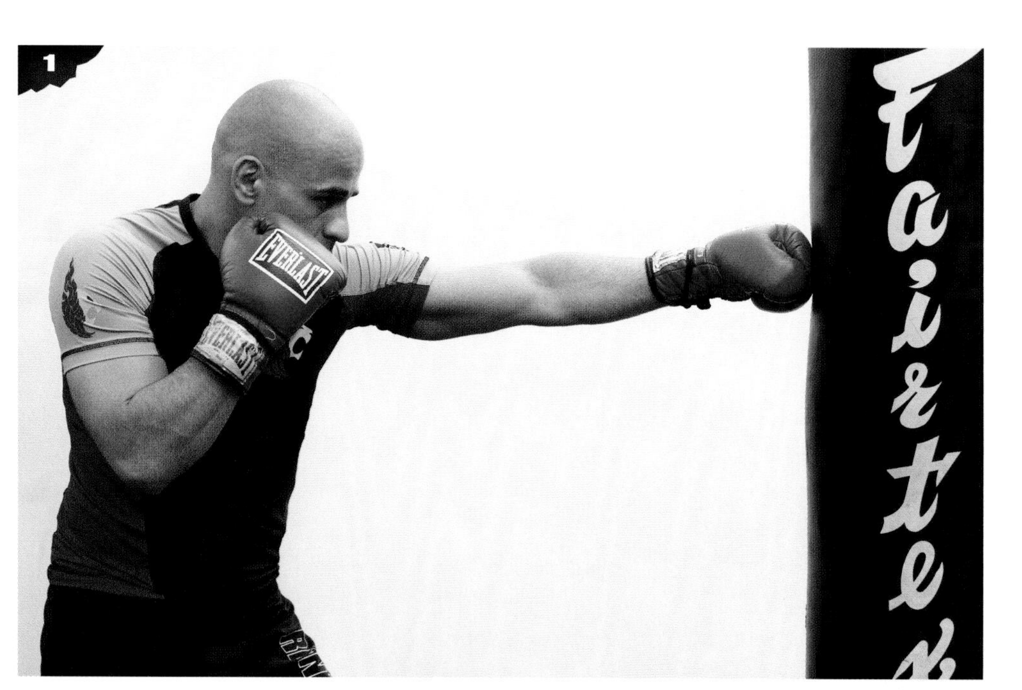

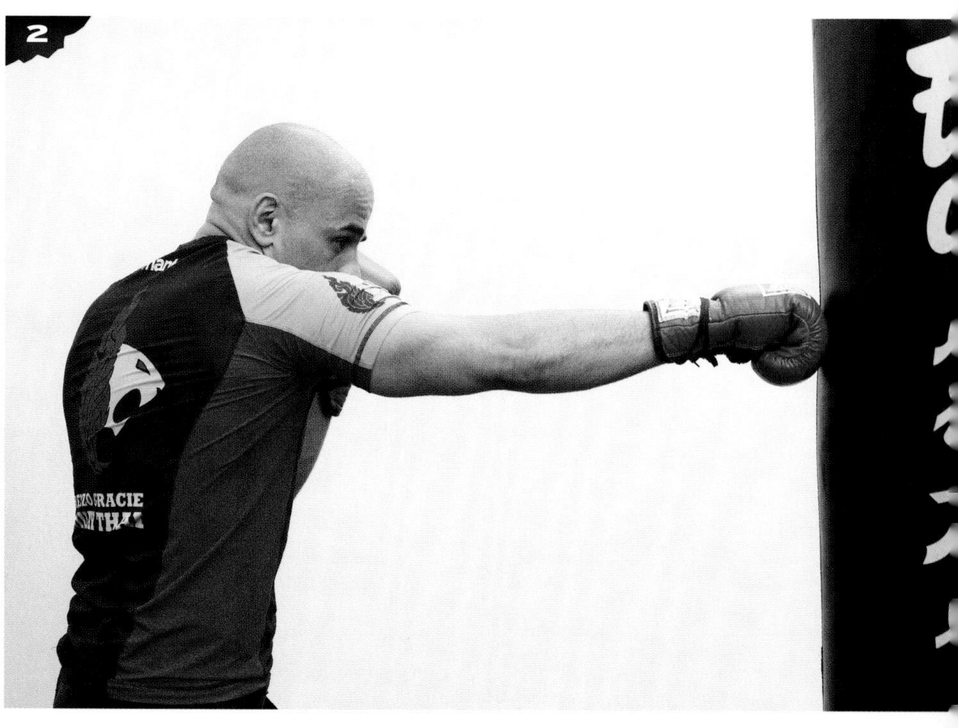

2. SPRAWLS

Begin standing in a good wrestling position with the hands out front and elbows at the sides. Drop to the ground while kicking the feet backward and landing on the hips, hands, and forearms. After the hip contacts the ground, jump back up to the original position.

1

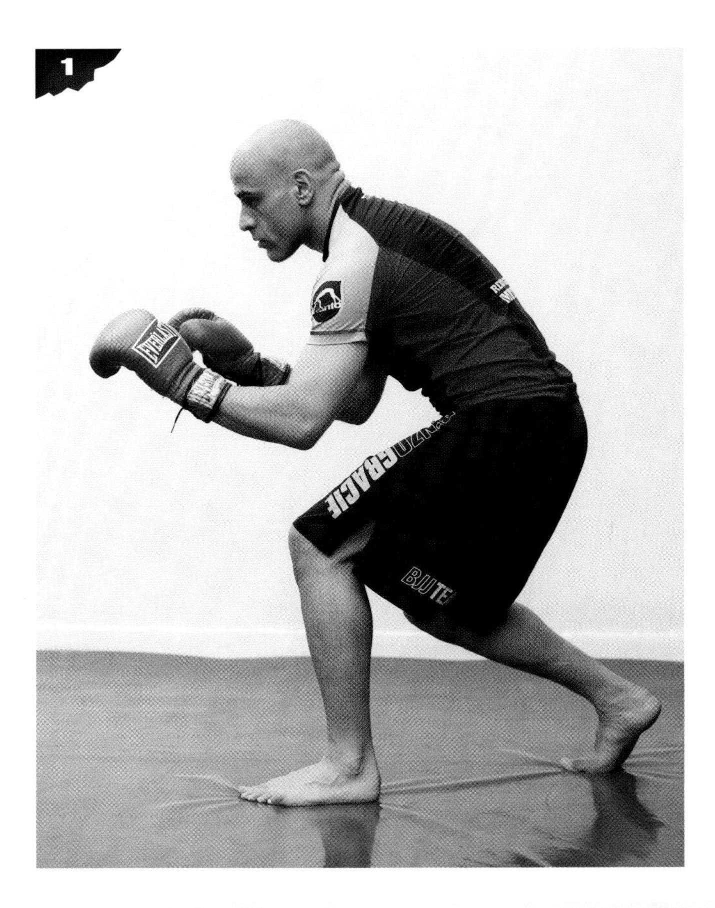

2

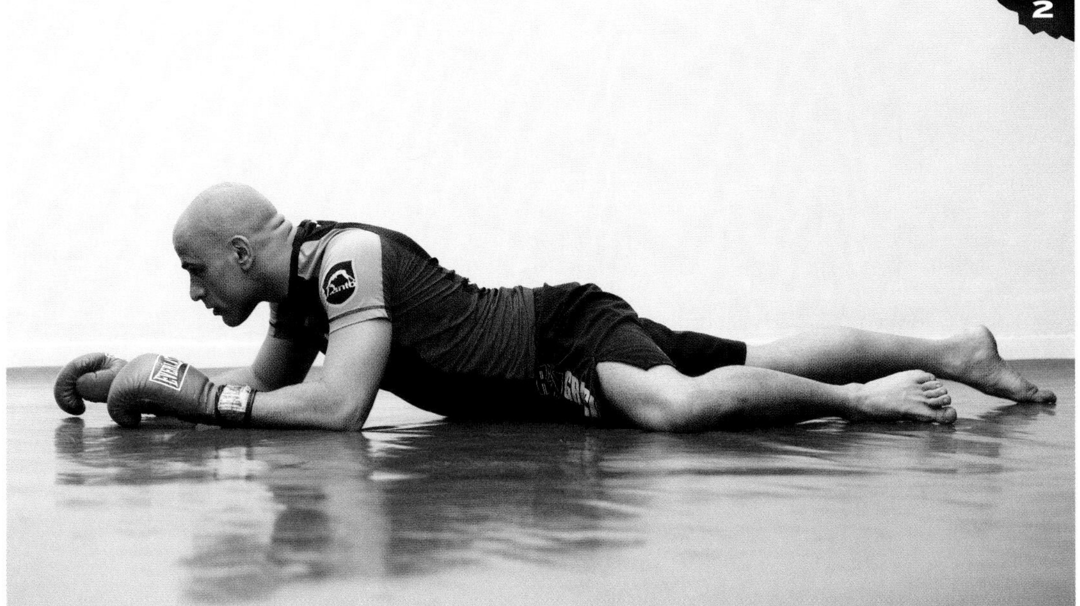

3. HEAVY BAG KNEES

Begin facing the heavy bag at a thigh's length away. Perform as many alternating knee strikes against the bag as possible for the required time. Keep the hands high as shown.

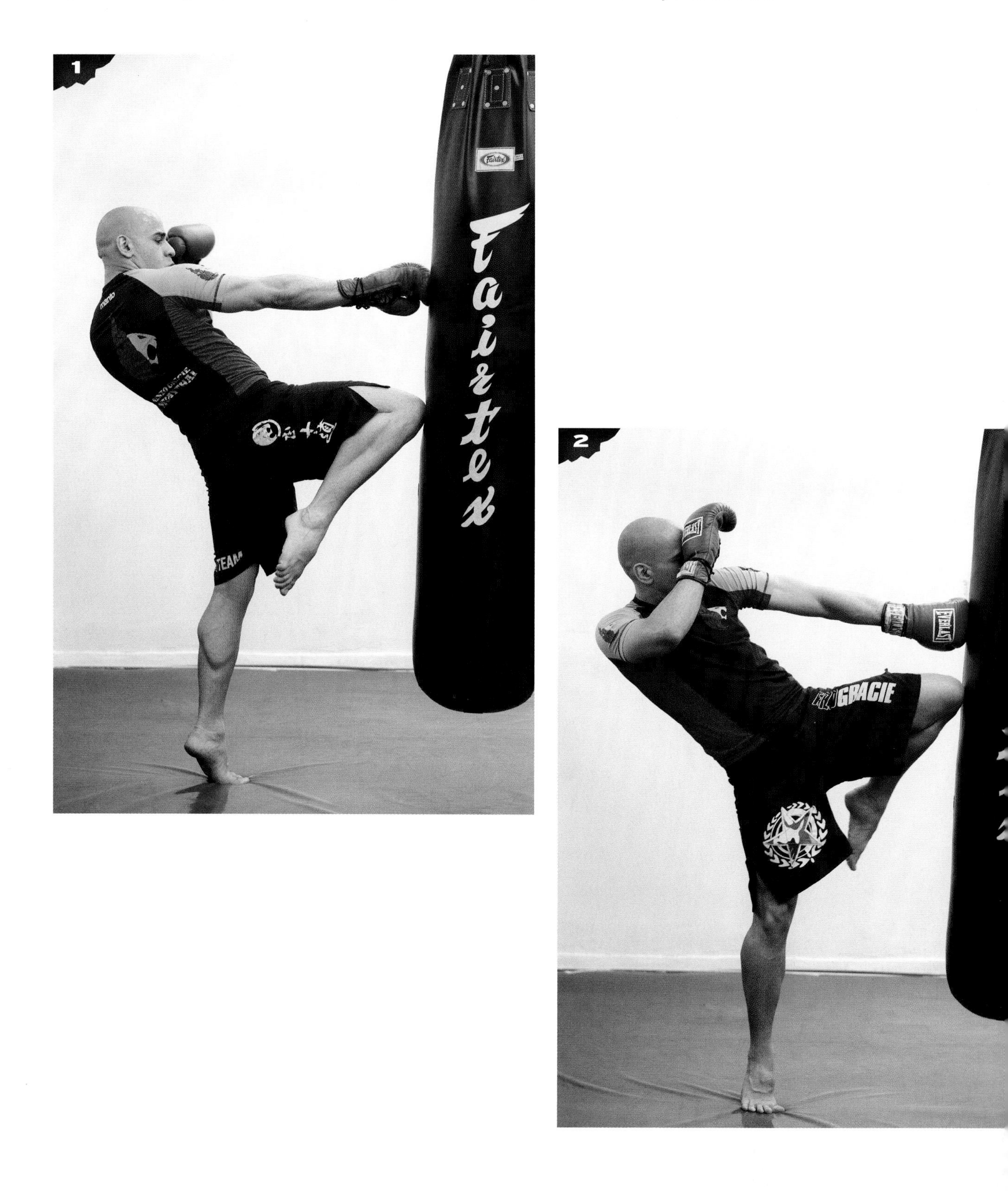

4. KNEE-ON-CHEST BAG DRILL

Begin with the heavy bag on the floor. One knee starts on the bag with the other leg out to the side. Support yourself with the arm on the same side as the supporting knee. Punch the bag with the opposite hand and then jump over the bag, switching the supporting knee and arm. Punch again and repeat as many times as possible for the required time.

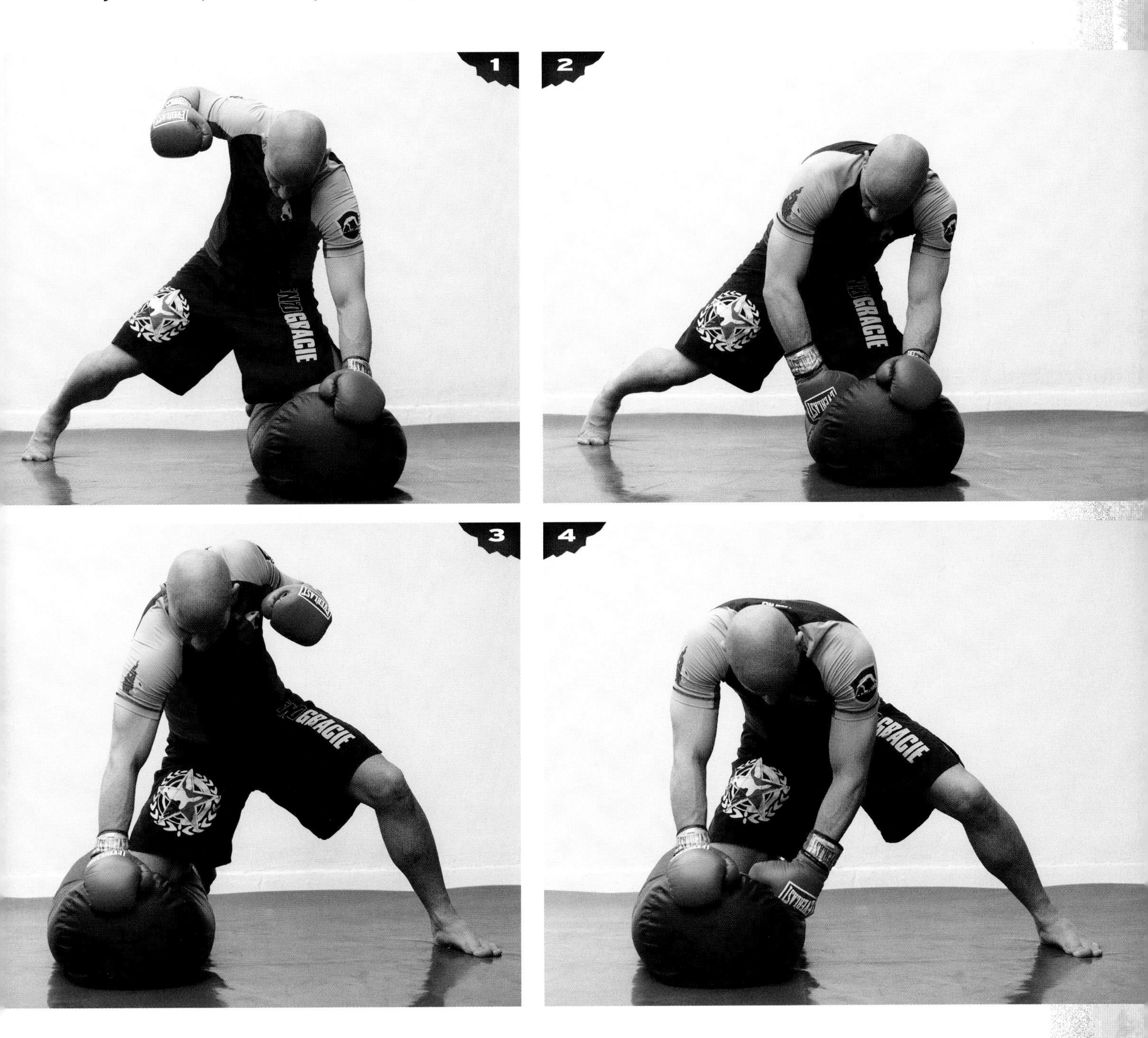

5. HEAVY BAG KICKS

Begin facing the bag in a fighting stance with both feet on the floor. Perform as many alternating kicks with each leg against the bag as possible for the required time. Keep the hands high as shown.

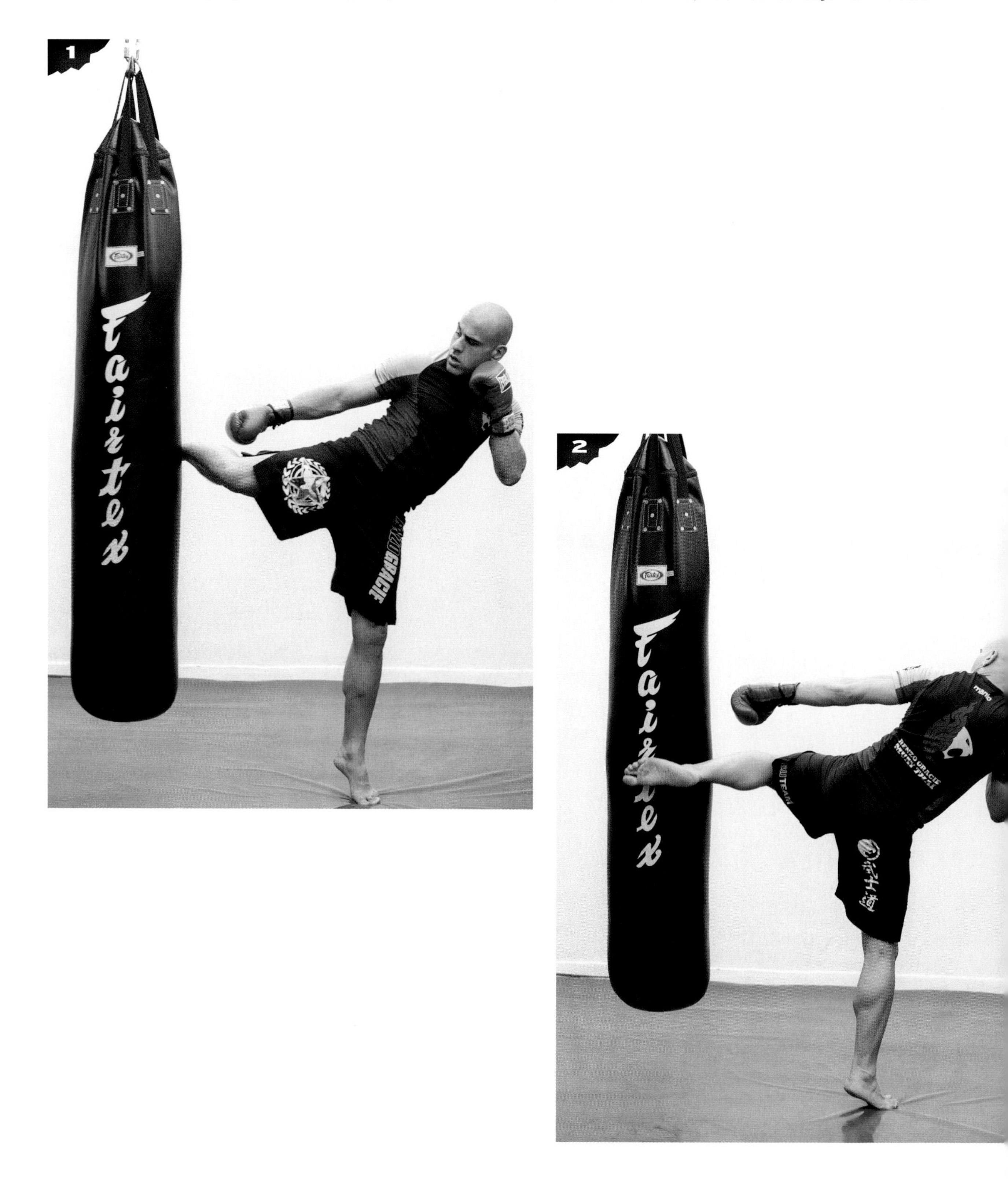

D. TIRE CIRCUIT

1. SLEDGEHAMMER SWINGS

Begin facing the tire with both feet pointed to the outside of the tire while holding the hammer. Bring the hammer back and over one side of the body and hit the tread of the tire as hard as possible. Return the hammer over the other side of the body and repeat as many times as possible in the alotted time.

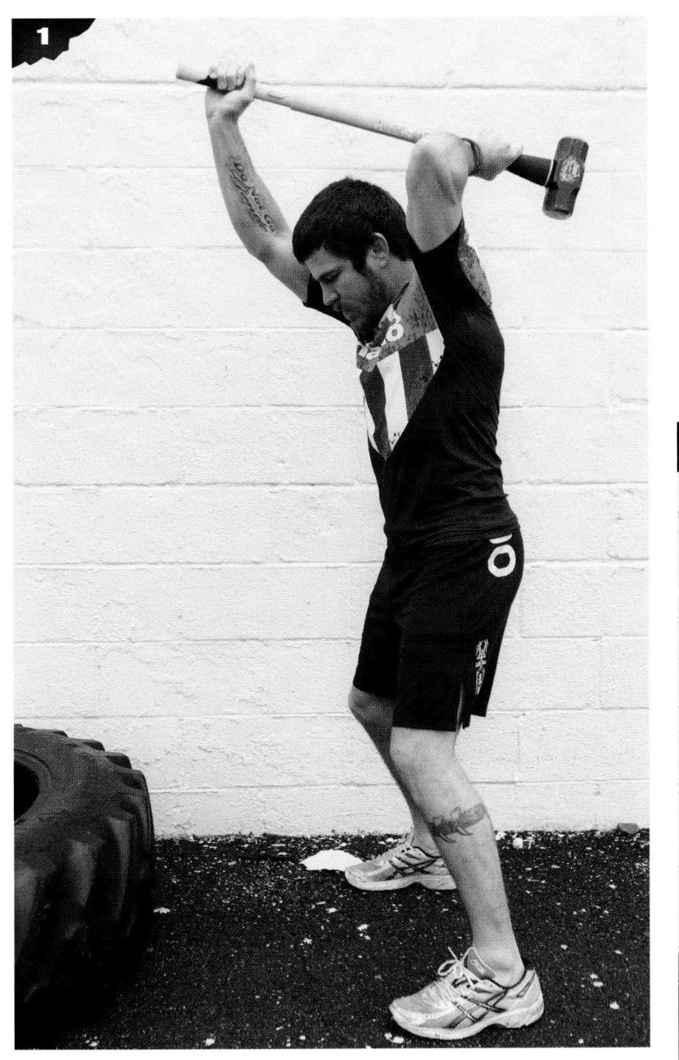

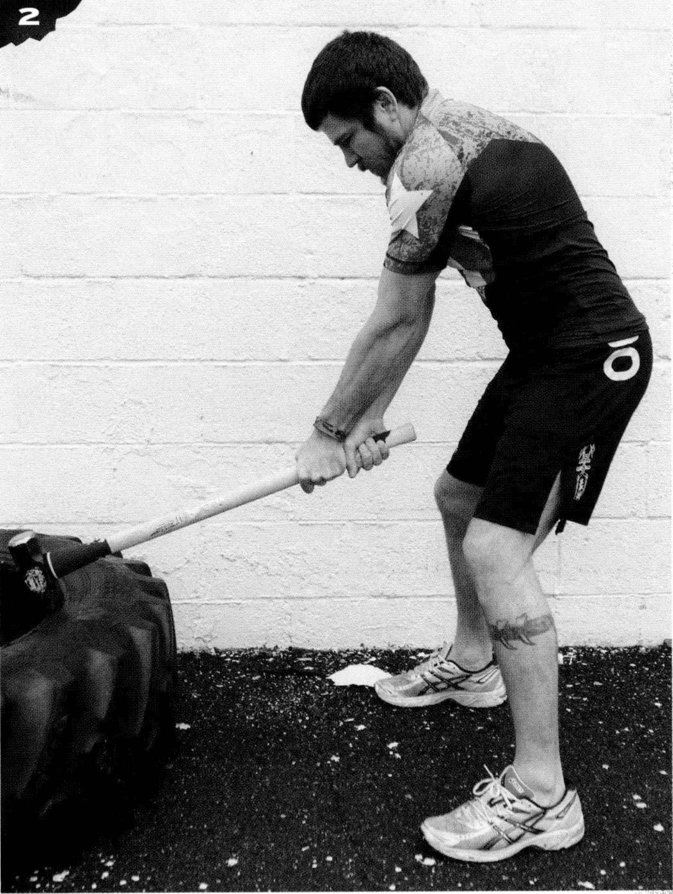

2. TOE TOUCHES

Begin standing with one foot on the tire and the other on the ground. Raise the opposite hand and arm of the foot on the tire. Hop in the air and switch the feet and arms. Repeat as quickly as possible in the allotted time.

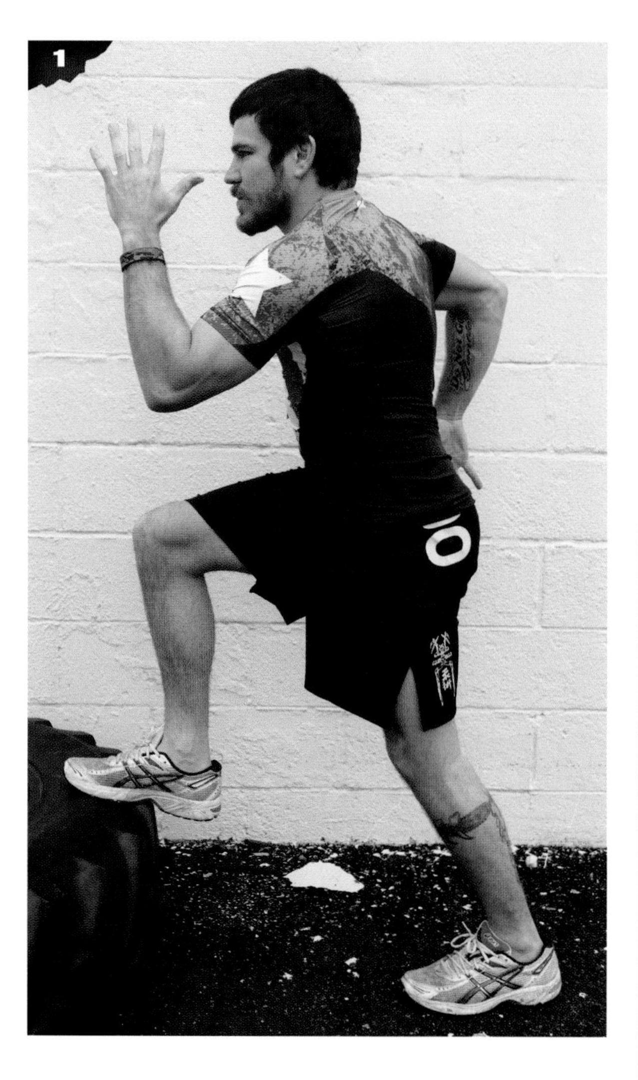

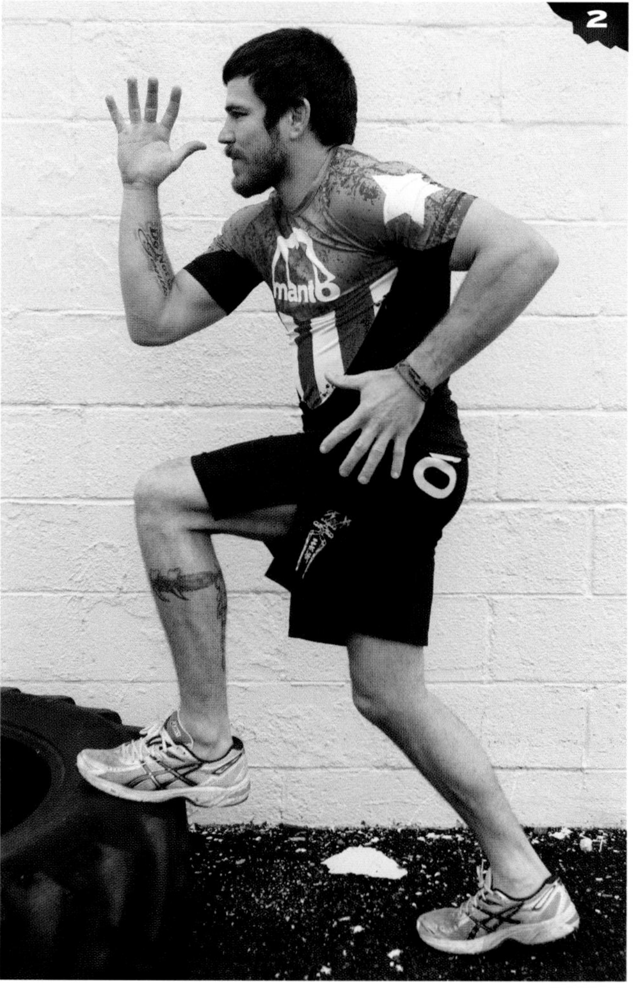

3. PLYO JUMPS

Begin standing outside the tire. Using both the arms and legs, jump up and into the tire. Land softly and then jump forward out of the tire. Turn quickly and repeat for as many jumps as possible in the allotted time.

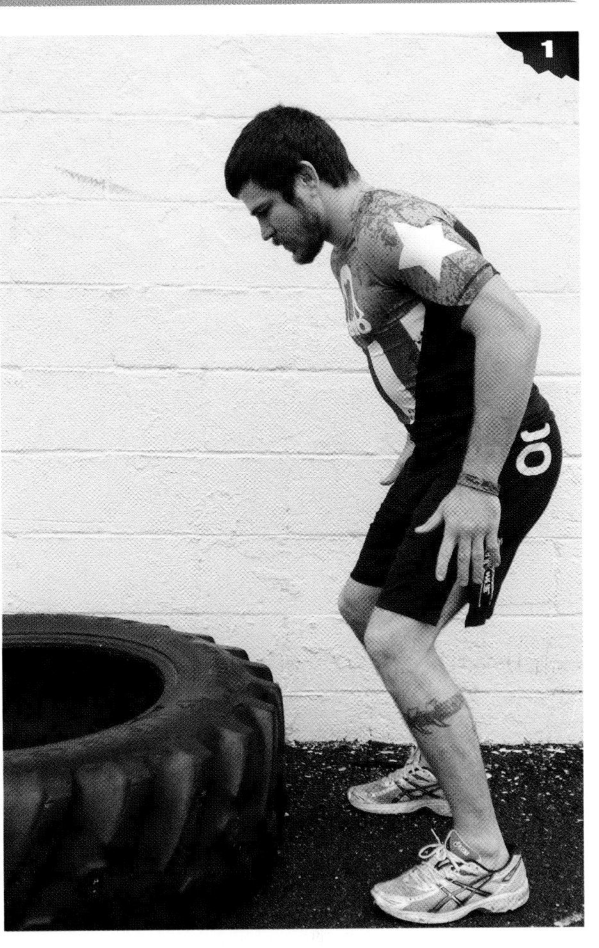

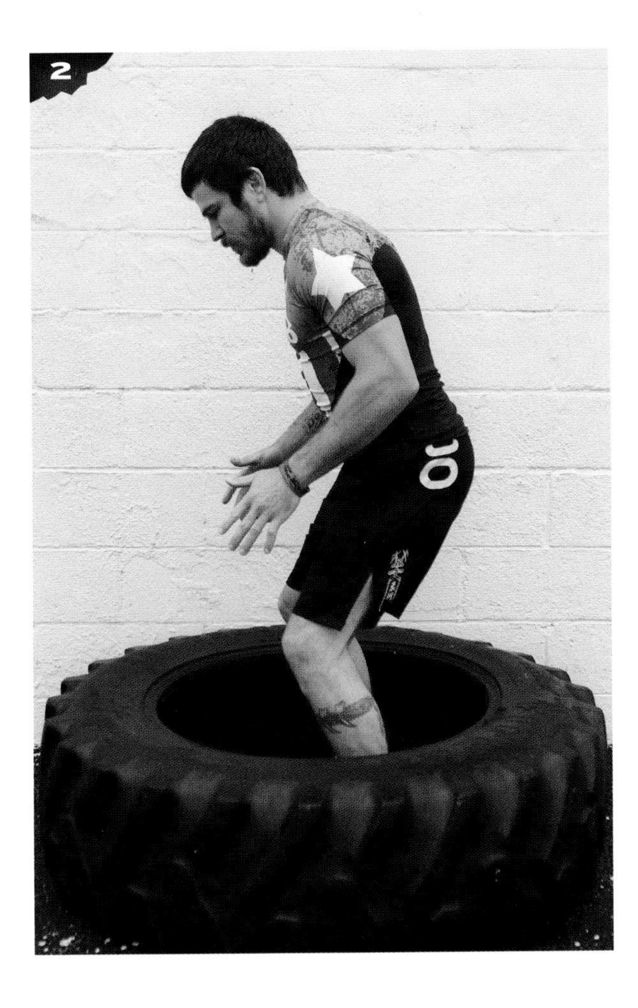

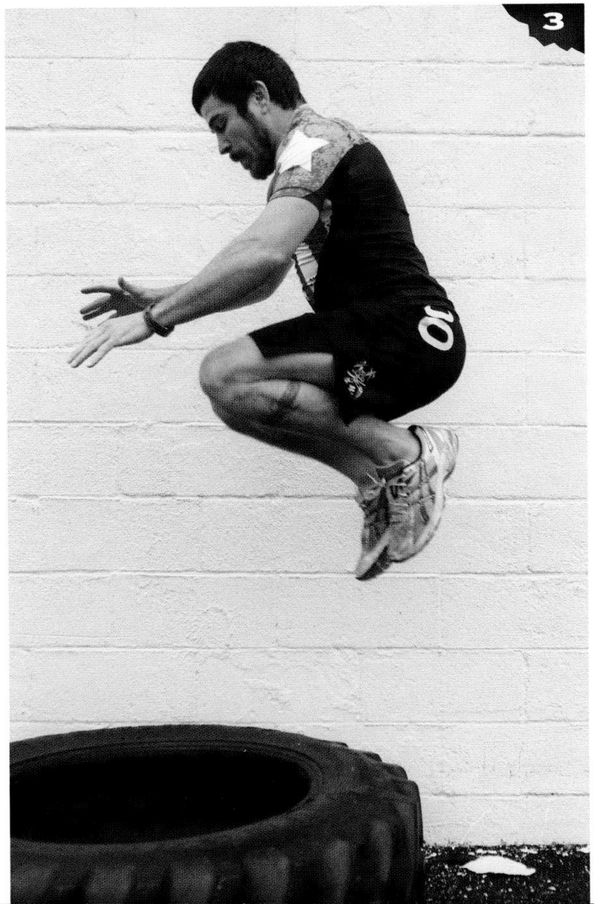

4. DEADLIFTS

Begin standing inside the tire. Bend down and grab the inside rim of the tire with both palms facing outward. Stand up by extending at the knees and lower back. Repeat as many times as possible in the allotted time.

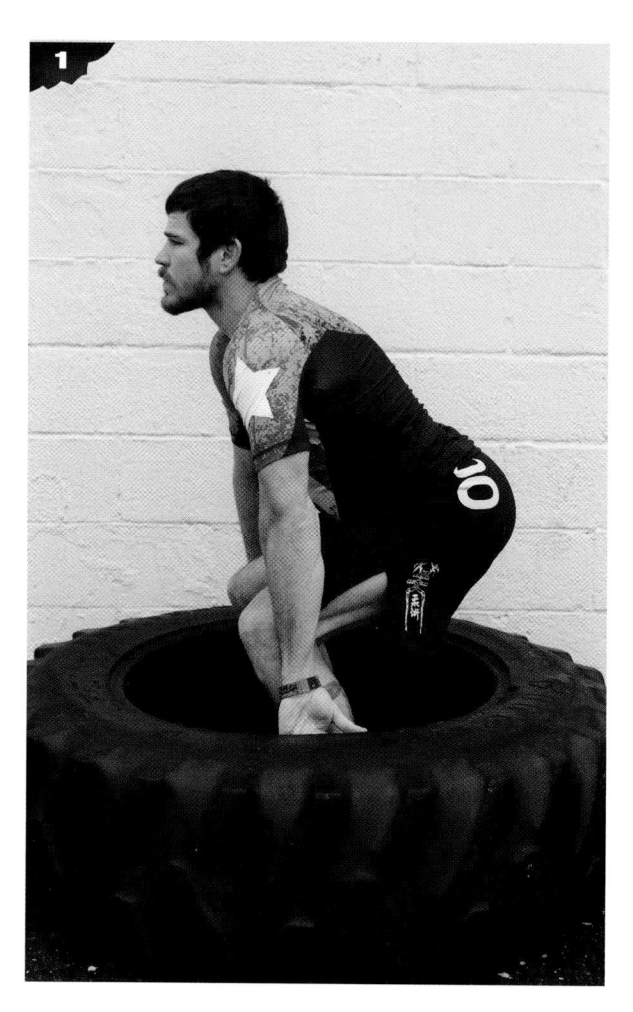

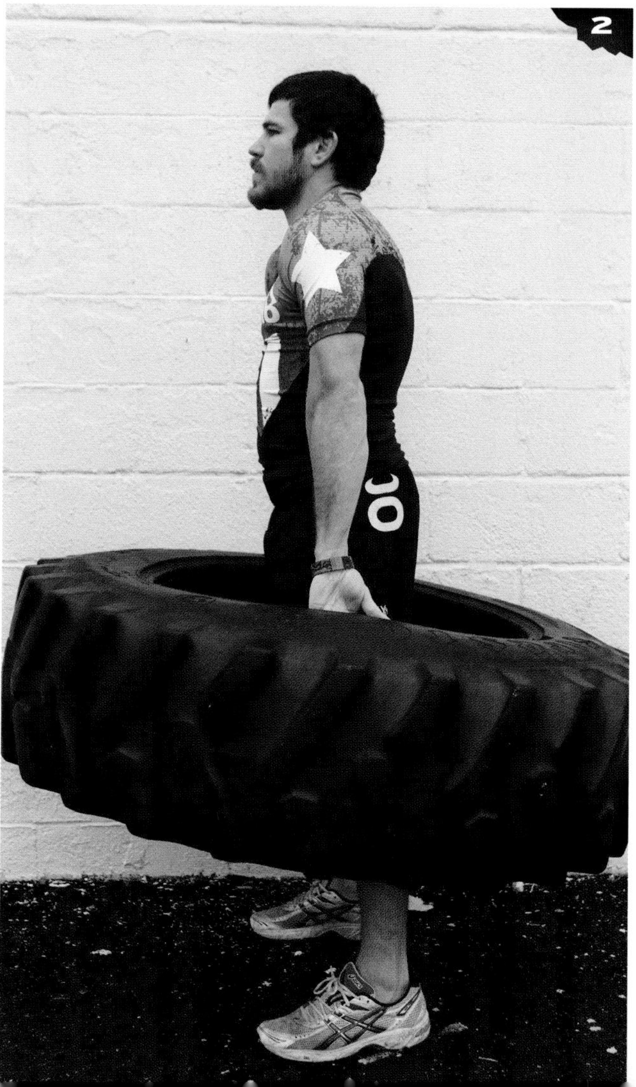

5. TIRE FLIP

Begin facing the tire. Bend down and grab both hands under the bottom rim. Using the legs, lift the tire onto one side while keeping the elbows extended. Turn the hands over and push the tire down as hard as possible.

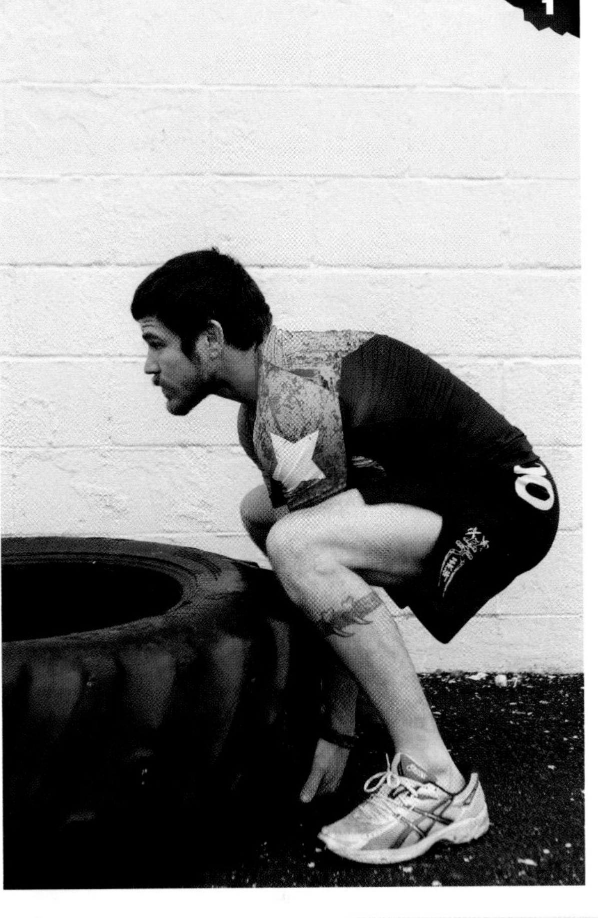

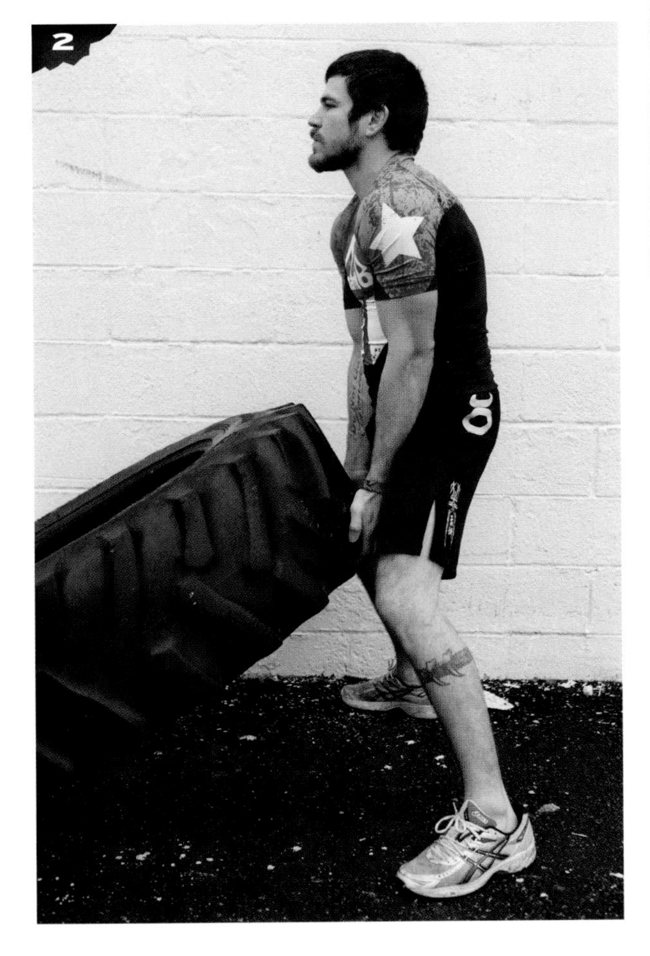

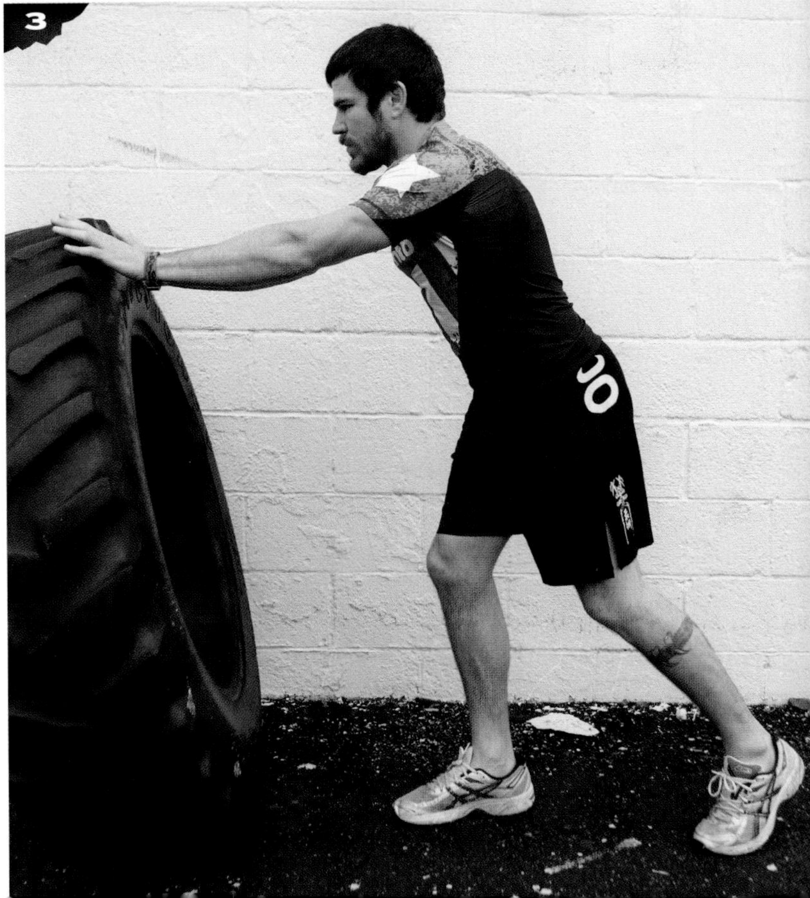

ENERGY CIRCUIT CHEATSHEET

Each exercise is 1 minute long, with 15 seconds for transitions. Allow 2 minutes between rounds.

A. STRONGMAN CIRCUIT

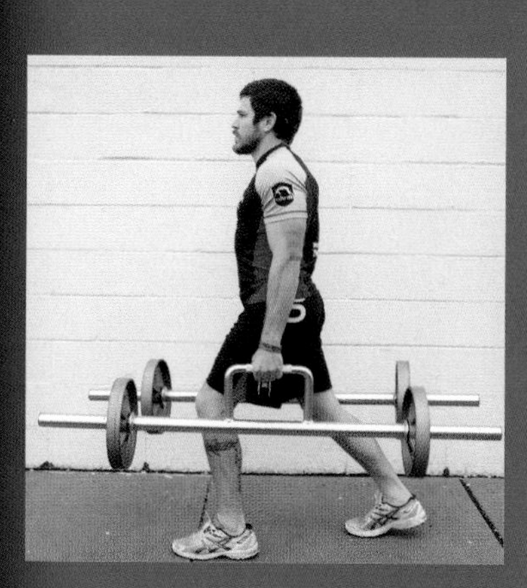

1. FARMER'S WALK

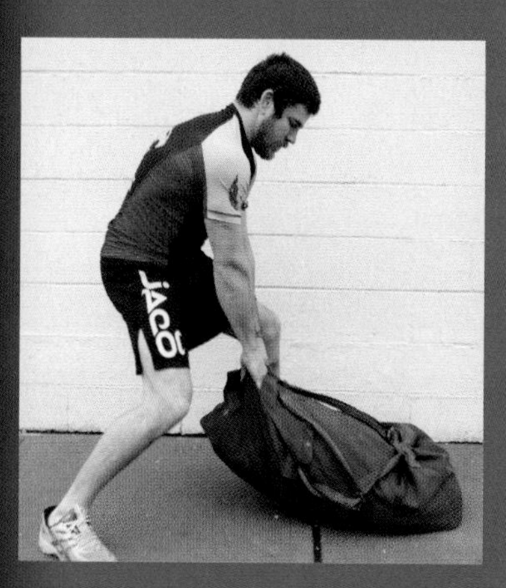

2. SANDBAG DRAG

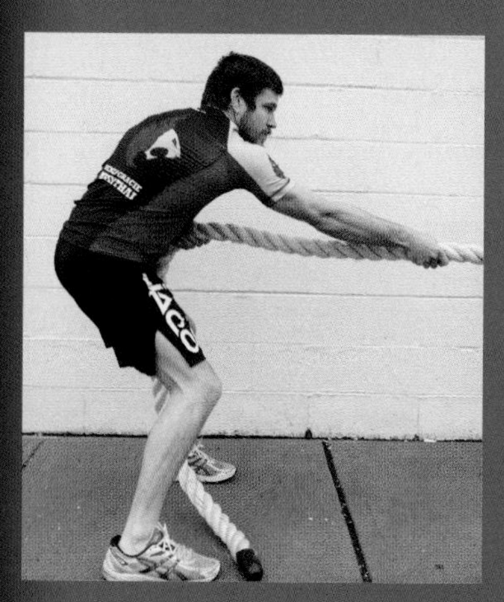

3. ARM-OVER-ARM ROPE PULL

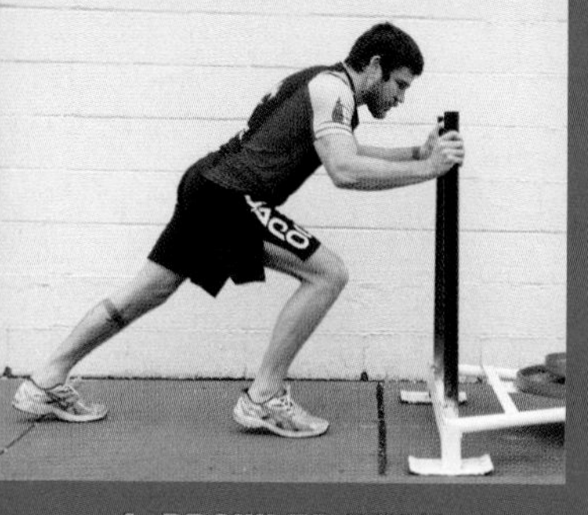

4. PROWLER PUSH

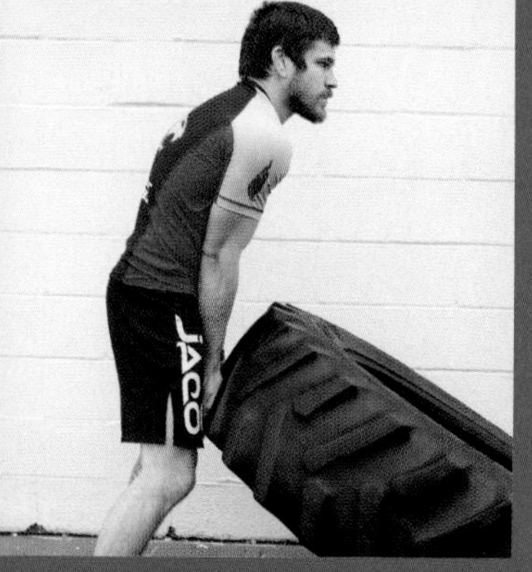

5. TIRE FLIP

B. POWER CIRCUIT

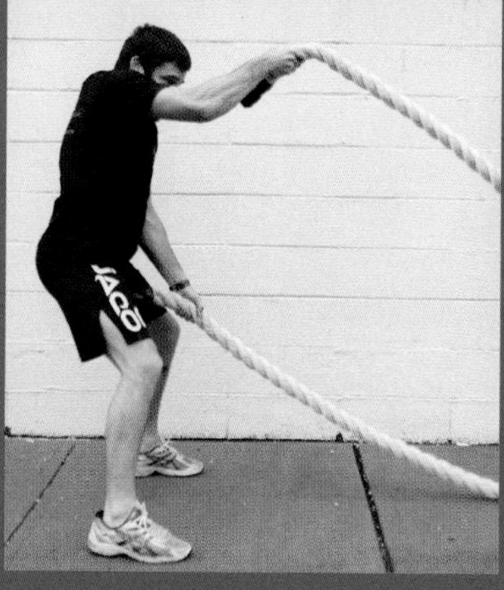

1. ROPE

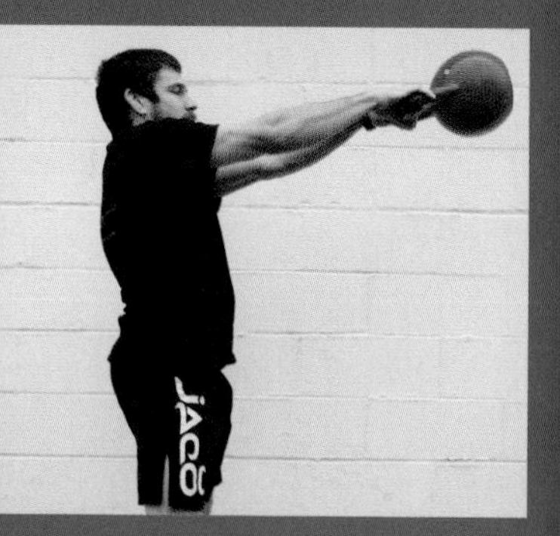

2. KETTLEBELL SWING

3. MED BALL SLAMS

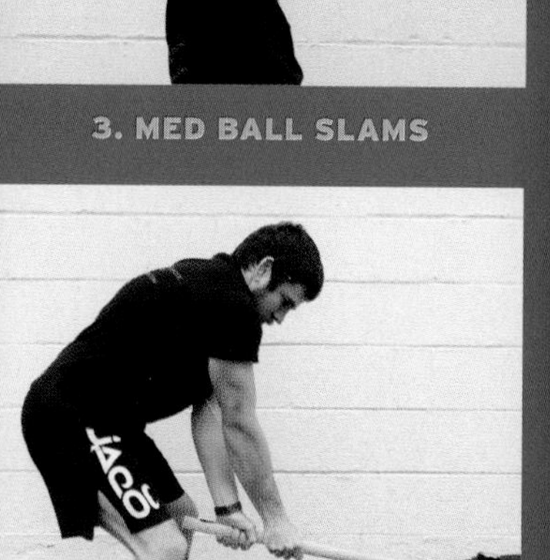

4. SLEDGEHAMMER SWINGS

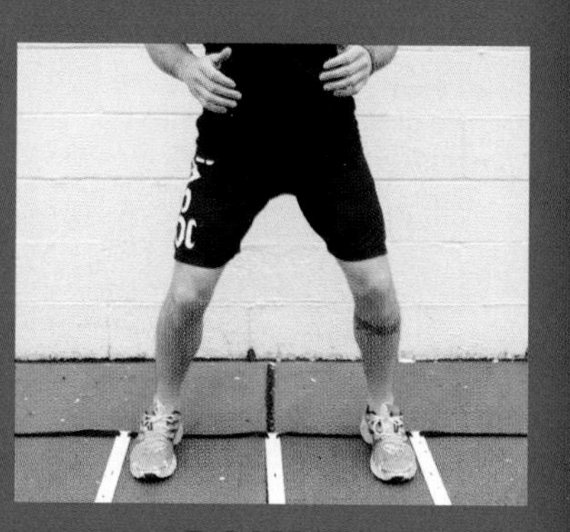

5. LADDER

C. FIGHTER CIRCUIT

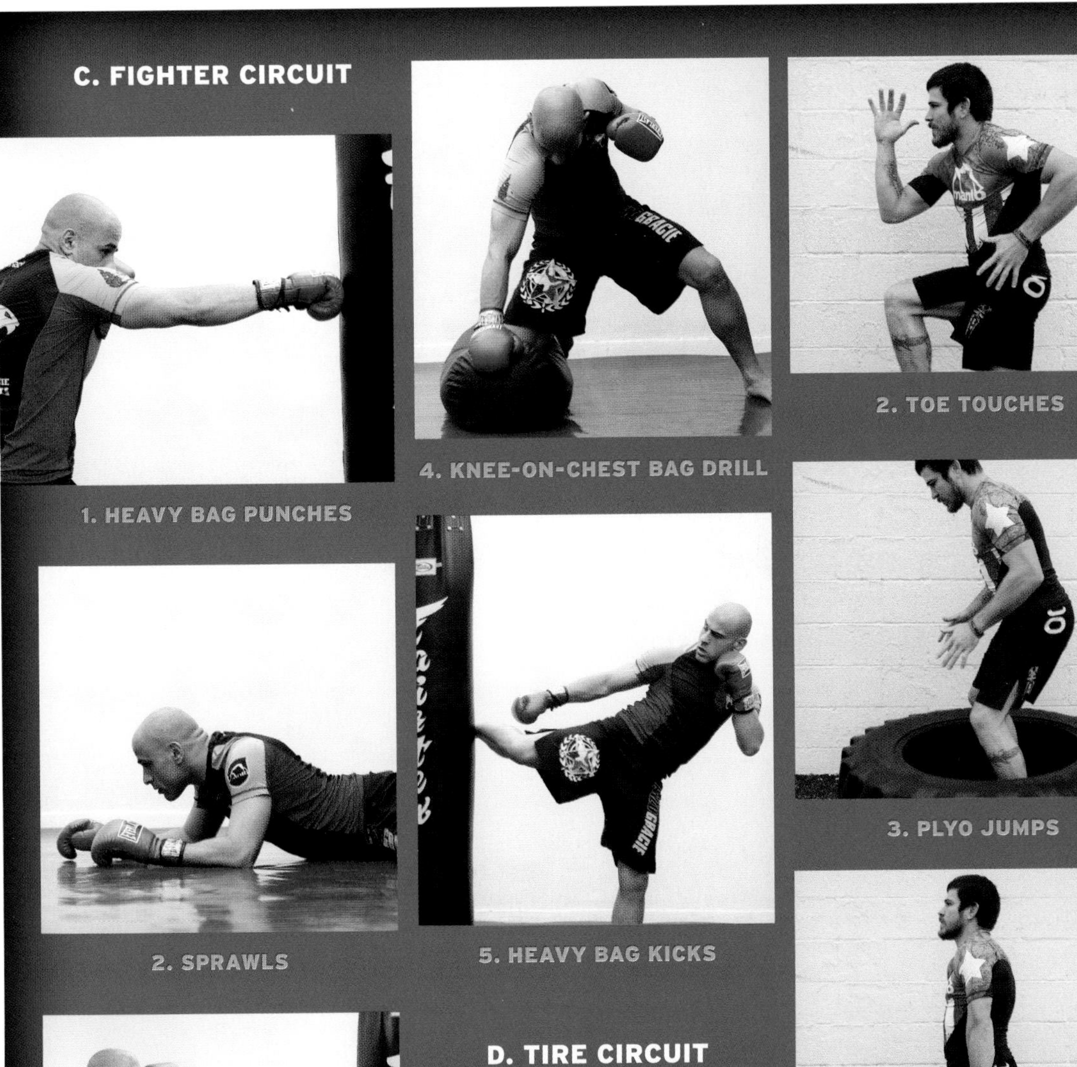

1. HEAVY BAG PUNCHES

2. SPRAWLS

4. KNEE-ON-CHEST BAG DRILL

5. HEAVY BAG KICKS

2. TOE TOUCHES

3. PLYO JUMPS

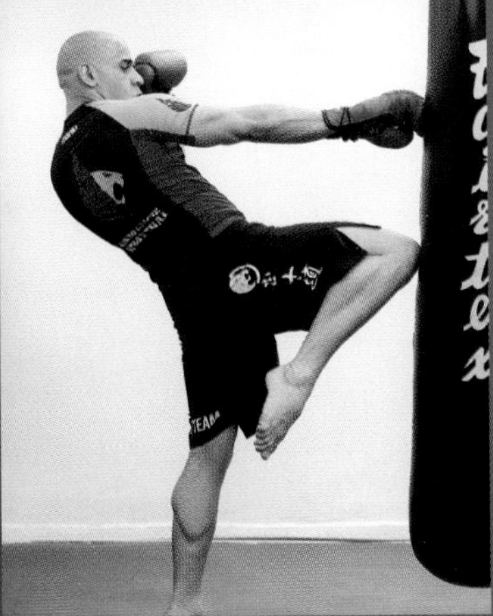

3. HEAVY BAG KNEES

D. TIRE CIRCUIT

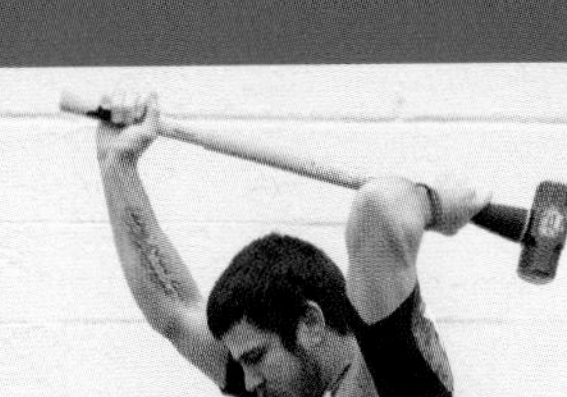

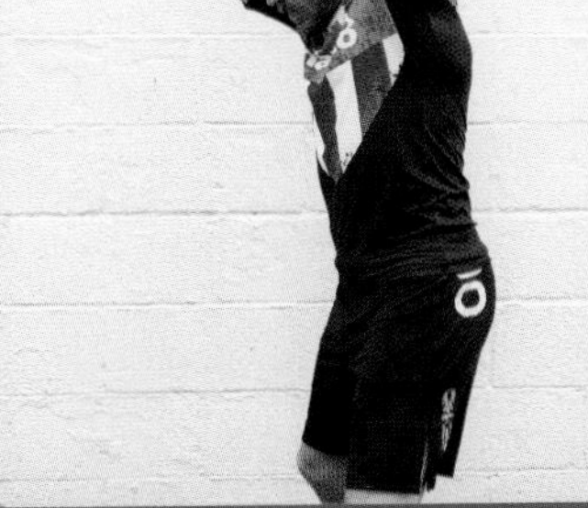

1. SLEDGEHAMMER SWINGS

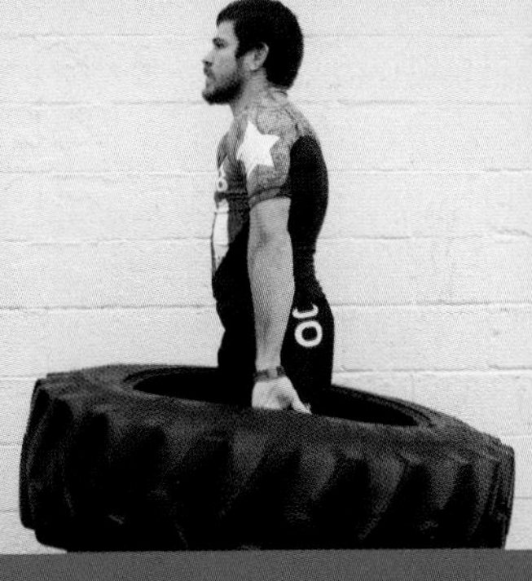

4. DEADLIFTS

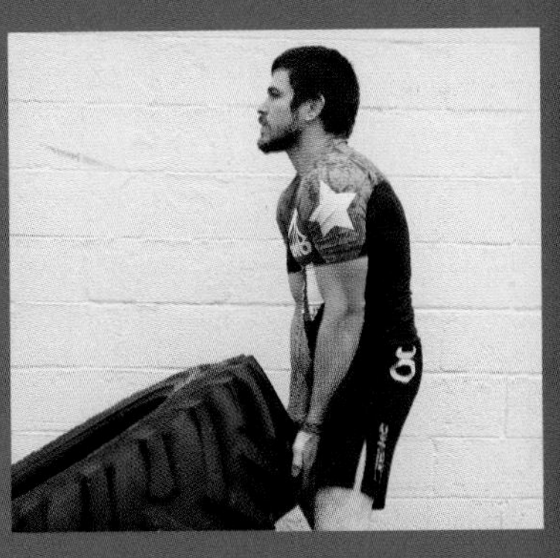

5. TIRE FLIPS

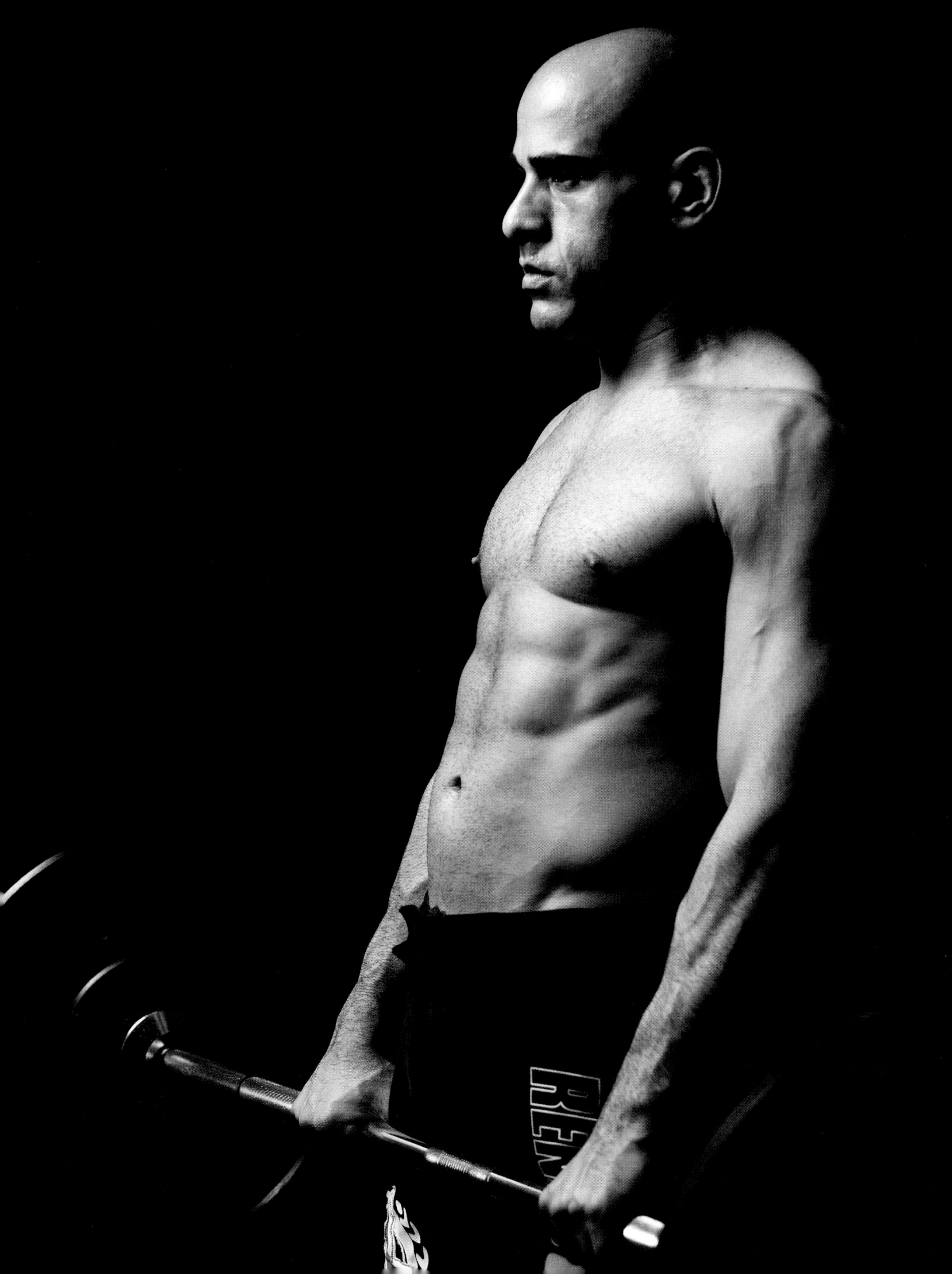

9

HURRICANE TRAINING

The Hurricane is the main form of Metabolic Training used in the TFW System. I've been developing this form of training over the last 12 years, as I was looking for a way to simulate the cardiovascular demands of a fight on an athlete while still building muscle. The name Hurricane came from the fact that this style of training is brief yet powerful, like a hurricane. Even before I understood the science behind why this style worked, I realized that just like after a real hurricane hits an area, there must be a period of rebuilding after the workout to get back to normal. Now, with the science to back up this style of training, I have come to recognize that the disruption caused by Hurricane Training creates the stimulus of rebuilding that burns fat and builds muscle.

The traditional Hurricane Training that I used for many years involved a treadmill and some form of either bodyweight- or equipment-based resistance. As people have performed the Hurricane around the world, I have recognized that not everyone has the luxury of a treadmill or a facility that has both a treadmill and weights close together. As a result of this, I have experimented with many other ways to create the same effect. While the treadmill is featured in the workouts in this chapter, you can replace it with regular sprinting, wall drives, resistance runs, and resistance biking for any of the exercises.

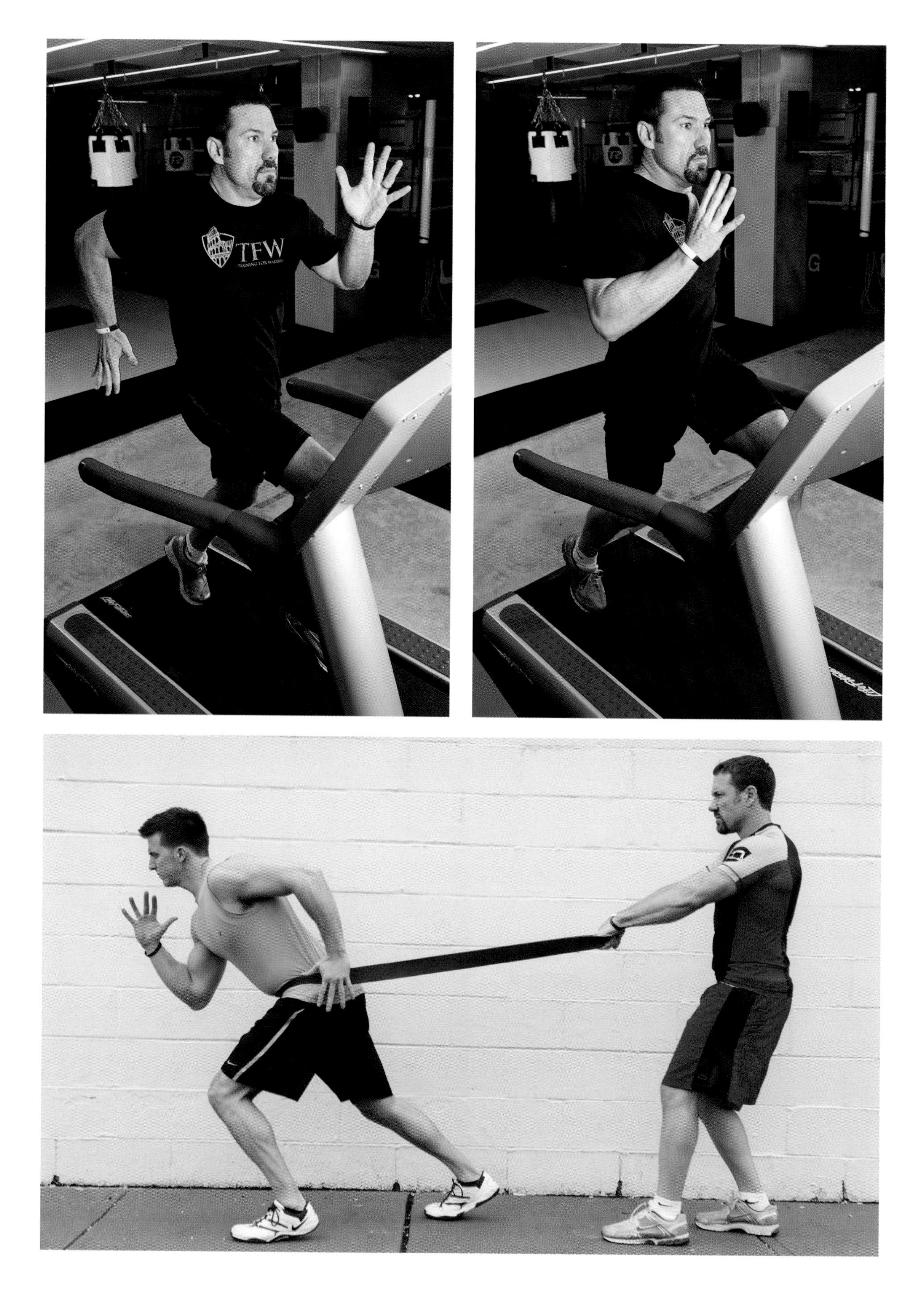
TFW
TRAINING FOR WARRIORS

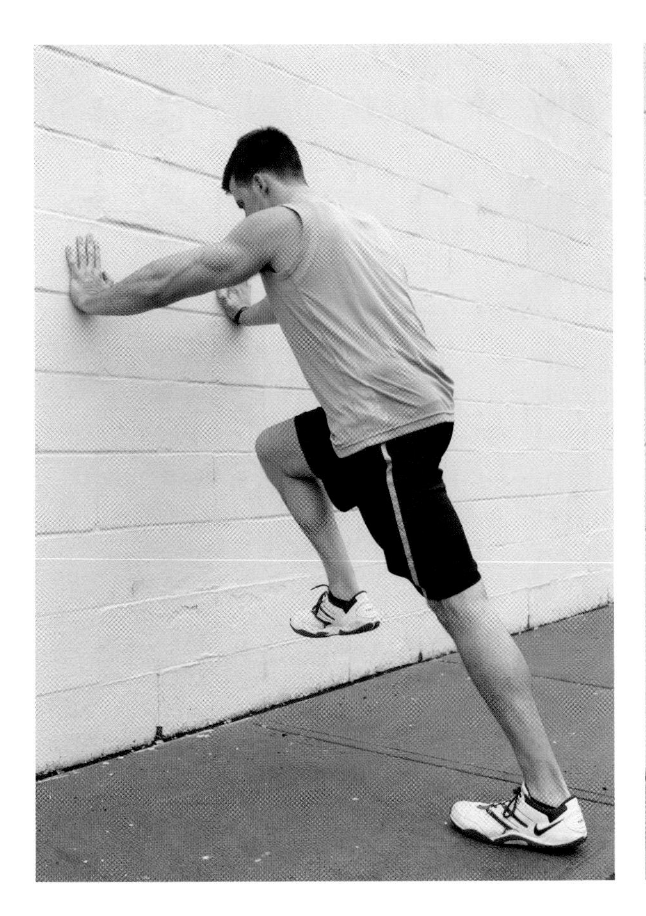

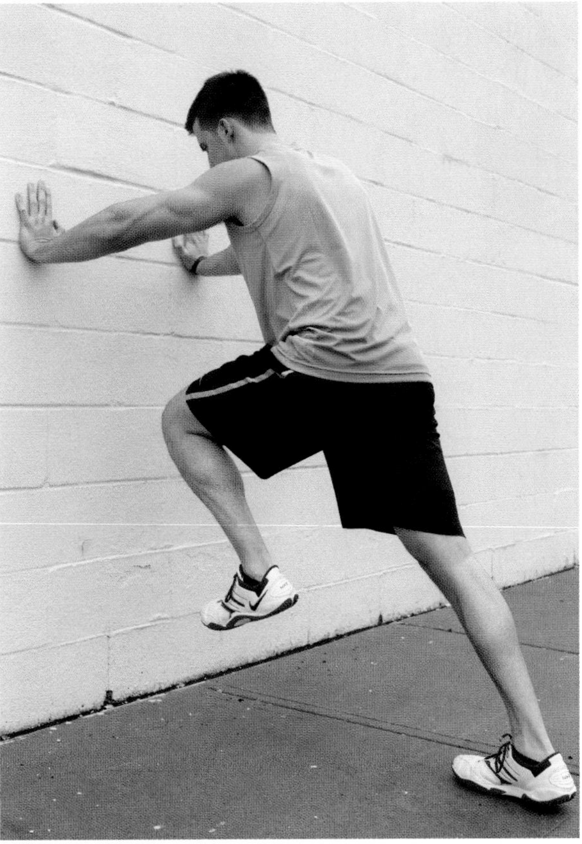

Even though there are a number of ways to utilize the Hurricane, I still prefer treadmill or regular sprinting since they involve coordination, work the entire body, build strength, and are very effective at raising the heart rate. I believe that sprinting is a fundamental human movement that is unfortunately rarely used by people after childhood. Excellent movements that mimic some of the demands of sprinting that can be used when a treadmill or longer sprints are not possible are wall drives and resisted running. These are especially excellent tools if you lack space to perform runs. Biking is another good choice, but often people may not have a resistance bike available. But regardless of your choice of heart-rate-increasing modality, I call that movement a sprint. This is because it is to be performed at maximum intensity for the prescribed distance or time.

There are two different ways that Hurricane Training can be applied in relation to overall approach. First, a Hurricane can be performed for a set time by monitoring work-to-rest ratios. Alternatively, it can be performed in order to achieve the shortest time possible according to the speed of the prescribed reps and sets.

WORK-TO-REST METHOD HURRICANE

When using the style that focuses on work-to-rest, you control the intensity of the Hurricane by controlling the rest periods and ultimately the length of the Hurricane. During this mode of Hurricane, you would attempt to perform as many repetitions as possible of the resistance exercises for the period of time that is set.

For instance, if you've decided that for a Category 3 Hurricane, you're going to use a

1:1 work/rest ratio, then the time of that Hurricane would look like one of these options:

For a 22-minute Hurricane (no rest period after the final set):

30-second sprint
30-second rest
15 seconds of curls
15 seconds rest
15 seconds of high pulls
15 seconds rest

One set would take 2 minutes.
One round would take 6 minutes.
Rest 2 minutes between rounds.
Repeat 3 times.

For a 19-minute Hurricane (no rest period after the final set):

30-second sprint
30-second rest
10 seconds of curls
10 seconds rest
10 seconds of high pulls
10 seconds rest

One set would take 1 minute, 40 seconds.
One round would take 5 minutes.
Rest 2 minutes between rounds.
Repeat 3 times.

There are many ways that the Hurricane can be manipulated according to the work/rest ratio. If the rest is increased, obviously the length of the Hurricane will increase.

BEST-TIME METHOD HURRICANE

In the Best Time scenario, it is up to you to determine the work/rest ratio in order to attempt to achieve a best time. In this case, you can employ what is called a negative work-to-rest ratio in that you jump from sprint to exercise to exercise (set to set) and also from round to round with little rest. This is a more demanding form of the Hurricane and must be employed only after experience is built with this style of training.

Here is how this model might look as compared to the Work-to-Rest Method.

30-second sprint
5-second rest
15 seconds of curls
5 seconds rest
15 seconds of high pulls
5 seconds rest
Repeat 3 times.

One set would take 1 minute, 10 seconds.
One round would take 3½ minutes.
Rest 1 minute between rounds.

Total time of the Hurricane: 12½ minutes (no rest period after the final set). As you can see, the density of this style is greatly increased and the workout is, as a result, much more intense.

Regardless of the method selected, every Hurricane has a similar format: nine total sets, each of which combines some form of training used to increase heart rate and some form of resistance training. These nine total sets are broken down into what we call three sets of three rounds. During the execution of a Hurricane, each individual round is composed of either different heart rate and resistance exercises or both.

There are five categories of Hurricanes. Each category increases in difficulty from Category 1 to 5. By learning the different demands of Hurricane Training, you can use the concept of undulating periodization to control the intensity of training throughout the week.

To properly execute Hurricane Training, it's necessary to understand the differences between the categories.

CATEGORY 1

This is the beginner's-level Hurricane and is used to prepare a trainee for the demands of future work. The Category 1 Hurricane is the only one to solely use exercises to increase heart rate and then wait for the heart rate to recover to a predetermined number of beats.

CATEGORY 2

This Hurricane differs from a Category 1 in that it uses two simple bodyweight activities in the place of recovery after each sprint, such as forms of pushups, sit-ups, or medicine ball drills.

CATEGORY 3

This Hurricane differs from a Category 2 in that it uses two light-resistance exercises after each sprint, such as barbell curls, dumbbell presses, barbell rows, and cable tricep pushdowns.

CATEGORY 4

This Hurricane increases in intensity from a Category 3 in that it uses two heavy-resistance exercises after each sprint. These activities might include barbell bench presses, chin-ups, and dips.

CATEGORY 5

This is the most demanding Hurricane as a result of the amount of muscle mass used and work performed. This Hurricane increases in intensity from a Category 4 in that it now uses two Strongman exercises after each sprint, such as tire flips, sledgehammer swings, and sled pushes.

In meteorology, Category 5 hurricanes are considered rare storms that result in the most catastrophic damage. This fact has important implications for the use of a Category 5 Hurricane in the TFW system. Although it is common for people to want to attempt the Category 5 first, this is something that must be built up to over time and should not occur too often in your training. Only use this category after a strong base of training has been attained.

HURRICANES: CATEGORY I

Perform the following for 9 sets: treadmill at 9 to 10 mph and 10% grade for 15-second sprints, with adequate recovery to reach 120 BPM before starting the next sprint.

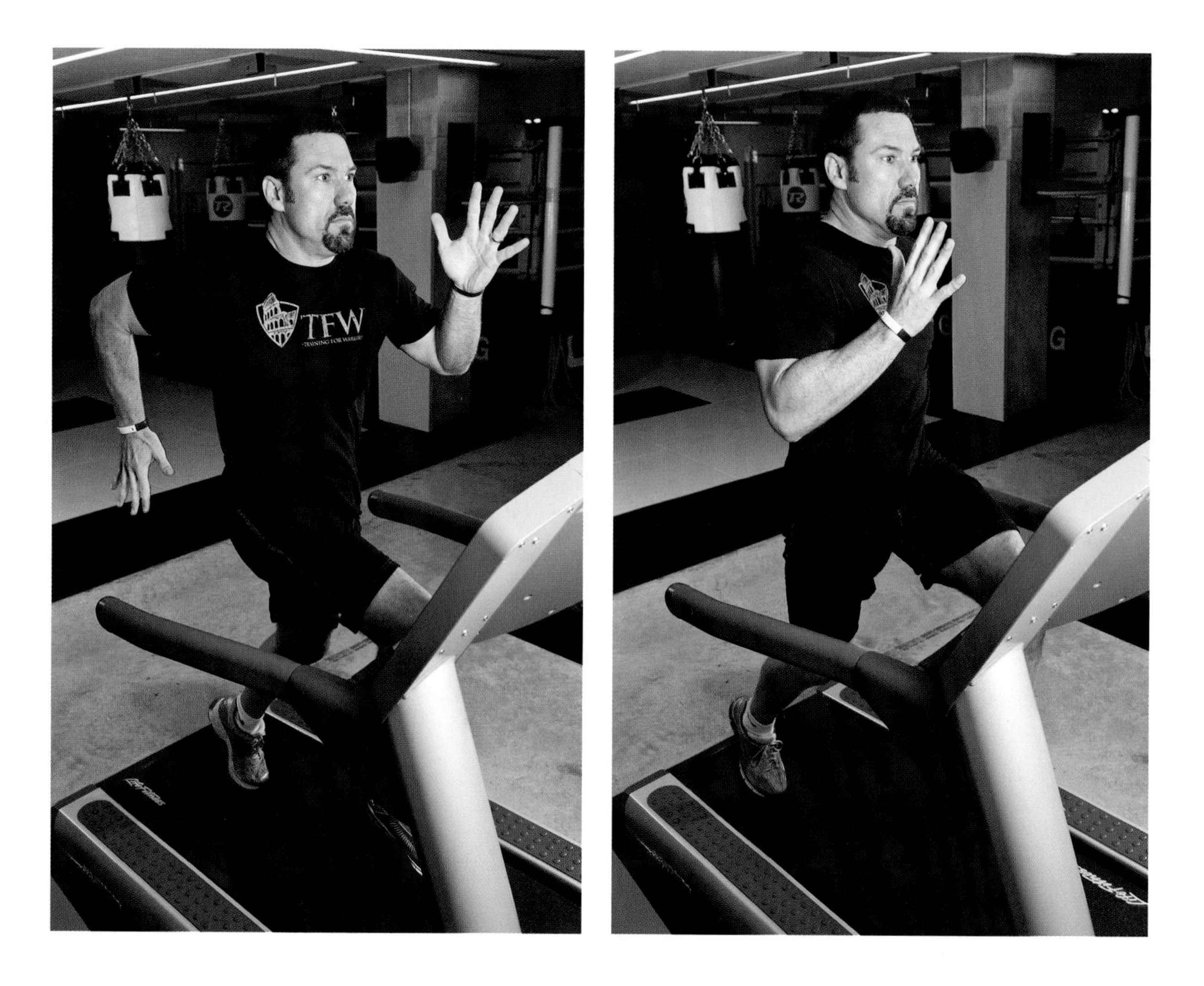

HURRICANES: CATEGORY 2

ROUND 1

Perform the following for 3 sets:
Treadmill at 9.0 mph x 10% grade for 20 seconds
Triangle Sit-ups x 8 each leg, Knee-to-Elbow Pushups x 10

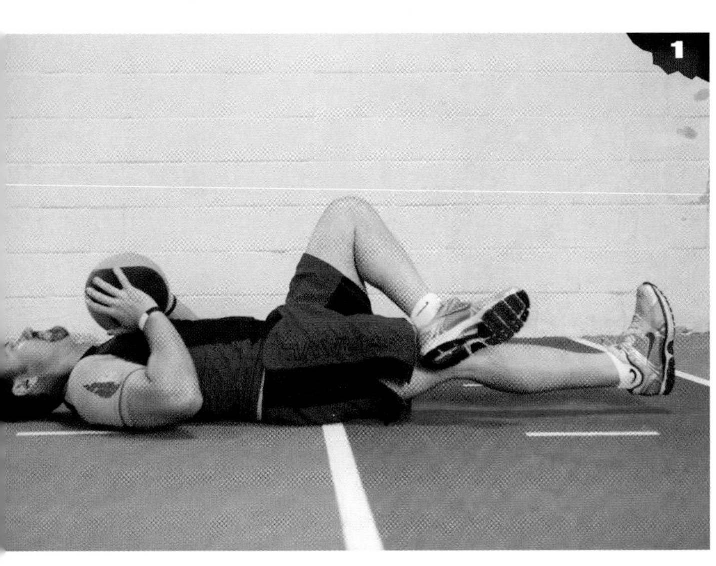

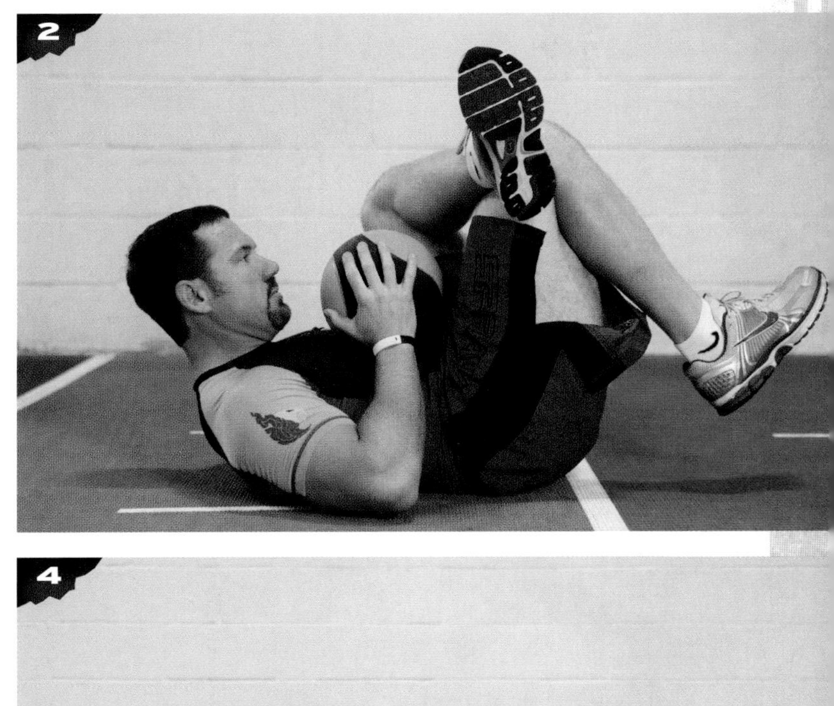

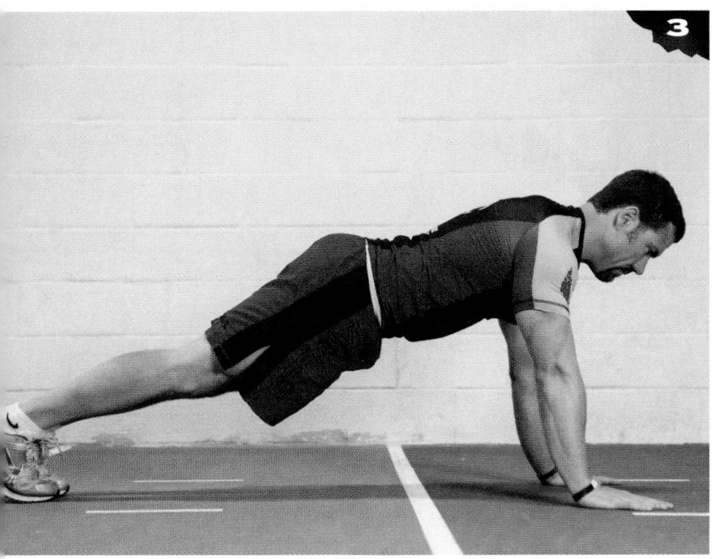

ROUND 2

Perform the following for 3 sets:
Treadmill at 10.0 mph x 10% grade for 20 seconds
Single-Leg Kicks x 8 each leg, Knee-to-Chest Pushups x 10

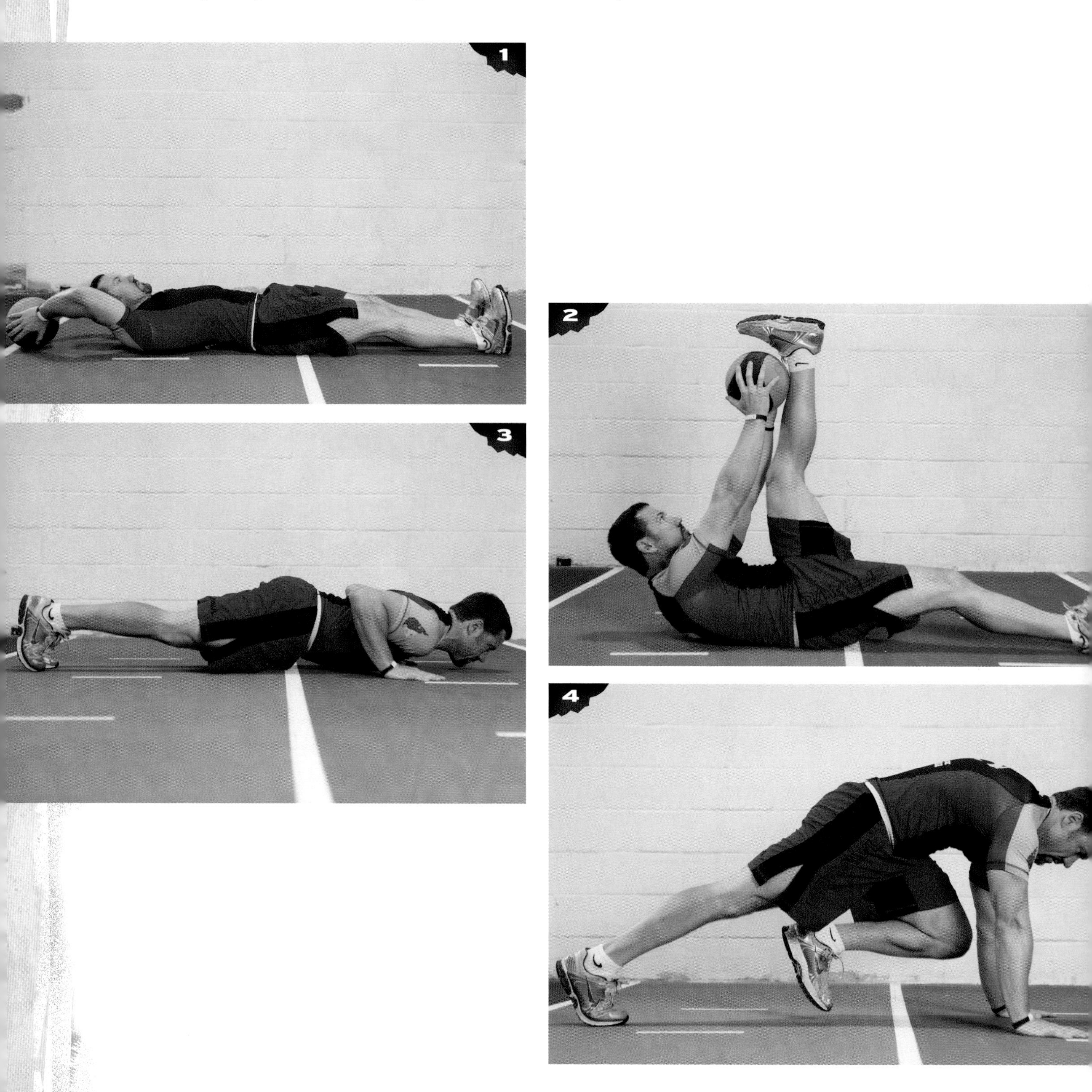

ROUND 3

Perform the following for 3 sets:
Treadmill at 10.5 mph x 10% grade for 20 seconds
Russian Twists x 50, Regular Pushups x 10

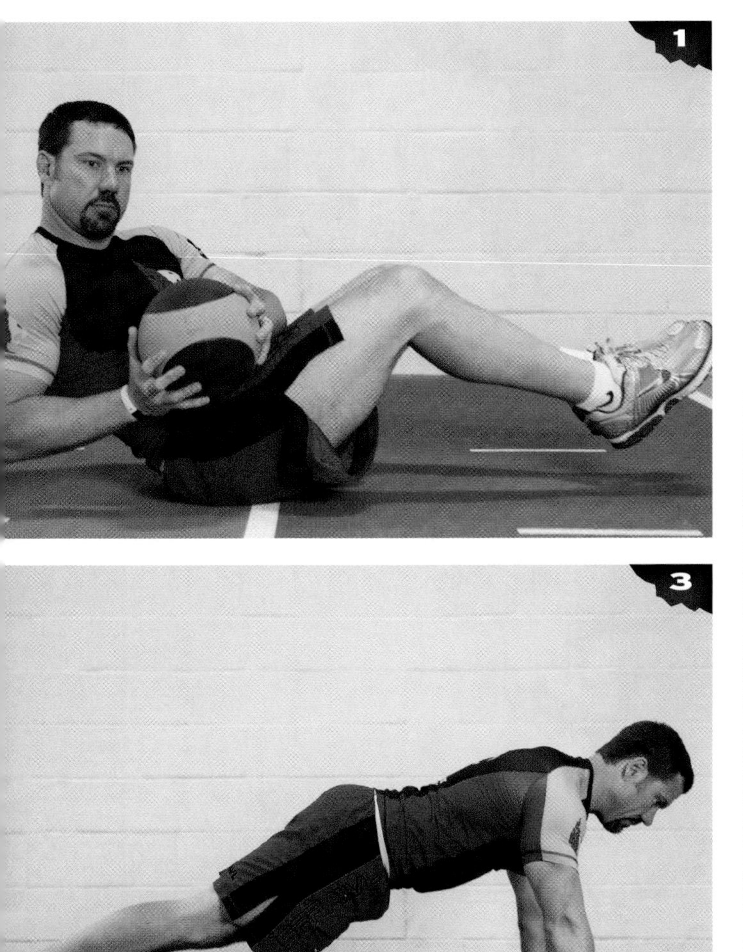

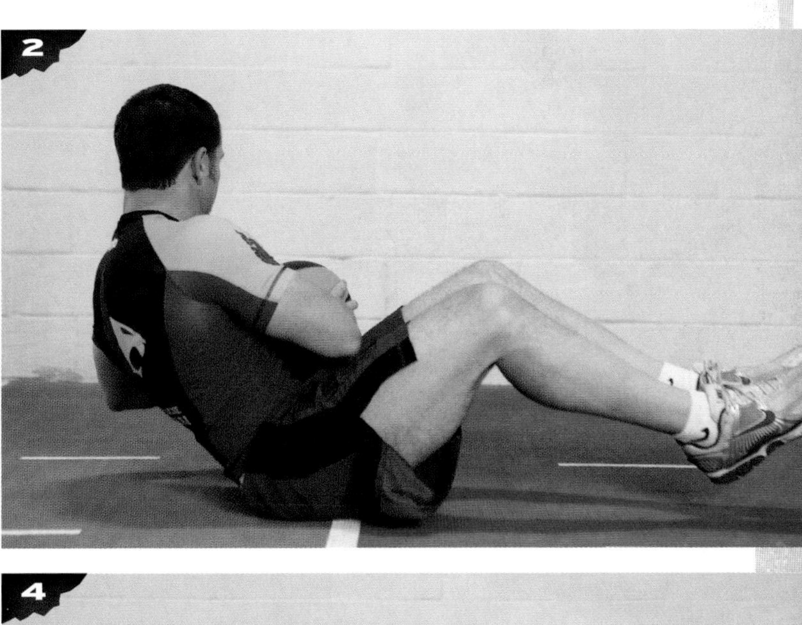

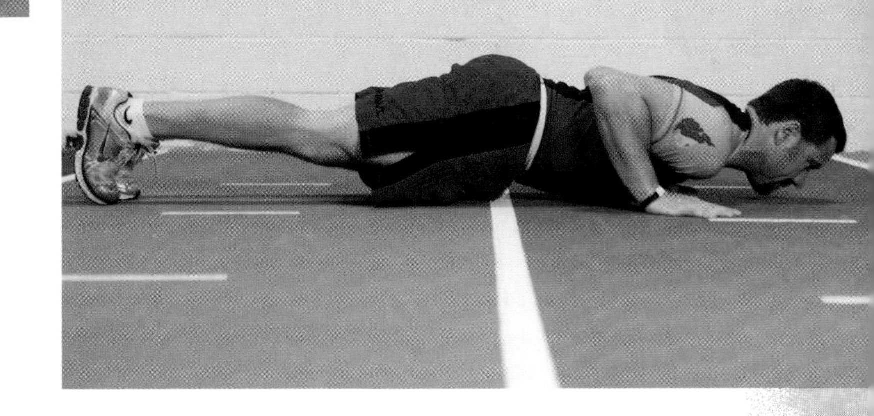

HURRICANES: CATEGORY 3

ROUND 1

Perform the following for 3 sets:
Treadmill at 9.5 mph x 10% grade for 25 seconds
Push Jerks x 10, Close Grip Snatch x 10

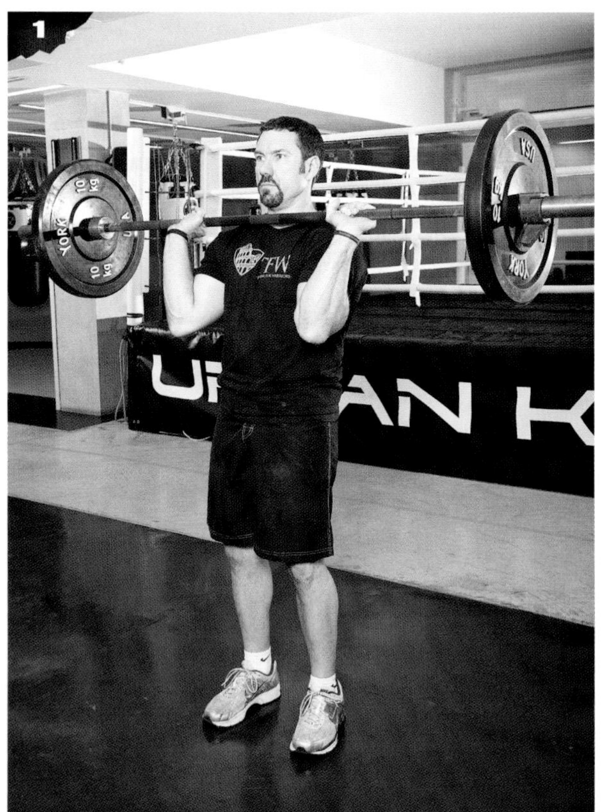

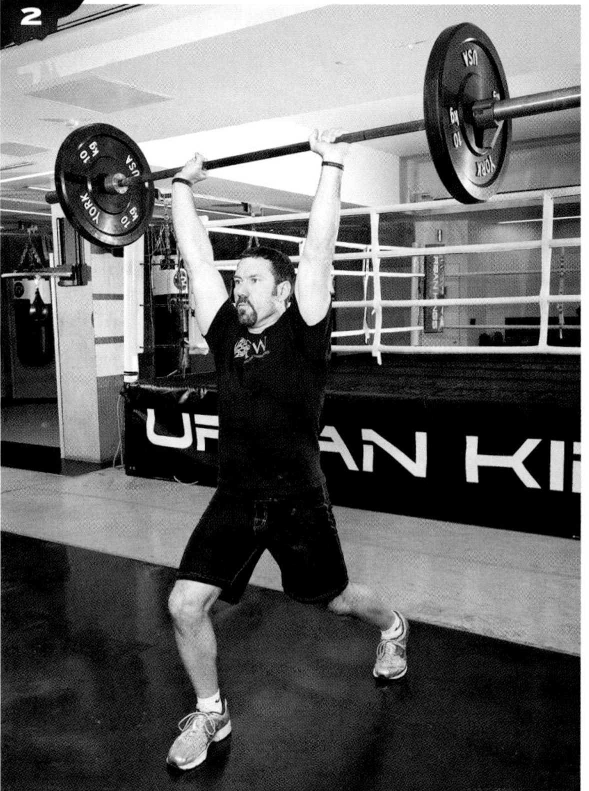

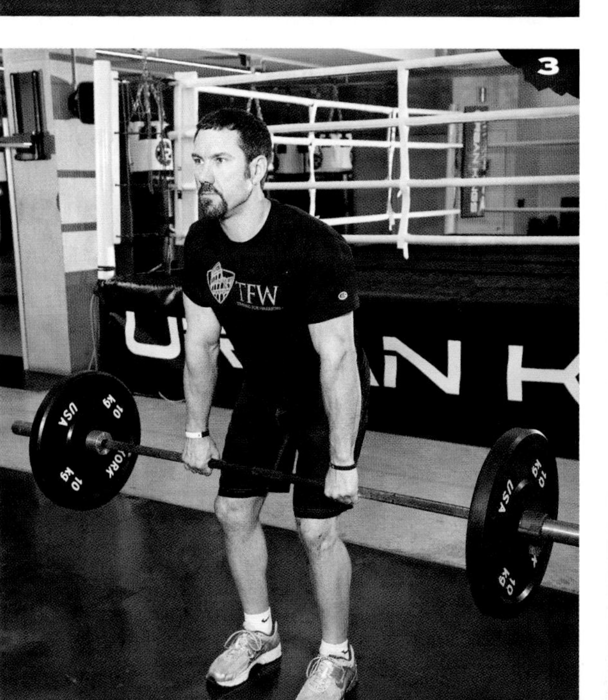

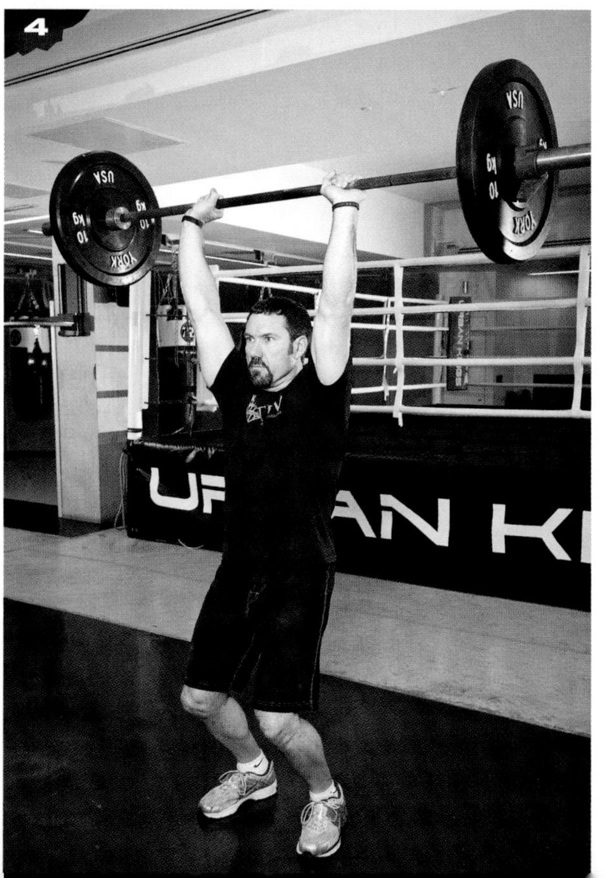

ROUND 2

Perform the following for 3 sets:
Treadmill at 10.5 mph x 10% grade for 25 seconds
Wide-Grip Bent-Over Row x 10, High Pull x 10

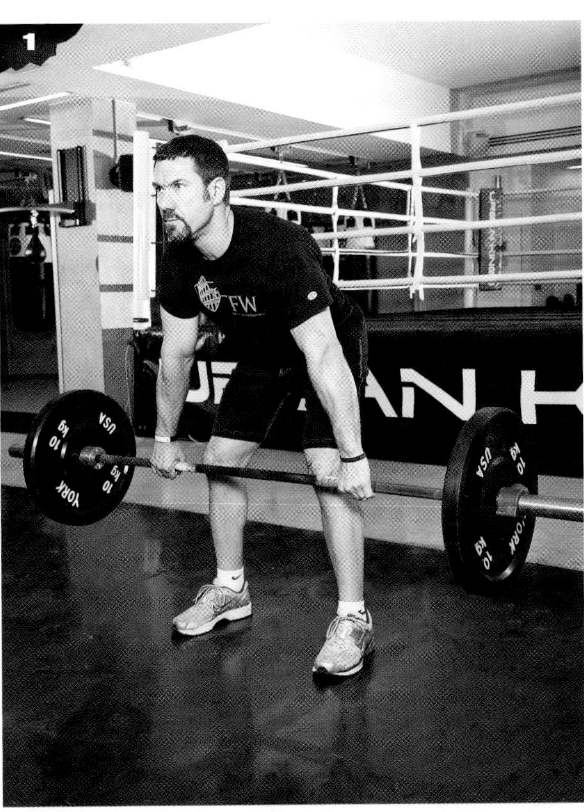

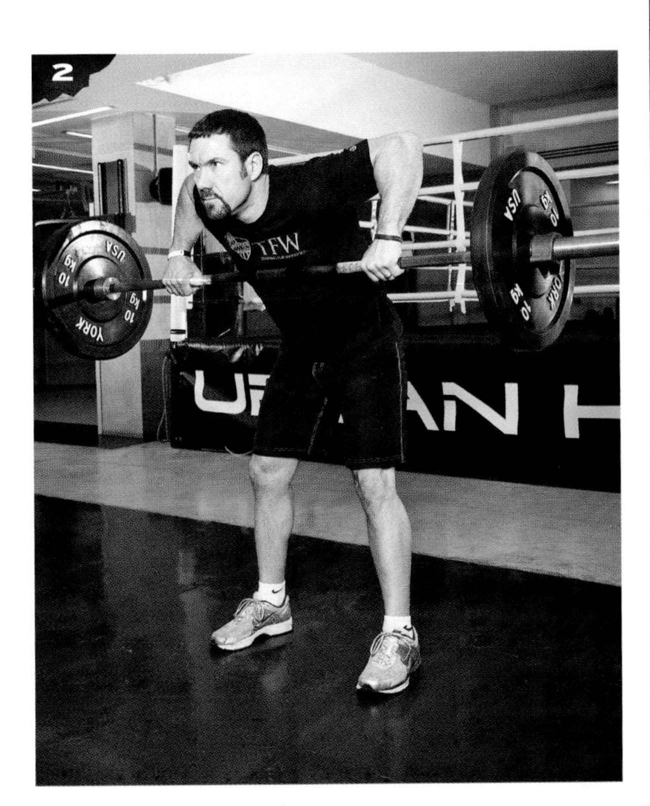

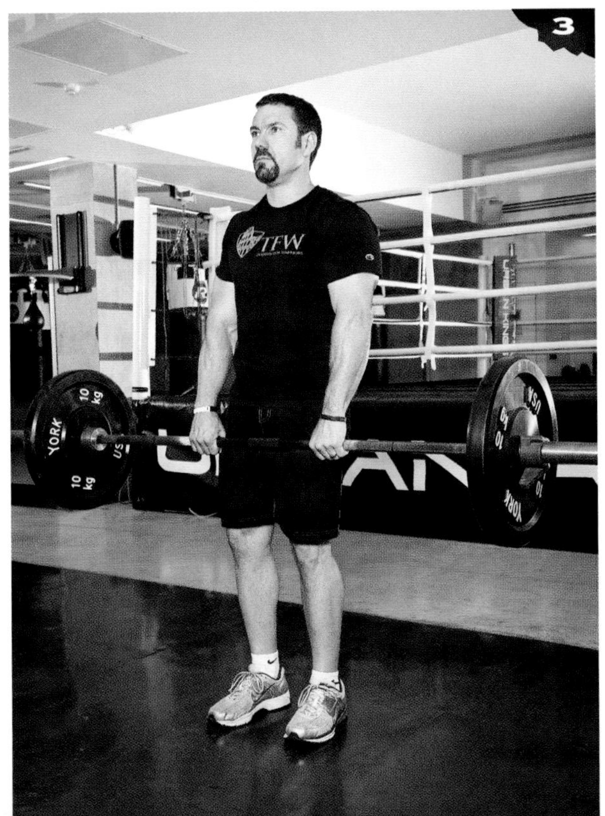

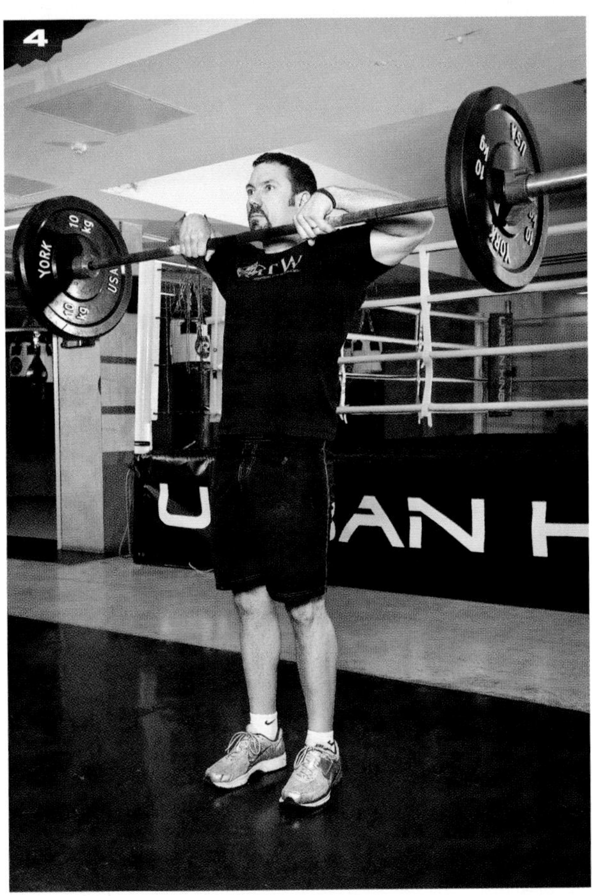

ROUND 3

Perform the following for 3 sets:
Treadmill at 11.5 mph x 10% grade for 25 seconds
Bicep Curl x 10, Triceps x 10

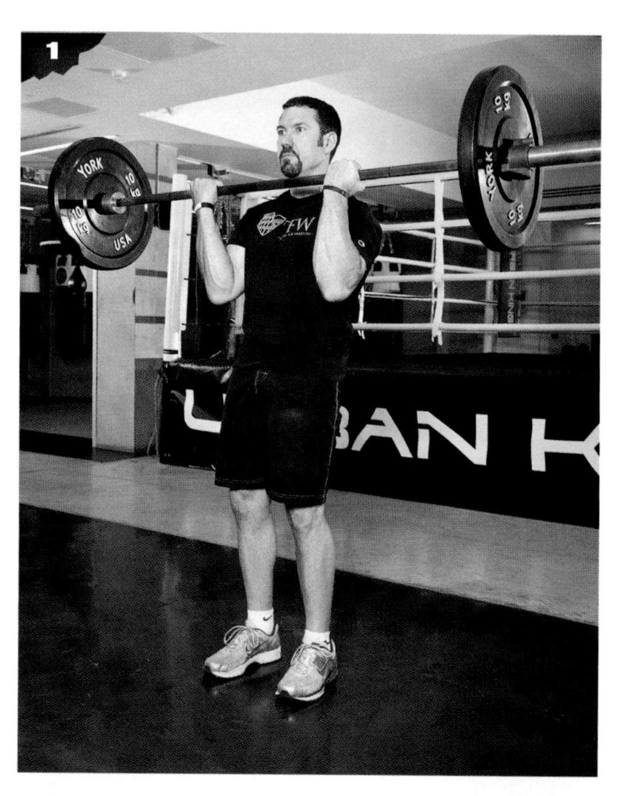

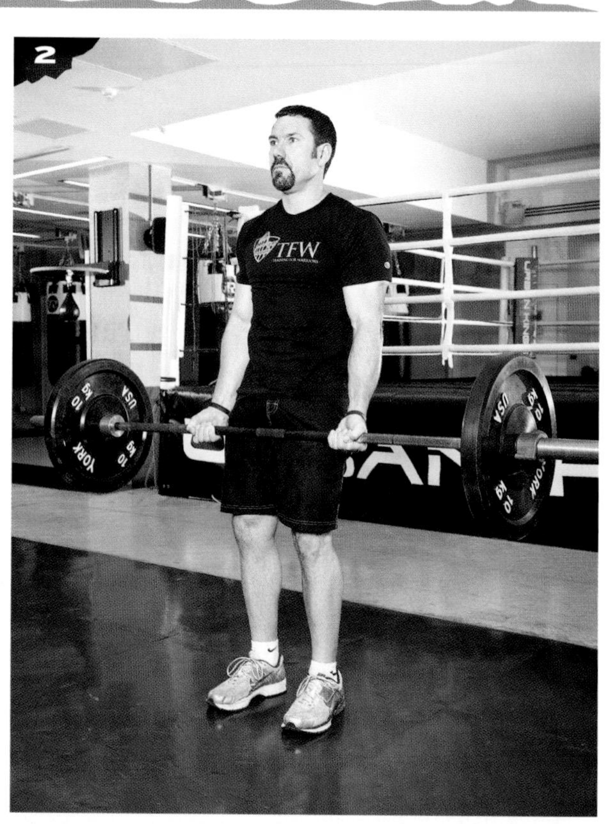

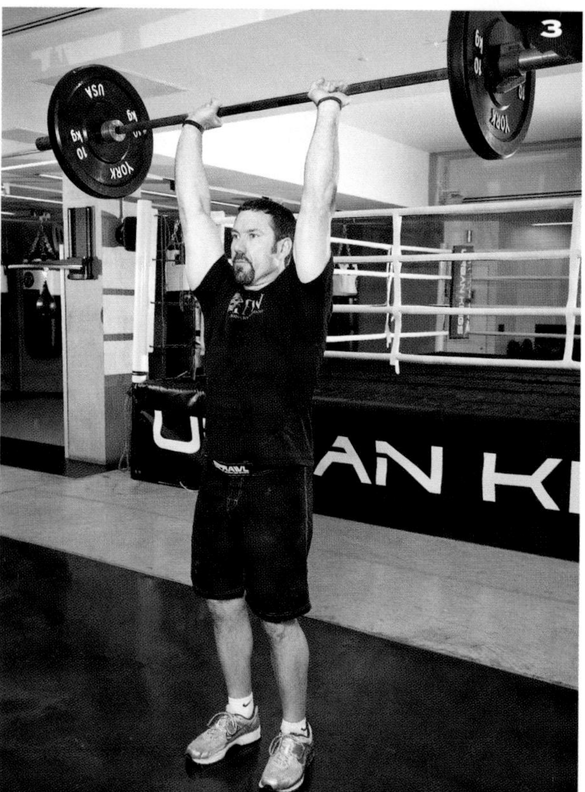

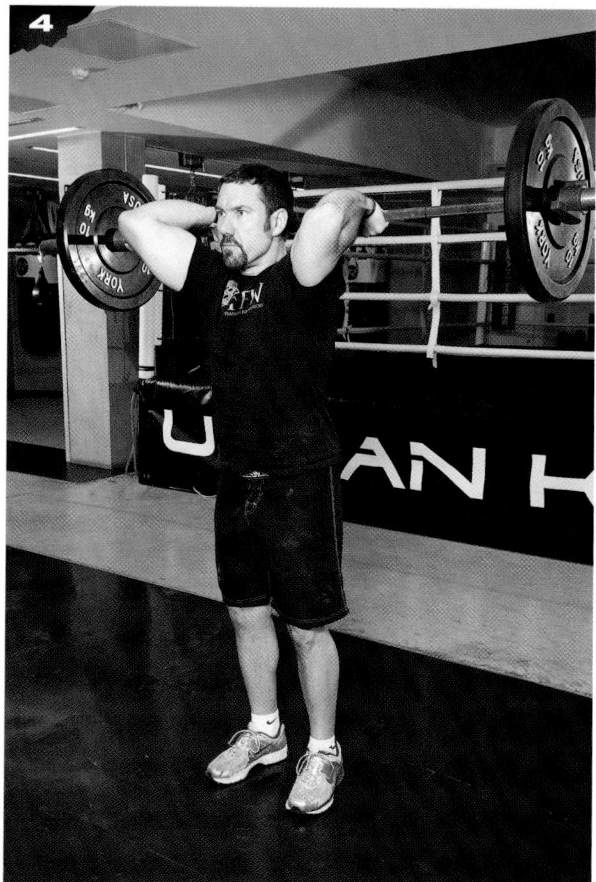

HURRICANES: CATEGORY 4

ROUND 1

Perform the following for 3 sets:
Treadmill at 10.5 mph x 10% grade for 30 seconds
Bench Press x 8, Chin-ups x 8

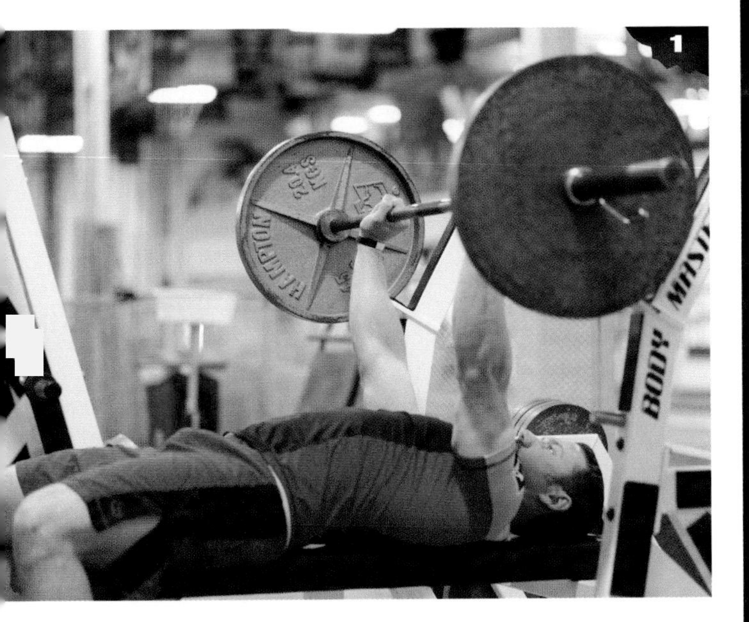

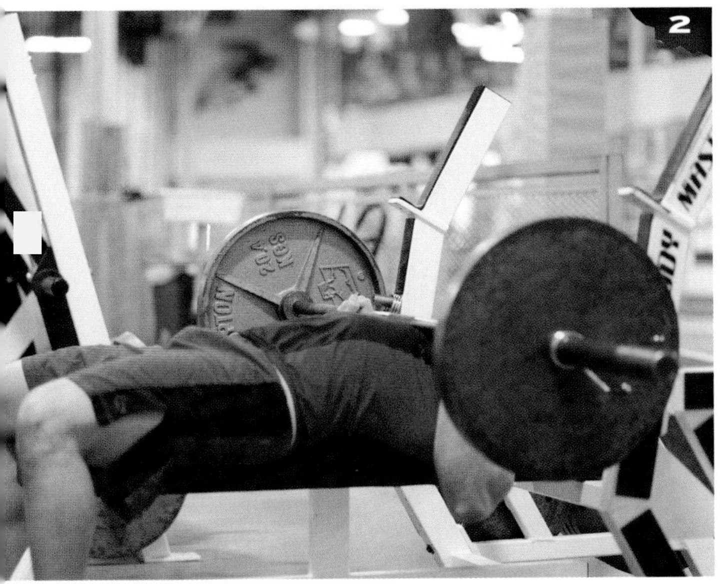

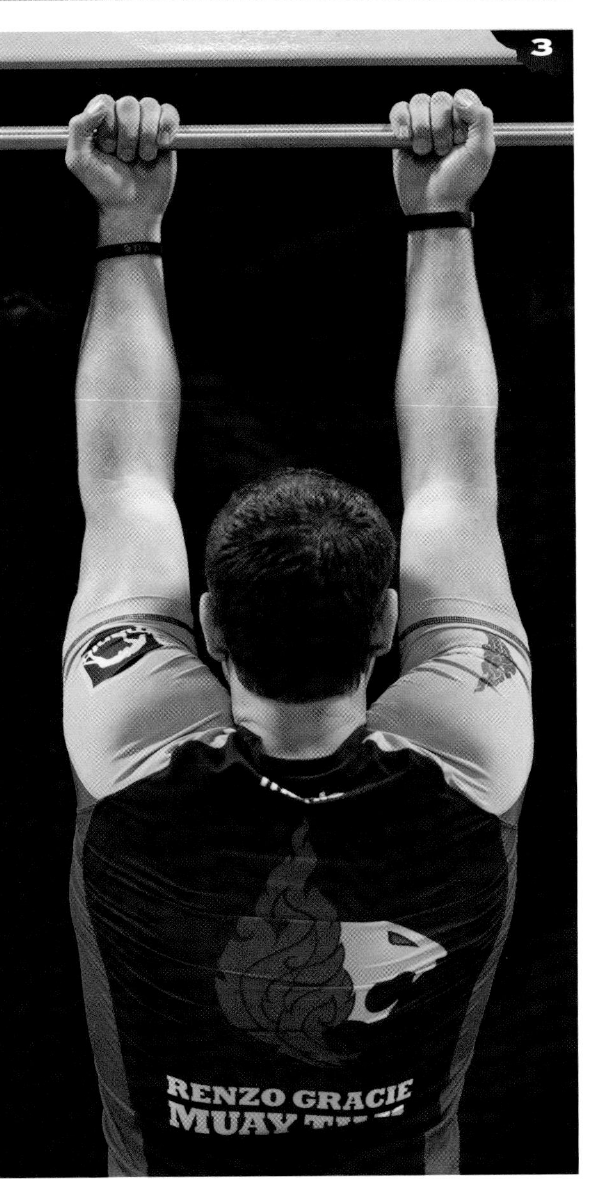

ROUND 2

Perform the following for 3 sets:
Treadmill at 12 mph x 10% grade for 30 seconds
Dips x 8, Overhead Press x 8

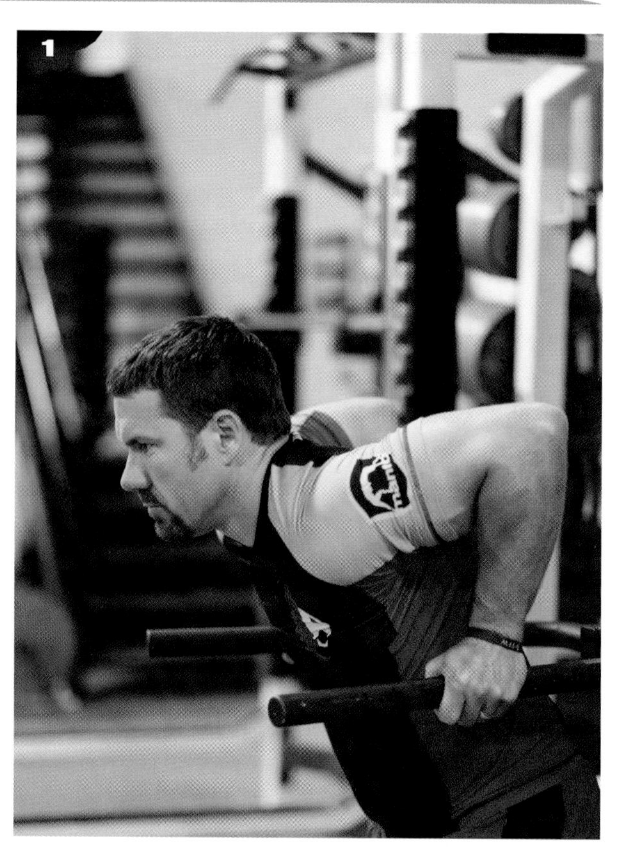

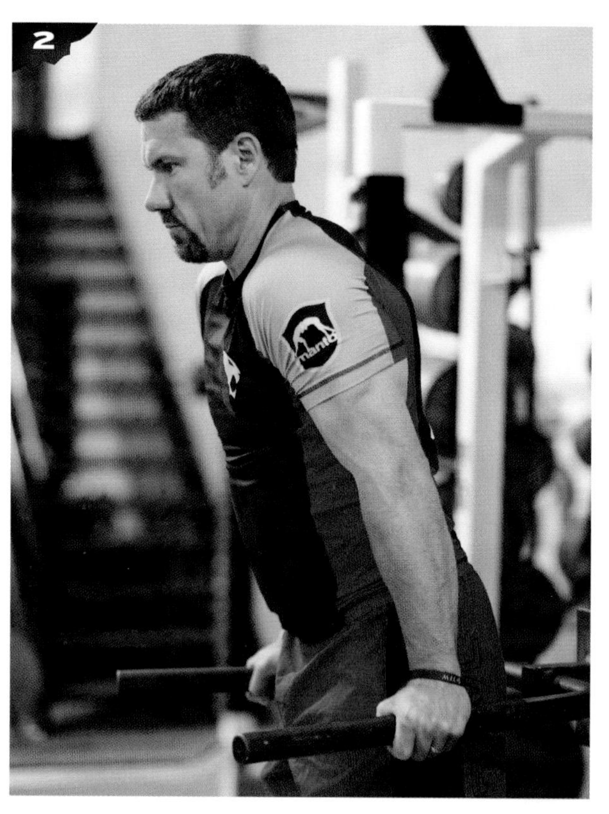

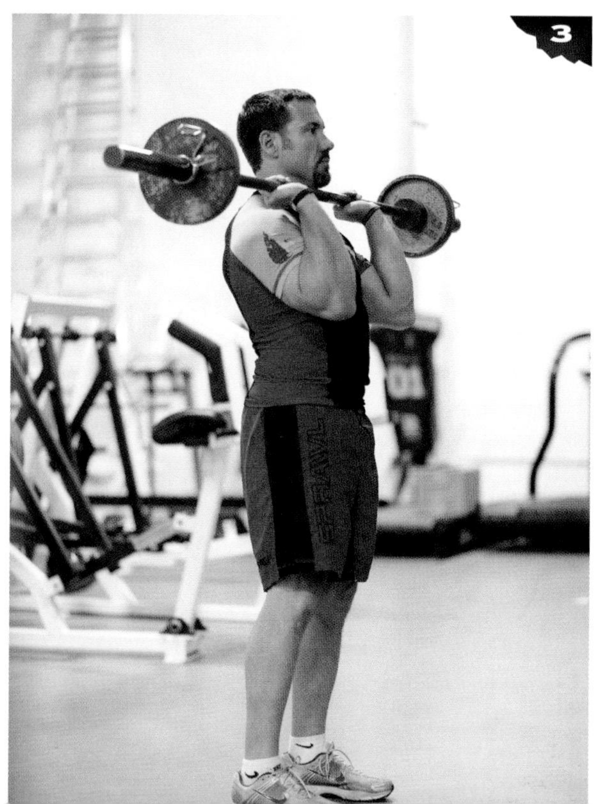

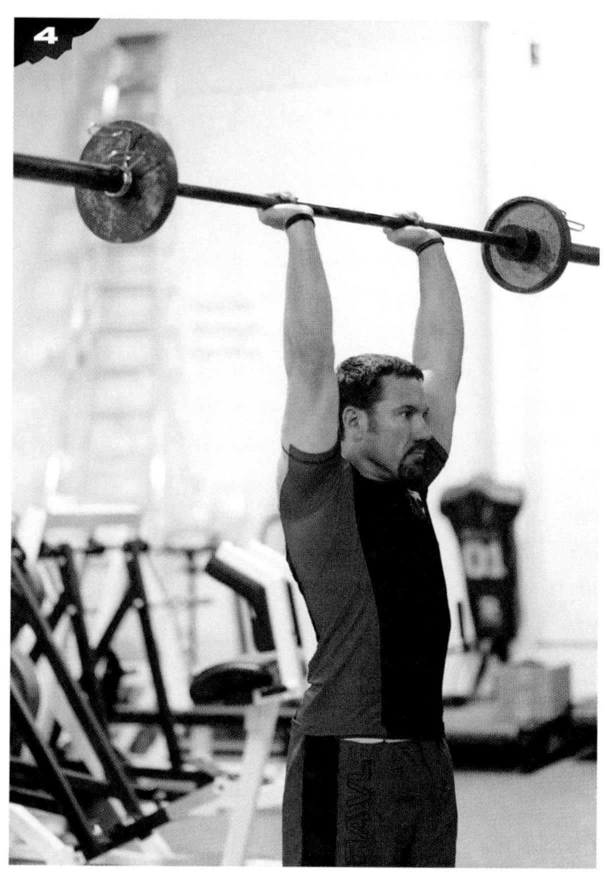

ROUND 3

Perform the following for 3 sets:
Treadmill at 13 mph x 10% grade for 30 seconds
Bent-Over Row x 10, Curls x 10

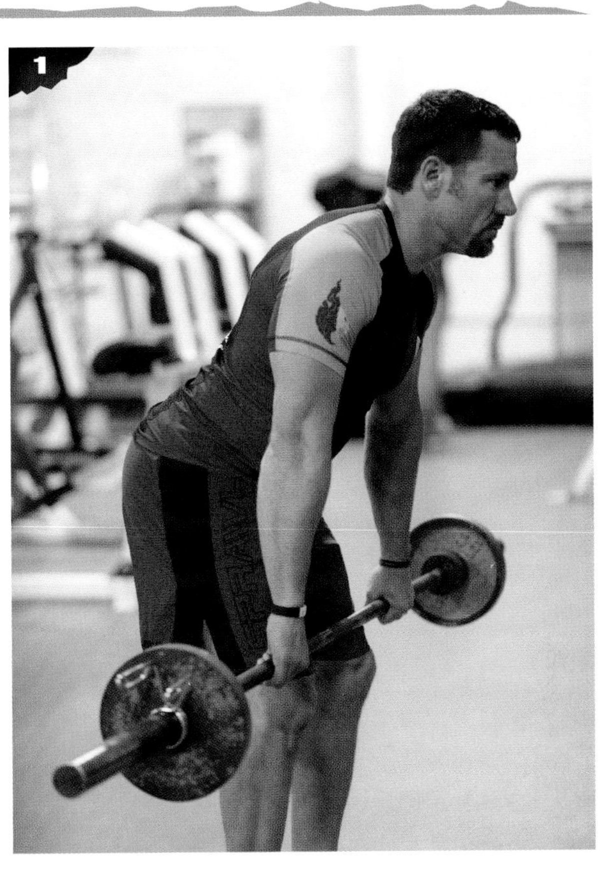
1

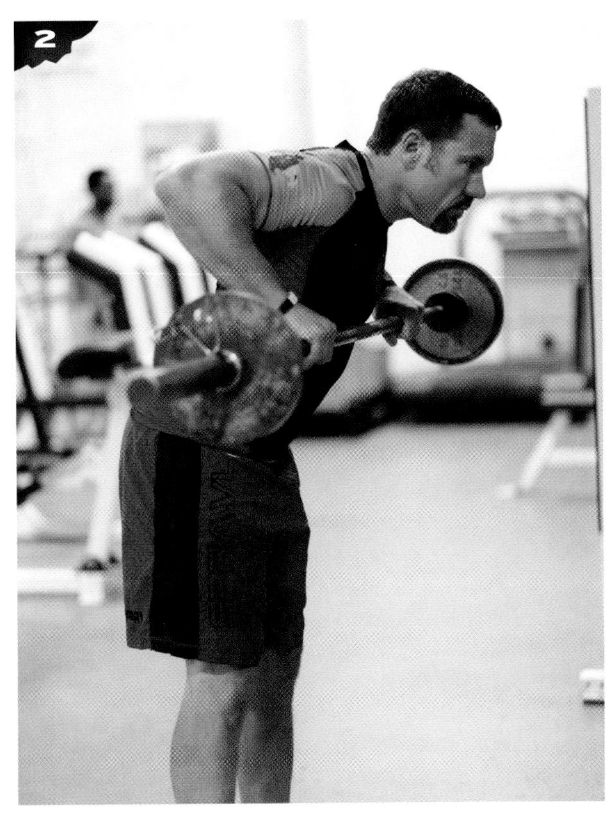
2

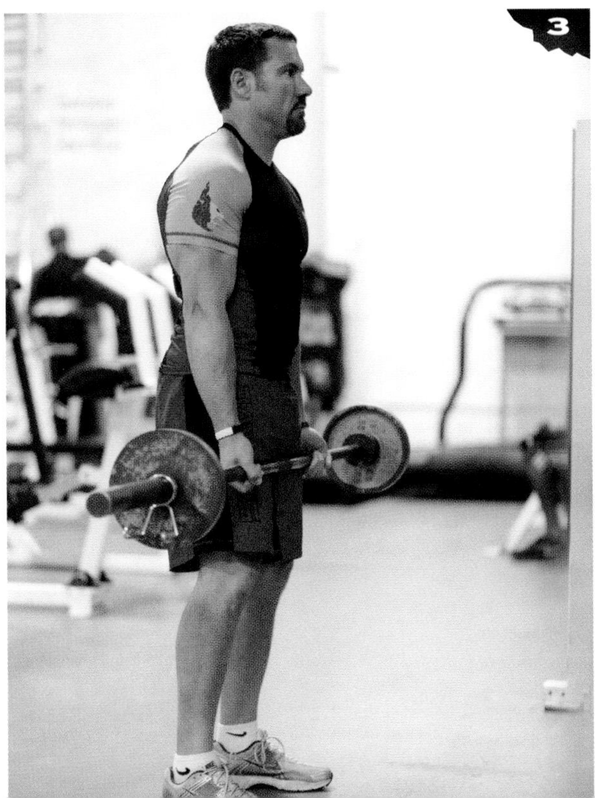
3

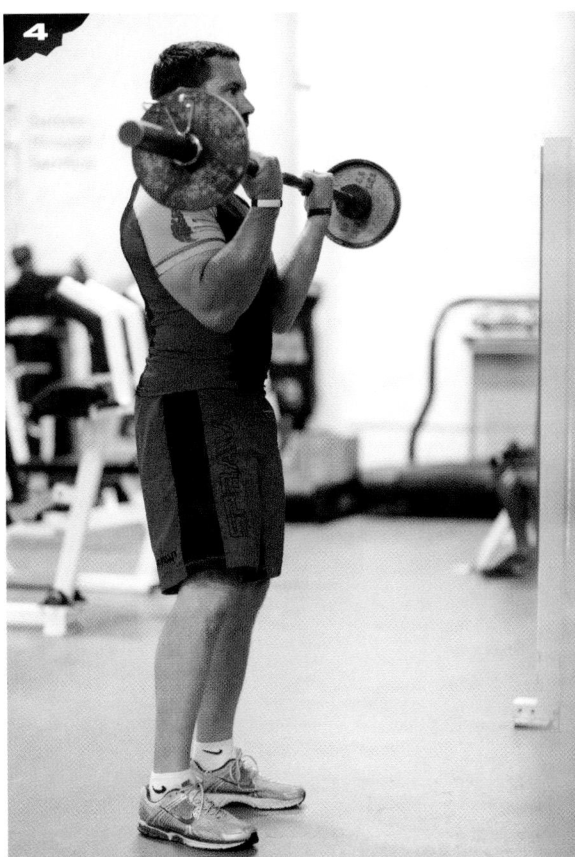
4

HURRICANE TRAINING CHEATSHEET

CATEGORY 1, TREADMILL

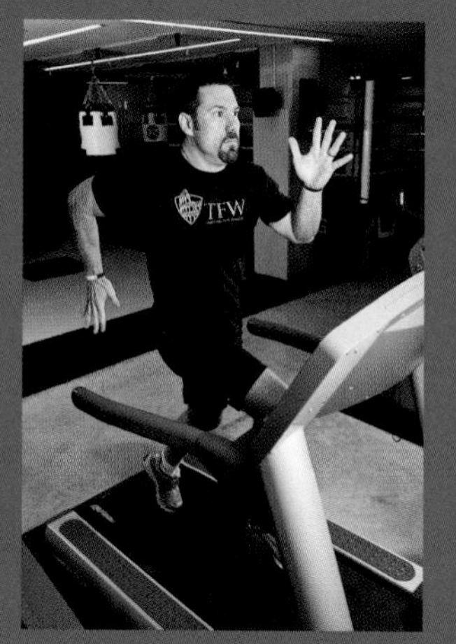

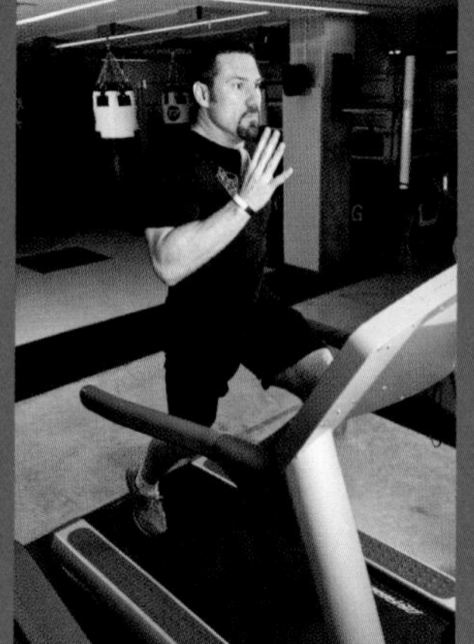

CATEGORY 2, ROUND 1

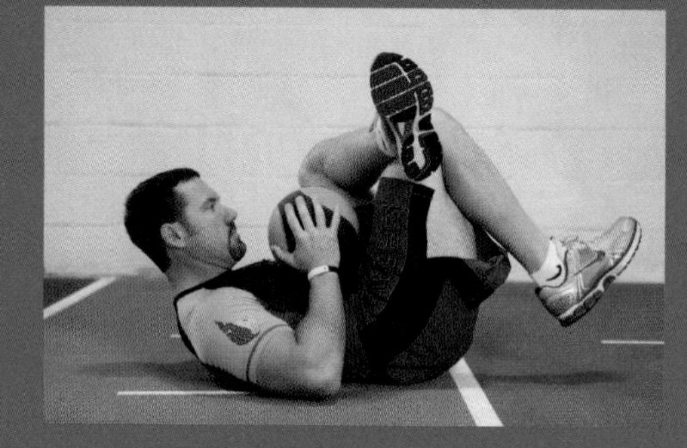

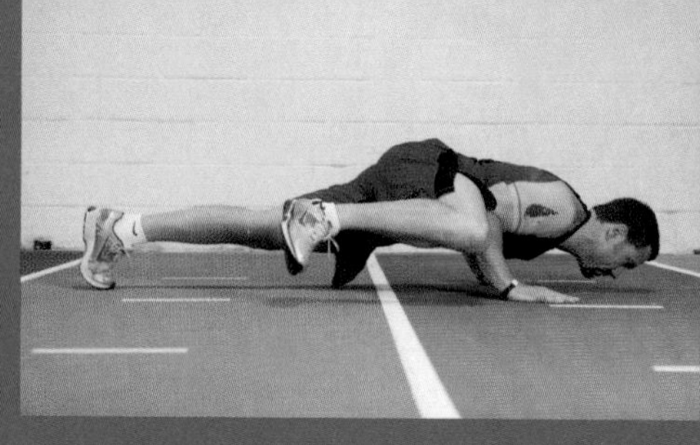

ROUND 2

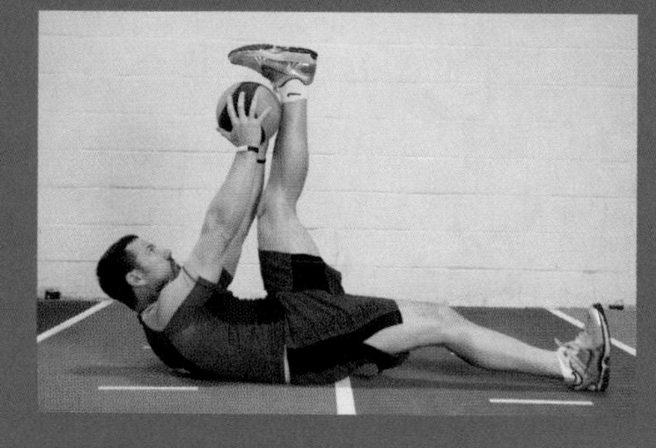

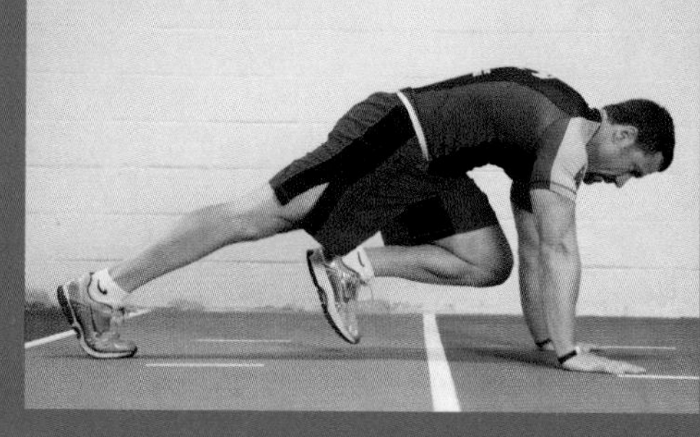

ROUND 3

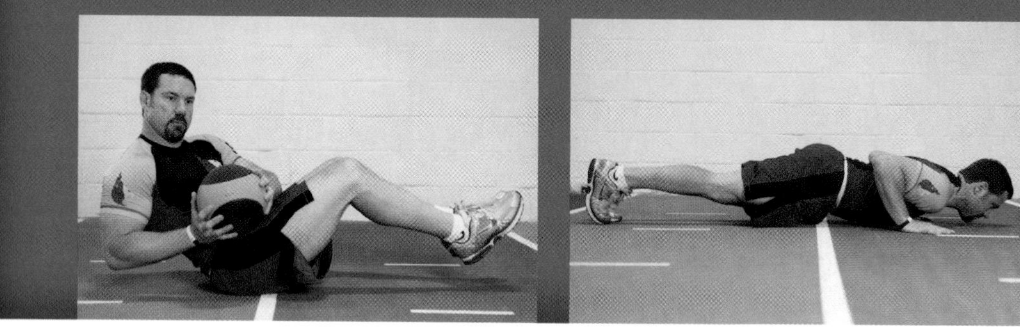

HURRICANE TRAINING CHEATSHEET

CATEGORY 3, ROUND 1

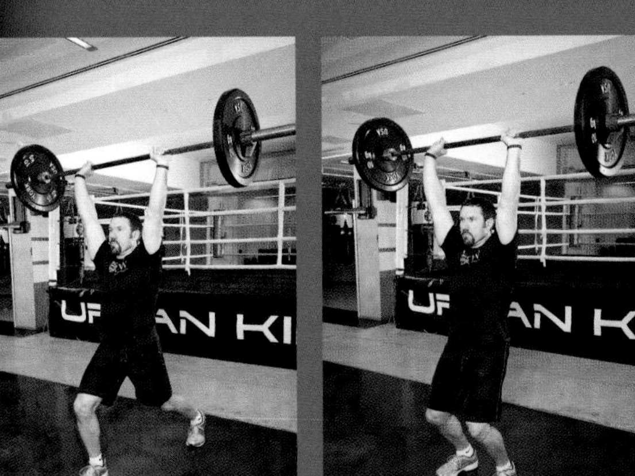

ROUND 2

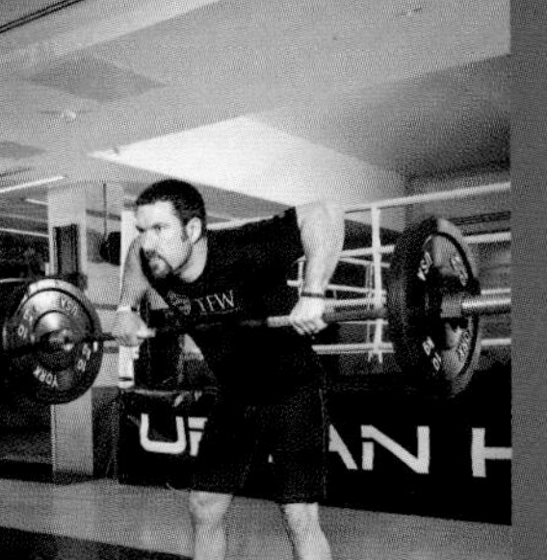

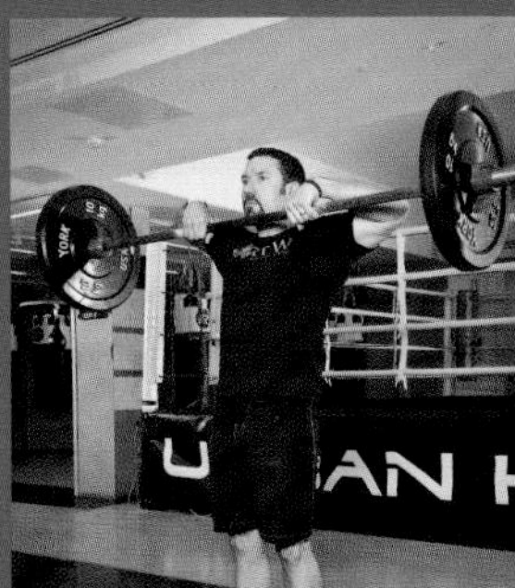

ROUND 3

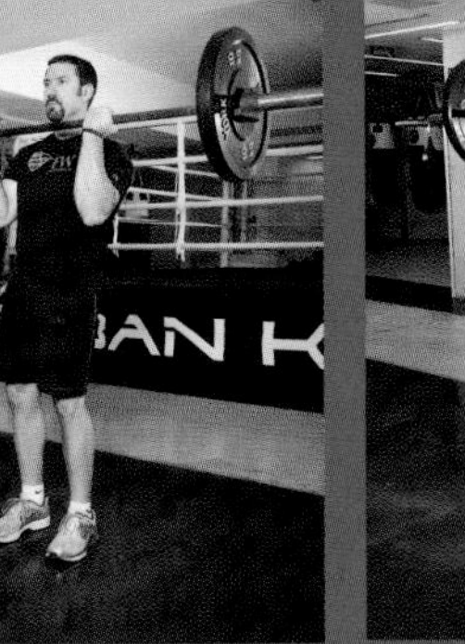

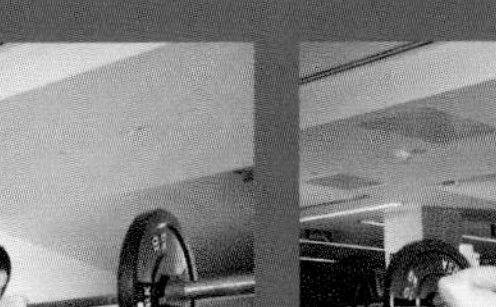

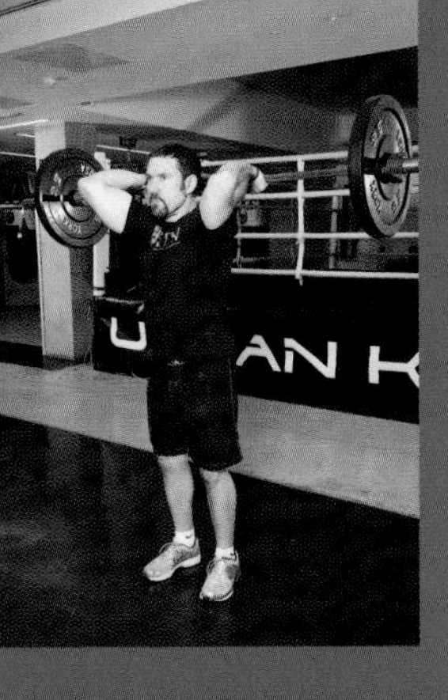

CATEGORY 4, ROUND 1

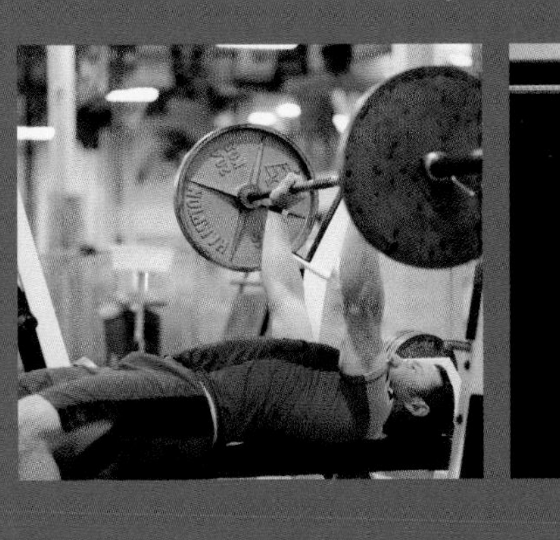

ROUND 2

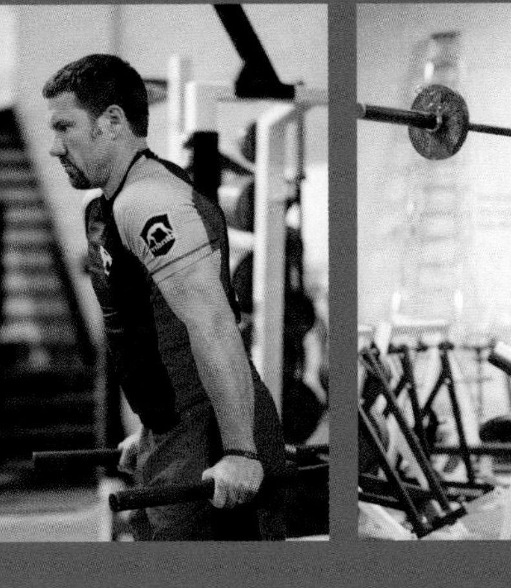

ROUND 3

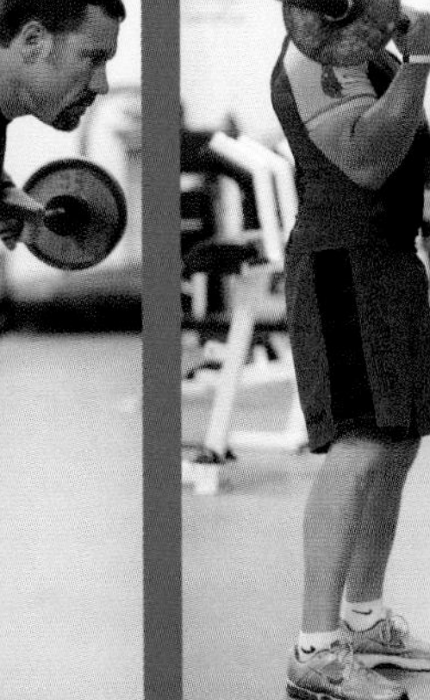

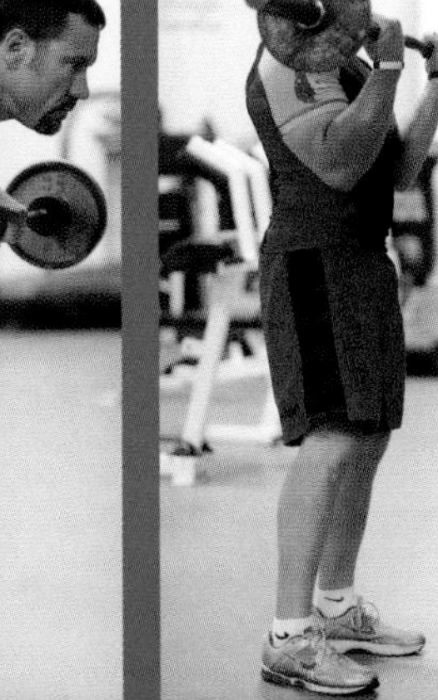

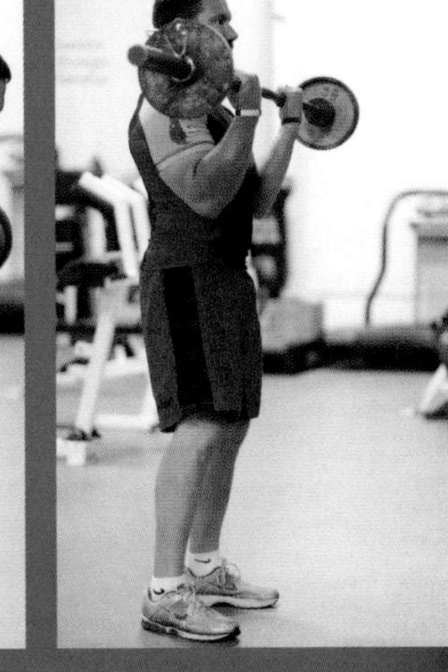

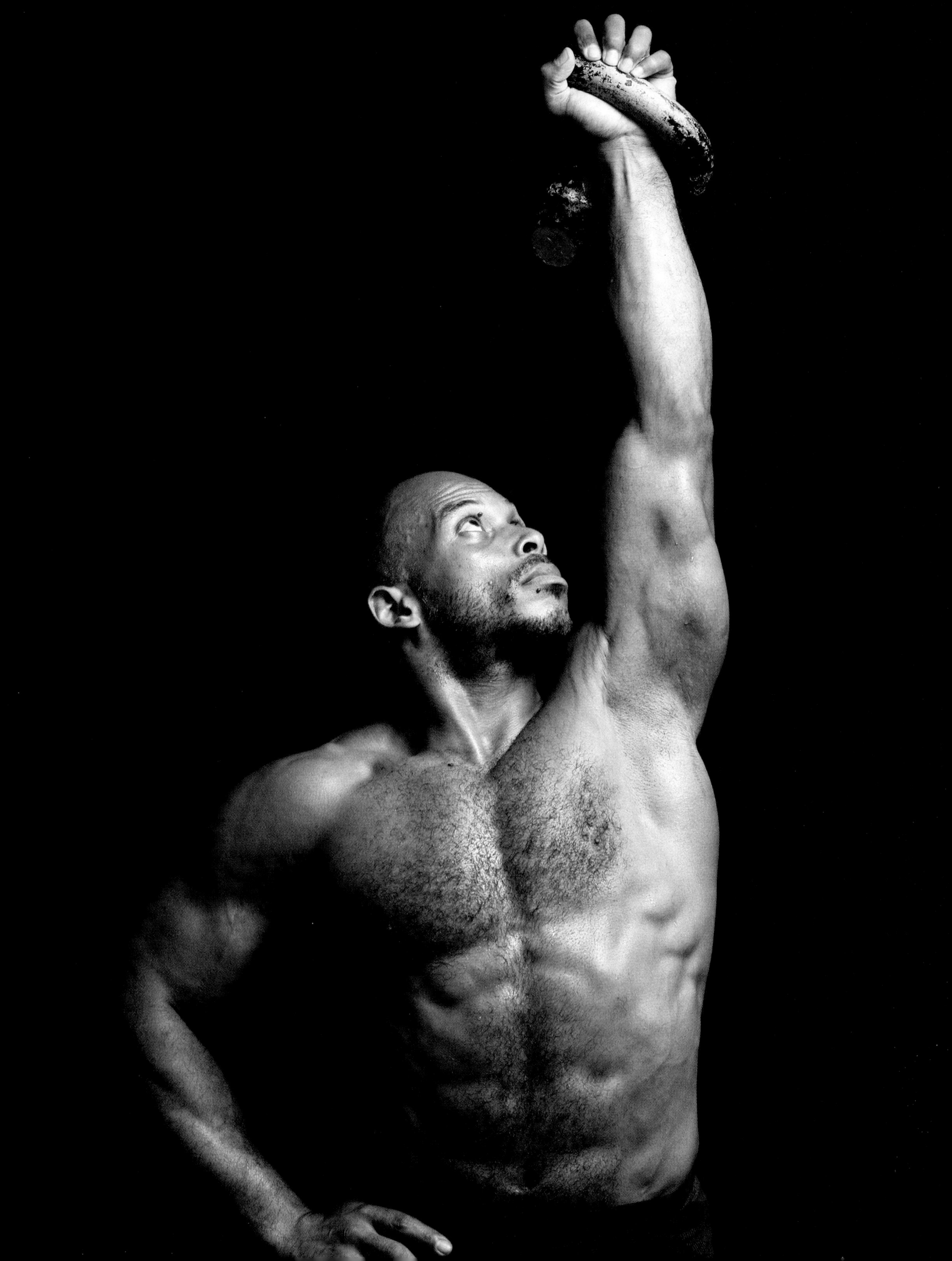

10

BARBELL, DUMBBELL, AND KETTLEBELL CIRCUITS

Using different training devices such as a barbell, dumbbell, or kettlebells in a continuous circuit is a popular form of Metabolic Training commonly known as complexes. Complexes are usually composed of two or more exercises that are performed in succession using the same exercise apparatus without stopping. A complex is usually measured according to volume, which is the total number of repetitions multiplied by the weight that is used. Historically, barbell and dumbbell complexes have been used sparingly over the last 20 years, but with the advent of the Internet and the explosion of other tools such as kettlebells, the use of complexes has become much more commonplace in training.

Since a complex can be used with a number of different pieces of equipment, a myriad of exercises, and practically any repetition scheme, the possibilities are endless. Usually when complexes are used, they differ in the exercise selection, number of exercises, or repetitions used. The difference in the way the TFW system utilizes complexes is that time is the main parameter for determining intensity.

More specifically, intensity is actually controlled in two ways. Since a TFW complex is required to be performed in a certain amount of time, the amount of weight (intensity) and speed of movement are affected. This is due to the fact that when a number of repetitions has to be performed in a certain amount of time, you are forced to increase the intensity of the performance. Without the element of time, although the complex may still be taxing, optimal results may not be produced. It also becomes more difficult to monitor an improvement in performance from one workout to the next. The use of time also ensures that the proper weight has been selected for certain lifts. Too much weight would slow the complex and since the goal of this style of training is to create a metabolic disturbance, there is no sense in using slower movements in order to use more weight. By performing sets for time, I have found the maximum metabolic disturbance can be created.

In order to use time to measure progress and also select training weights for maximum intensity, the TFW system uses 30 or 60 seconds as the set maximums for the barbell and dumbbell complexes contained in this chapter. This means that your goal is to perform the entire complex in under 30 or 60 seconds. Once you are able to do this, you are allowed to increase the weight of the exercise. If you are unable to do this, you remain at that weight or lessen the weight until you can still hit the goal time. This way, you will be able to monitor records in terms of time at every weight in which you perform a complex. This makes it easy to assess progress and control your training program.

Work/rest ratios for complexes are ultimately up to you, but I would recommend at least a 1:2 ratio and a maximum of five total complexes per workout. The larger the muscles utilized in a complex, the longer you may wish to make your work/rest ratio. For instance, a complex of barbell curls, high pulls, and overhead presses is much less stressful than back squats, lunges, and front squats.

You will notice that when performing a complex, there will be one exercise that is often the "limiting" exercise of the set. This means that there may be one exercise in which the weight selected is the most difficult to perform. The limiting exercise ensures the use of lighter weight and that the goal time can be achieved. For instance, a barbell curl is the limiting exercise when compared to the deadlift when they are both within the same complex.

Since the barbell, dumbbell, and kettlebell are versatile tools, there are a wide range of exercises that can be selected to create a complex. As with every form of Metabolic Training featured in this book, practitioners are often culprits of poor technique during the use of complexes. Although the weight is often reduced during a complex, this does not give you license to utilize poor form as a result of fatigue, increased speed, or lack of prior practice. In the Training for Warriors system, the 10 Commandments of Metabolic Training clearly state that the goal is to use excellent form while still performing high volumes of work. This consistency of execution will allow you to recognize whether you are making progress from one complex to another by making sure that form is kept to a high standard.

The intensity of a complex can be altered in the following ways: exercise selection, number of exercises performed, number of repetitions performed, amount of weight selected, total volume of the complex, duration of the complex, speed of movement, rest periods, and total number of complexes performed.

A. BARBELL COMPLEXES: LOWER BODY

This complex is to be completed in 30 seconds. Each exercise is to be performed for 10 repetitions.

1. ZERCHER SQUAT

Begin standing while holding the barbell in the crook of the elbows. While maintaining posture, squat down until the elbows almost touch the knees. Press down with both feet and return to the original position.

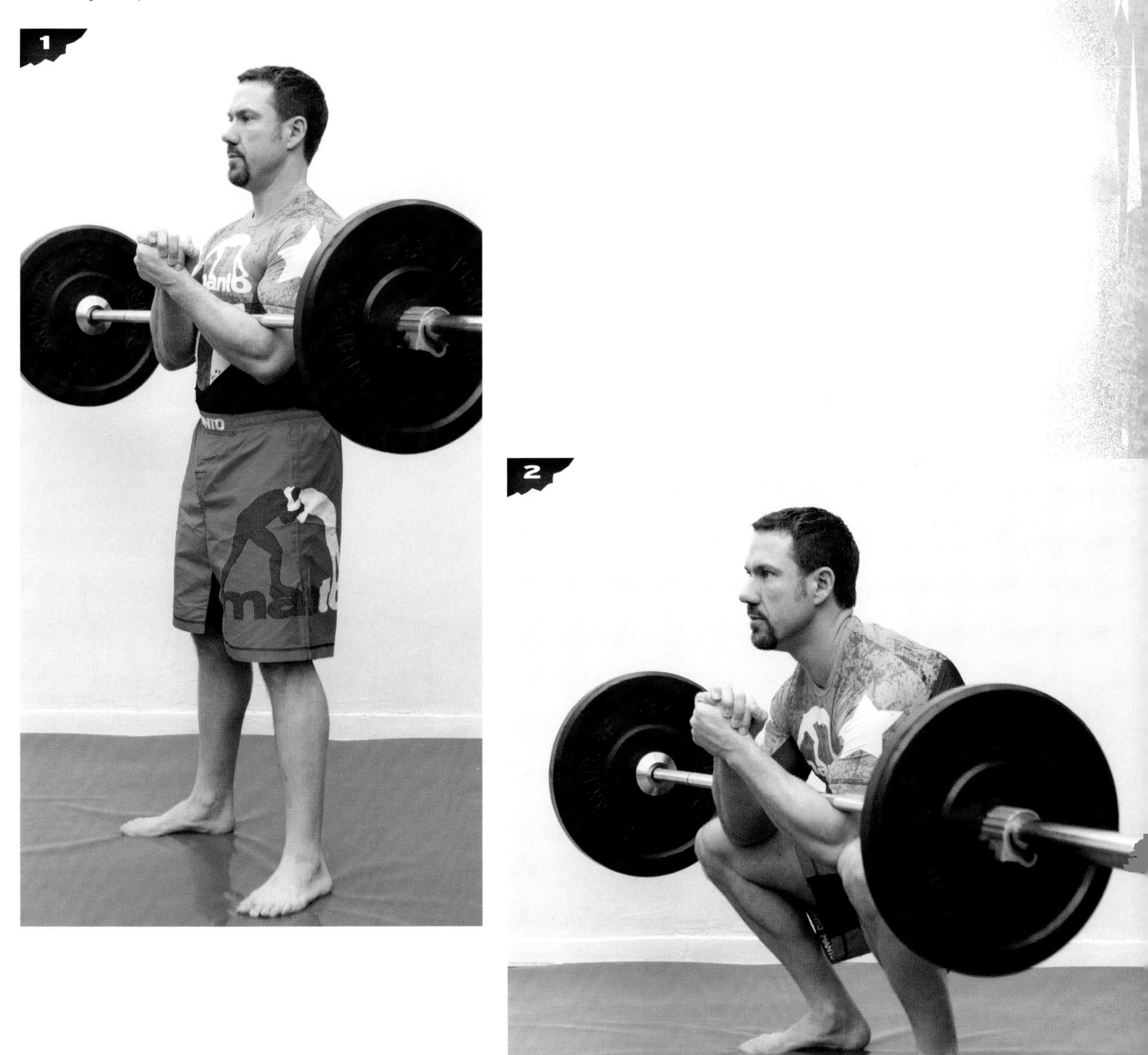

2. ZERCHER LUNGE

Begin standing while holding the barbell in the crook of the elbows. Step forward with one leg and lower the body so that the back knee almost touches the ground. Press back into the ground with the front foot and return to the original position.

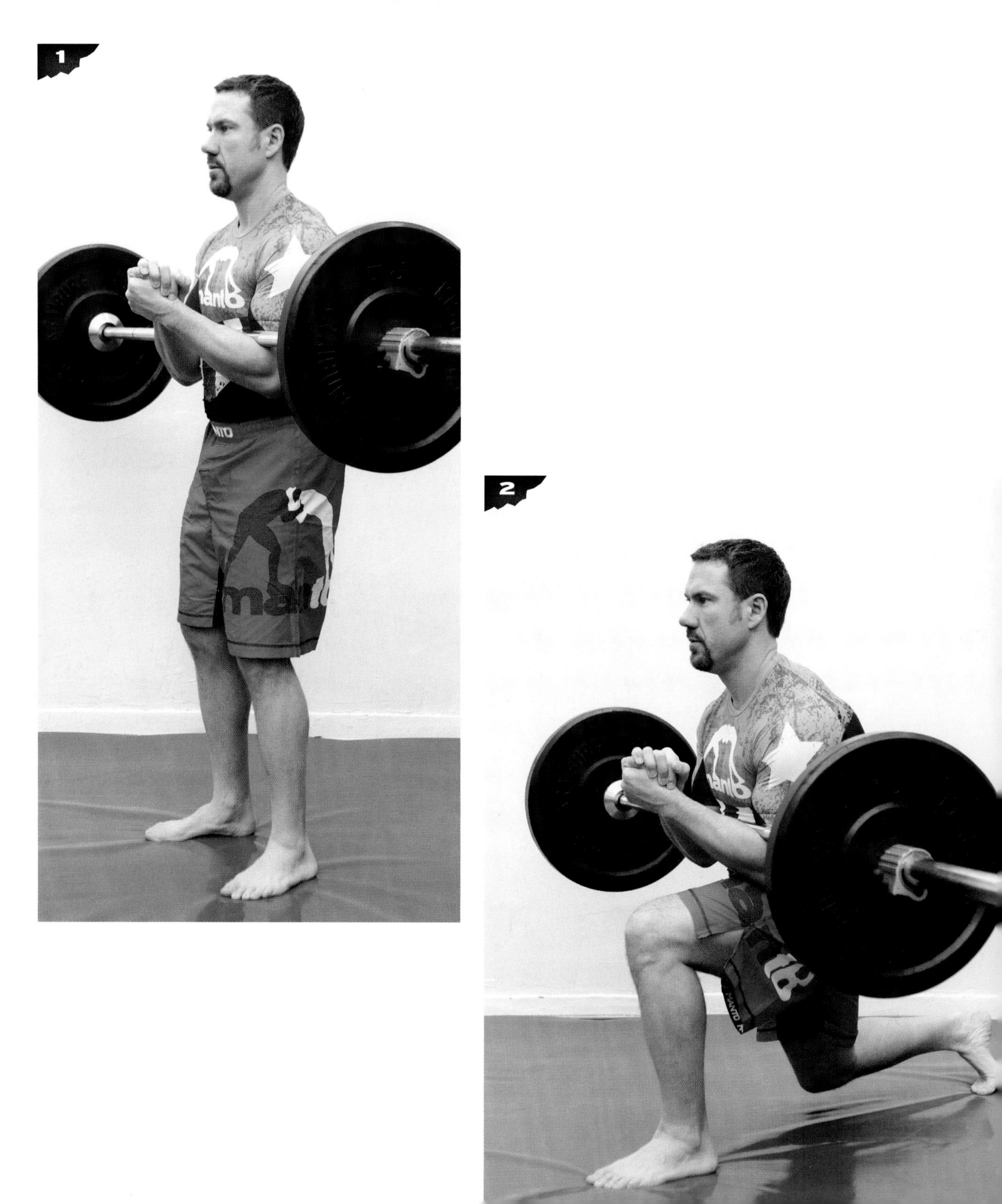

3. ZERCHER GOOD MORNING

Begin standing while holding the barbell in the crook of the elbows. Lean forward at the waist while slightly bending the knees. Extend at the lower back and return to the original position.

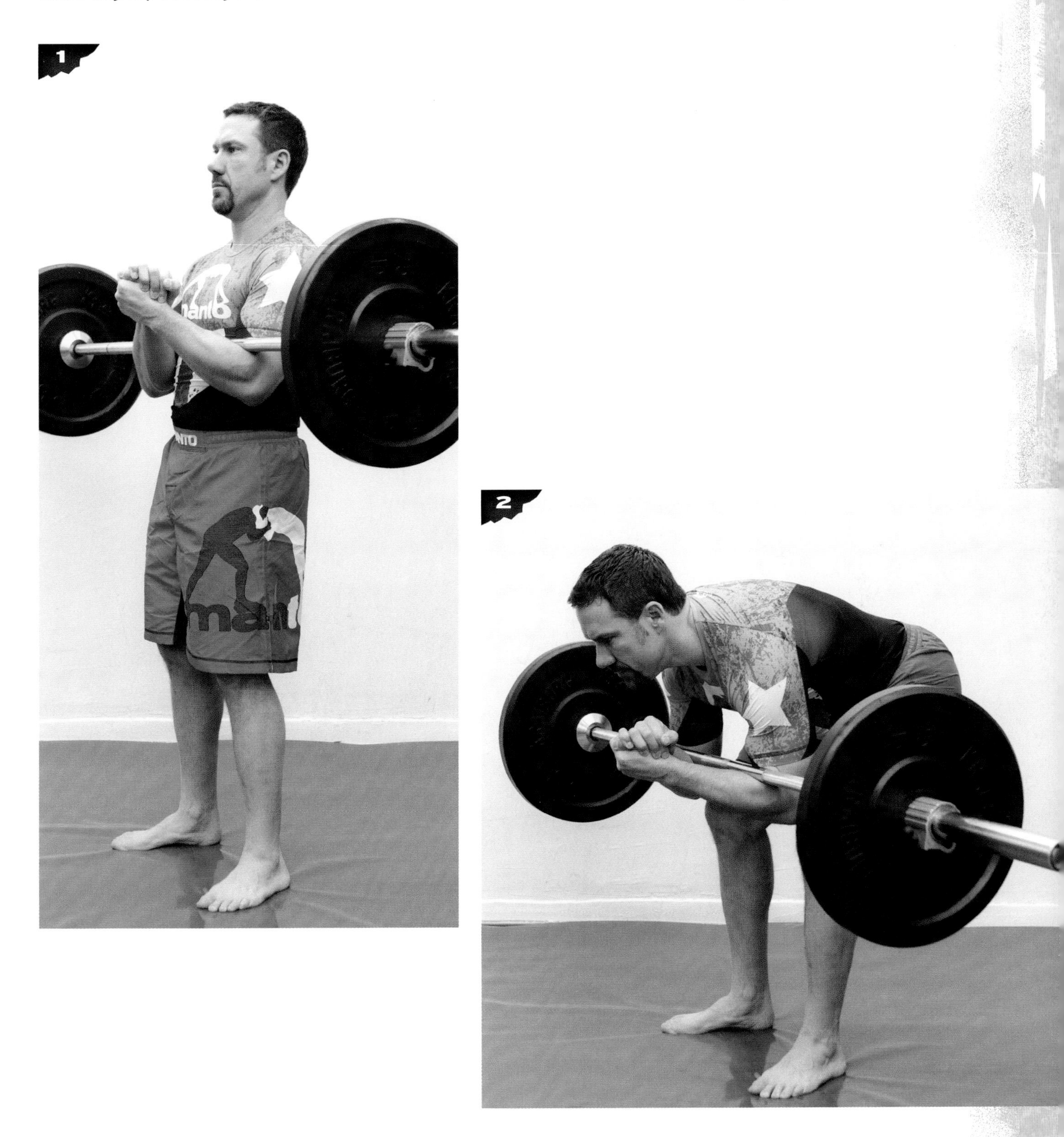

B. BARBELL COMPLEXES: UPPER BODY

This complex is to be completed in 30 seconds. Each exercise is to be performed for 10 repetitions.

1. BENT-OVER ROW

Begin by leaning forward and holding the bar at knee height with a shoulder-width grip. Pull the elbows back so that the bar touches the chest at nipple level. Lower to the original position and repeat.

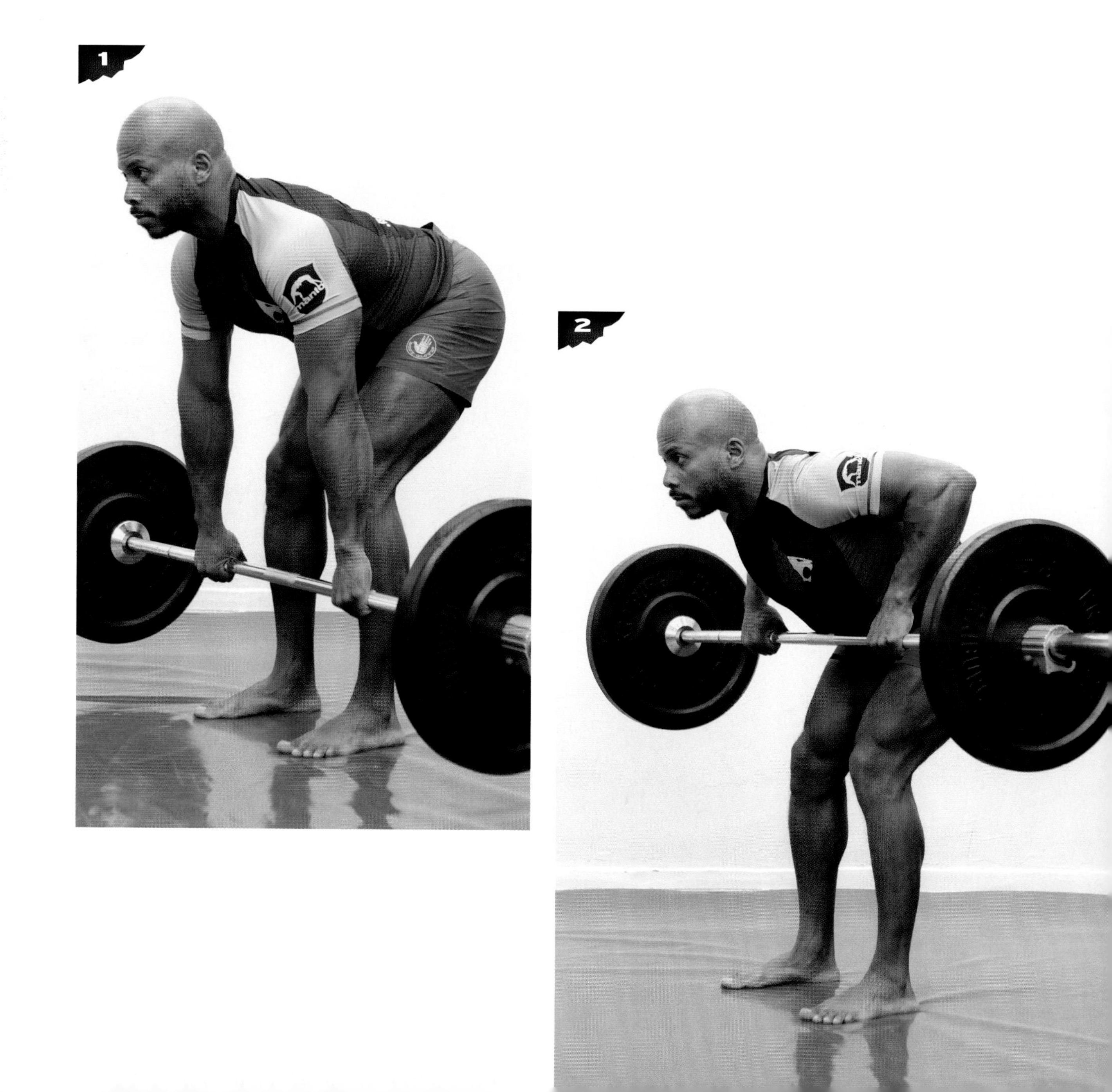

2. HIGH PULL

Stand up and switch the hands to a grip slightly narrower than shoulder width. Bring the bar from the height of the waist up to the chest by pulling the elbows up to ear height. Lower to the original position and repeat.

1

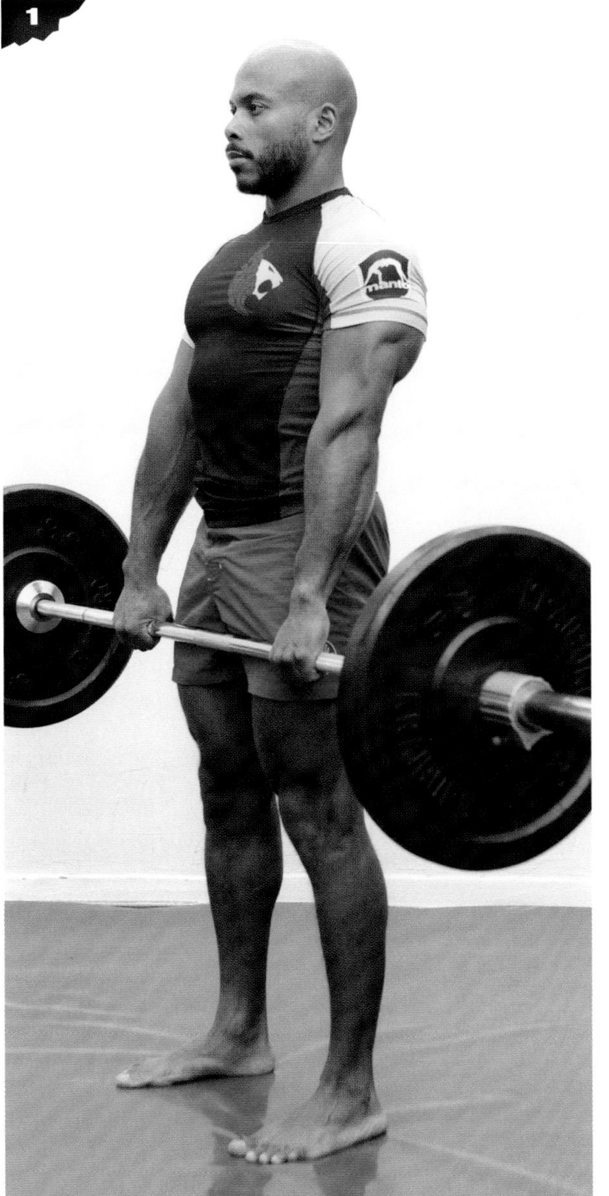

2

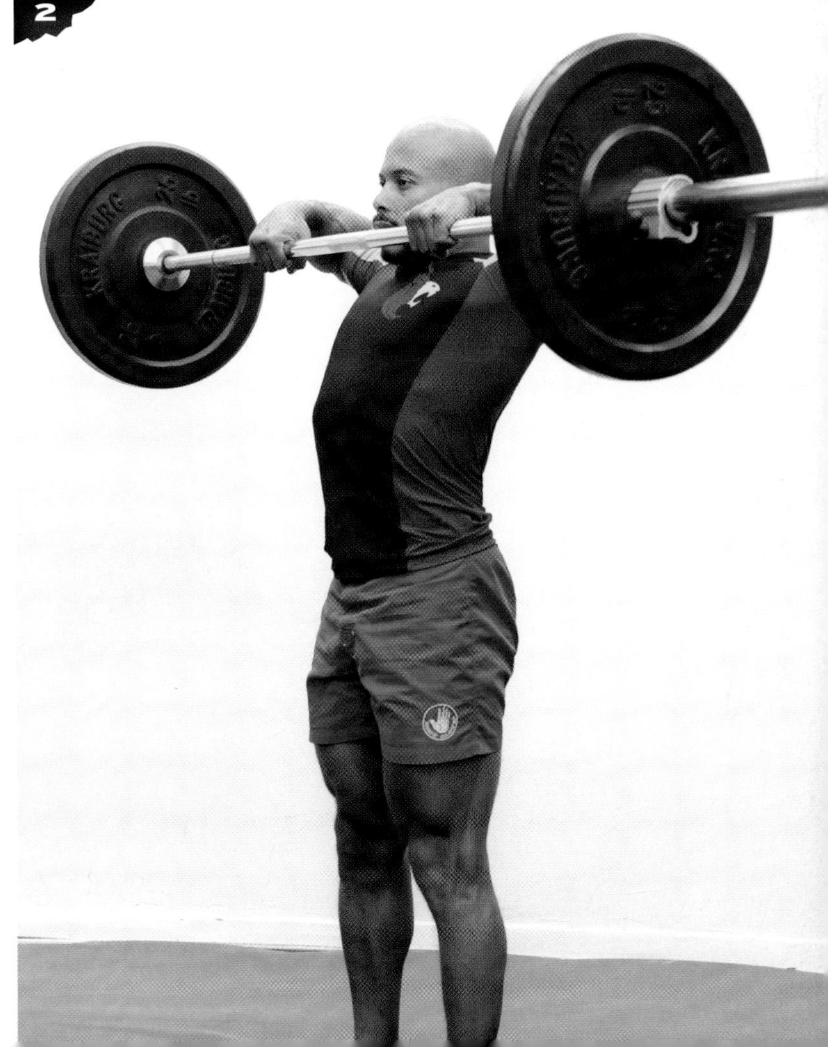

3. OVERHEAD PRESS

Hold the bar at chest height with a shoulder-width grip. Press the bar overhead by extending at the elbows. Lower the bar to the chest and repeat.

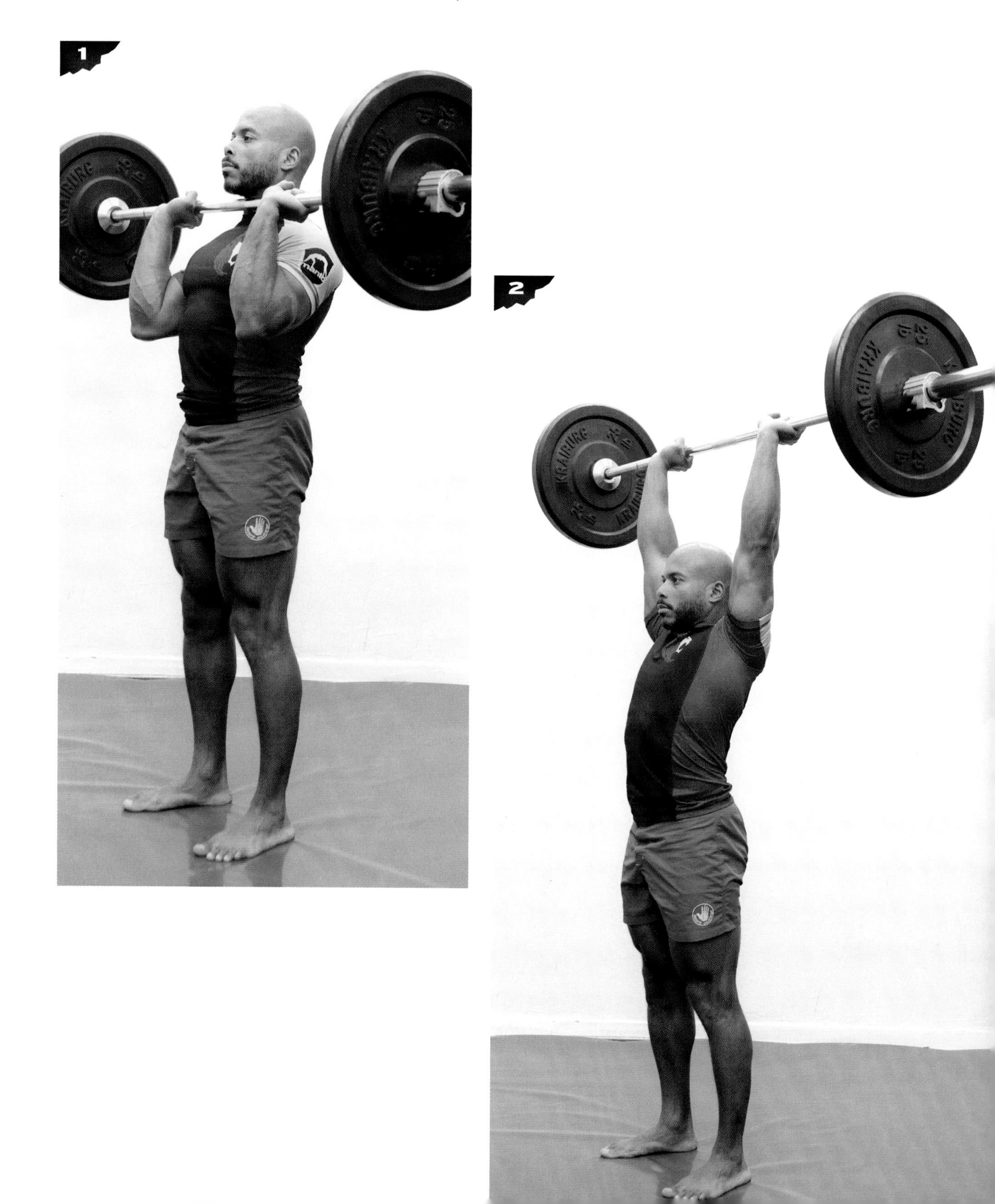

C. BARBELL COMPLEXES: FULL BODY

This complex is to be completed in either 30 or 60 seconds. Each exercise is to be performed for either 5 or 10 repetitions depending on the time frame selected.

1. STIFF-LEGGED DEADLIFT

Start by standing with the bar held in a shoulder-width grip at the height of the hips. While keeping the lower back flat and the knees slightly bent, bend forward at the waist so that the bar passes more than halfway down the shin. Extend at the lower back and return to the original position.

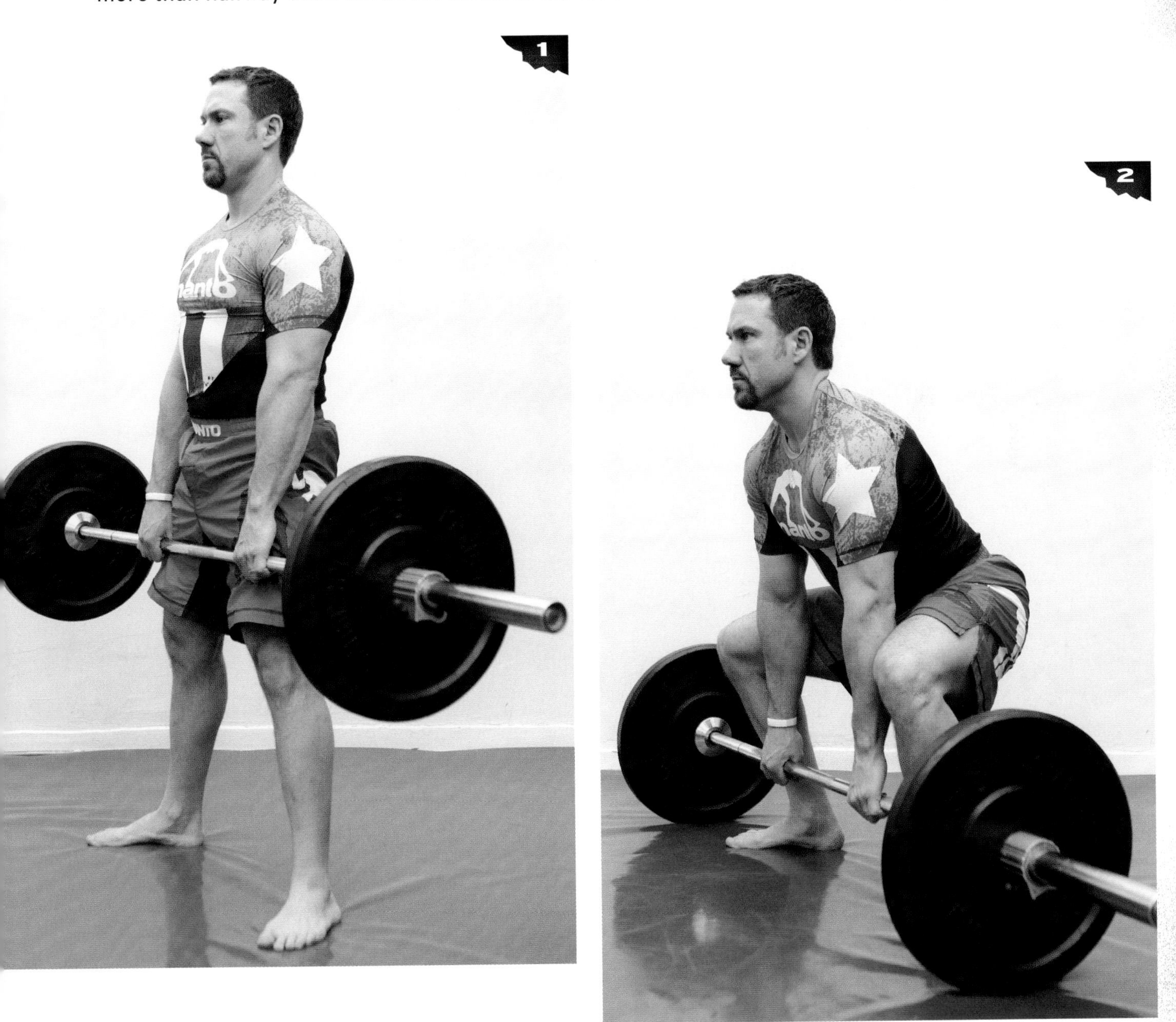

2. WIDE-GRIP BENT-OVER ROW

Begin by leaning forward and holding the bar at knee height with a wider than shoulder-width grip. Pull the elbows back so that the bar touches the chest at nipple level. Lower to the original position and repeat.

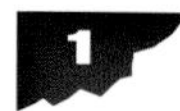

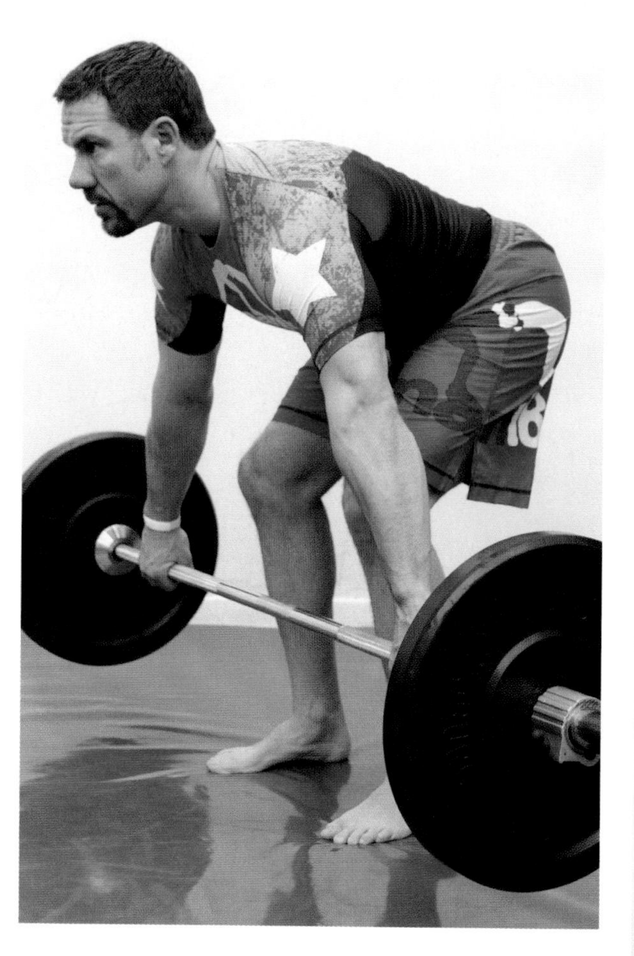

2

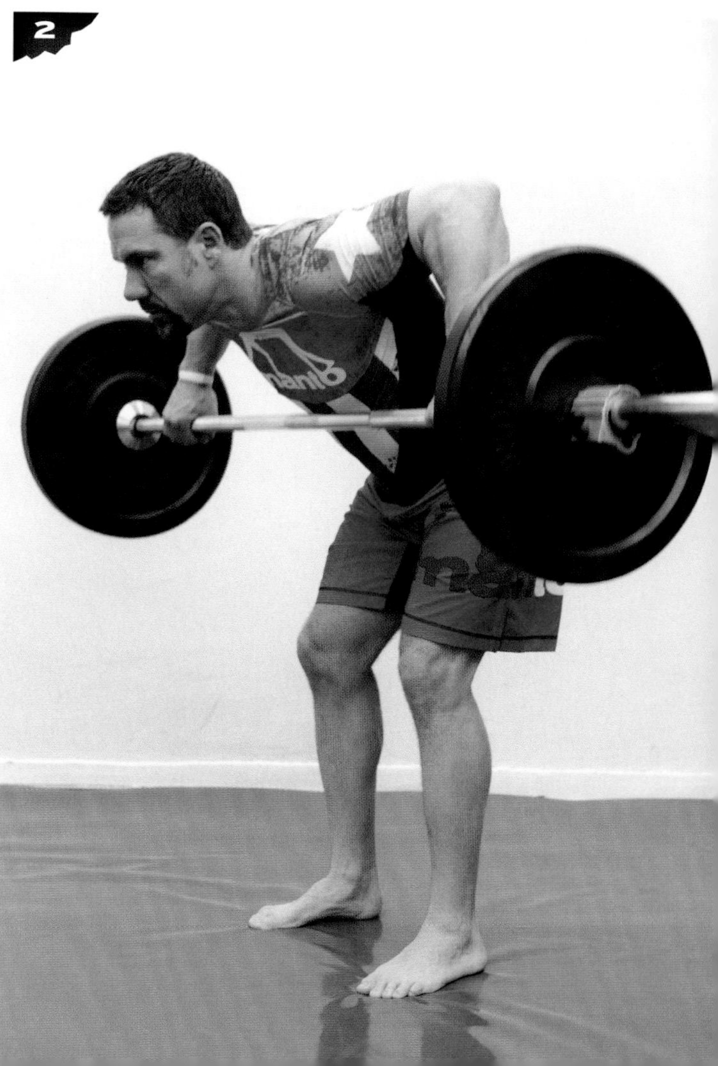

3. HIGH PULL

Stand up and switch the hands to a grip slightly narrower than shoulder width. Bring the bar from the height of the waist up to the chest by pulling the elbows up to ear height. Lower to the original position and repeat.

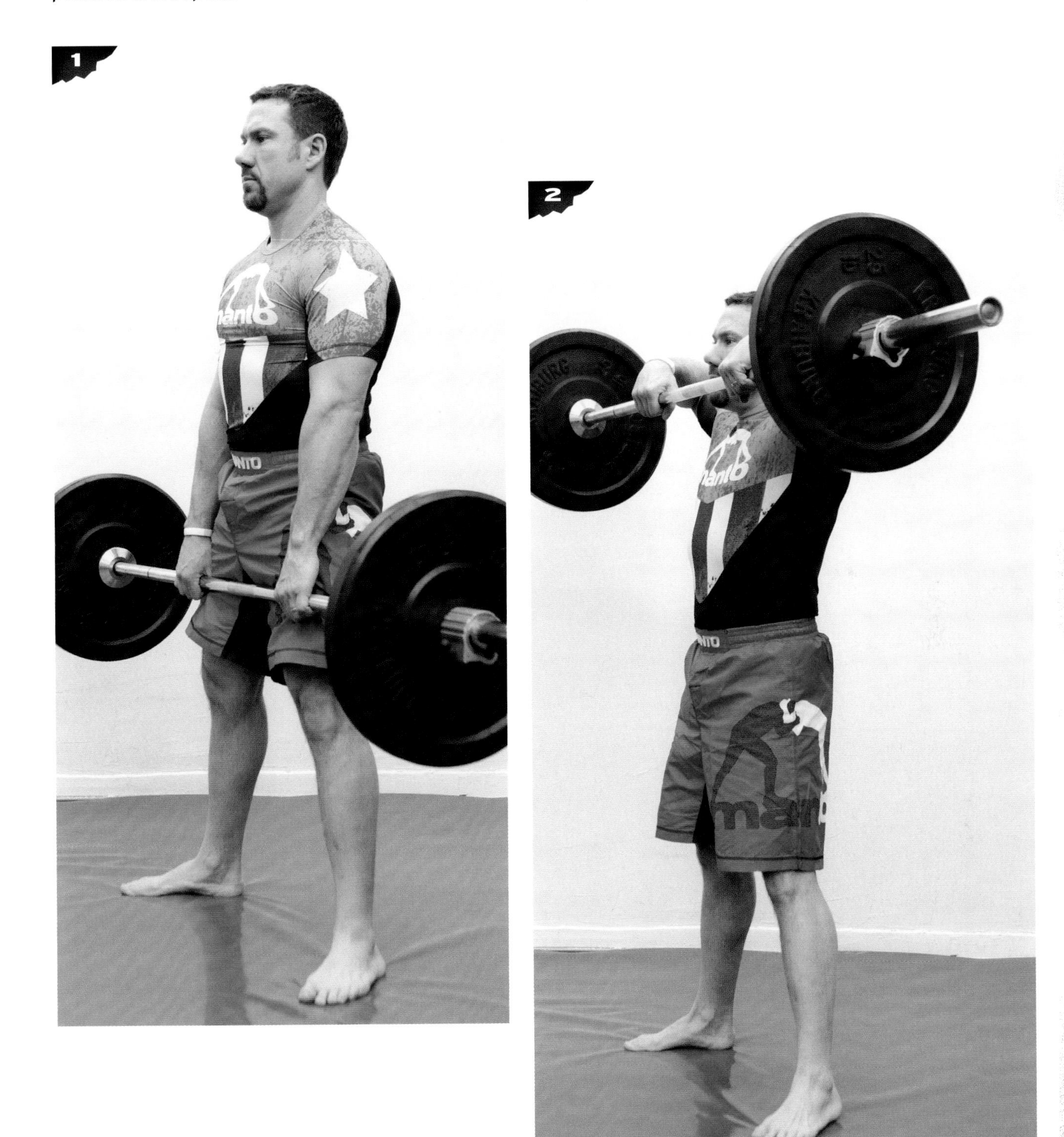

4. FRONT SQUAT

Bring the bar to the clean position at the height of the shoulders. Lower the hips to the parallel-squat position by bending at the knee. Press up by extending at the knees, hips, and low back.

1

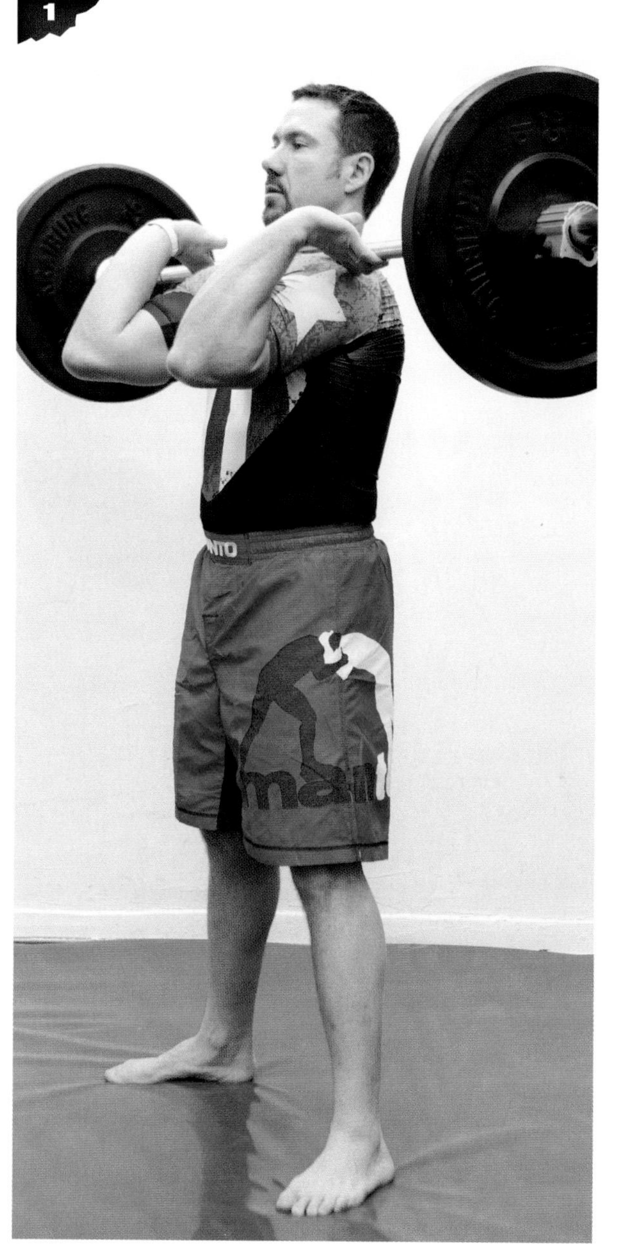

2

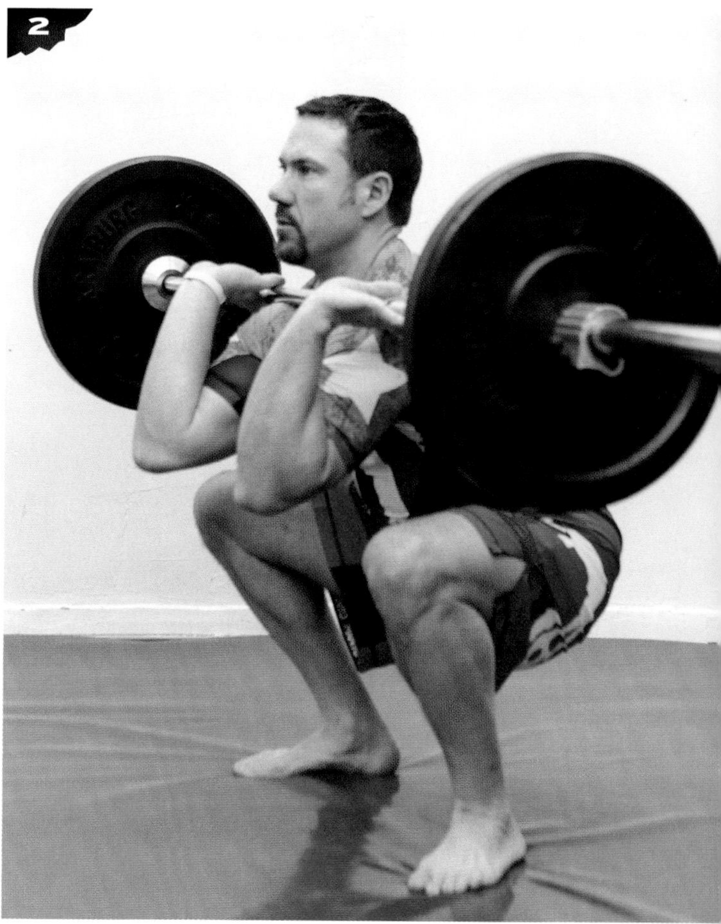

5. OVERHEAD PRESS

Hold the bar at chest height with a shoulder-width grip. Press the bar overhead by extending at the elbows. Lower the bar to the chest and repeat.

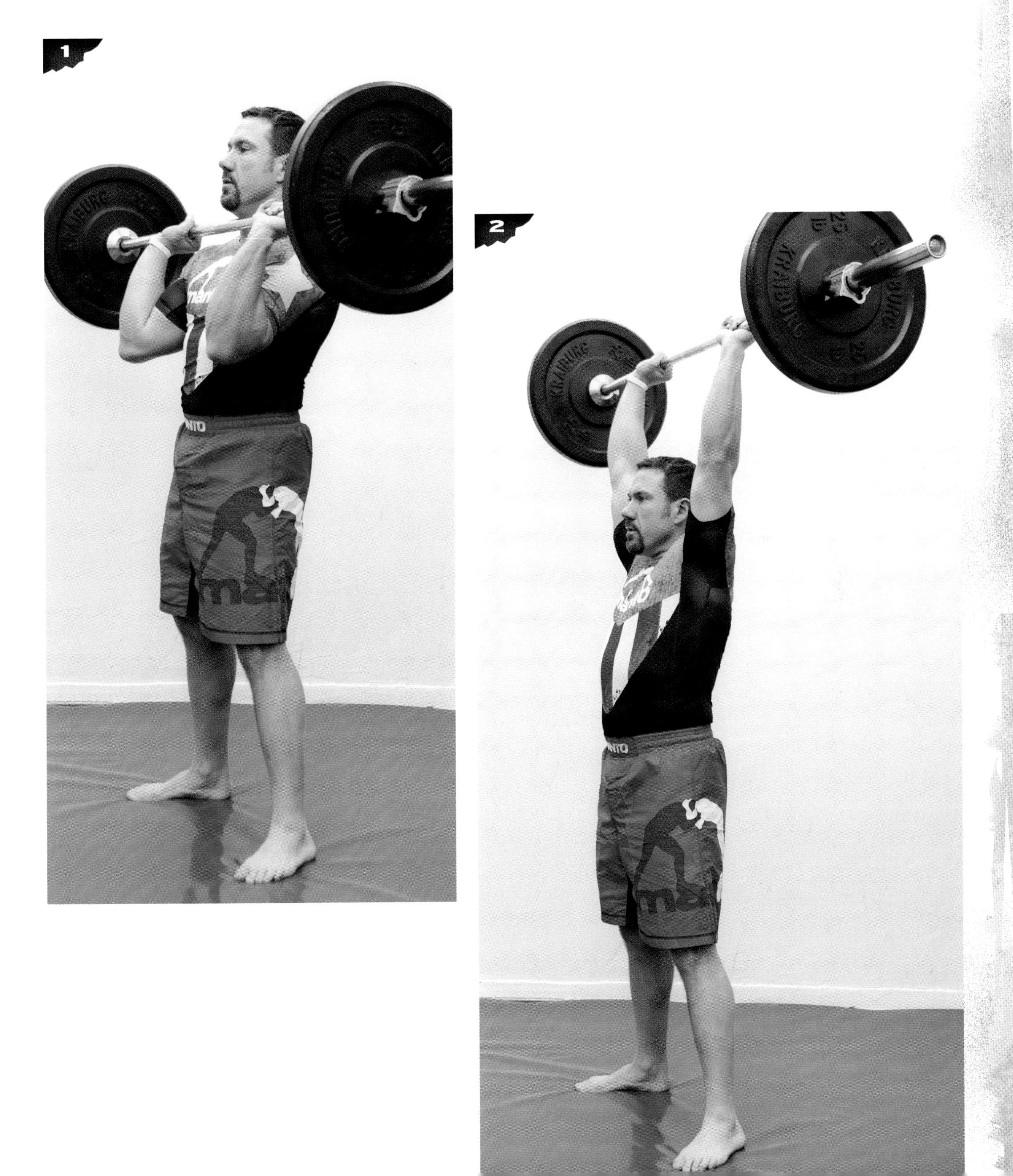

6. BACK SQUAT

Bring the bar overhead and place it behind the neck. Lower the hips to the parallel-squat position by bending at the knee. Press up by extending at the knees, hips, and lower back.

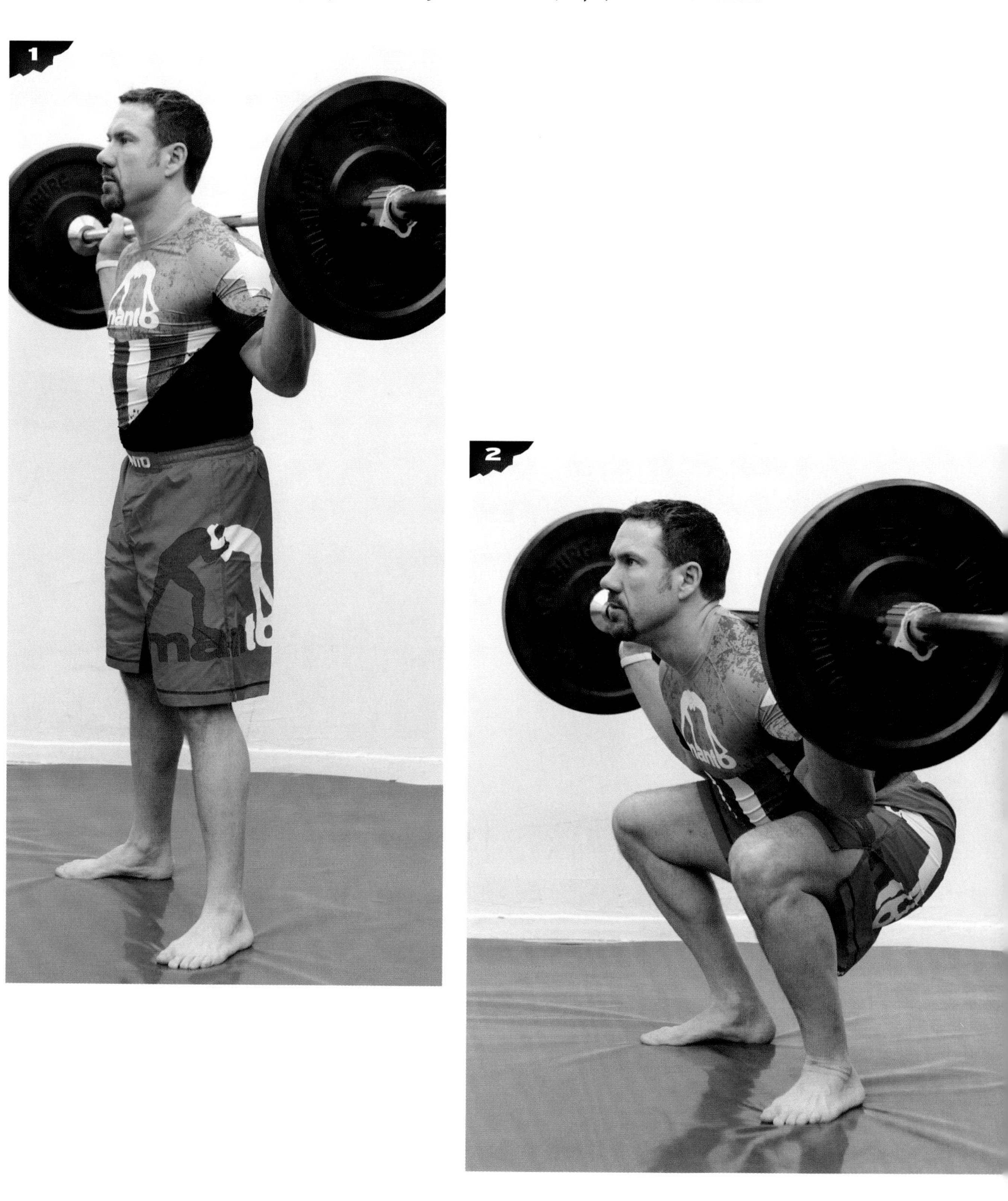

D. BARBELL COMPLEXES: 10-EXERCISE CIRCUIT

This complex is to be completed in either 30 or 60 seconds. Each exercise is to be performed for either 3 or 6 repetitions depending on the time frame selected.

1. STIFF-LEGGED DEADLIFT

Start by standing with the bar held by a shoulder-width grip at the height of the hips. While keeping the lower back flat and the knees slightly bent, bend forward at the waist so that the bar passes more than halfway down the shin. Extend at the lower back and return to the original position.

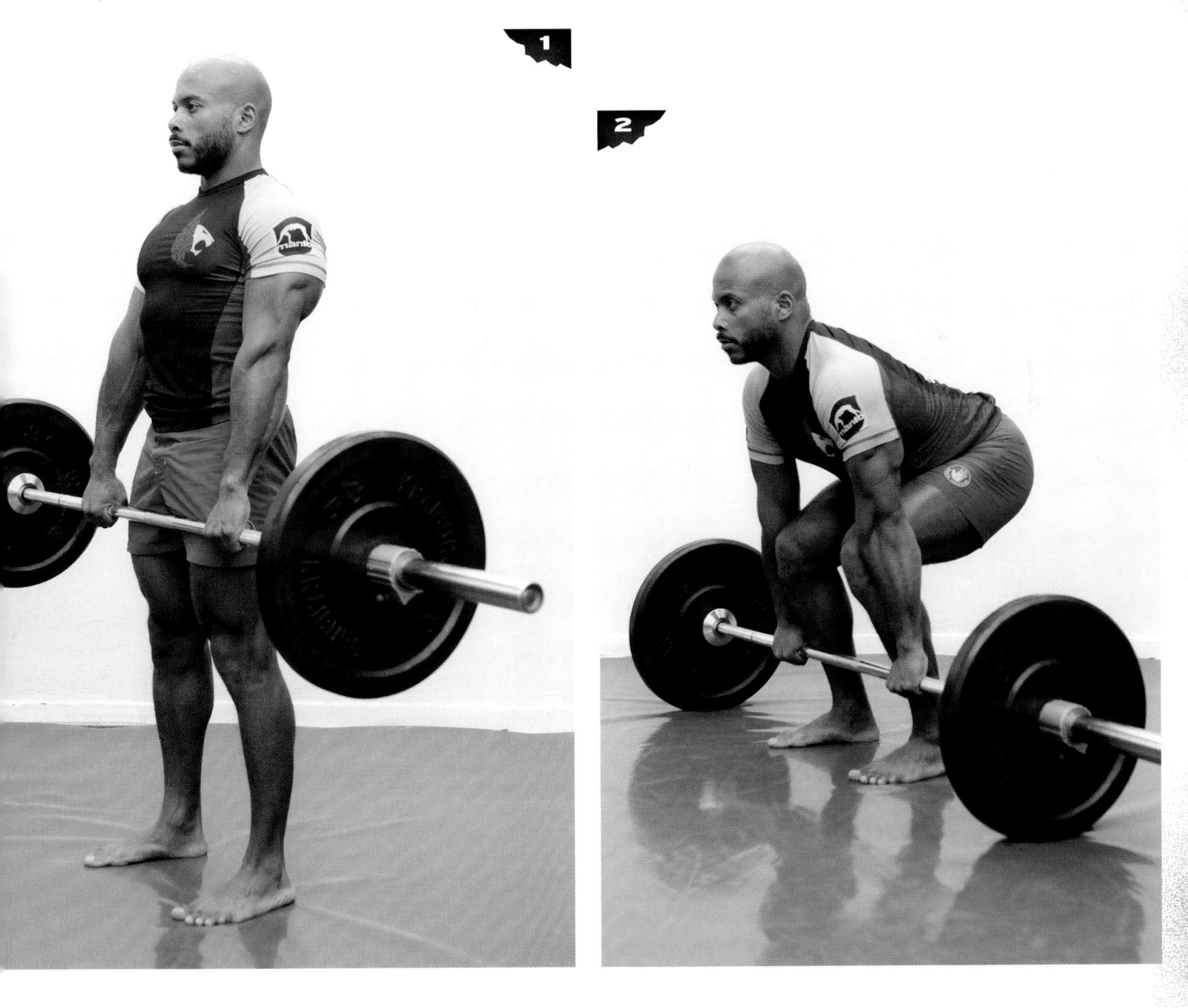

2. SHRUG

Begin with the bar held by a shoulder-width grip at the height of the hips. Pull the shoulders up toward the ears while keeping the elbows extended. Lower back to the original position.

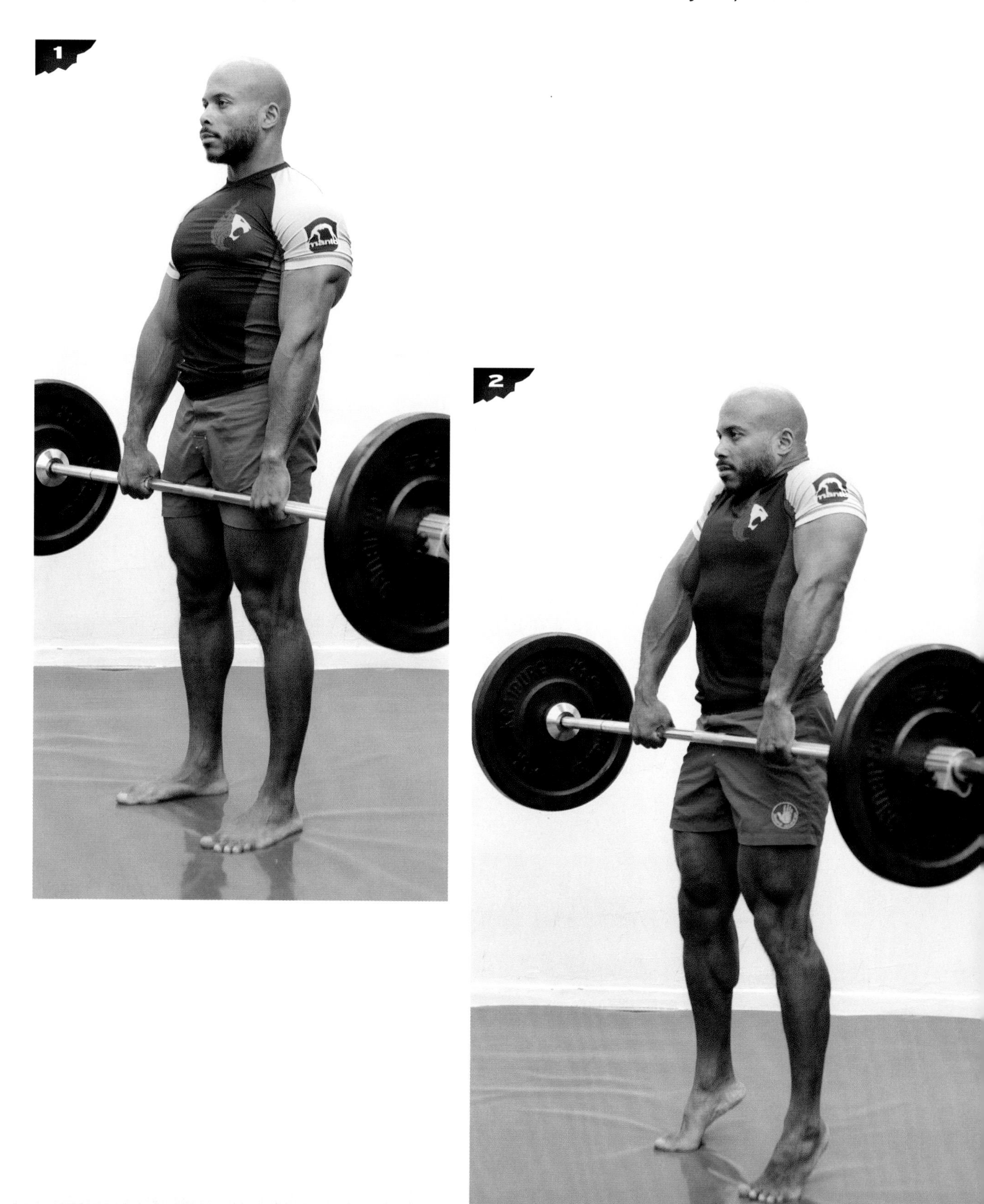

3. CLEAN

Start by standing with the bar held by a shoulder-width grip at the height of the mid-thigh. Quickly jump and shrug the bar up to the clean position. Lower the weight back to the start position and repeat.

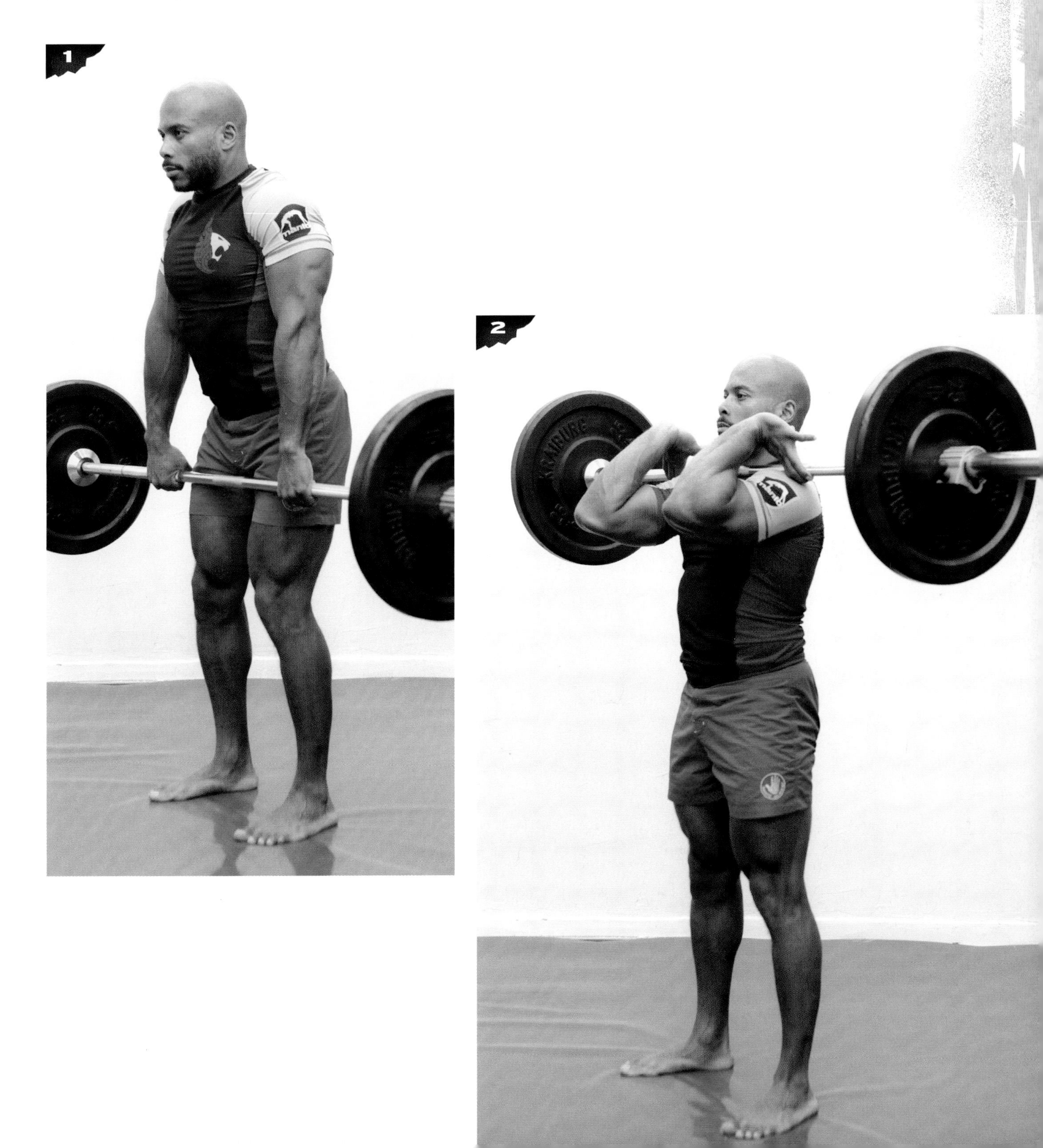

4. PUSH JERK

Hold the bar at chest height with a shoulder-width grip. Press the bar overhead by extending at the elbows and using the legs for power. Lower the bar to the chest and repeat.

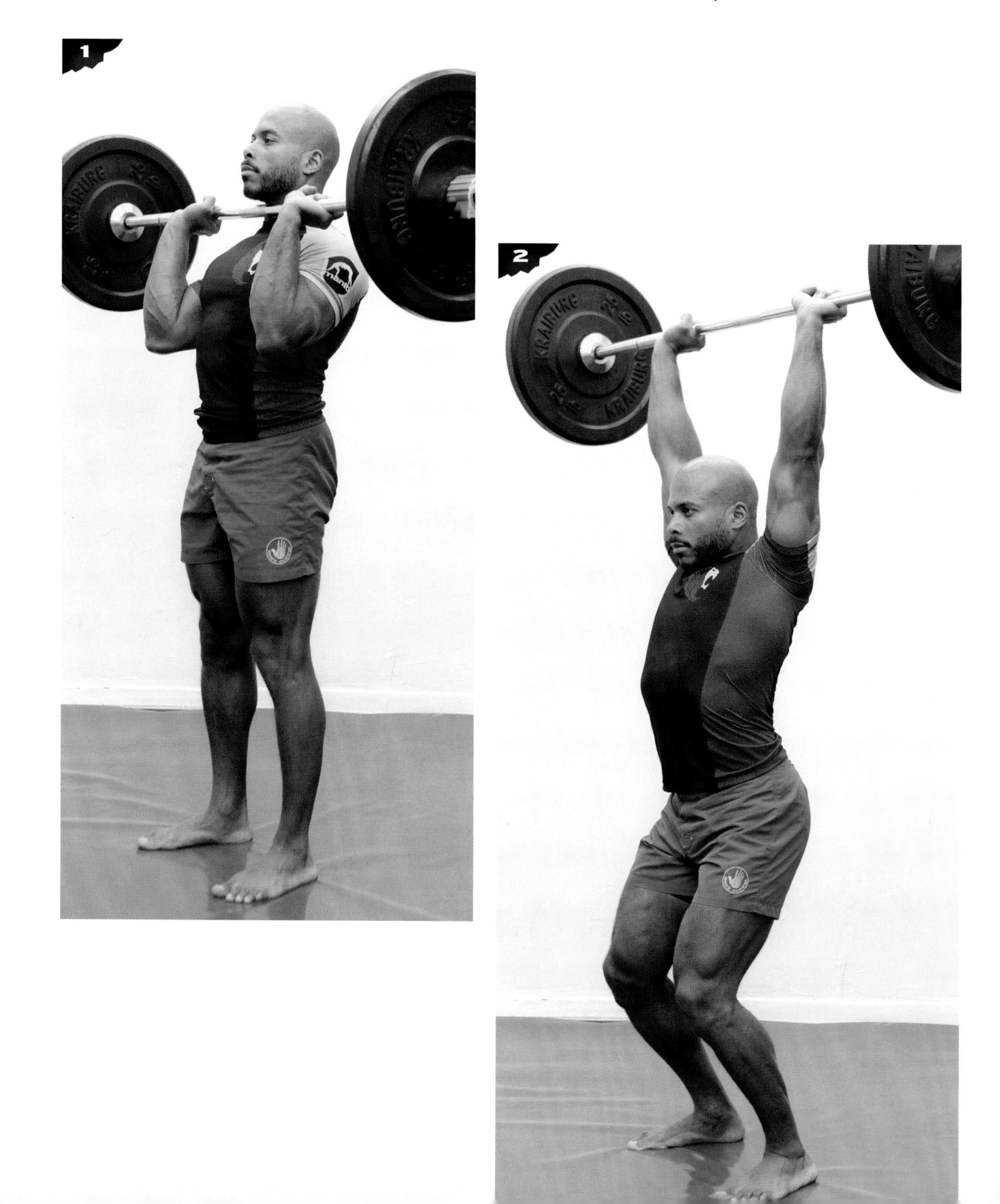

5. HIGH PULL

Stand up and switch the hands to a grip slightly narrower than shoulder width. Bring the bar from the height of the waist up to the chest by pulling the elbows up to ear height. Lower to the original position and repeat.

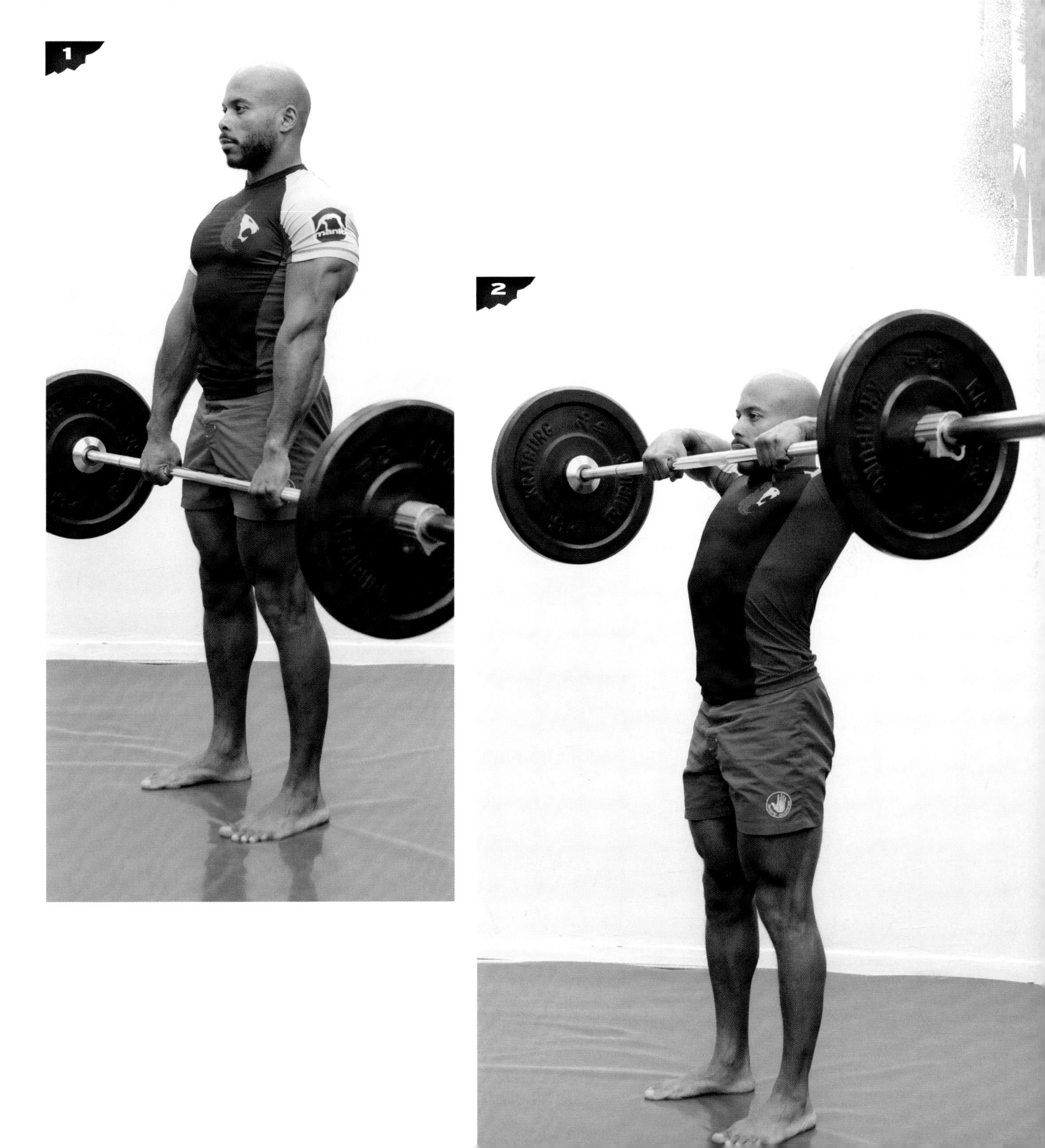

6. BENT-OVER ROW

Begin by leaning forward and holding the bar at knee height with a wider than shoulder-width grip. Pull the elbows back so that the bar touches the chest at nipple level. Lower to the original position and repeat.

1

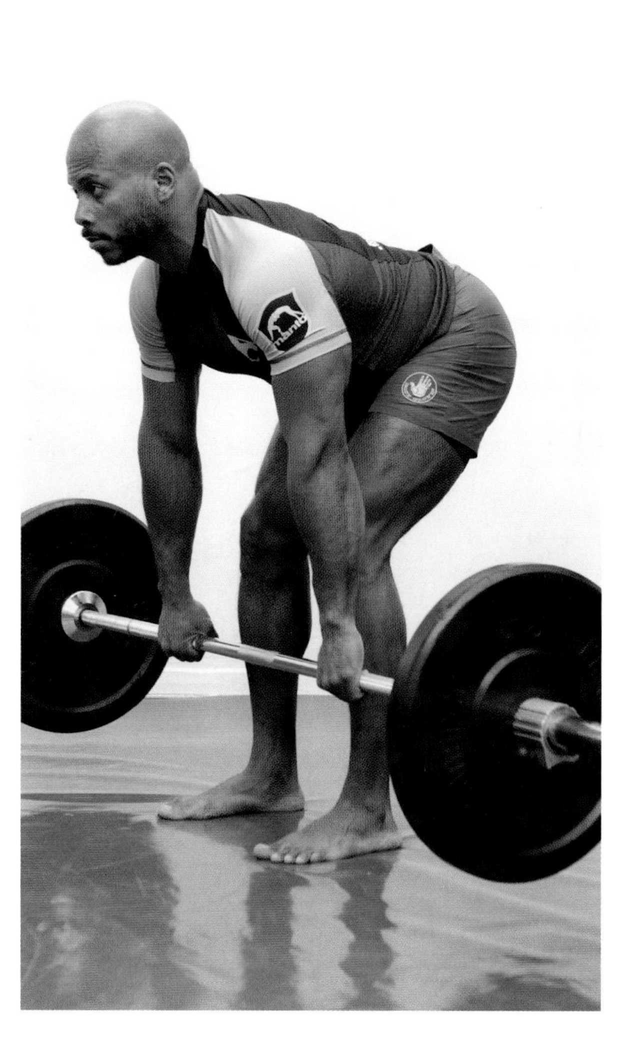

2

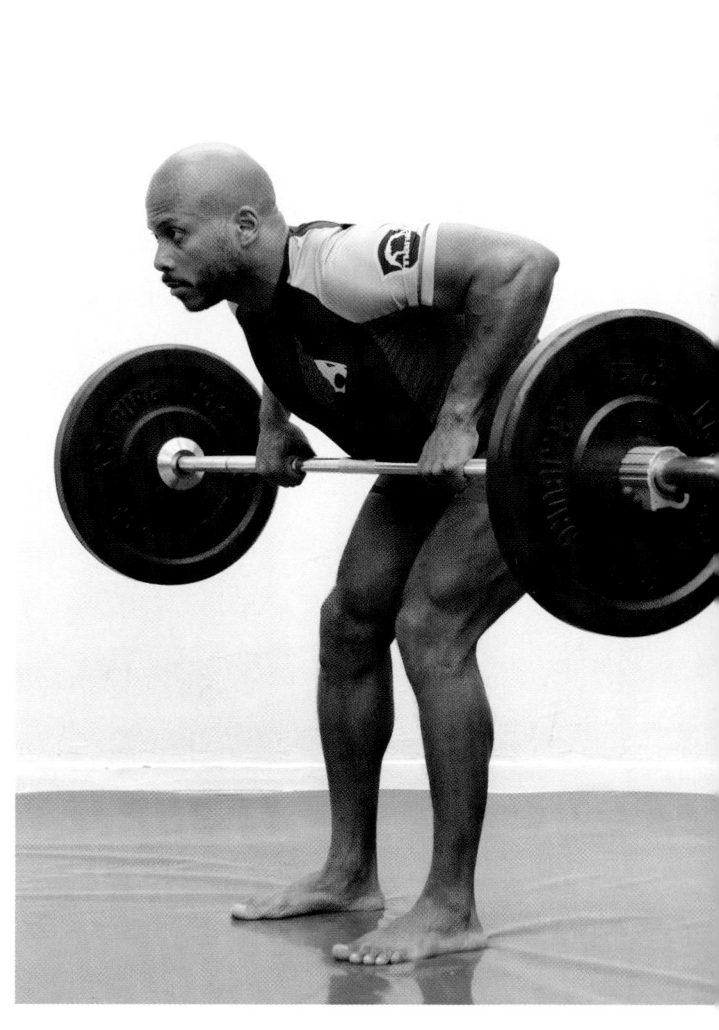

7. JUMP SQUAT

Bring the bar overhead and place it behind the neck. Lower the hips to the parallel-squat position by bending at the knee. Jump by quickly extending at the knees, hips, and lower back. Land softly and repeat.

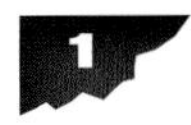

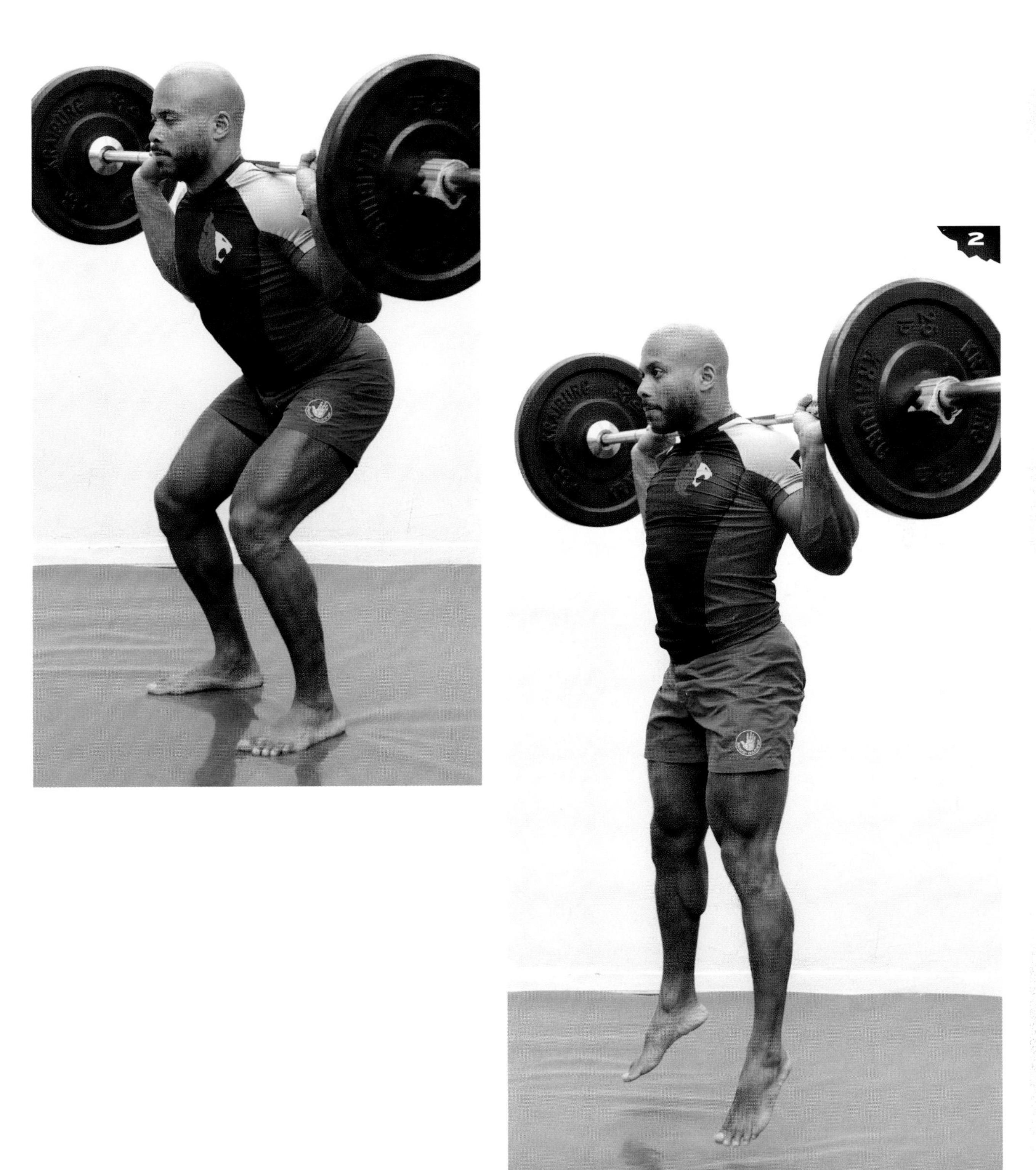

8. GOOD MORNING

Keep the bar placed behind the neck. Lean forward at the waist while keeping the lower back flat and the knees slightly bent.

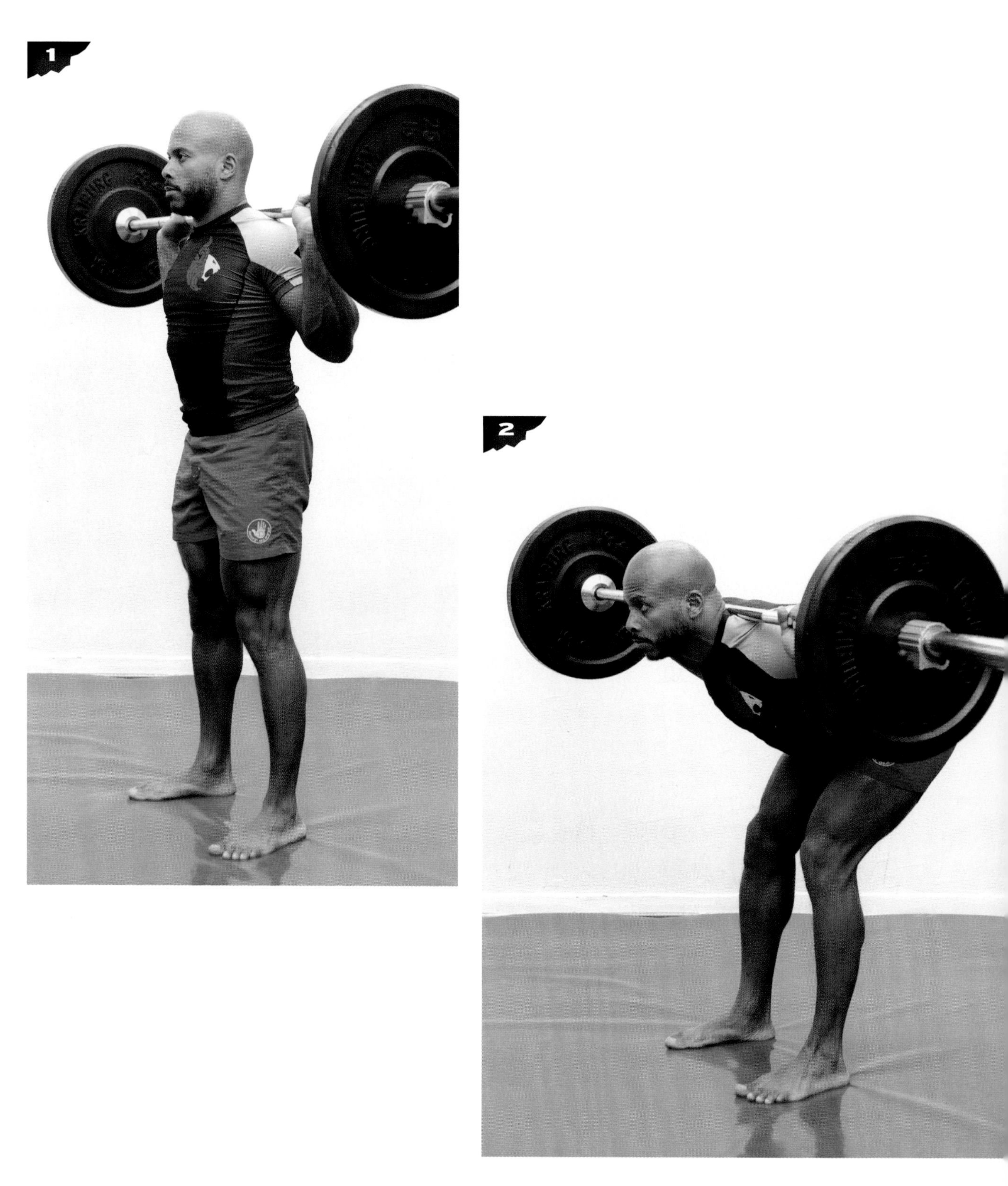

9. TRICEP EXTENSION

From the behind-the-neck position, press the bar overhead. Bend at the elbows to lower the bar back behind the head.

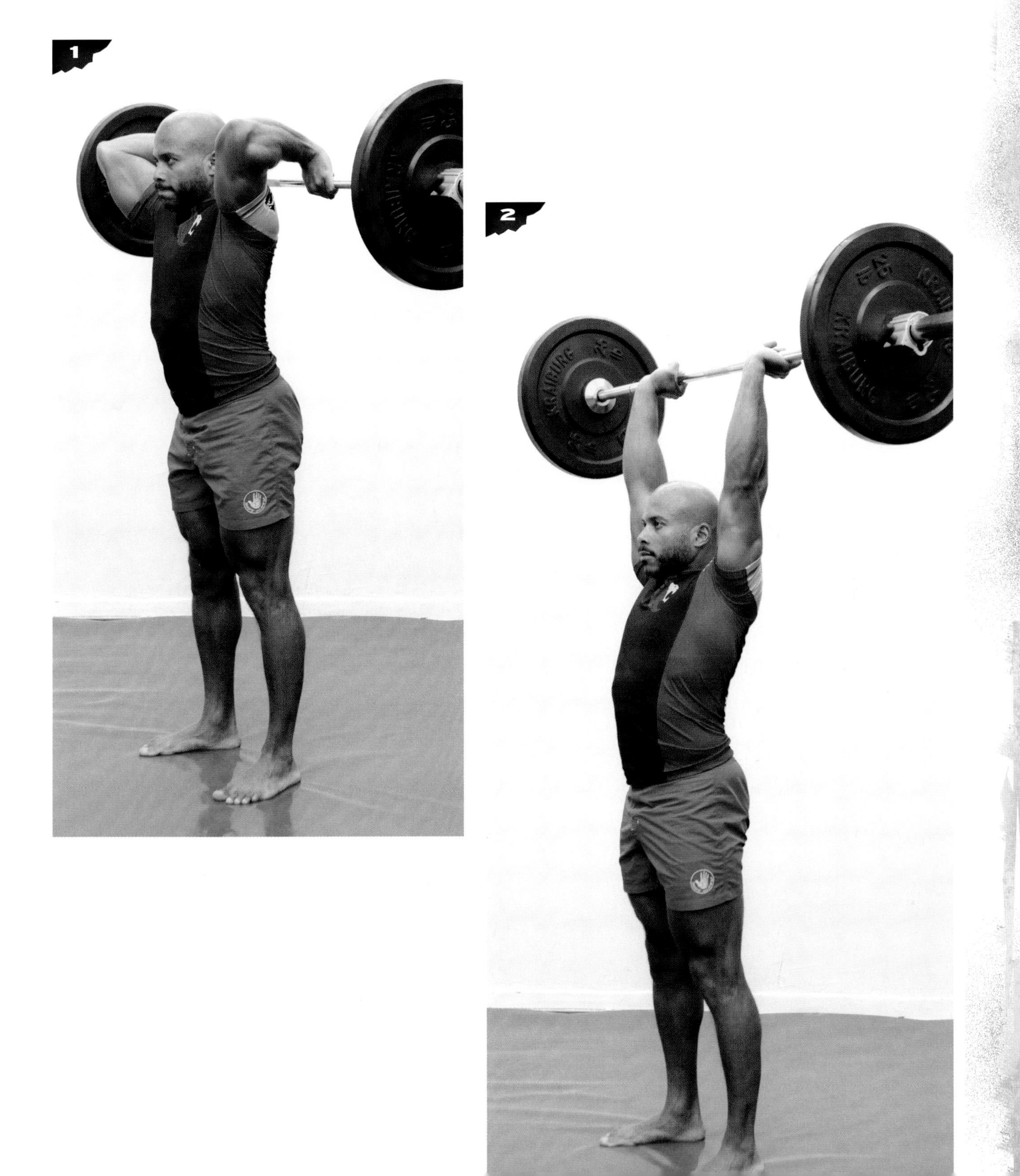

10. BICEP CURL

Bring the bar back in front of the body and switch to an underhand grip. Starting from hip height, curl the bar up to the height of the chin. Lower back to the start position.

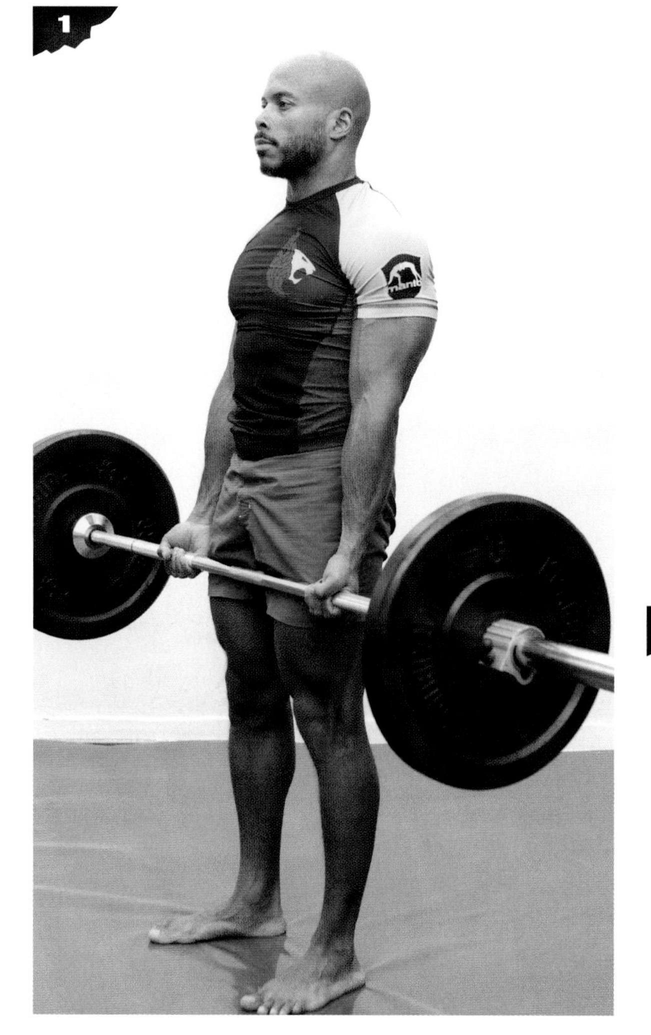

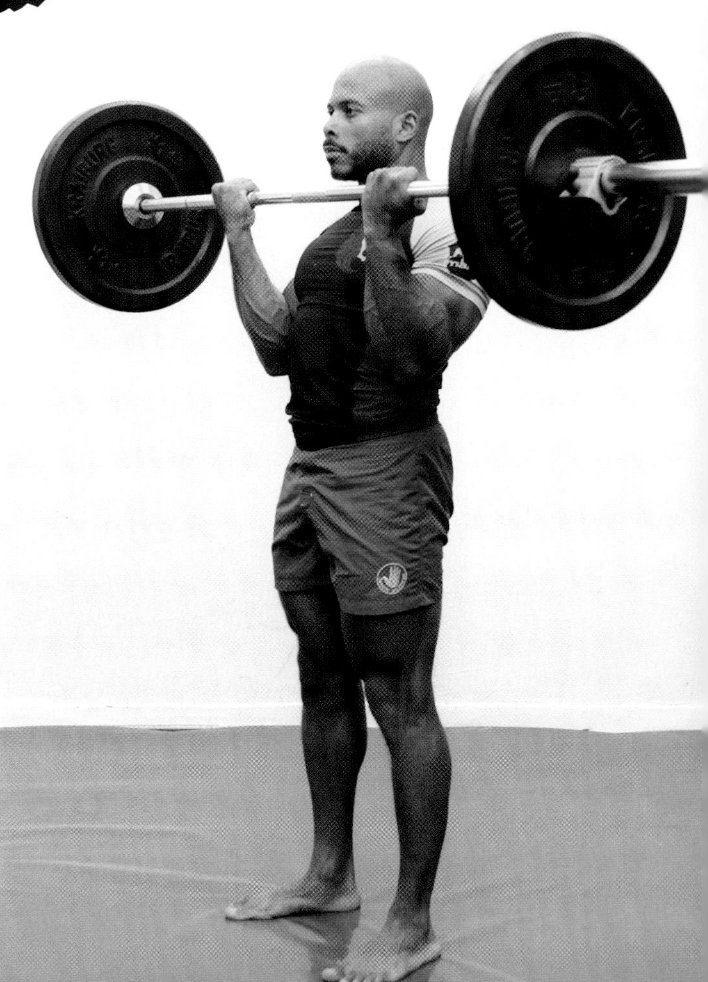

A. DUMBBELL COMPLEXES: UPPER BODY

This complex is to be completed in 30 seconds. Each exercise is to be performed for 10 repetitions.

1. DUMBBELL CURL

Hold the dumbbells at mid-thigh with the palms facing forward. Curl the dumbbells up to the height of the chin. Lower to the original position.

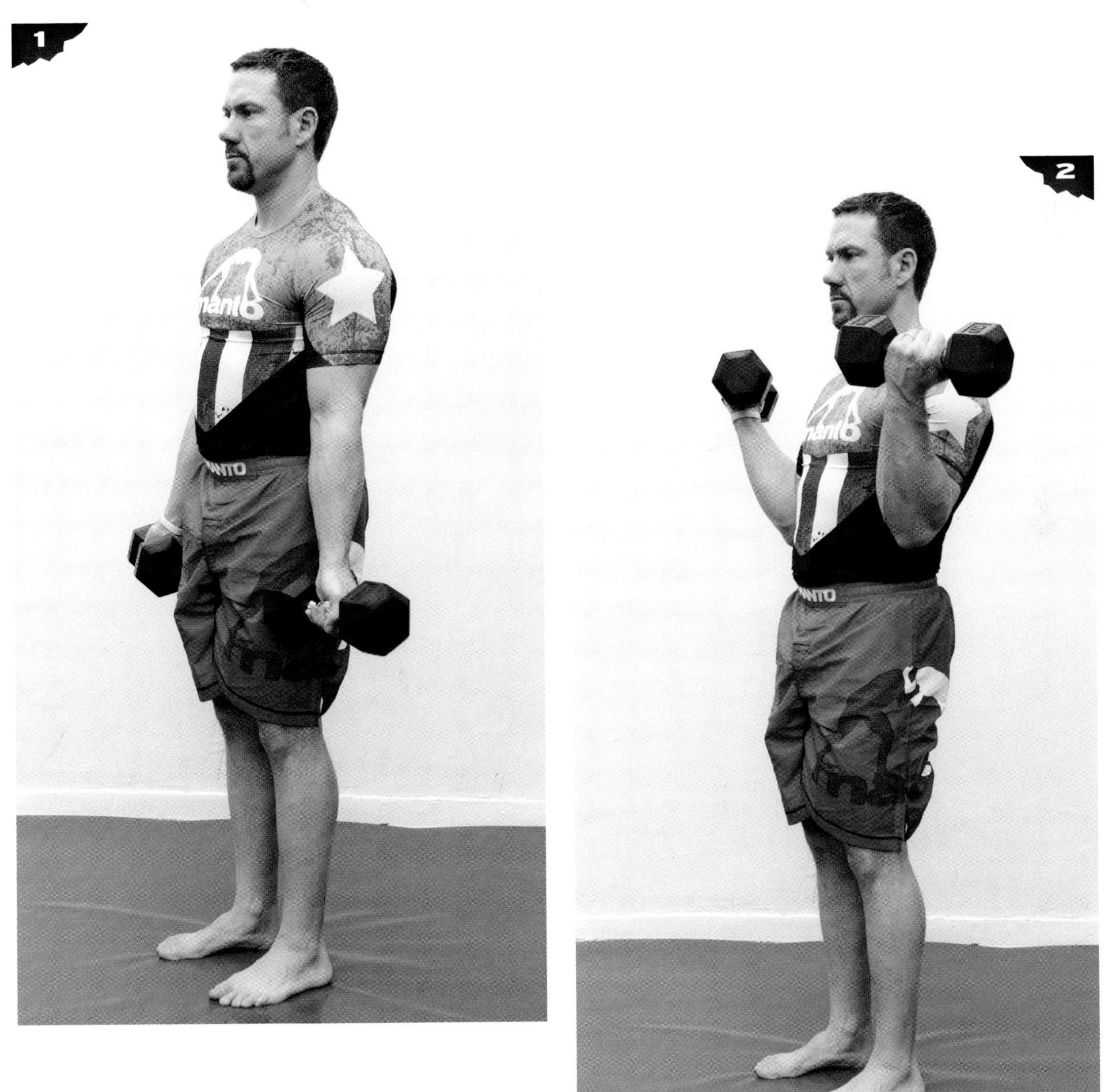

2. UPRIGHT ROW

Hold the dumbbells at mid-thigh with the palms facing backward. Lift the dumbbells by raising the elbows and hands to the height of the chin. Lower to the original position.

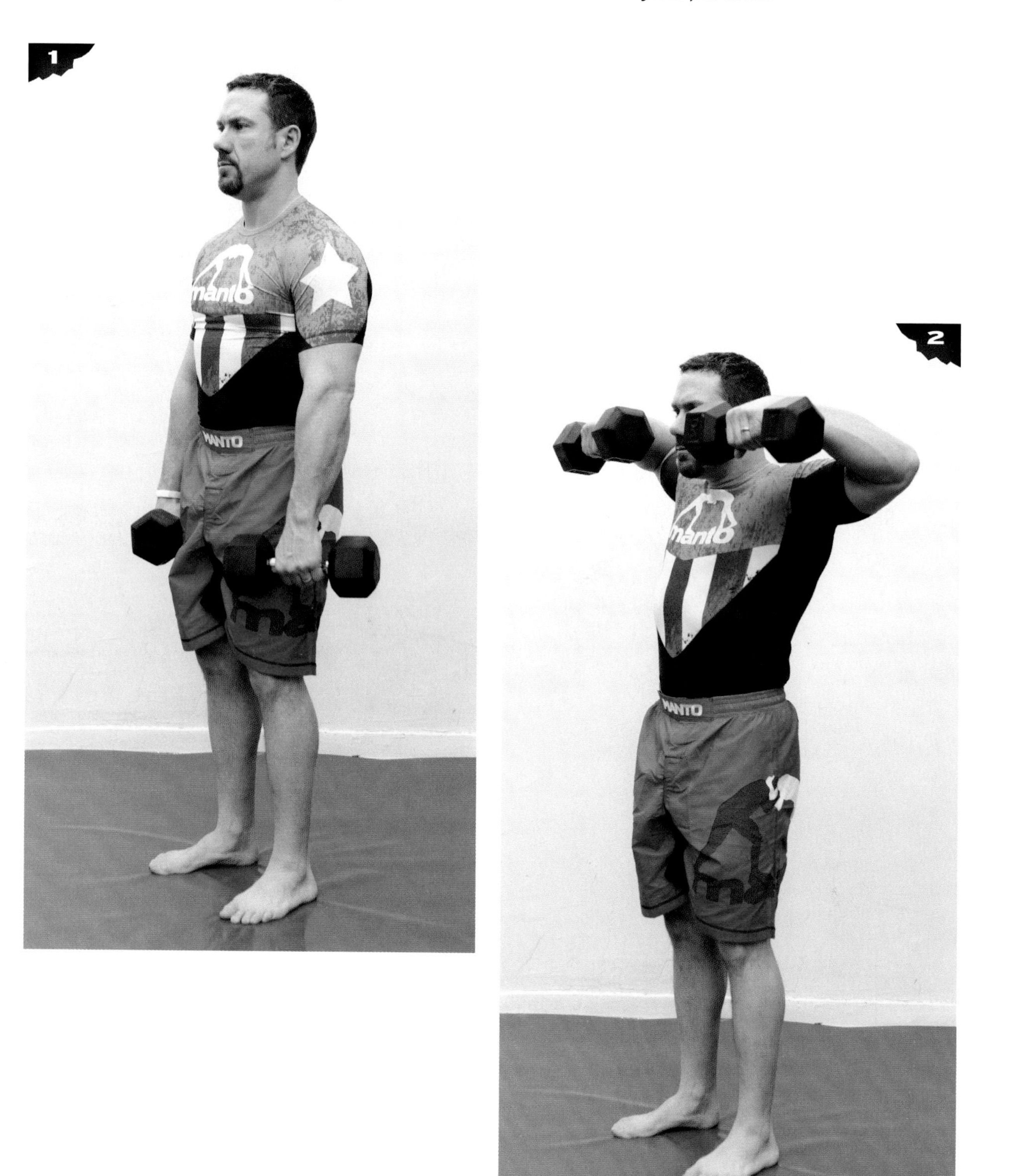

3. FRONT SQUAT TO PRESS

Bring the dumbbells up and rest them on the shoulders. Lower the hips to the parallel-squat position by bending at the knees. Press up by extending at the knees, hips, and lower back. As you reach the standing position, press the dumbbells overhead by extending at the elbows. Lower them to the chest and repeat.

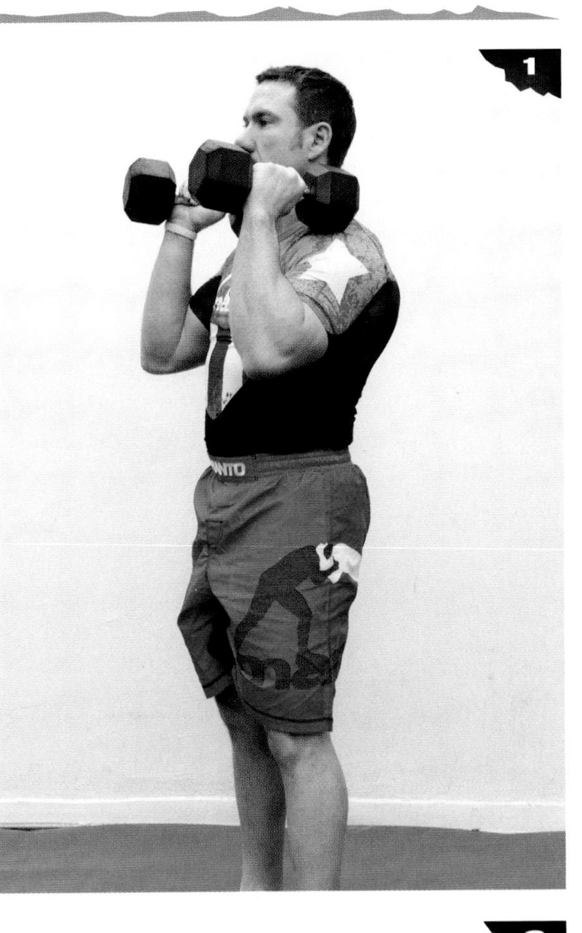

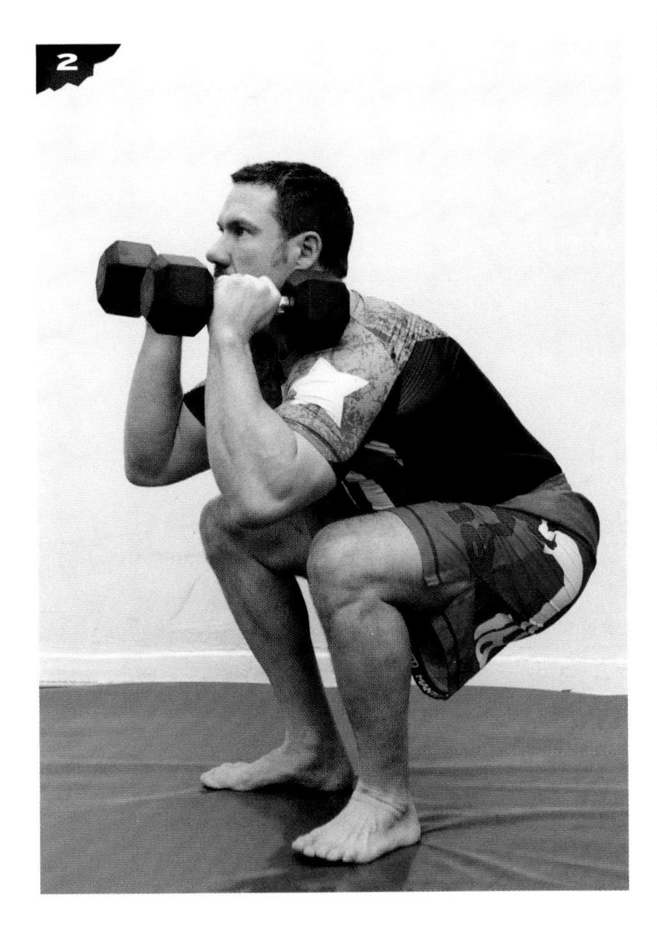

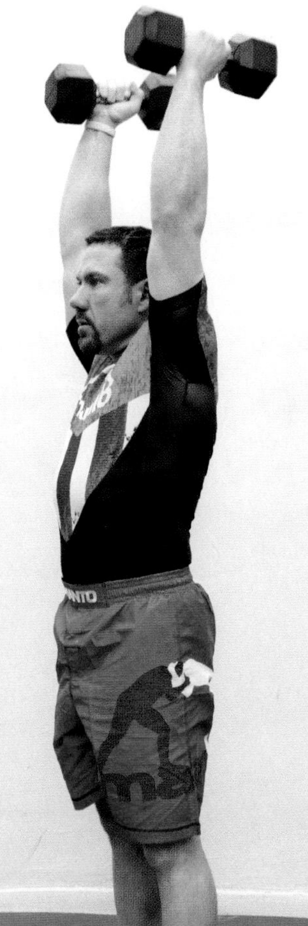

B. DUMBBELL COMPLEXES: LOWER BODY

This complex is to be completed in either 30 or 60 seconds. Each exercise is to be performed for either 5 or 10 repetitions depending on the time frame selected.

1. DEADLIFT

Begin standing with the dumbbells at mid-thigh and the palms facing backward. While keeping the lower back flat and the knees slightly bent, bend forward at the waist so that the dumbbells pass more than halfway down the shin. Extend at the lower back and return to the original position.

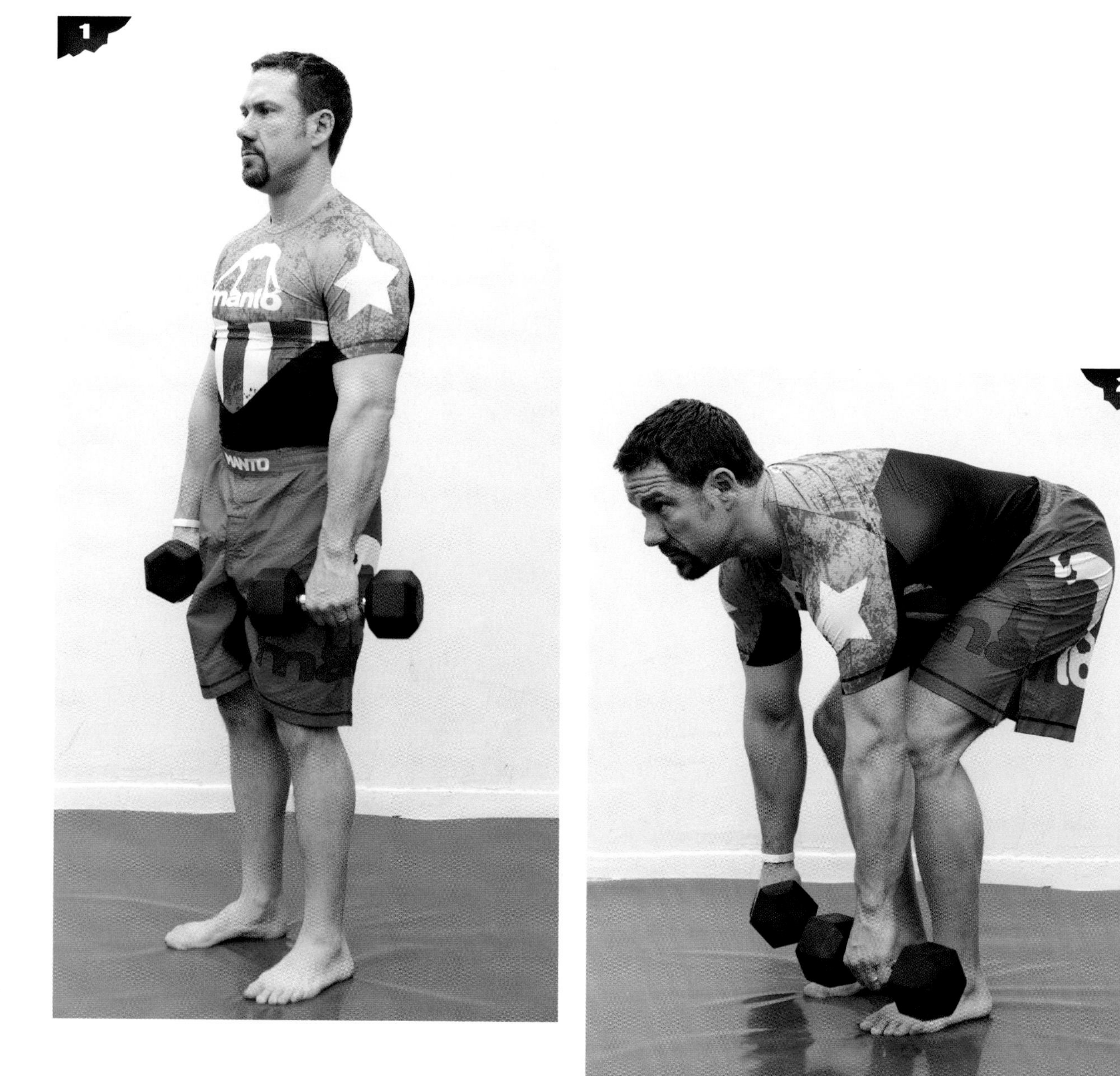

2. HAMMER CURL

Hold the dumbbells at mid-thigh with the palms facing the hips. Curl the dumbbells up to the height of the chin. Lower to the original position.

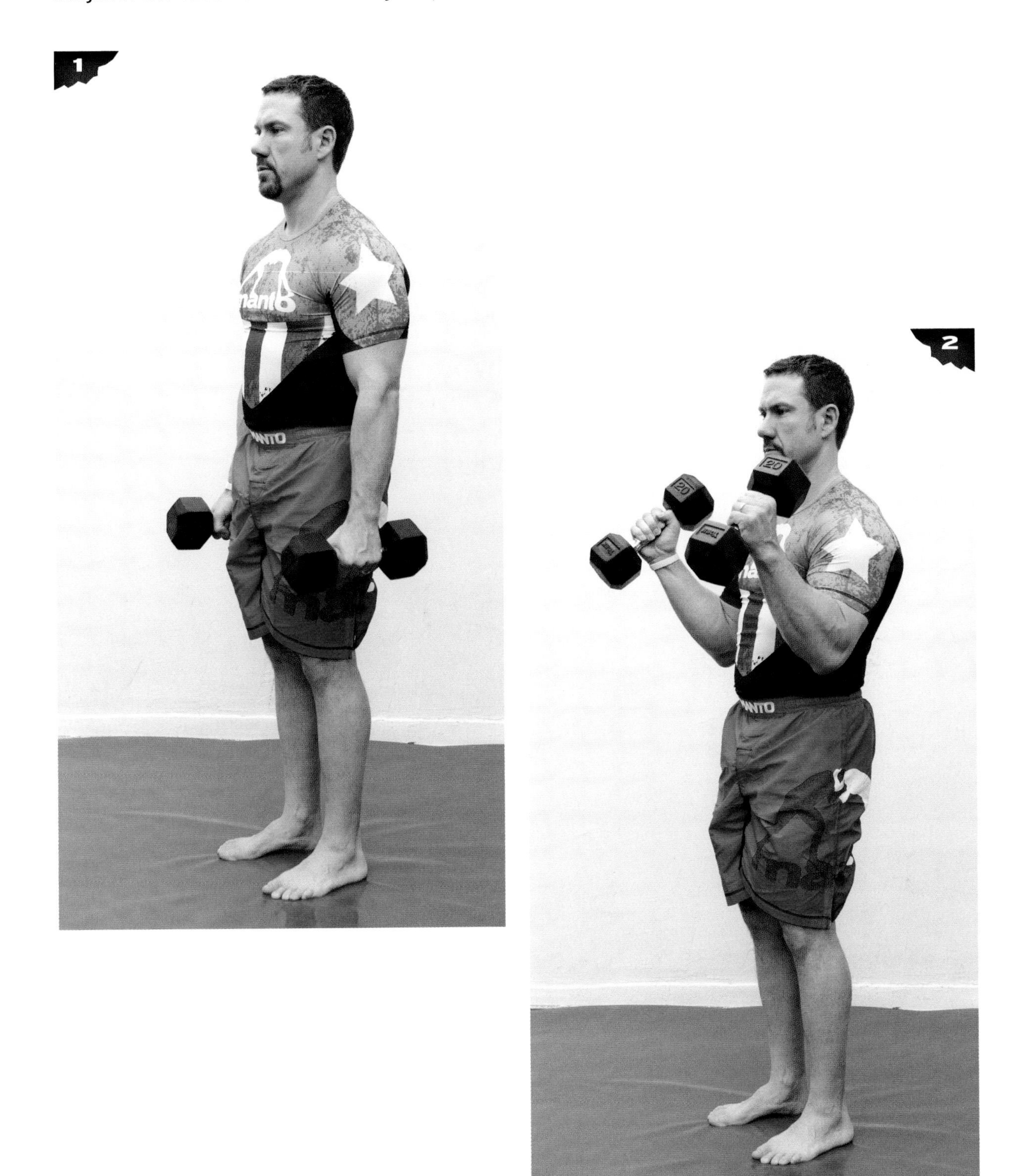

3. BENT-OVER ROW

Bend over so that the dumbbells are at mid-shin height and the palms are facing backward. While keeping a flat lower back, row the dumbbells up to the chest. Lower to the original position.

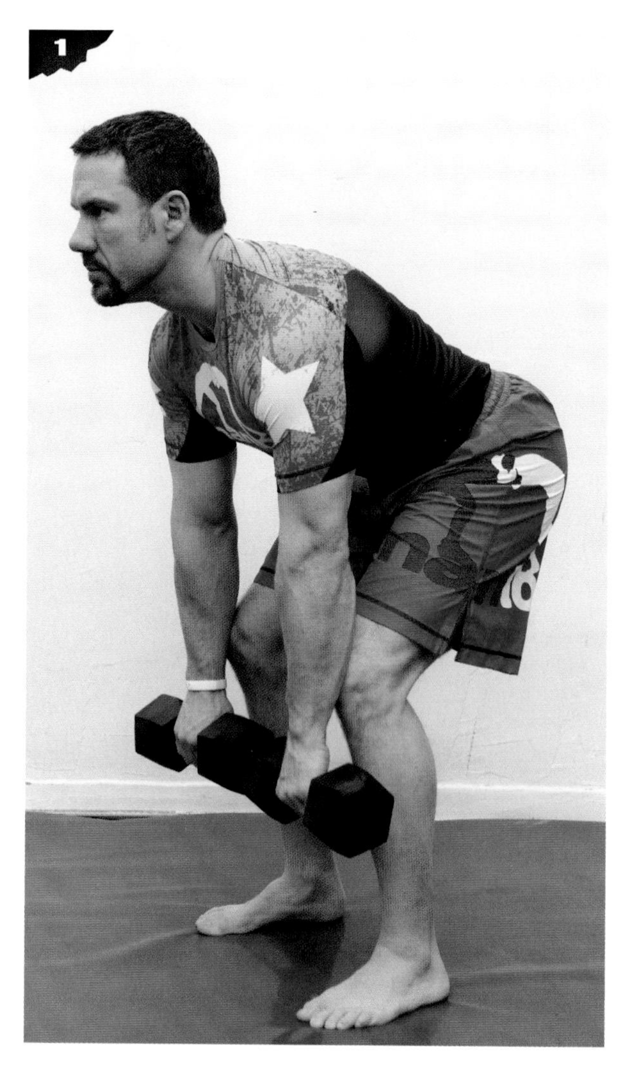

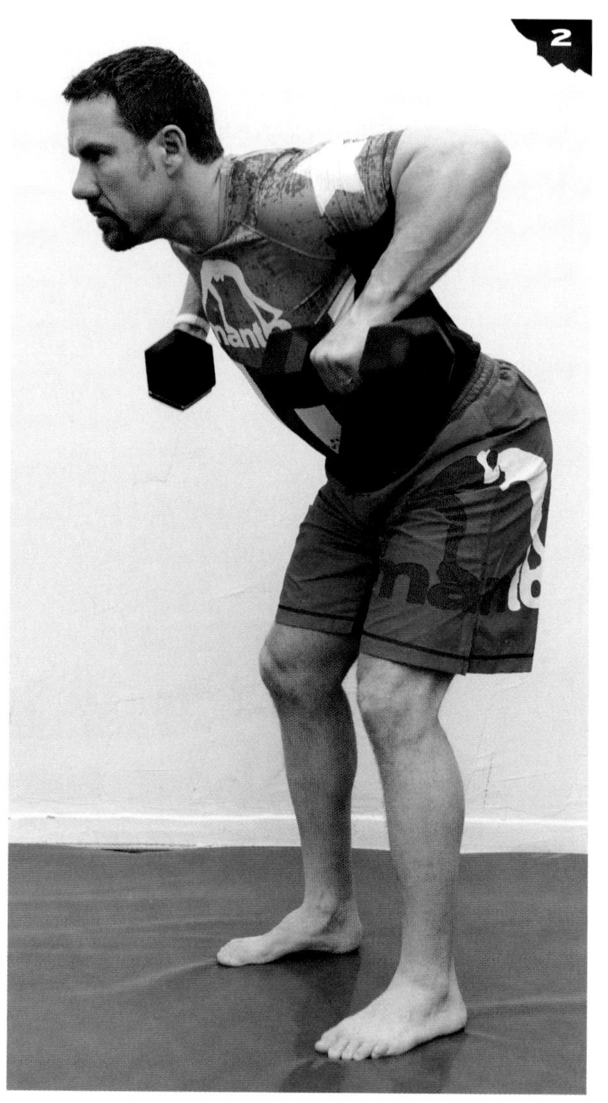

4. SNATCH

Bend over so that the dumbbells are at mid-shin height and the palms are facing backward. While keeping a flat lower back, jump and bring the elbows overhead. Lower them back to the original position.

1

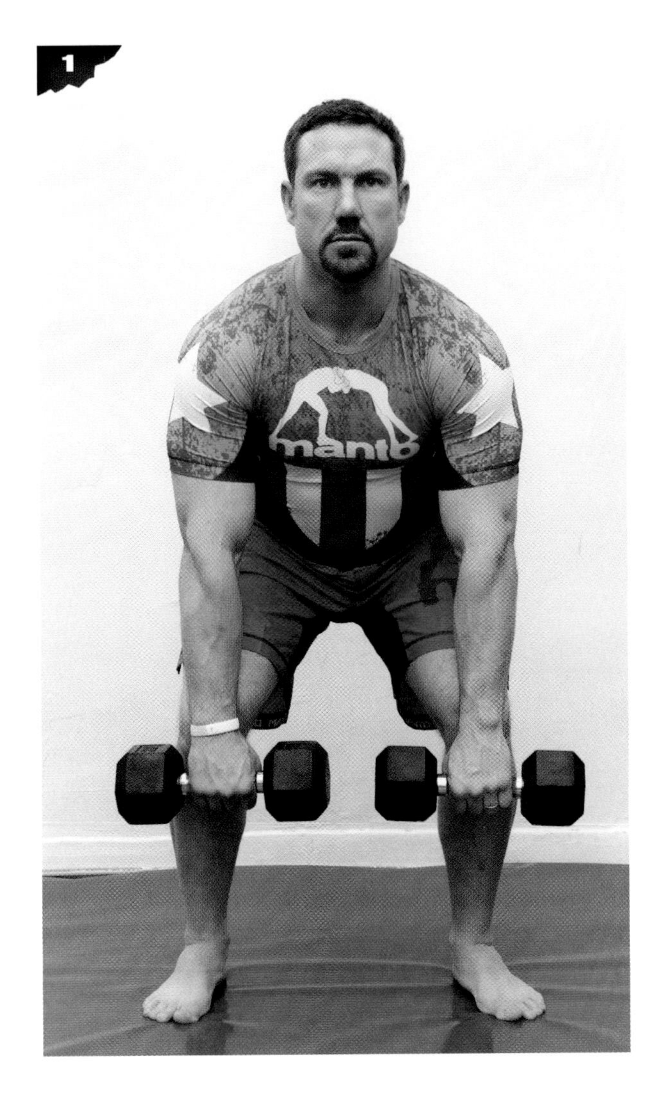

2

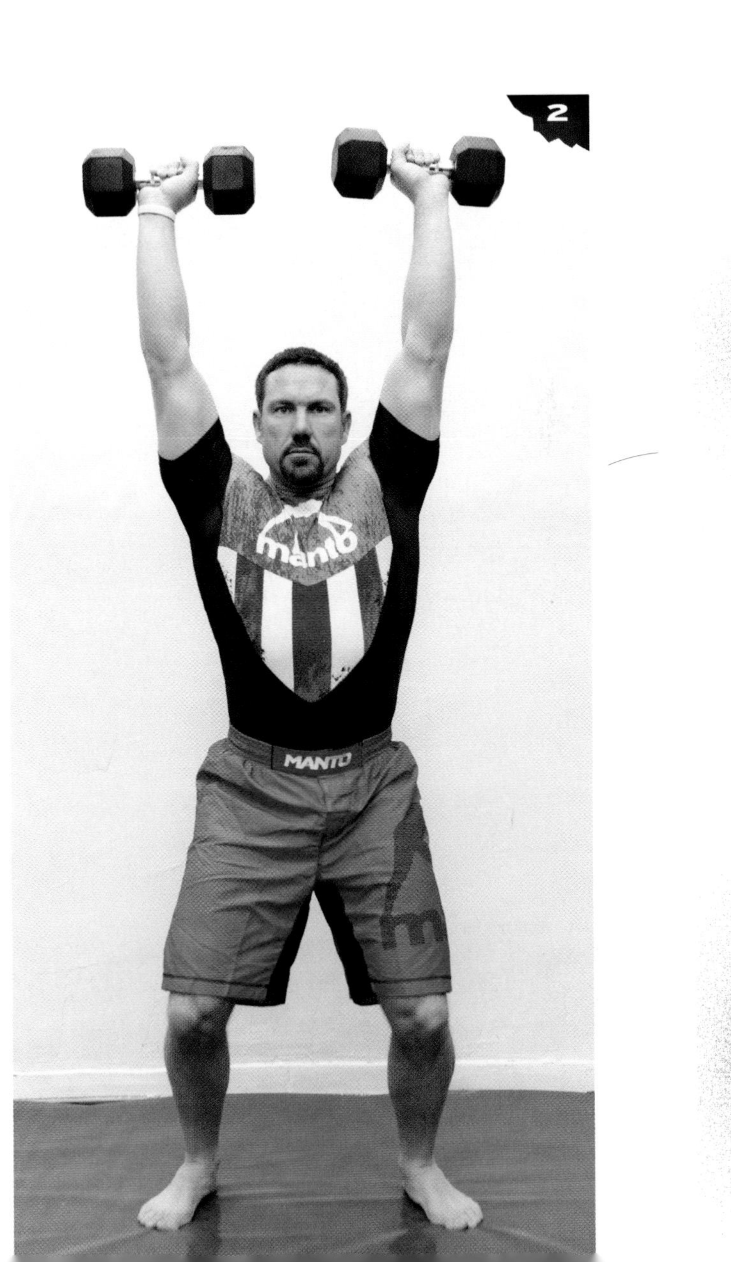

5. SQUAT

Hold the dumbbells at mid-thigh with the palms facing the hips. Lower the hips to the parallel-squat position by bending at the knee. Press up by extending at the knees, hips, and lower back.

1

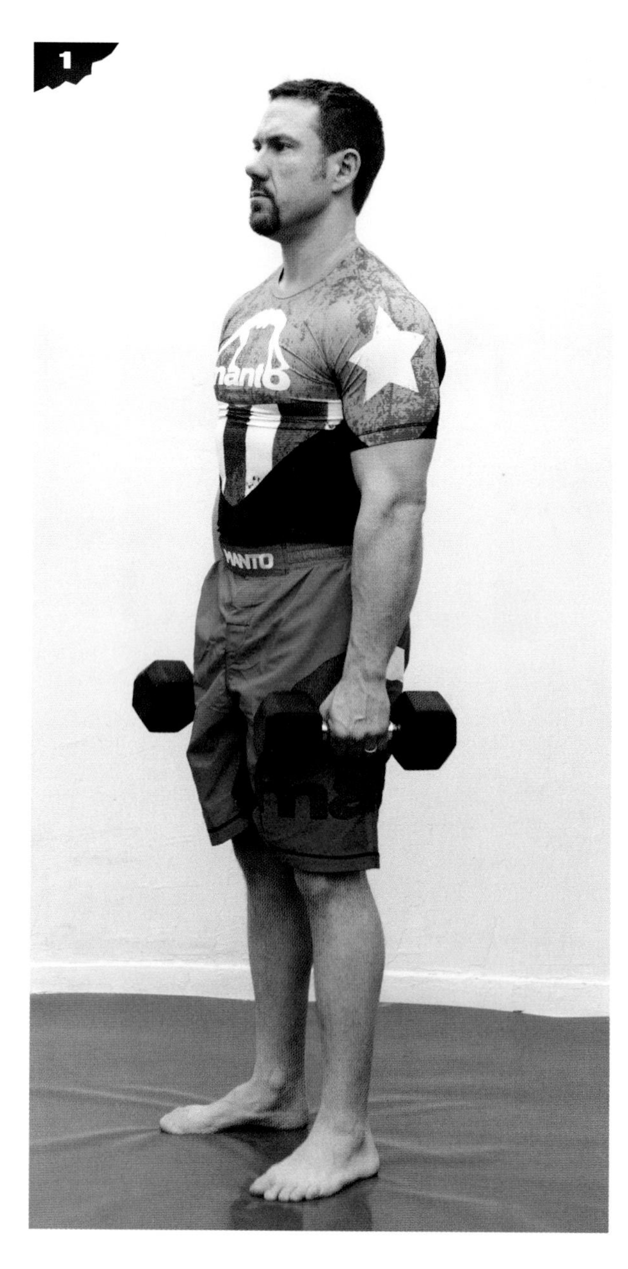

2

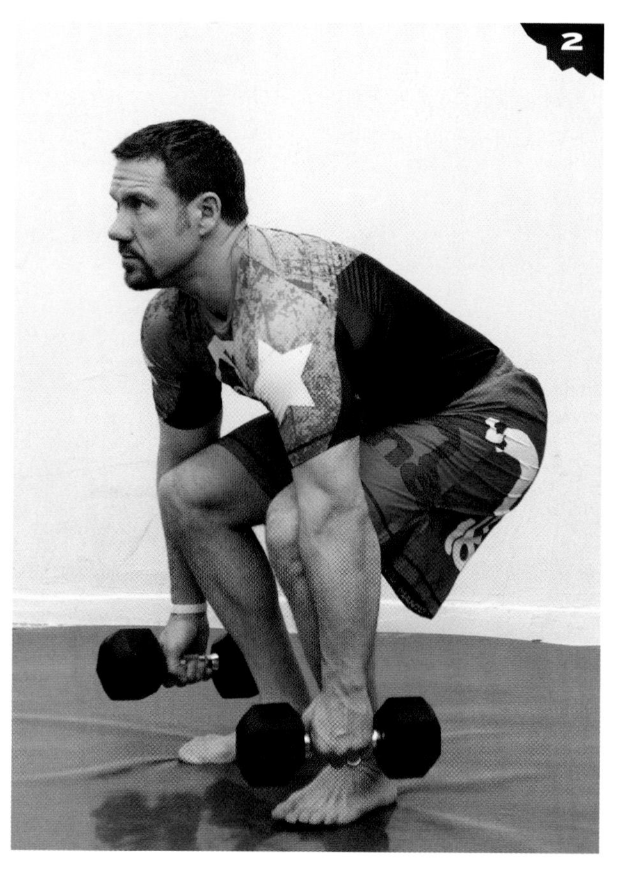

6. LUNGE

Hold the dumbbells at mid-thigh with the palms facing the hips. Step forward with one leg and lower the back knee almost to the ground. Press back up to the original position.

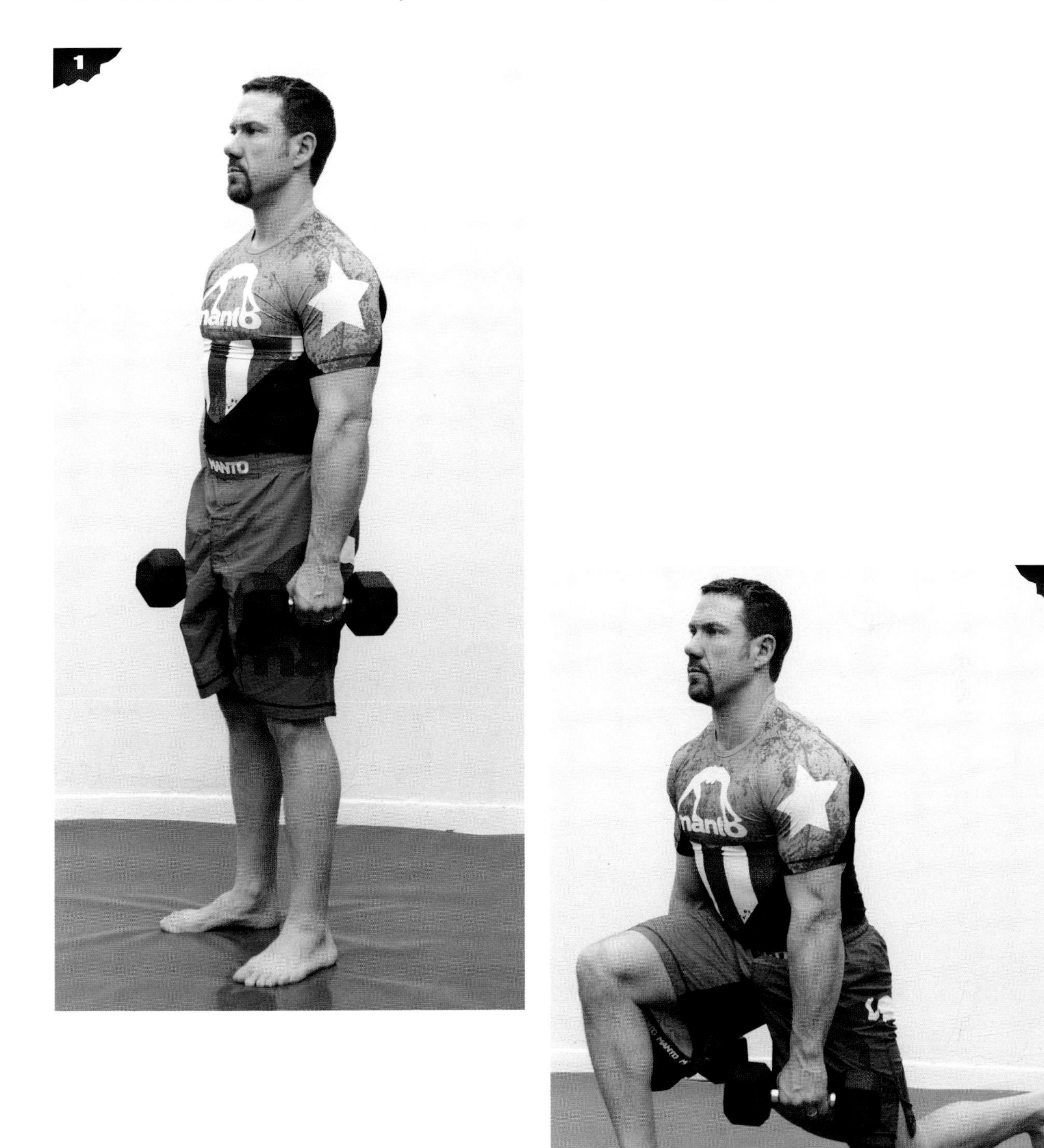

C. DUMBBELL COMPLEXES: SINGLE

This complex is to be performed in the best time possible. Each exercise is to be performed for 6 repetitions.

1. SINGLE-ARM ROW

Begin bent over with one hand supporting the thigh and the other holding the dumbbell. Bring the elbow up and back, and row the dumbbell to the chest. Lower under control and repeat.

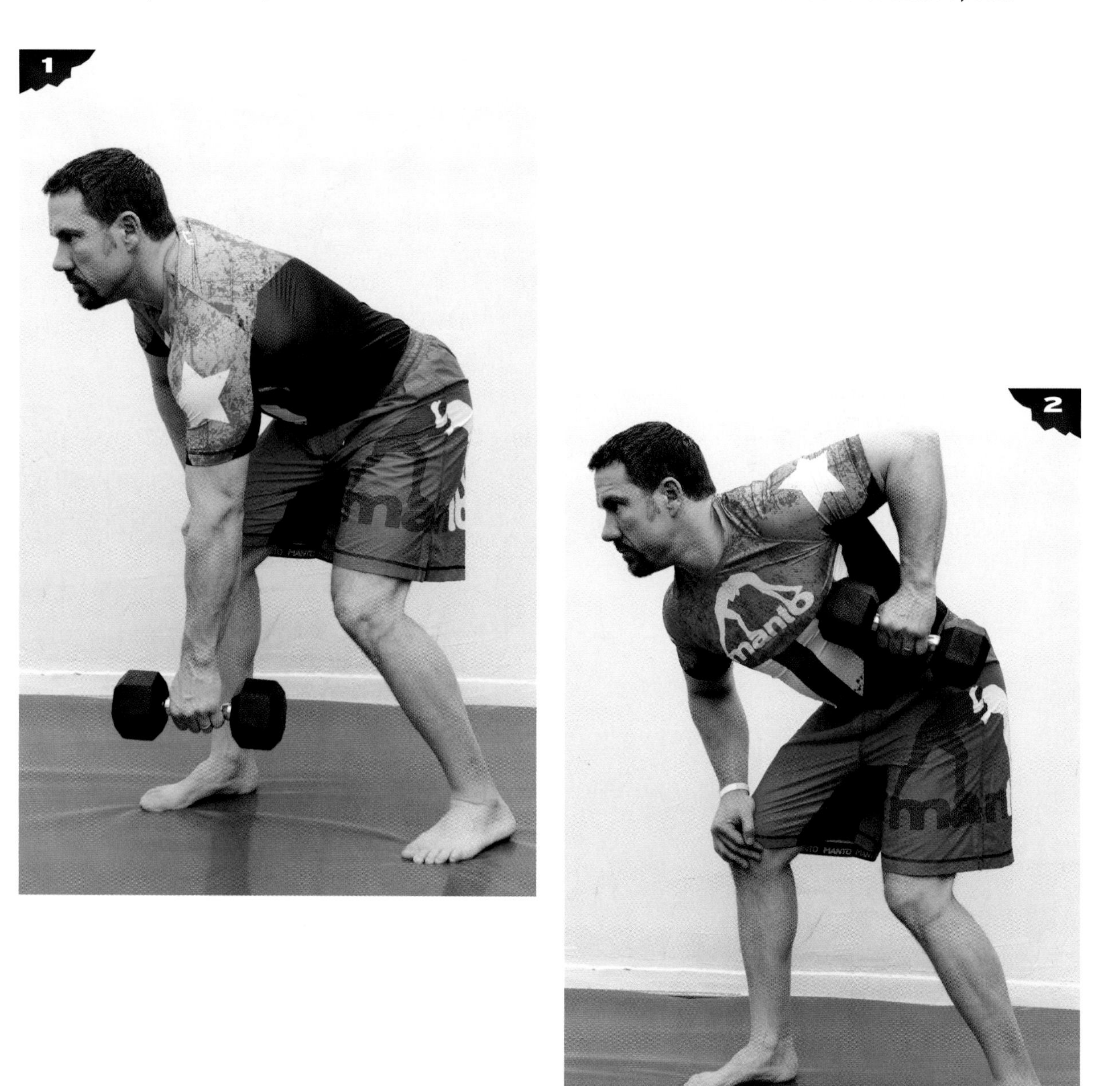

2. LUNGE ON SHOULDER

Begin standing with the dumbbell resting on one shoulder. Lunge forward with the chest tall until the back knee almost touches the ground. Press back up to the start position and repeat with other leg.

1

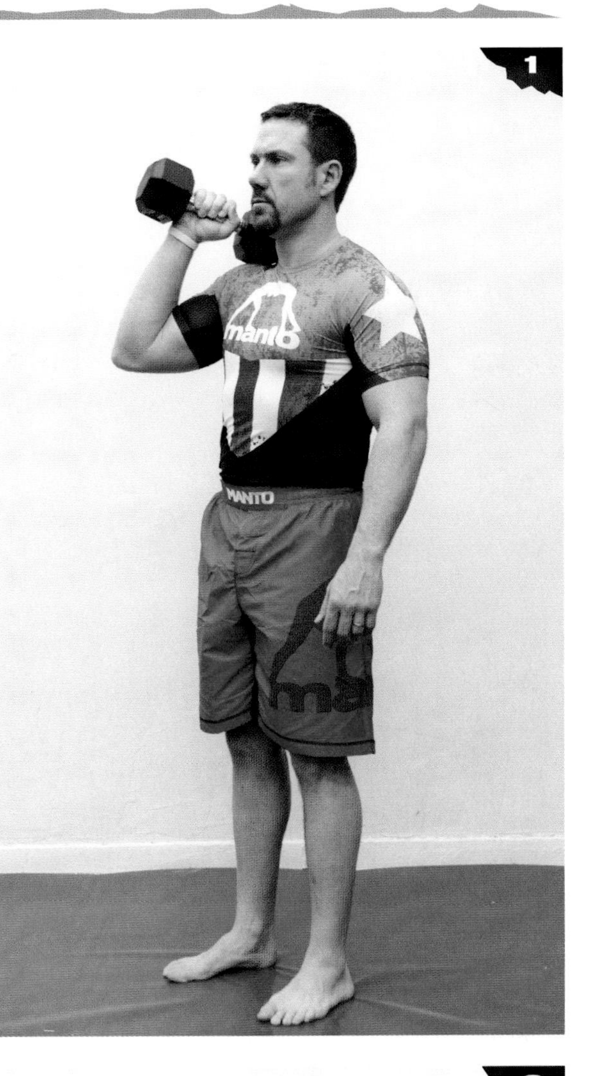

2

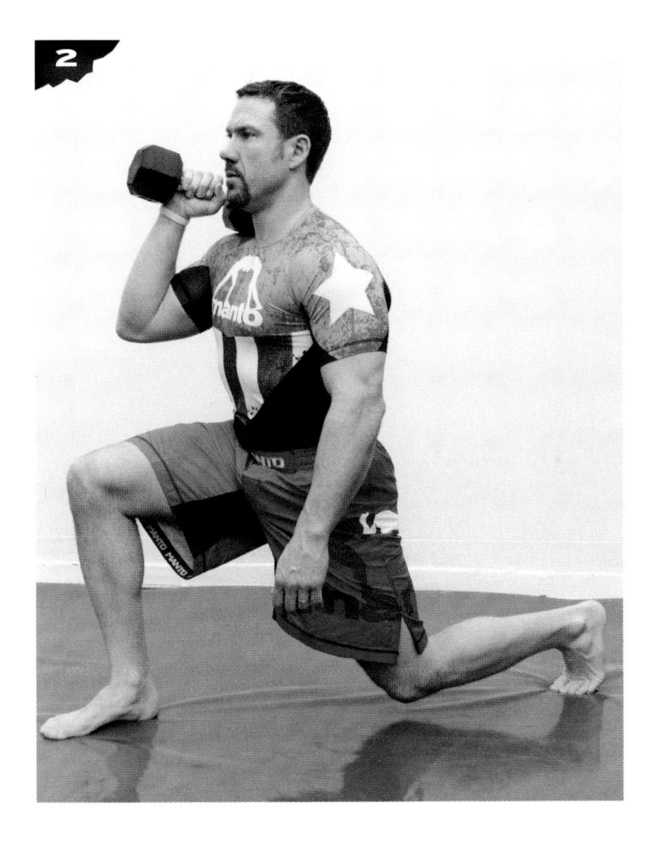

3

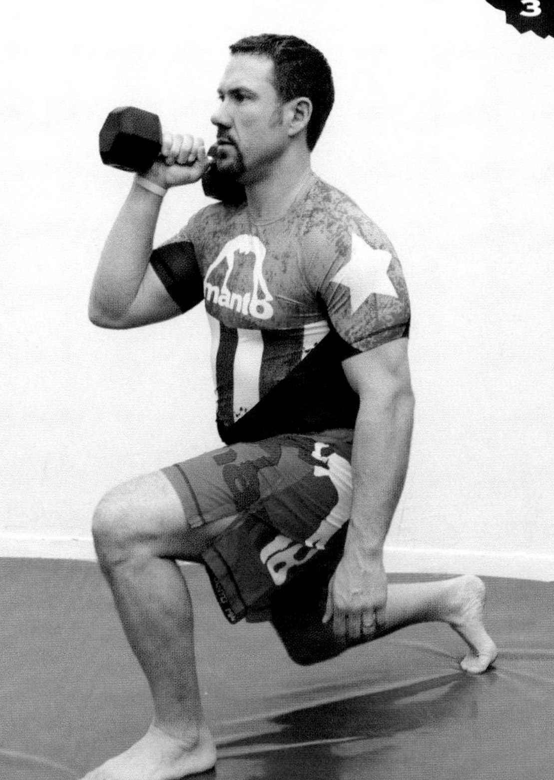

3. SNATCH

Begin bent forward with the dumbbell held between the legs. Jump using the legs and bring the dumbbell explosively overhead. Reverse the motion and lower under control and repeat.

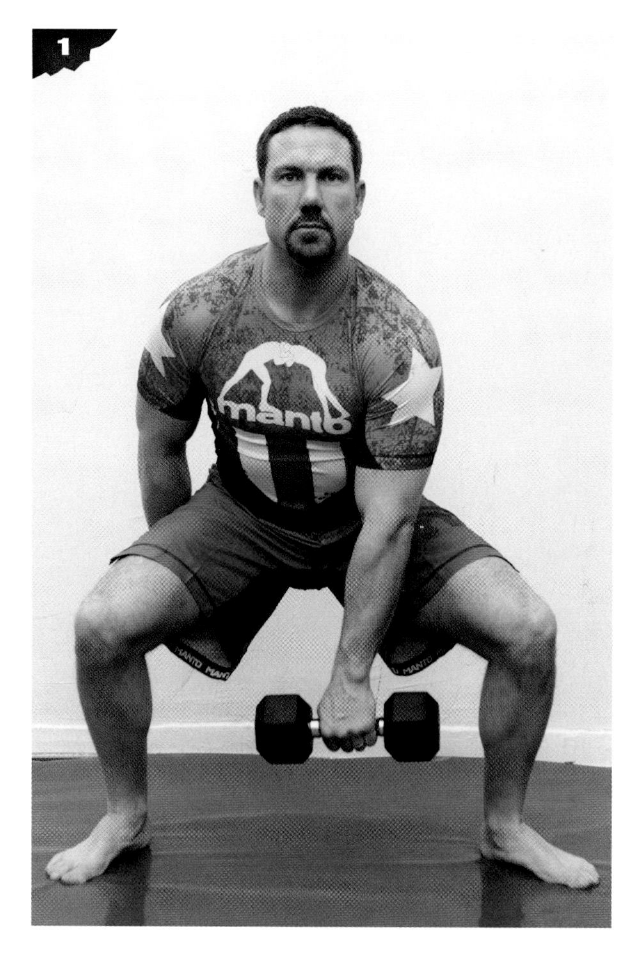

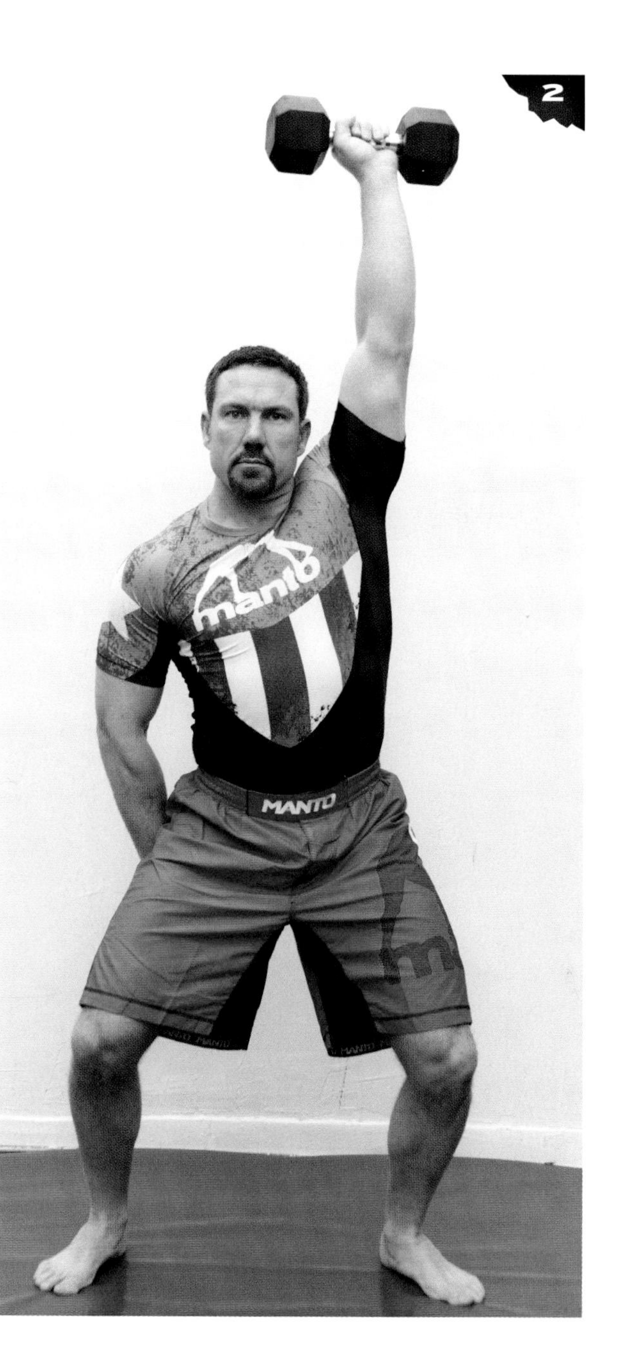

4. OVERHEAD LUNGE

Begin standing with one dumbbell held overhead. Lunge forward with the chest tall until the back knee almost touches the ground. Press back up to the start position and repeat.

1

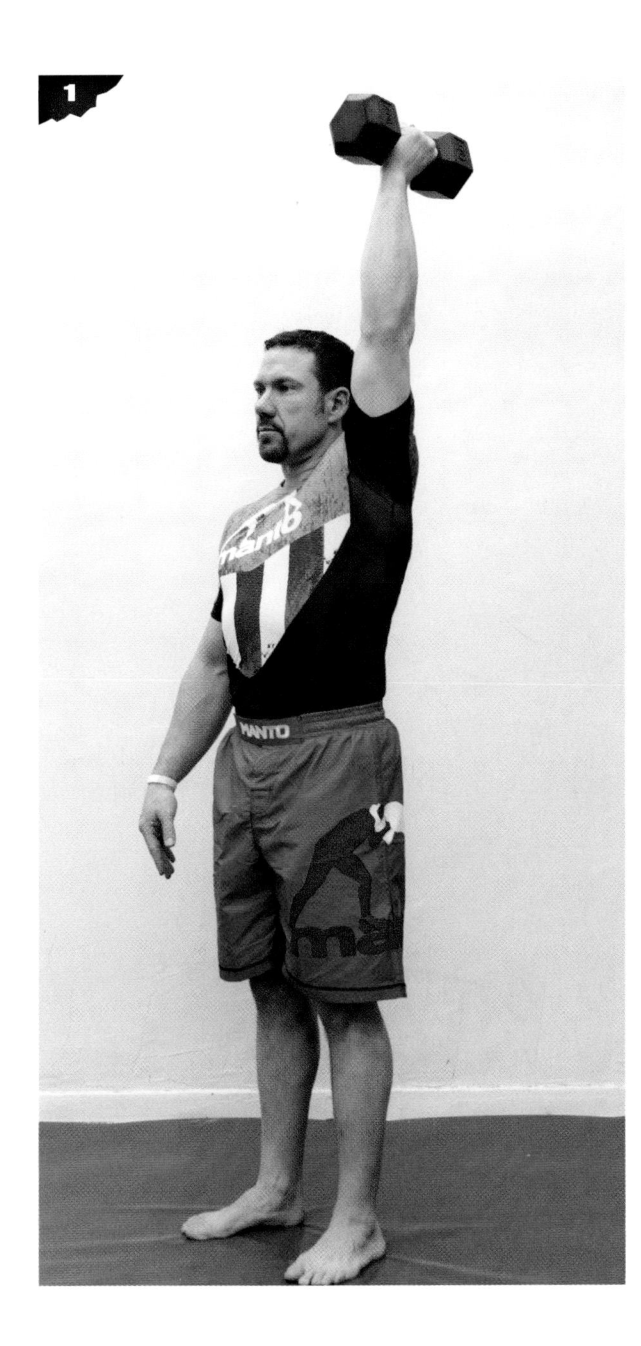

2

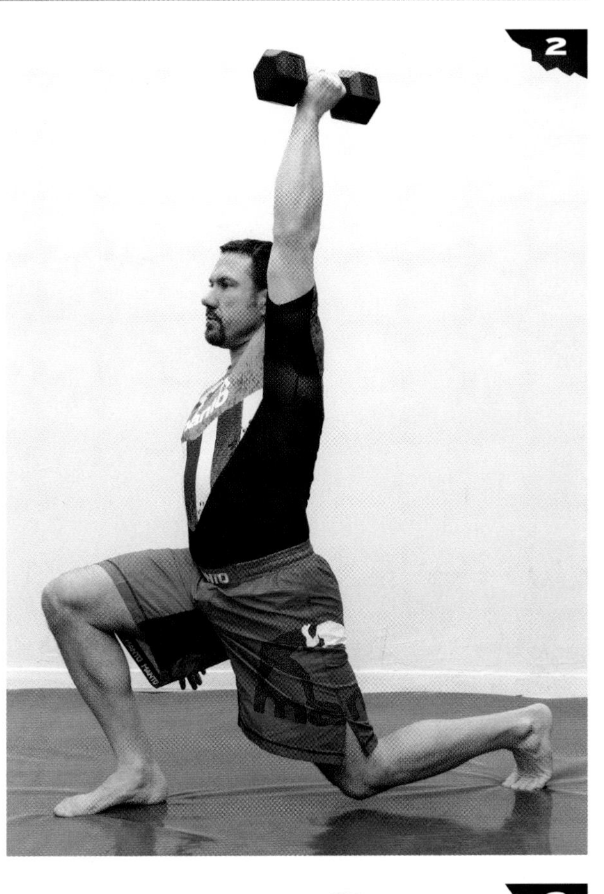

3

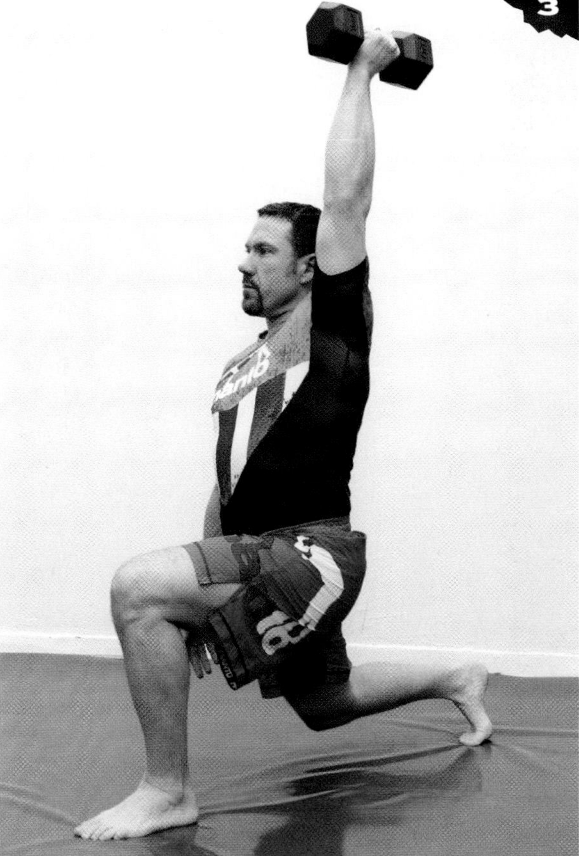

5. DUMBBELL SWING

Begin standing with the dumbbell held between the legs. Extend at the knees and hips and swing the dumbbell overhead. Lower under control and repeat.

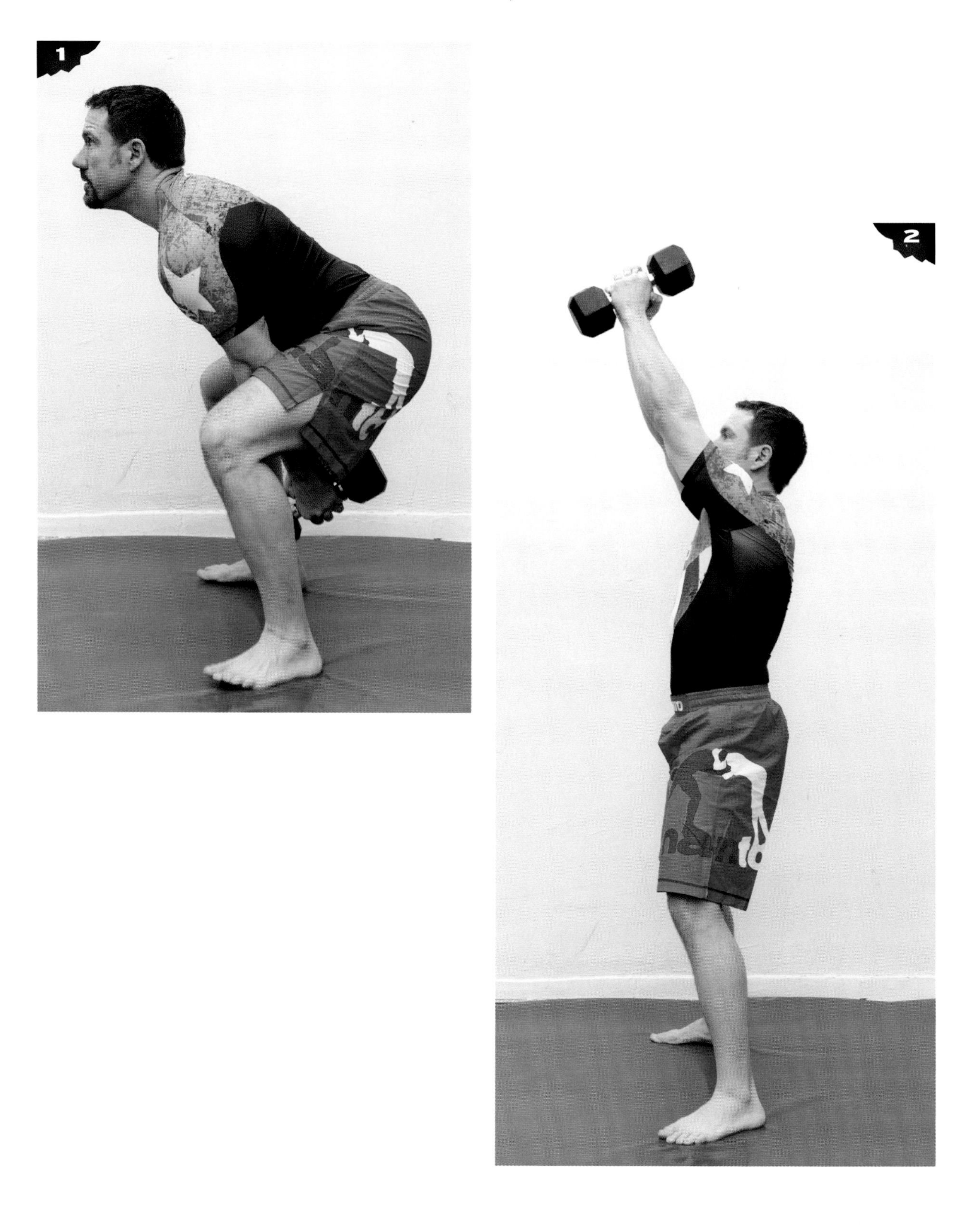

6. SIDE LUNGE

Begin standing, holding one end of the dumbbell in each hand. Step out to one side and lower the dumbbell to the floor. Press back up and repeat on the other side.

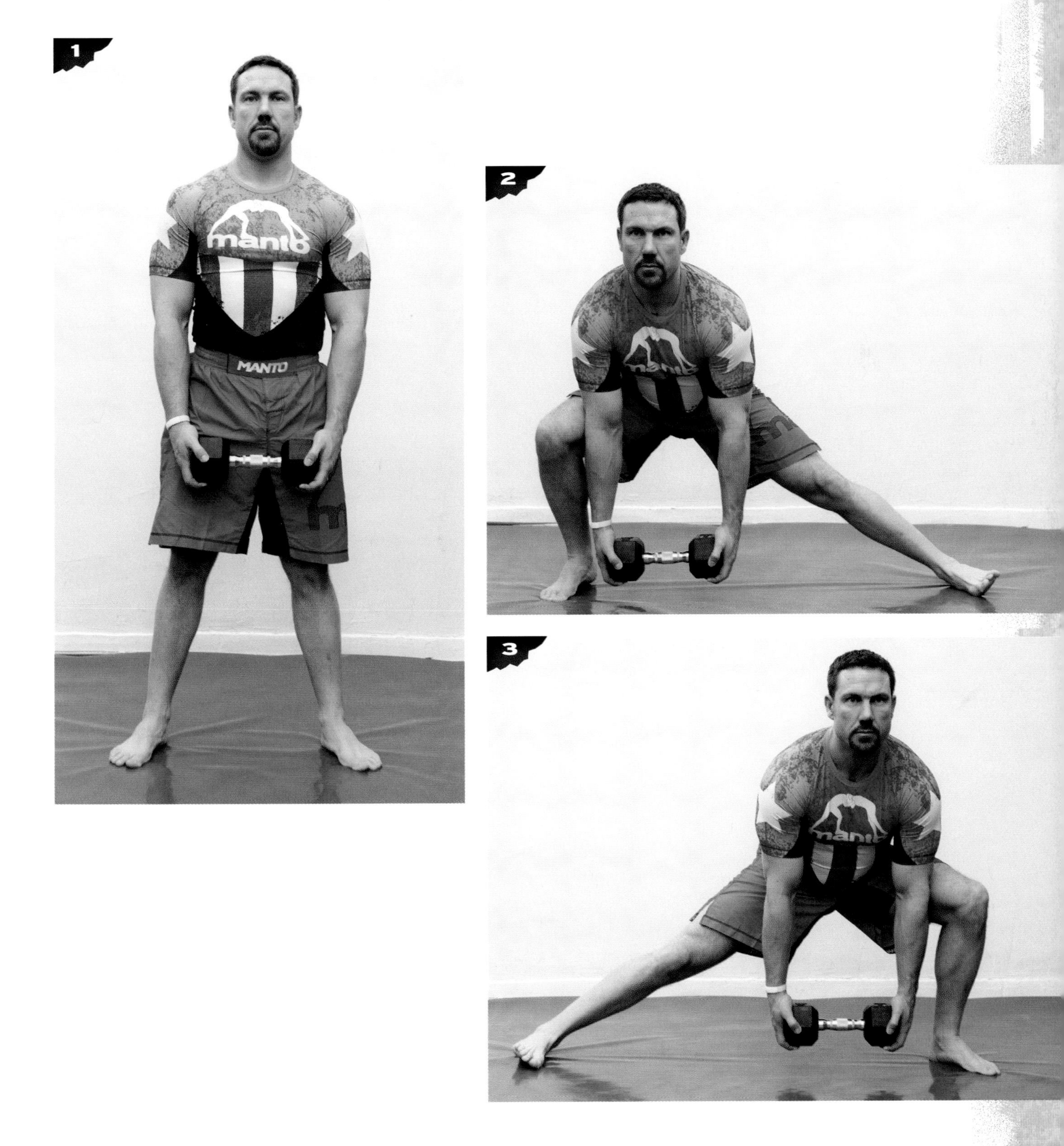

Since many of the kettlebell exercises cannot be used as rapidly as those using the barbell and dumbbell due to the nature of the performance of many of the exercises, I commonly use these complexes for best time, not with a time limit. The key is to perform each exercise as fast as possible while still maintaining proper form.

A. KETTLEBELL COMPLEX I

Perform each exercise for 10 repetitions.

1. FRONT SWINGS

Begin holding a bell in each hand. Squat down as you swing the bells between the legs and then stand up by extending at the hips to swing the bells up to shoulder height.

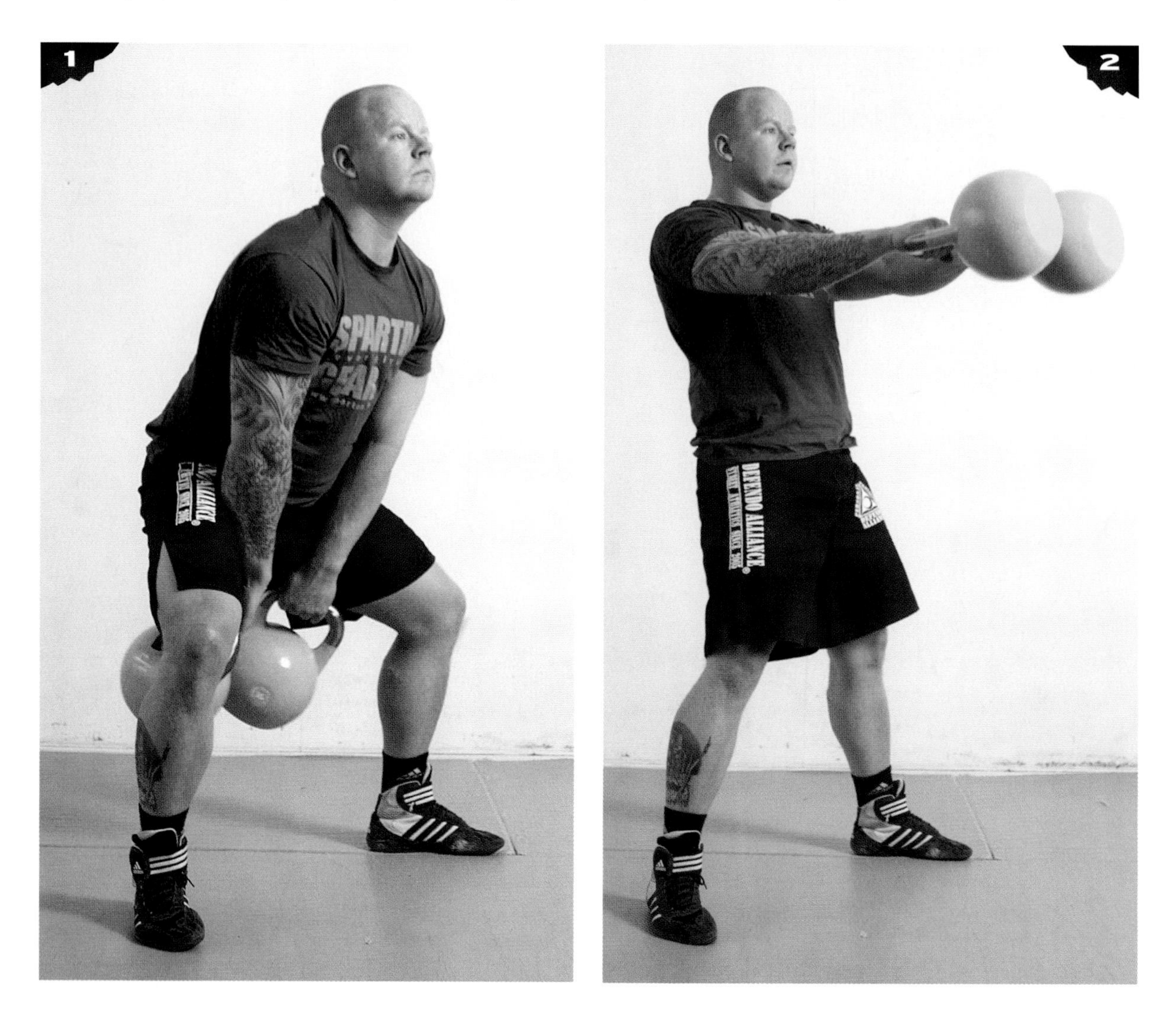

2. FRONT SQUAT

Begin standing with the bells racked on the forearms. While keeping the torso upright, squat down by bending at the knee and hips. Stand back up by extending at the knees and hips.

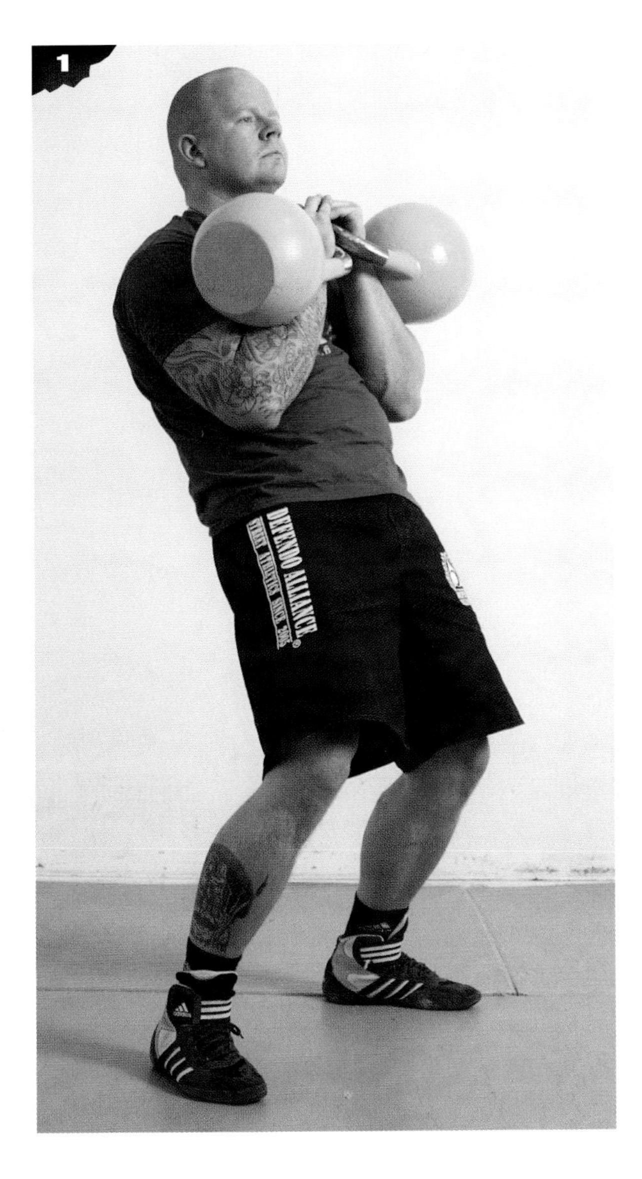

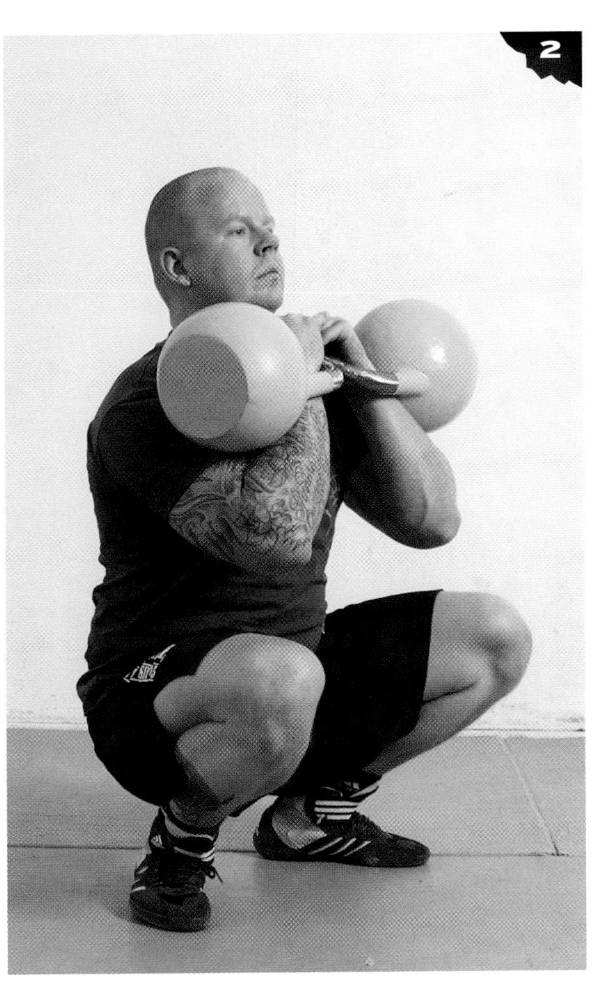

3. PUSH JERKS

Begin standing with the bells racked on the forearms. Squat down slightly and then drive into the ground with the feet and explosively press the bells overhead. Lower to the original position and repeat.

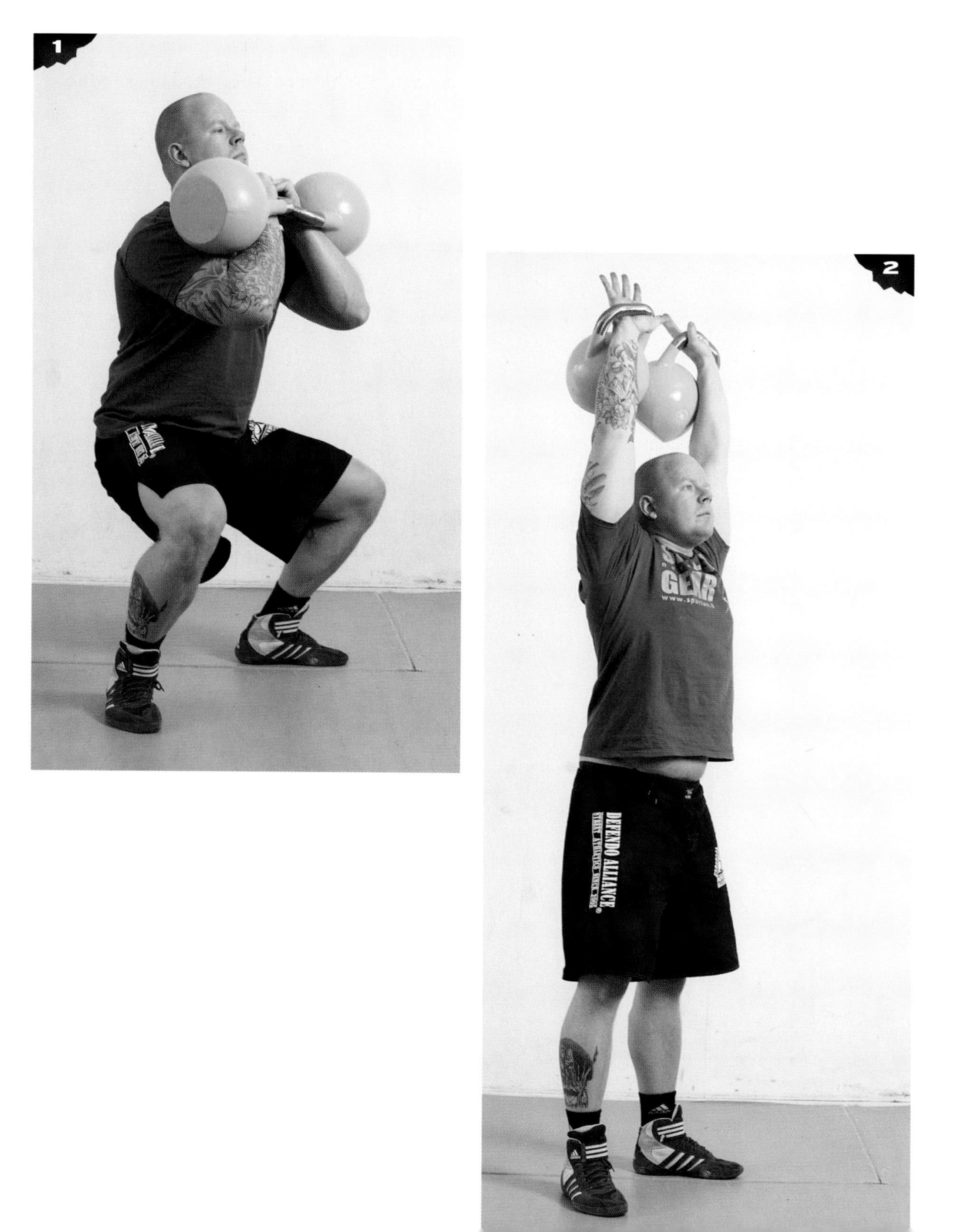

B. KETTLEBELL COMPLEX 2

Perform each exercise for 10 repetitions.

1. FRONT SWINGS

Begin holding a bell in each hand. Squat down as you swing the bells between the legs and then stand up by extending at the hips to swing the bells up to shoulder height.

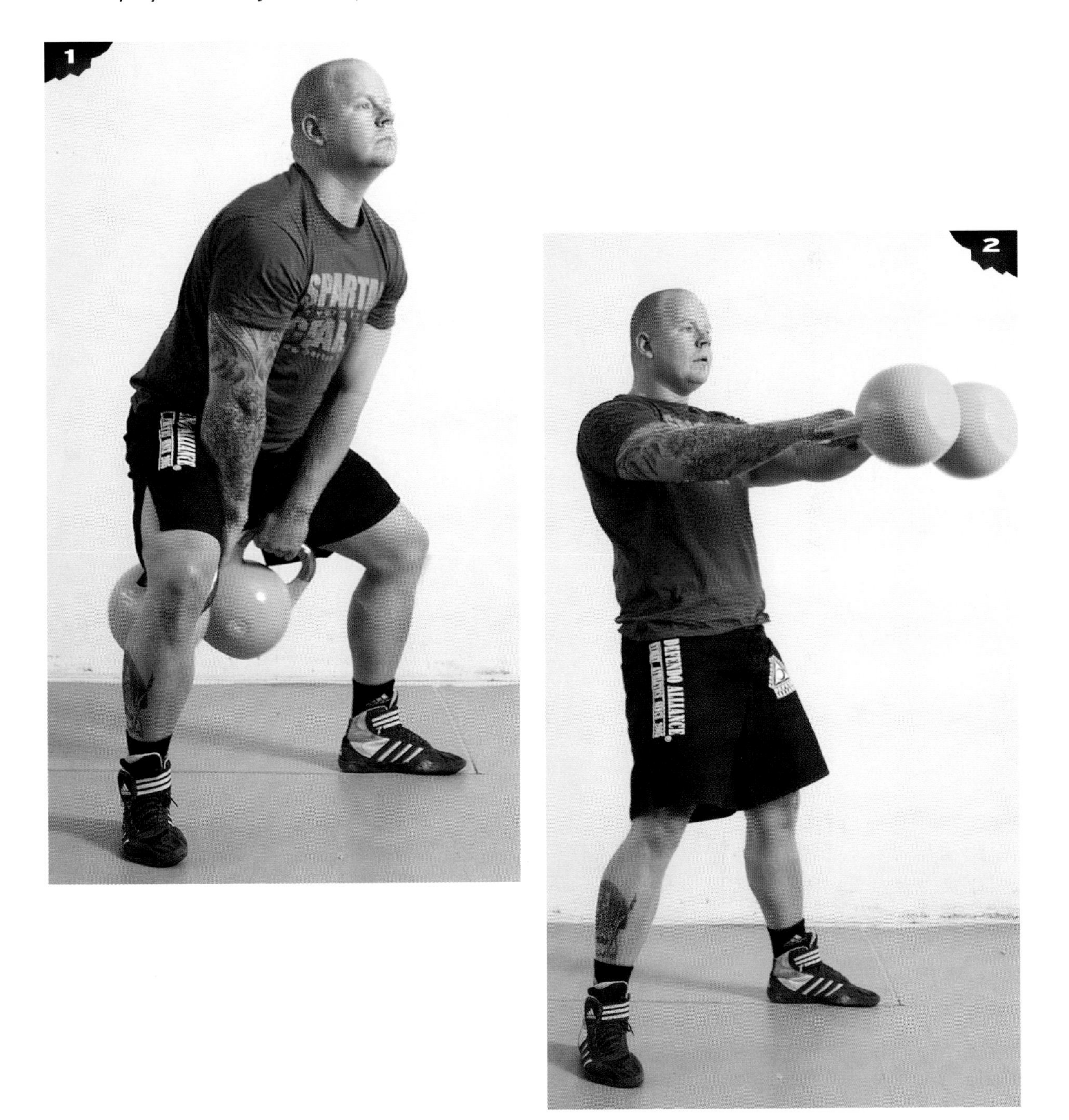

2. SWING TO ROW

Begin holding a bell in each hand. Squat down as you swing the bells between the legs and then stand up by extending at the hips. At the top of the swing, row the bells back by raising and pulling the elbows backward.

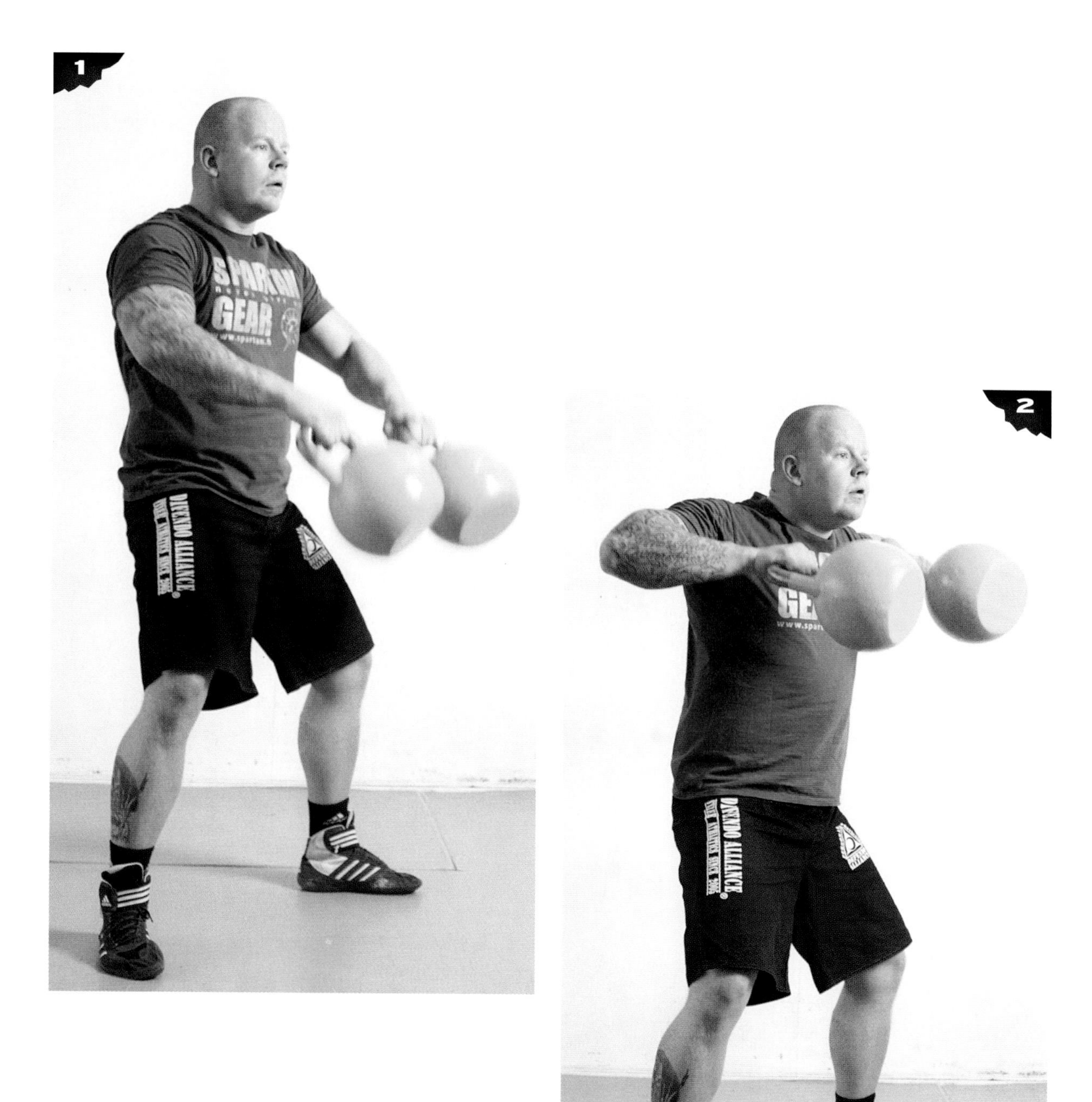

3. SQUAT BACK SWINGS

Begin holding a bell in each hand. Squat down as you swing the bells outside of the legs and then stand up by extending at the hips to swing the bells up to shoulder height with the palms facing each other.

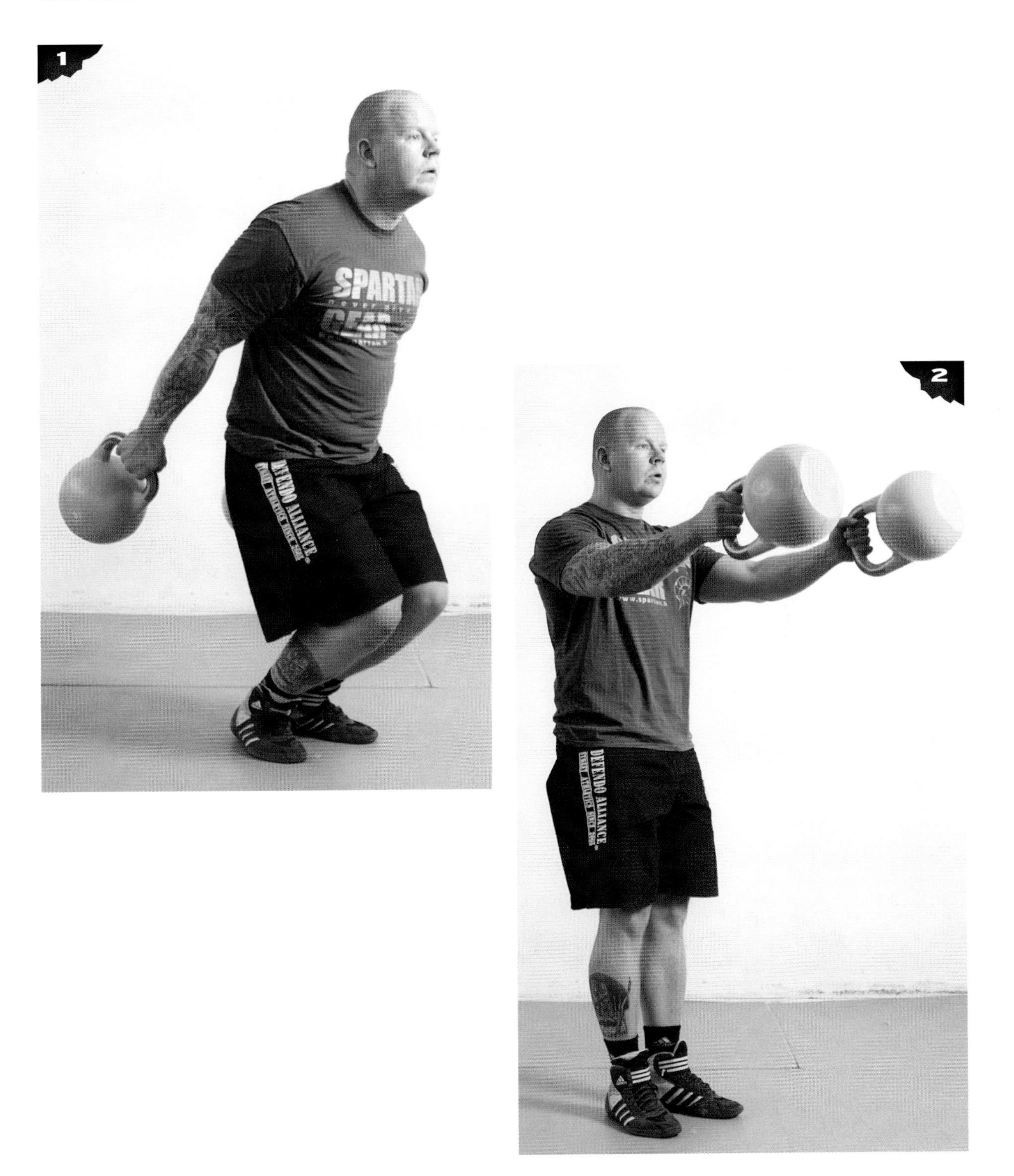

4. ALTERNATING SWINGS

Begin holding a bell in each hand. Swing one bell back and the other one forward. At the end of the motion, switch direction with each arm.

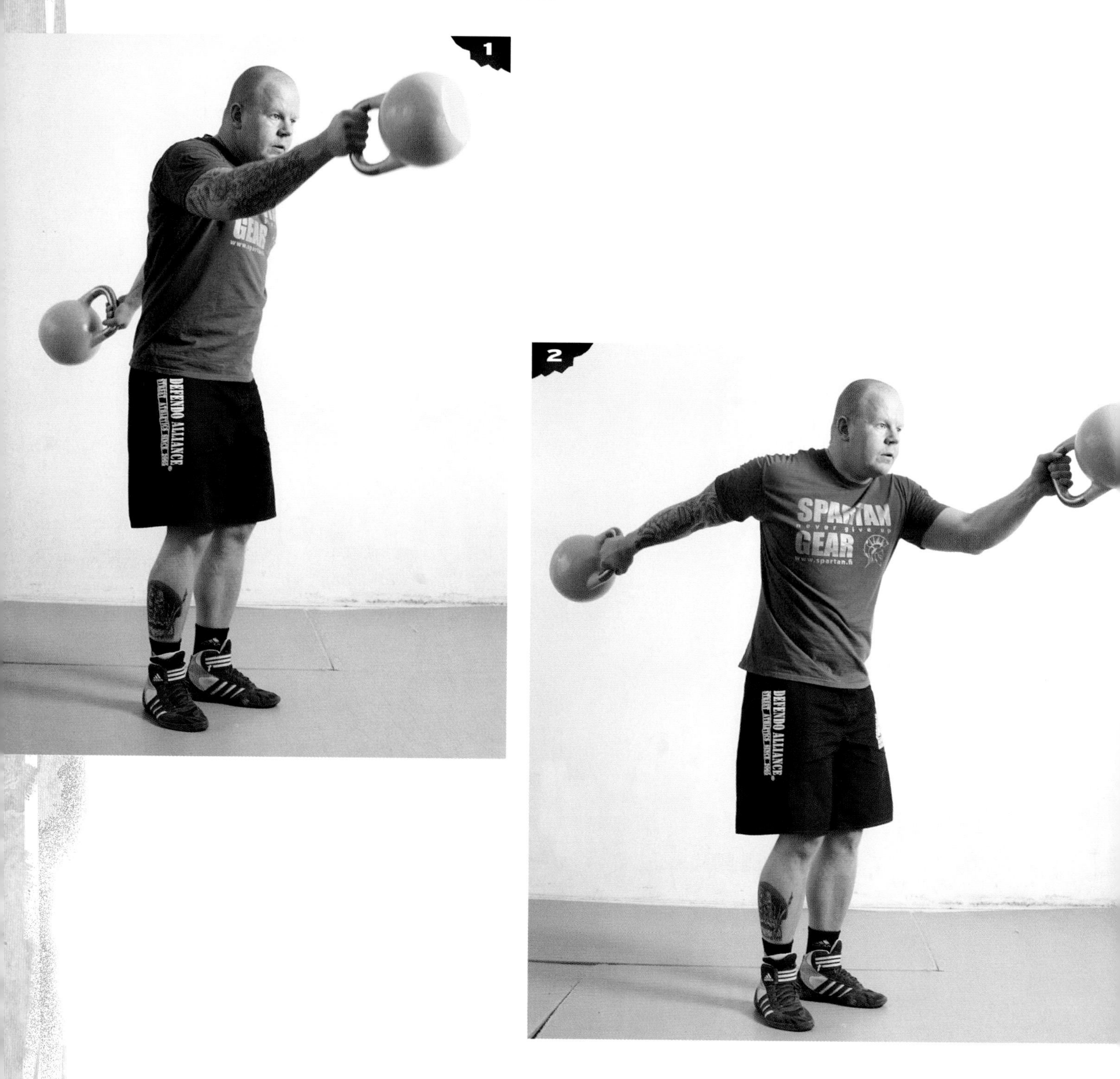

C. KETTLEBELL COMPLEX 3

Perform each exercise for 10 repetitions.

1. SINGLE-BELL FRONT SWING

Begin holding one bell with both hands. Squat down as you swing the bell between the legs and then stand up by extending at the hips to swing the bell up to shoulder height.

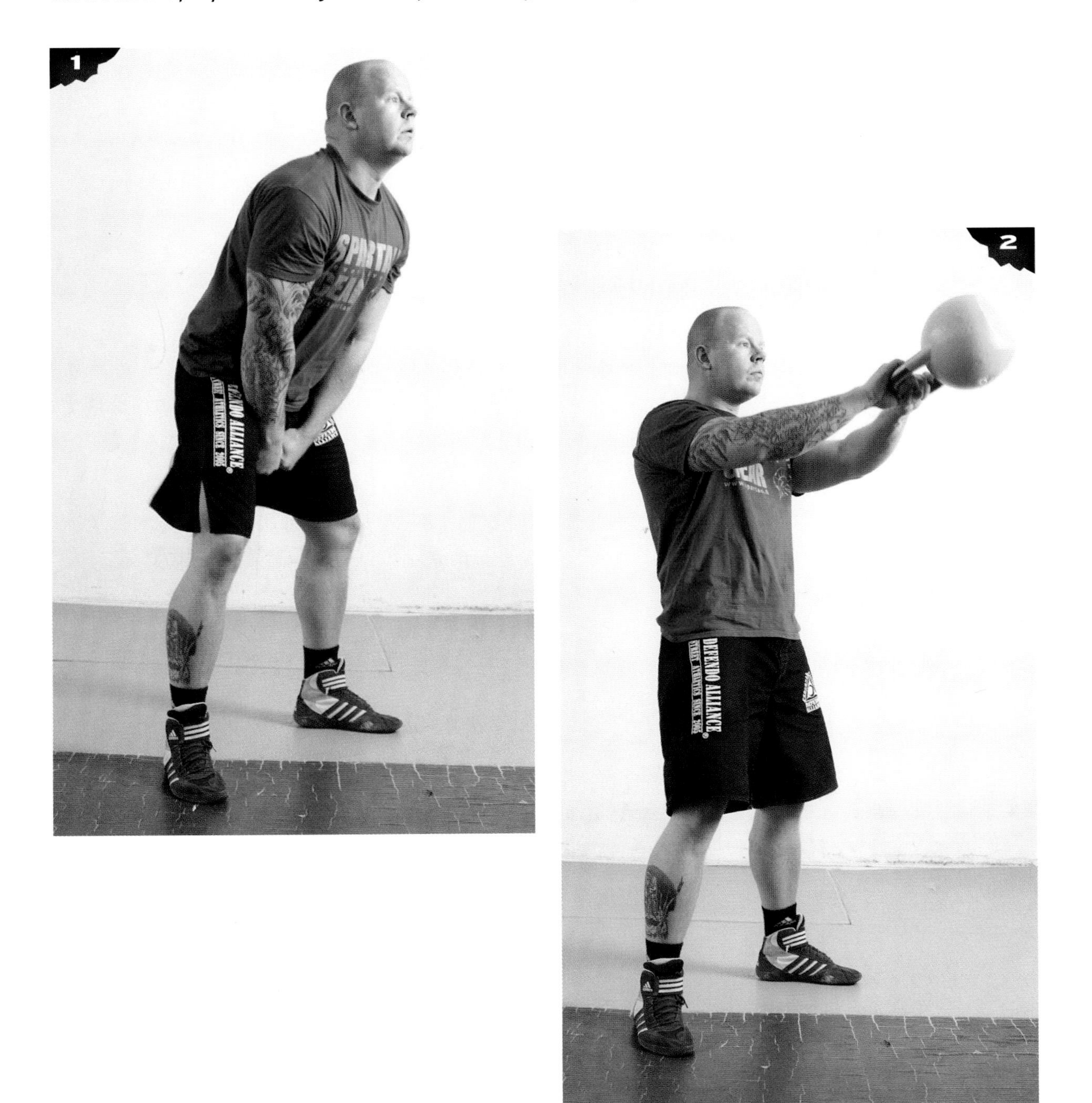

2. SINGLE-BELL CURL

Begin holding one bell with both hands at the hips. Curl the bell upward by flexing at the elbows. Lower the bell back down under control to the original position.

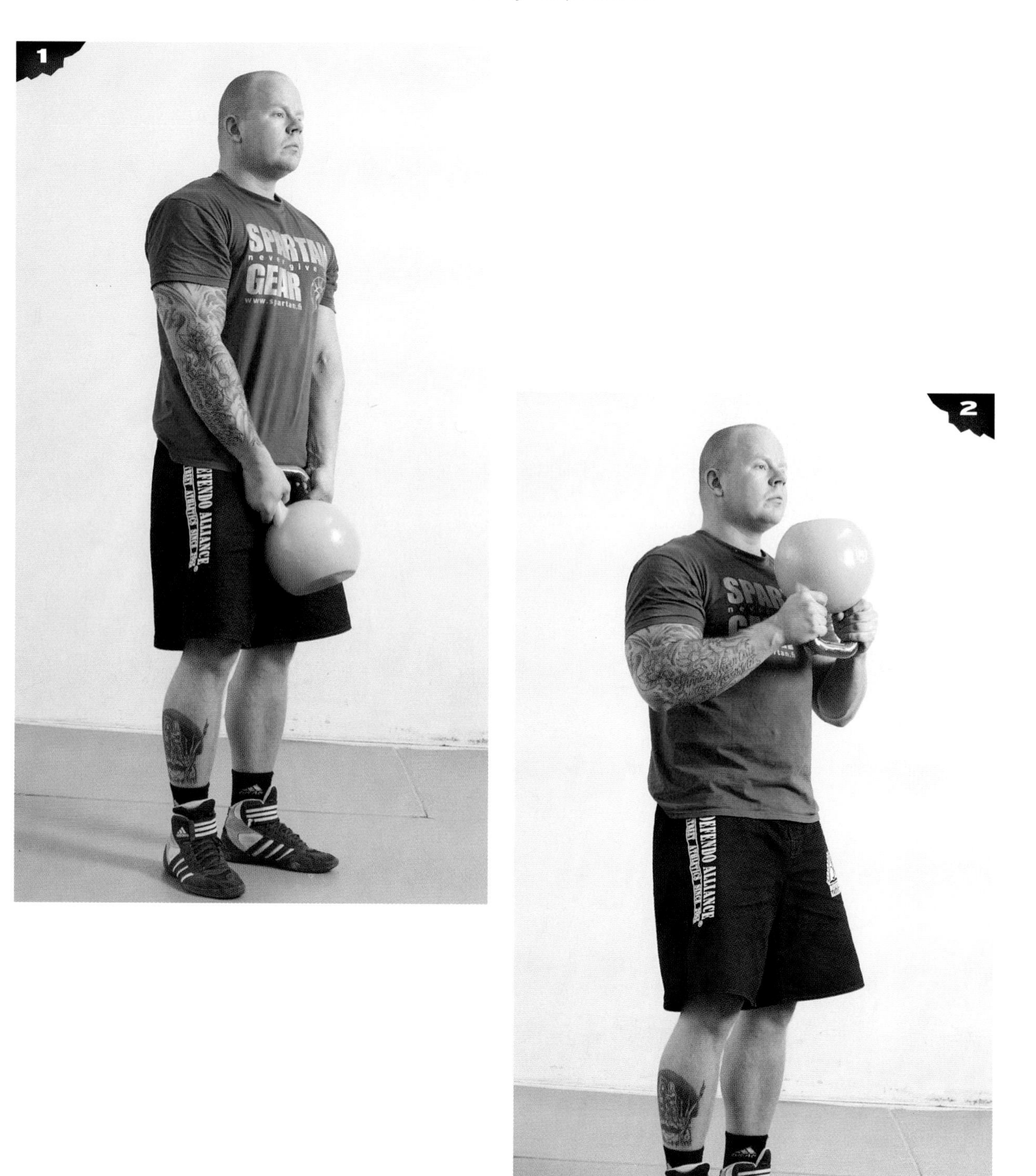

3. SINGLE-BELL TRICEP

Begin holding one bell with both hands overhead. Lower the bell behind the head until it almost touches the back of the neck. Extend at the elbows to bring the bell back to the original position.

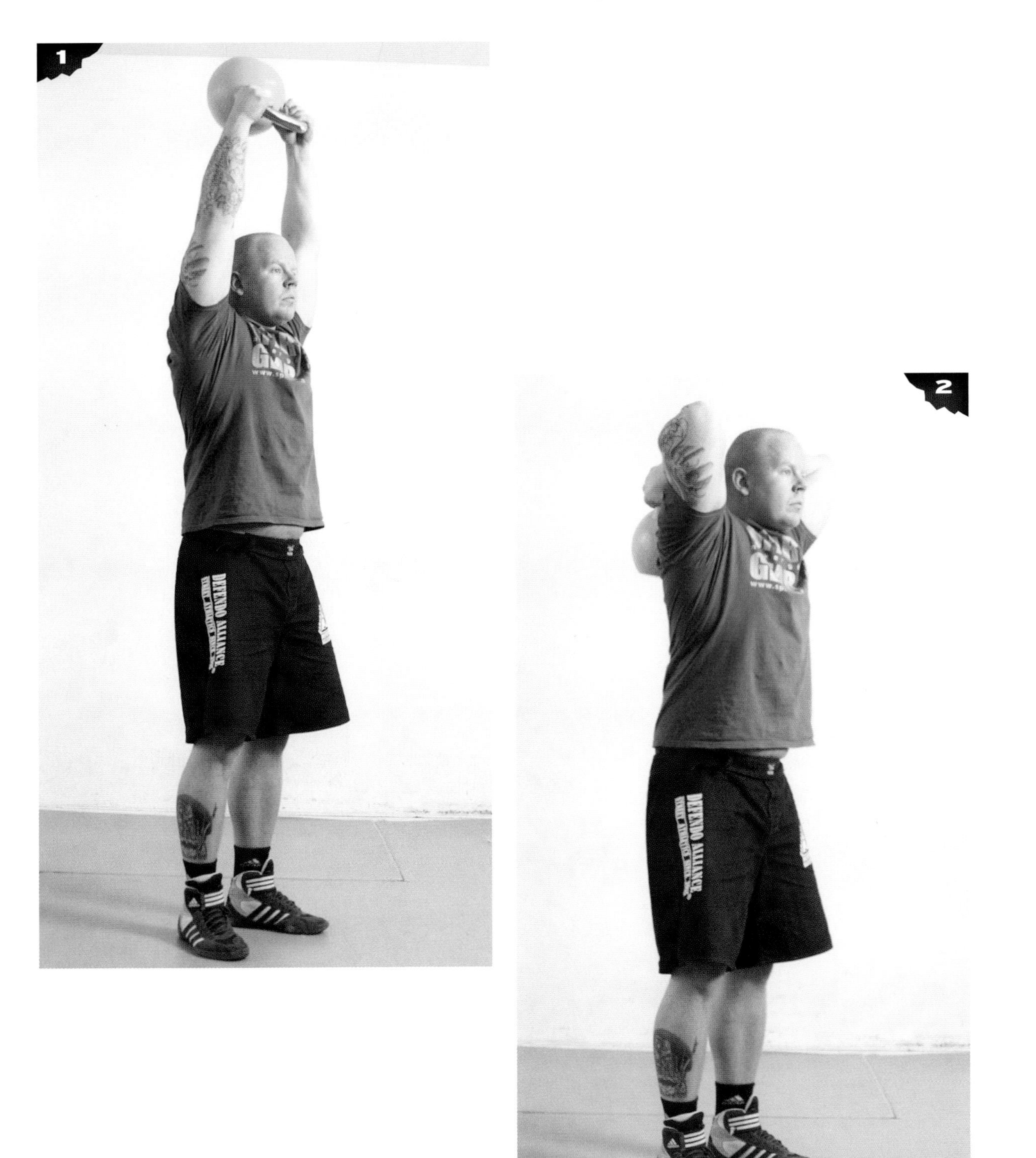

D. KETTLEBELL COMPLEX 4

Perform each exercise for 10 repetitions. On the last exercise of this complex, make sure to use each leg five times.

1. OVERHEAD SQUAT

Begin with the bells held overhead with the elbows extended. Lower the torso by bending at the hips and knees. Extend the knees and return to standing.

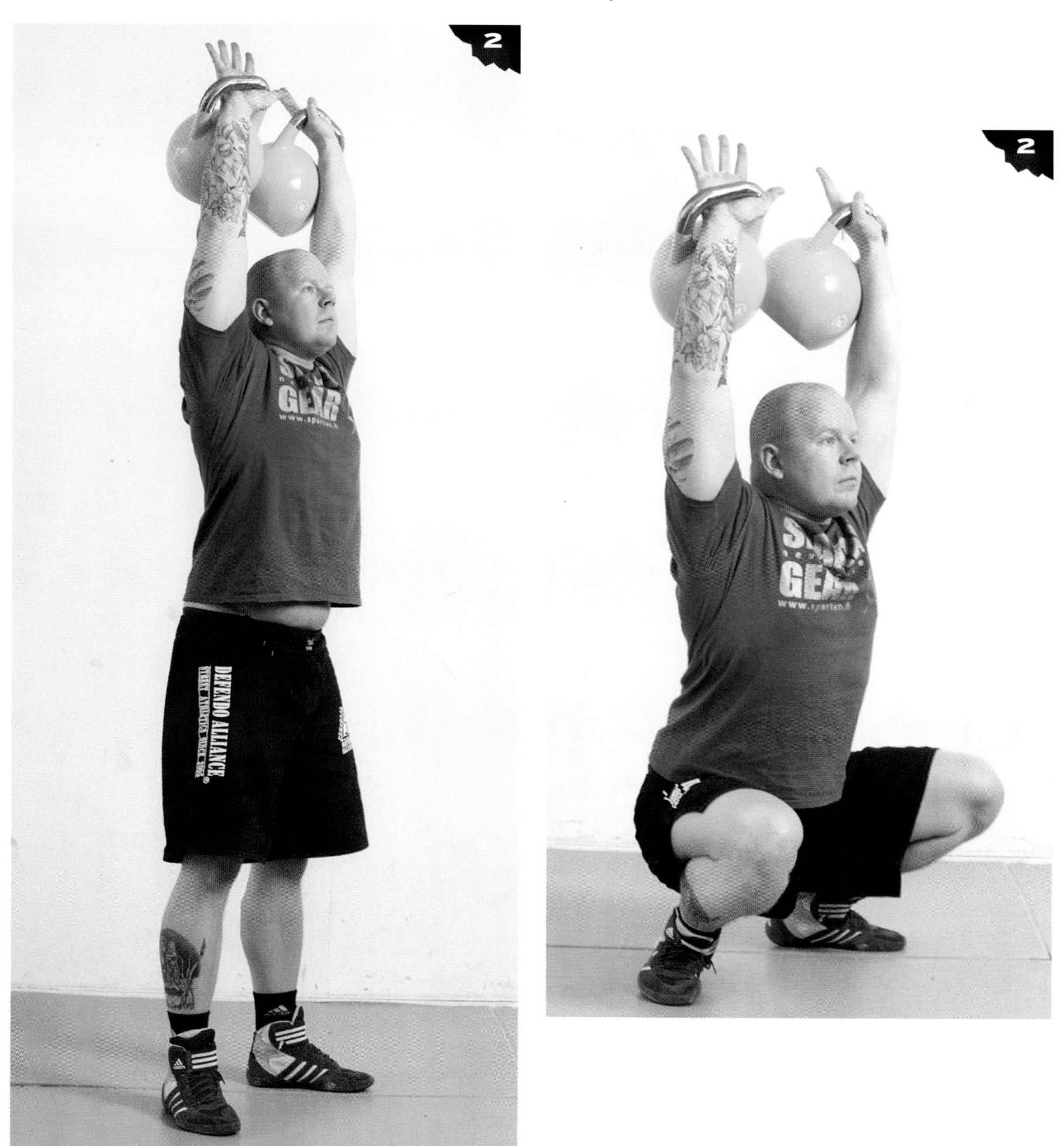

2. ALTERNATING SQUAT AND OVERHEAD PRESS

Begin with one bell held overhead and the other racked on the forearm. As you begin to squat, reverse the positions of the bells so that they are opposite at the bottom of the squat. Again reverse the positions once you come to standing.

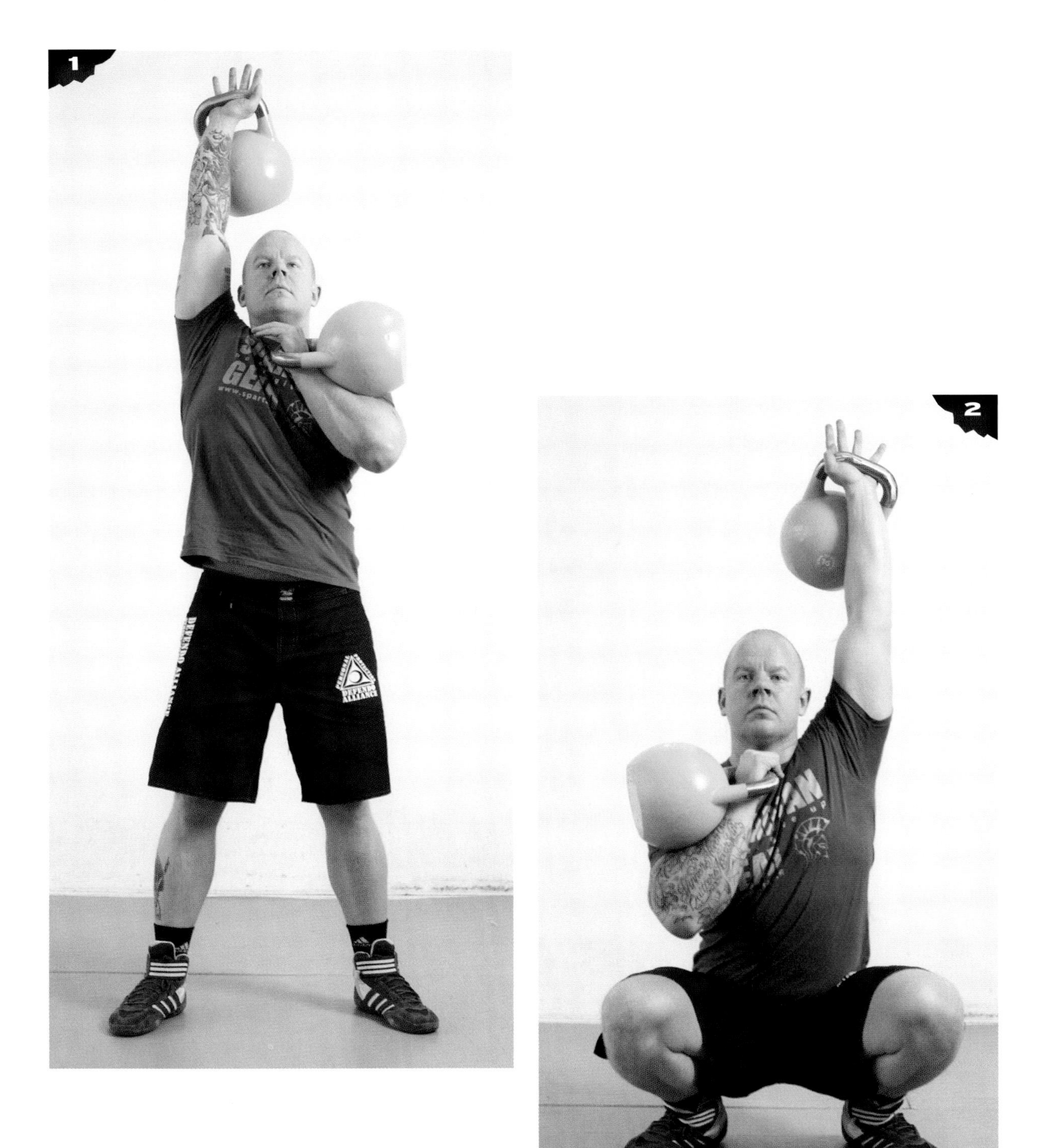

3. LUNGE AND OVERHEAD PRESS

Begin squatting with the bells in the racked position on the forearms. Step forward with one foot so that the back knee almost touches the ground. Press the bells overhead from the front lunge position. Return the bells to the forearms and press back up with the leg to the original position.

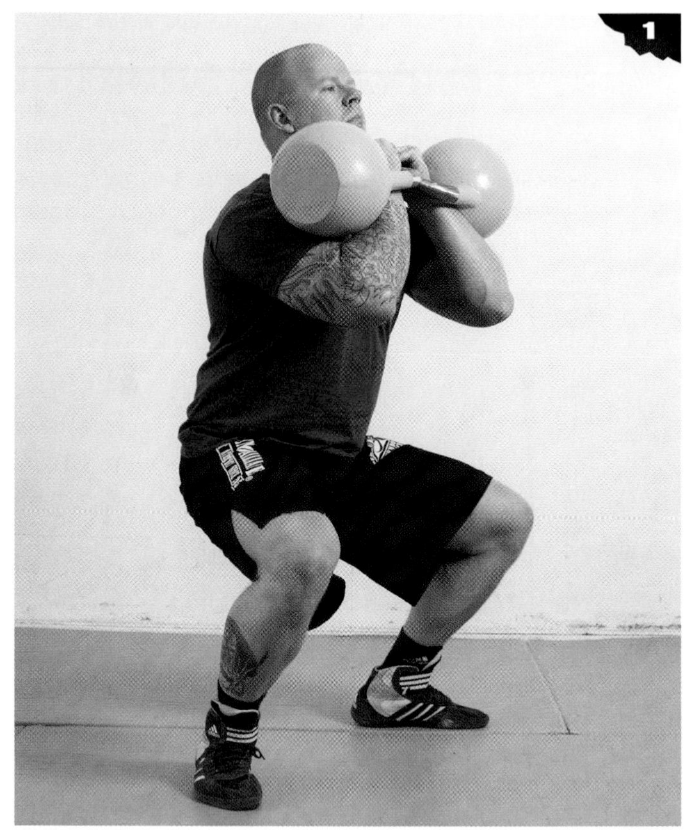

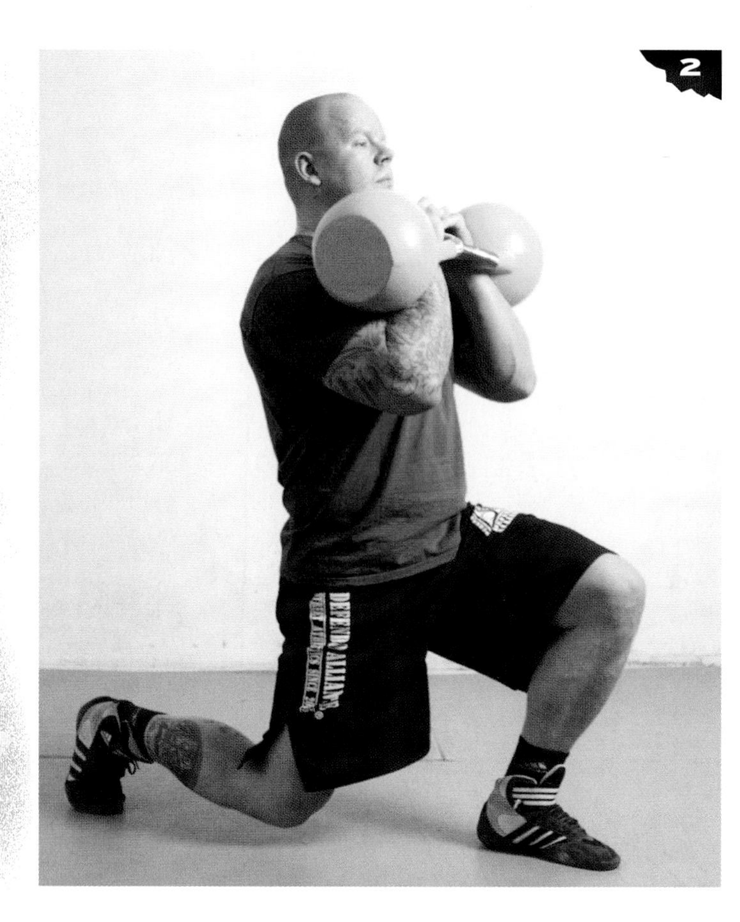

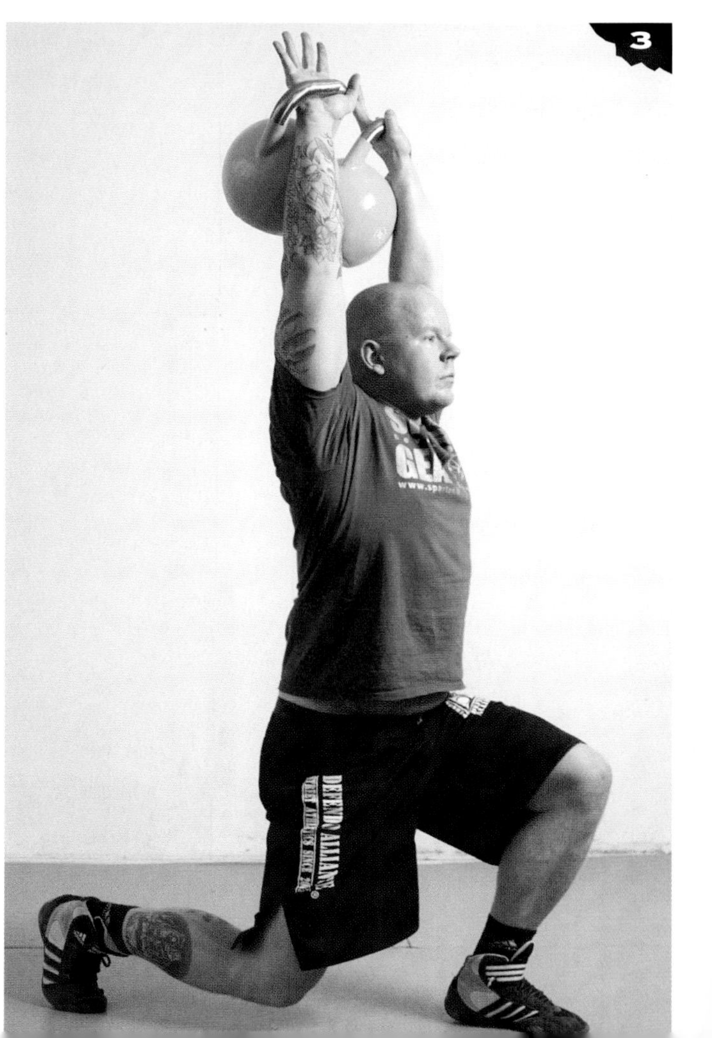

E. KETTLEBELL COMPLEX 5

Perform 10 repetitions of each exercise. For the lunge and side lunge, make sure to perform 5 repetitions on each leg.

1. SQUAT

Begin standing with the bells racked on the forearms. Squat down to the parallel-squat position so that the knees are at 90 degrees. Extend back at the knees and hips to return to the original position.

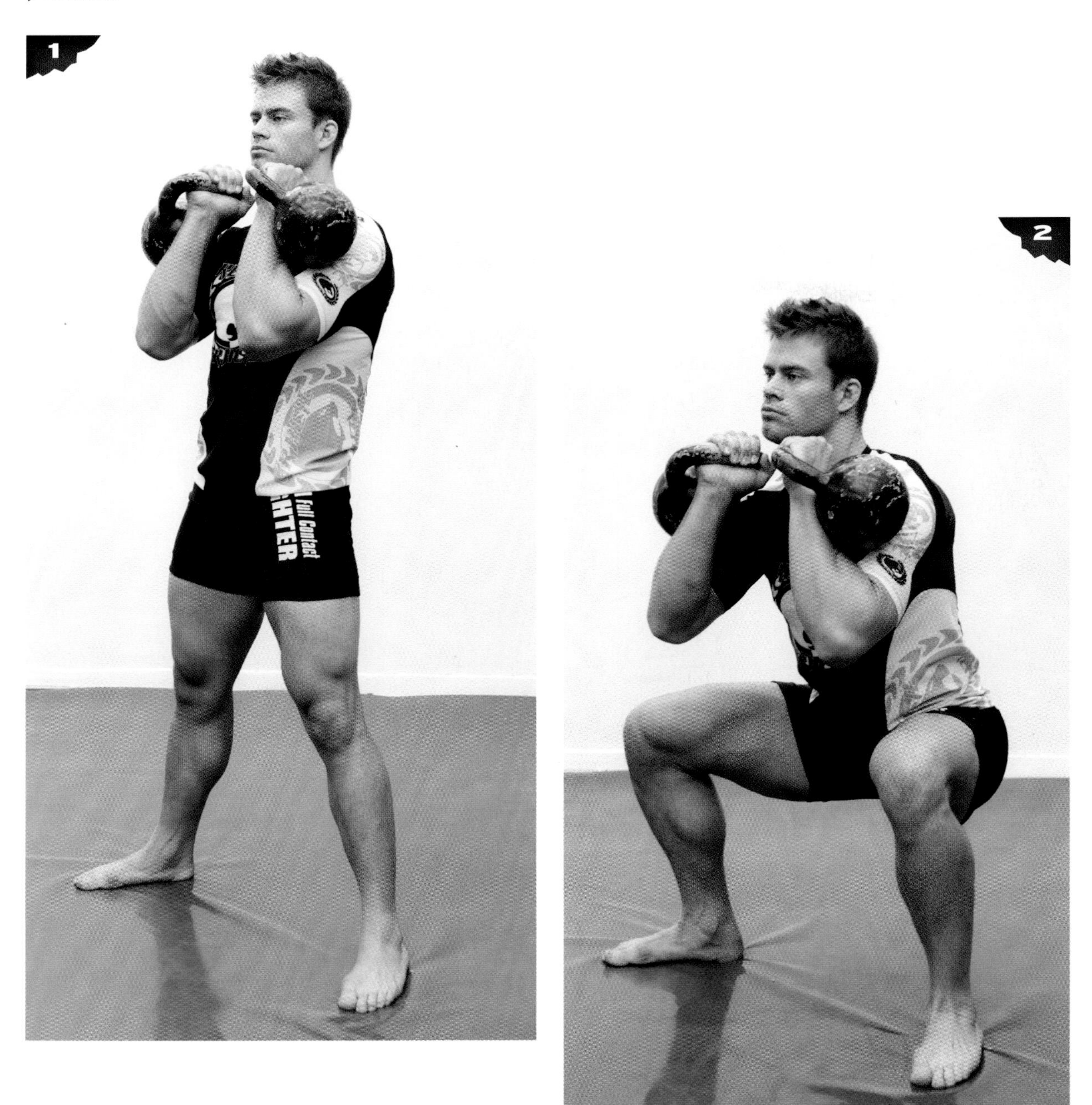

2. HIGH PULL

Begin standing in a half-squat position with the bells between the legs. Stand up and pull the elbows up to the height of the chin. Lower the bells under control to the start position.

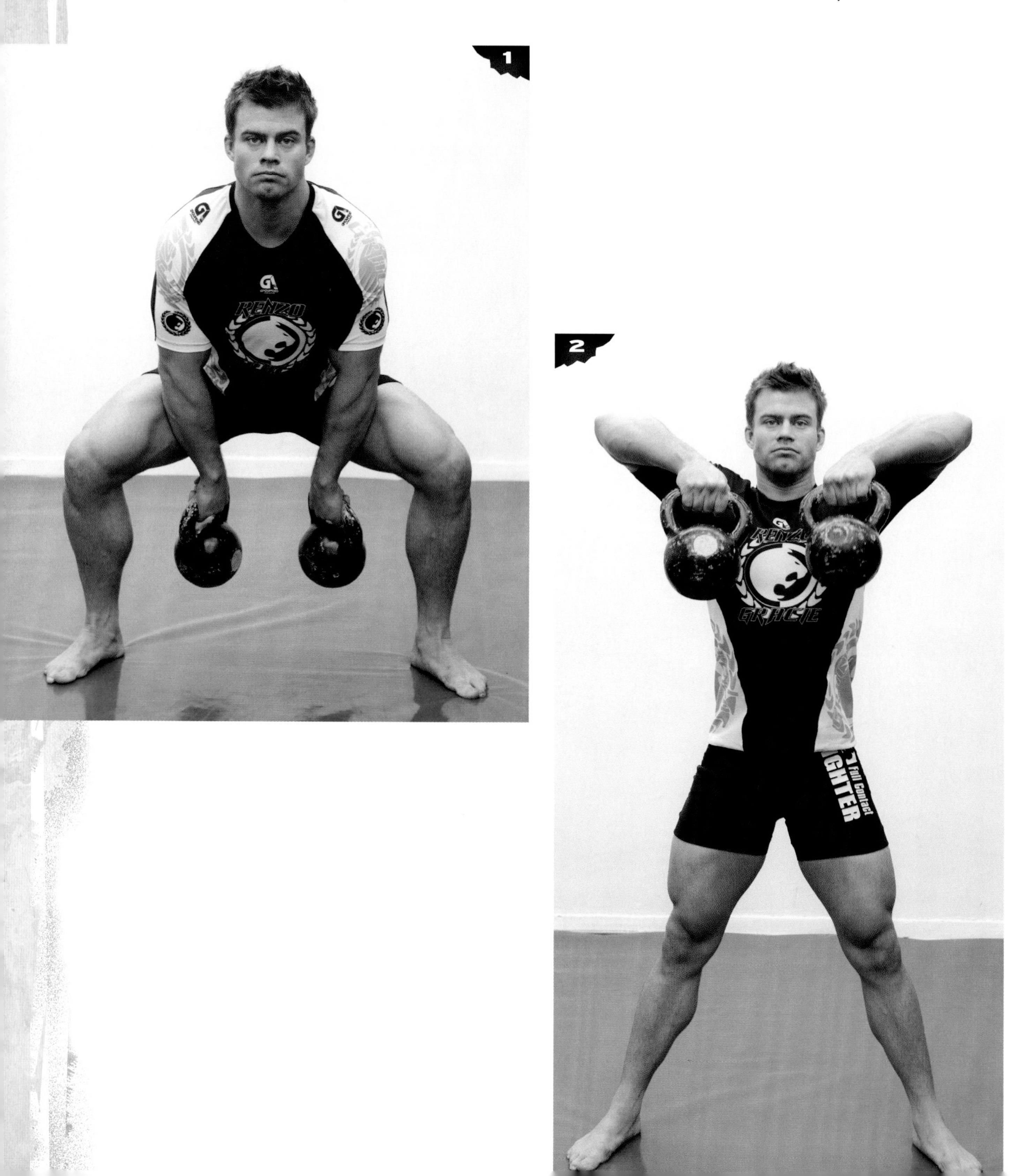

3. BENT-OVER ROW

Begin standing in a half-squat position with the bells between the legs. Pull the elbows to the sides and raise the bells to the chest. Lower the bells under control to the start position.

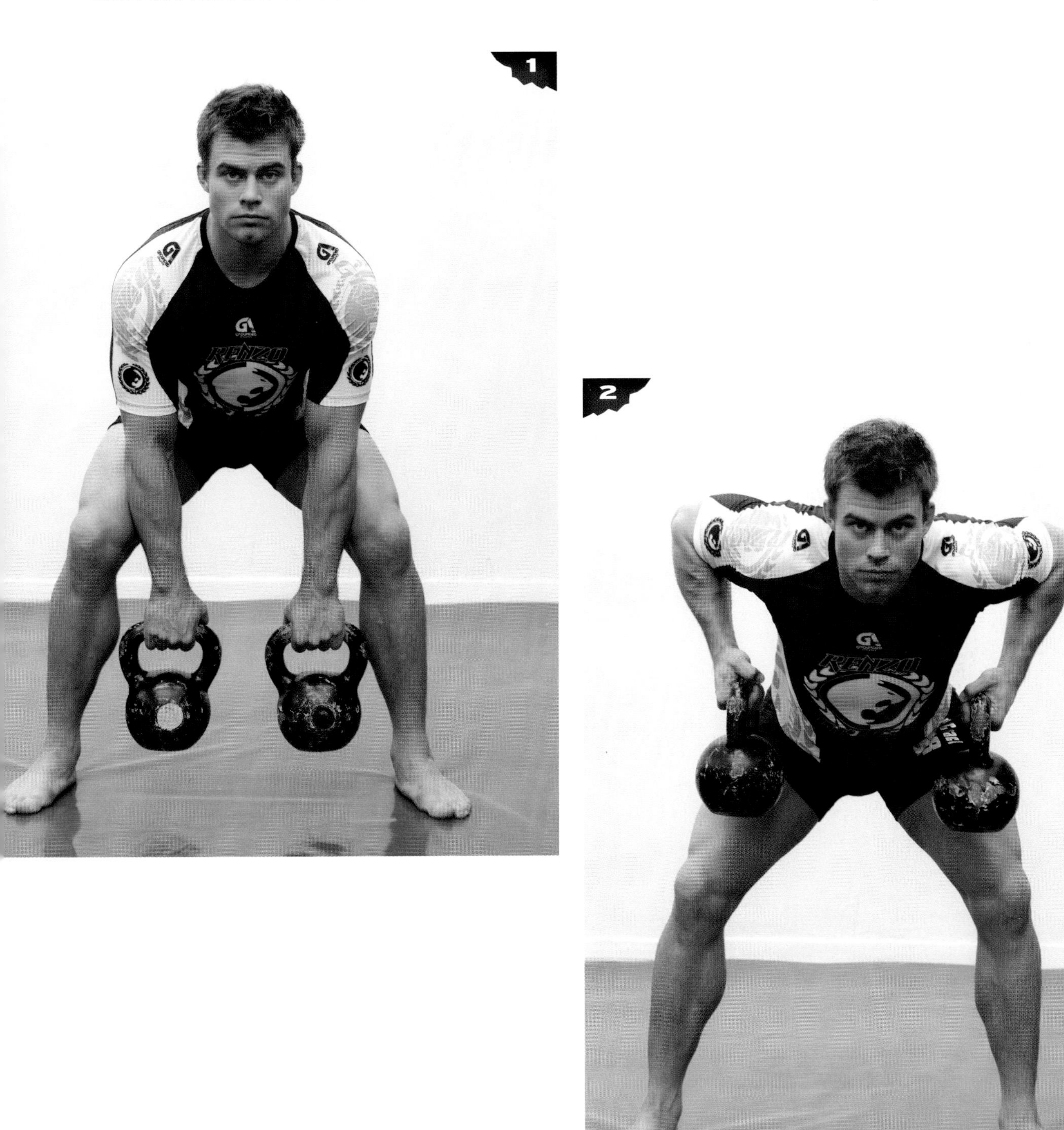

4. DEADLIFT

Begin standing with the bells held at the height of the hips. Bend forward at the waist and lower the bells past halfway down the shin. Extend at the hips to return to the start position.

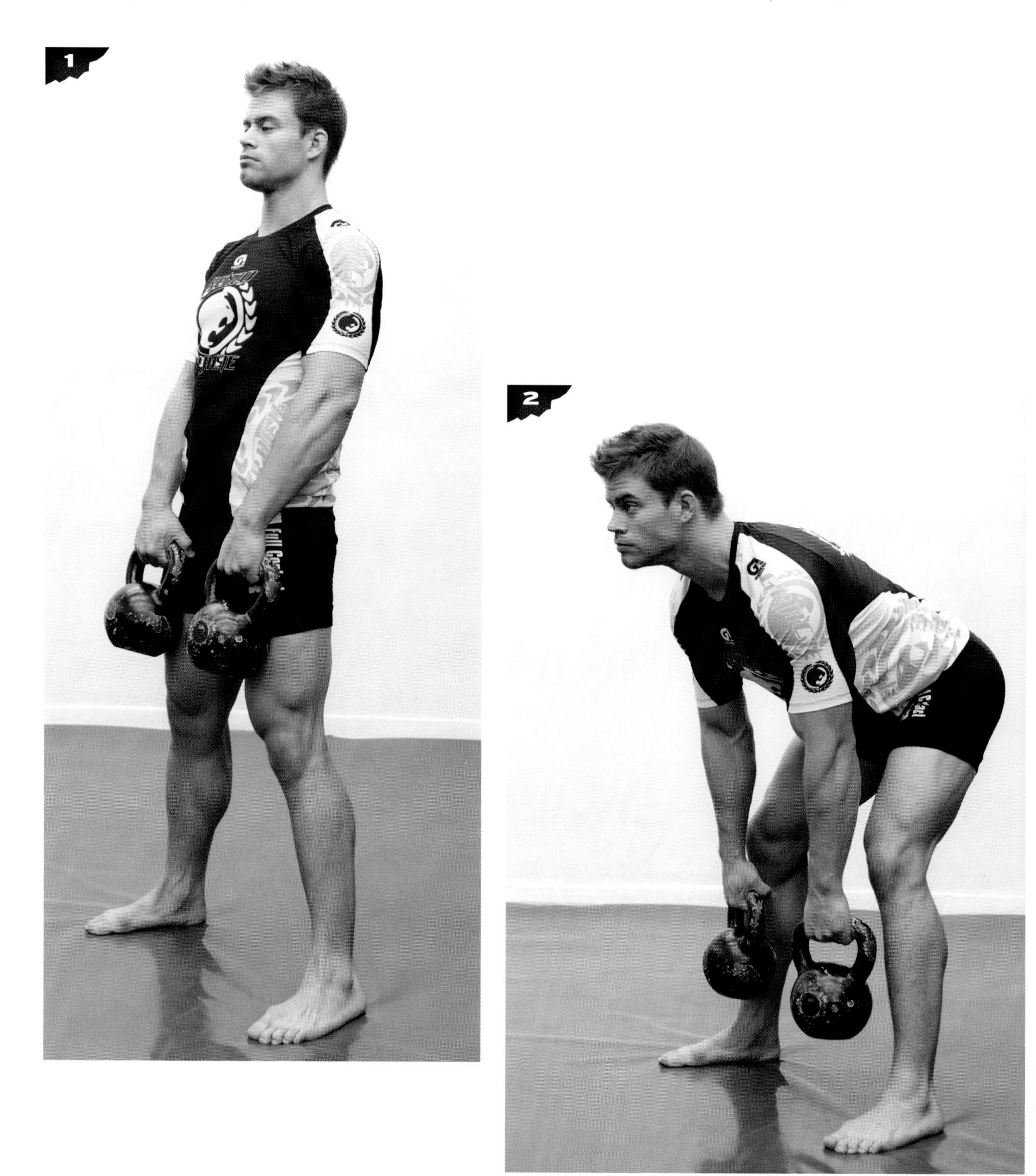

5. LUNGE

Begin standing with the bells in the racked position on the forearms. Step forward with one foot so that the back knee almost touches the ground. Press back into the ground with the leg to return to the original position. Repeat on the other leg.

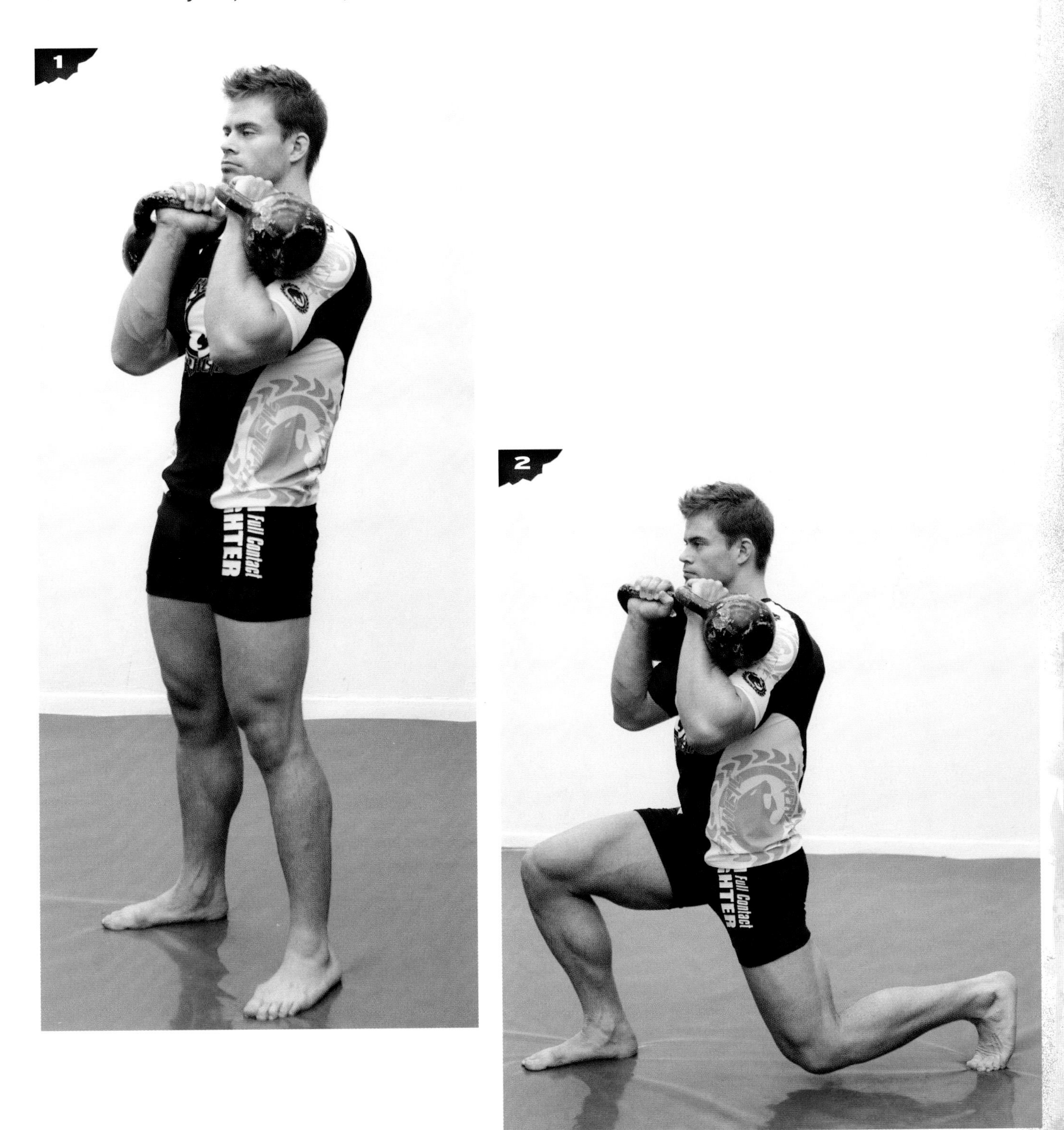

6. GOOD MORNING

Begin standing, holding one bell (or both bells) behind the neck. Bend forward at the waist with only a slight bend at the knees and keep the lower back flat. Extend at the hips to return to the original position.

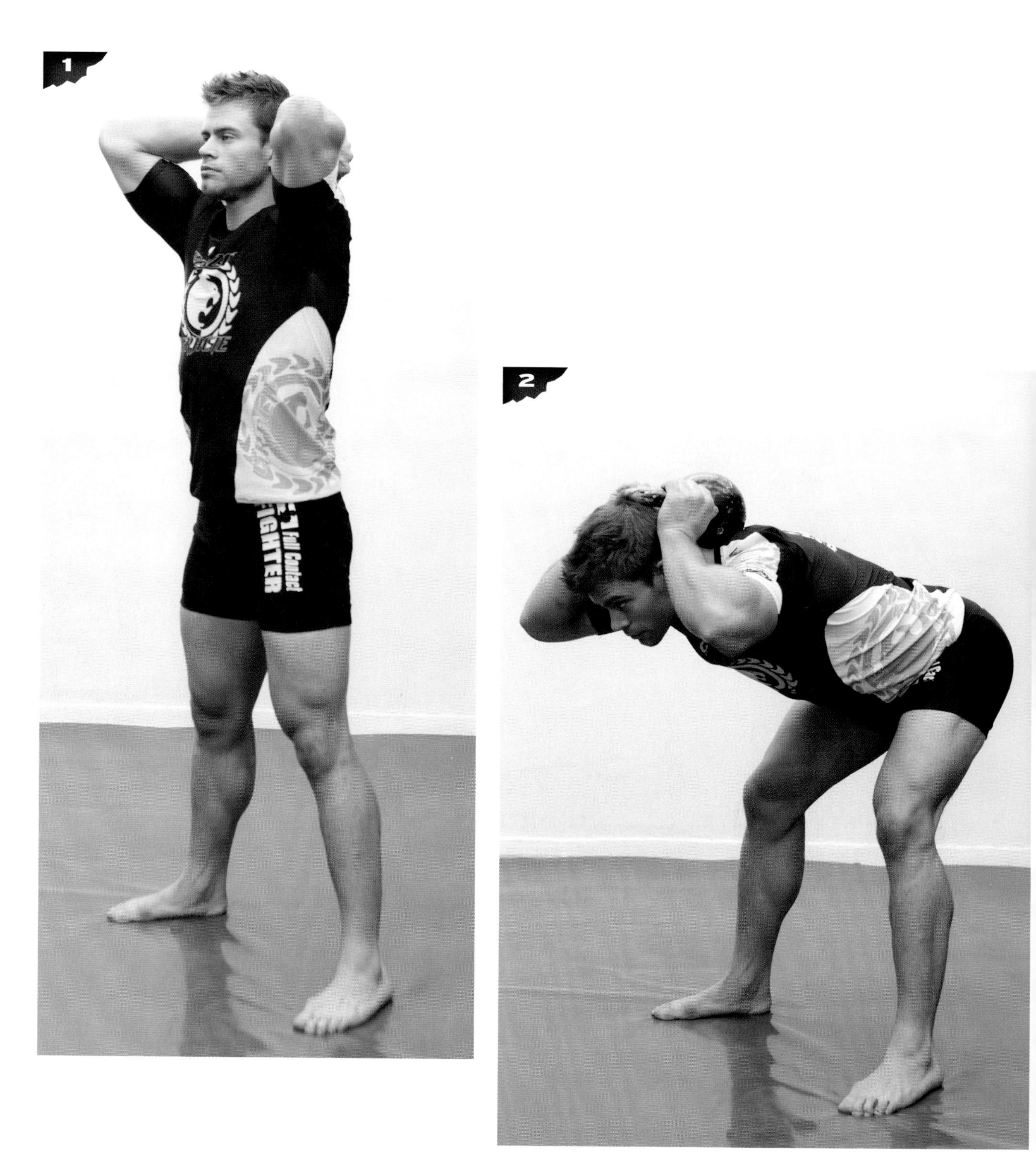

7. SIDE LUNGE

Begin standing with the bells racked on the forearms. Step out to one side and lower the hips by bending at the knee and waist. Press back with the lead foot to get to the original position. Repeat on the other leg.

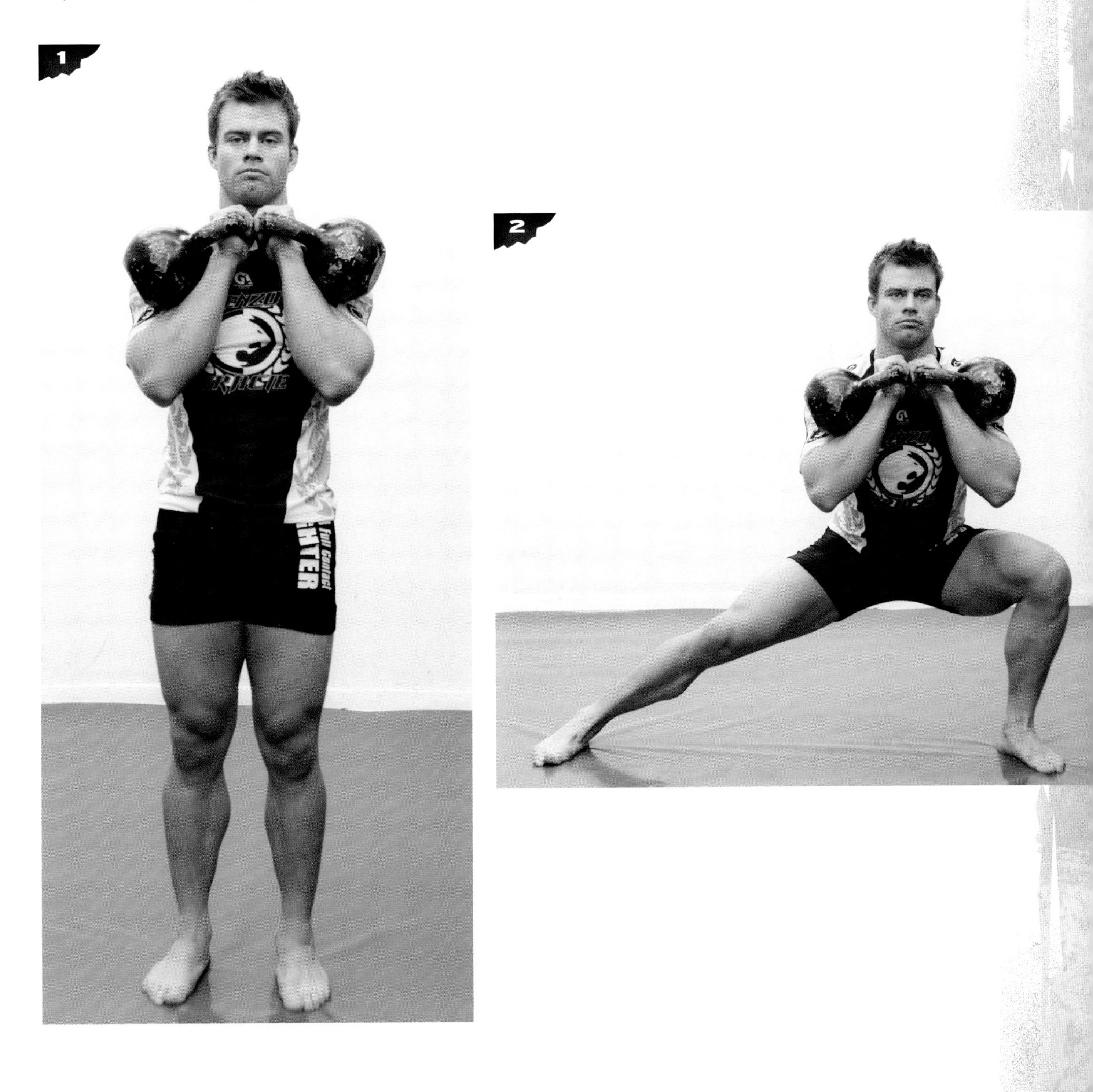

8. SWING TO ROW

Begin holding a bell in each hand. Squat down as you swing the bells between the legs and then stand up by extending at the hips. At the top of the swing, row the bells back by raising and pulling the elbows backward.

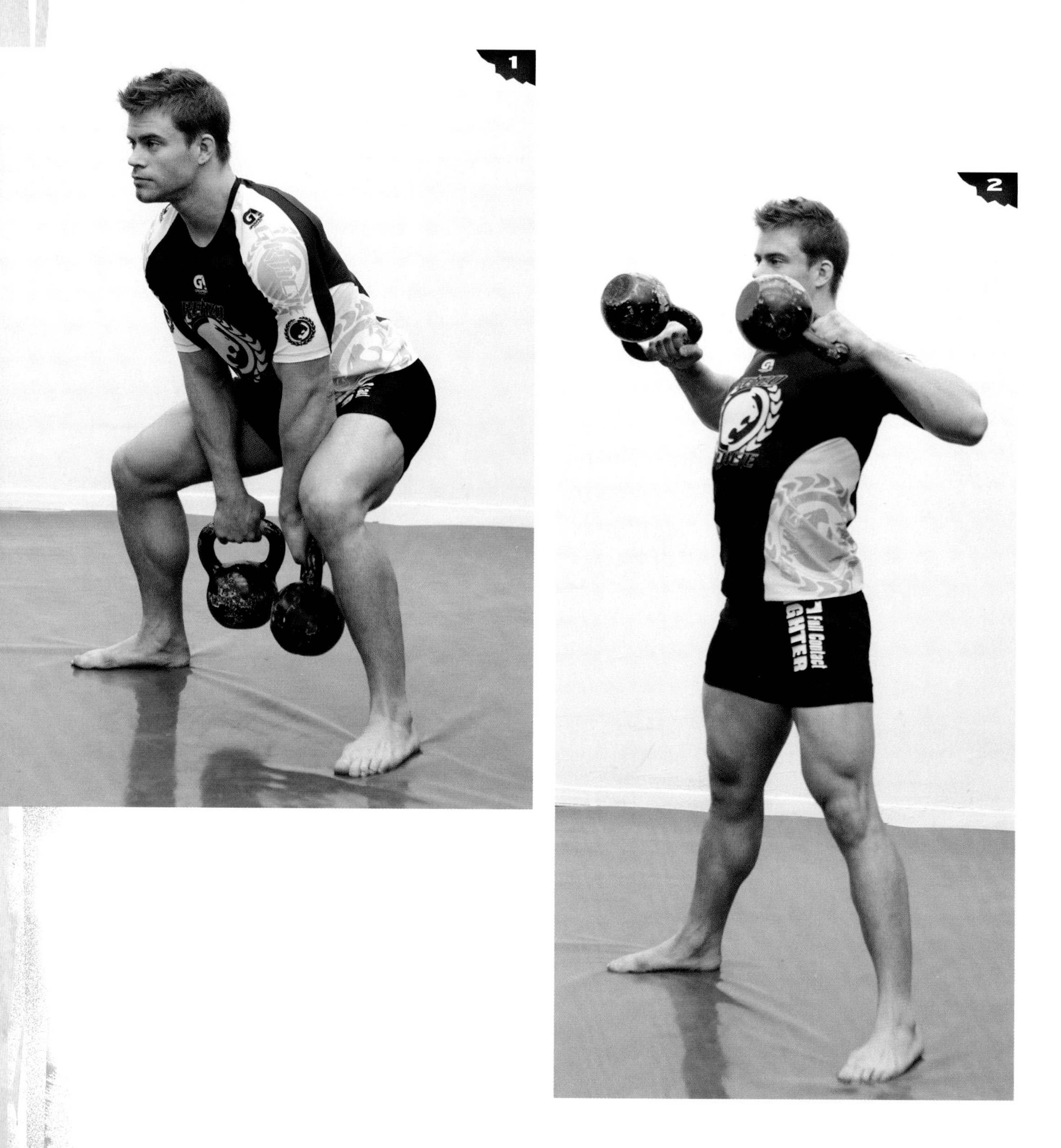

FULL-BODY BARBELL COMPLEX CHEATSHEET

1. STIFF-LEGGED DEADLIFT

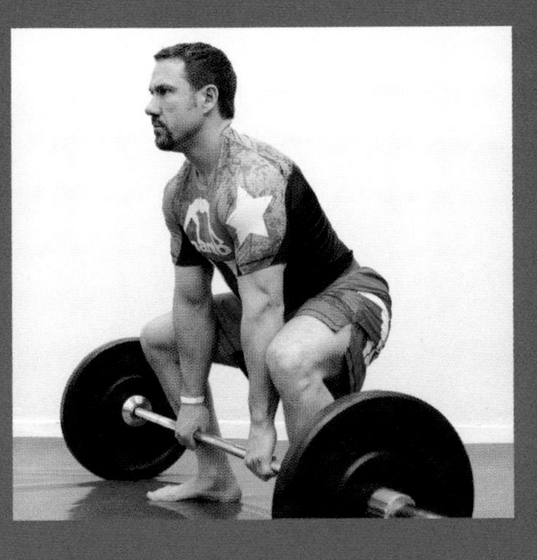

2. WIDE-GRIP BENT-OVER ROW

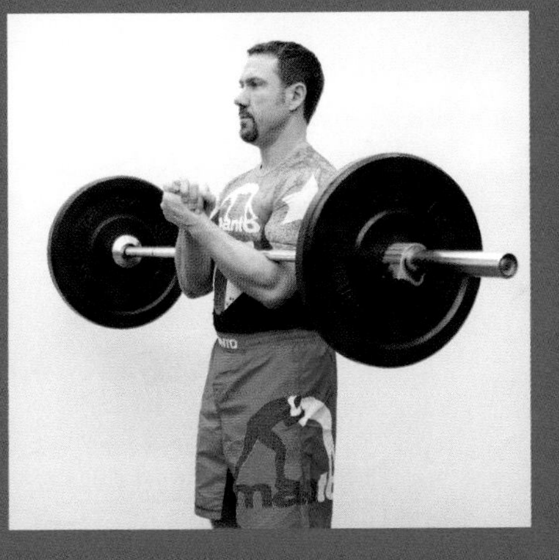

3. HIGH PULL

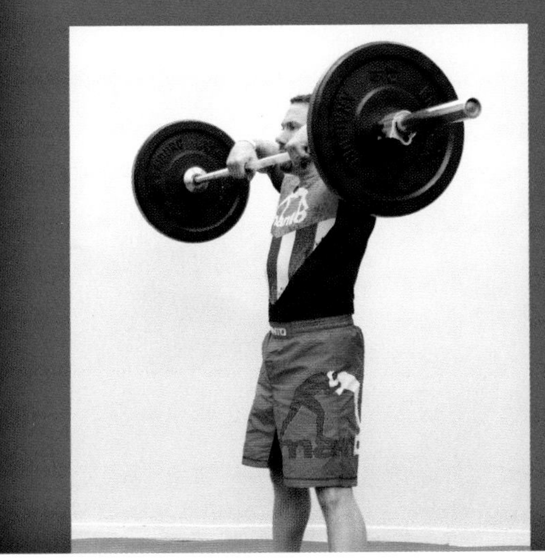

4. FRONT SQUAT

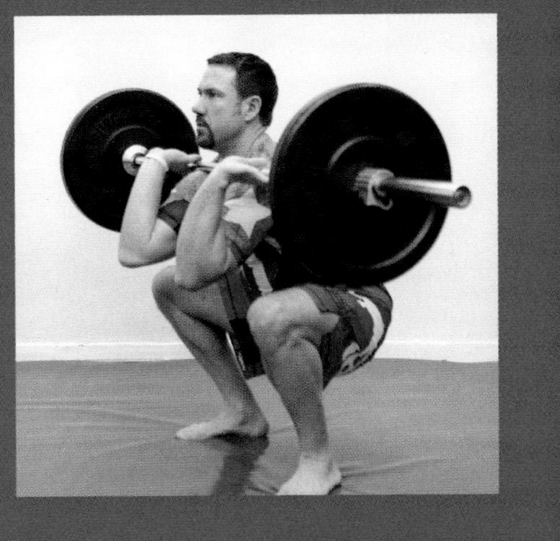

5. OVERHEAD PRESS

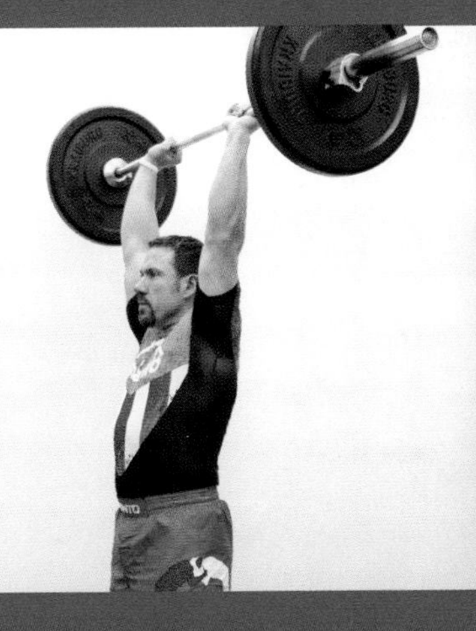

6. BACK SQUAT

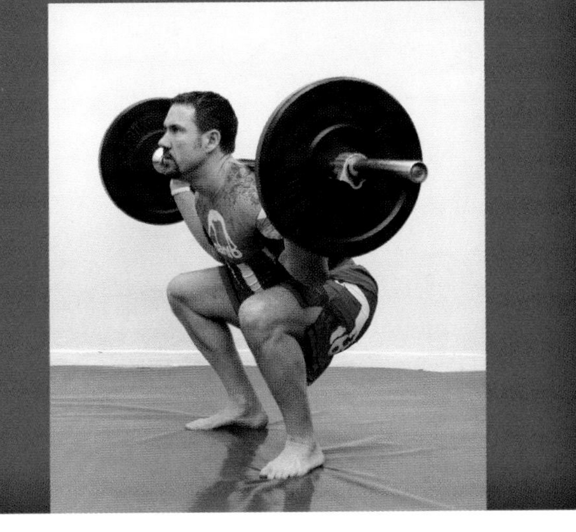

10-EXERCISE BARBELL COMPLEX CHEATSHEET

1. STIFF-LEGGED DEADLIFT

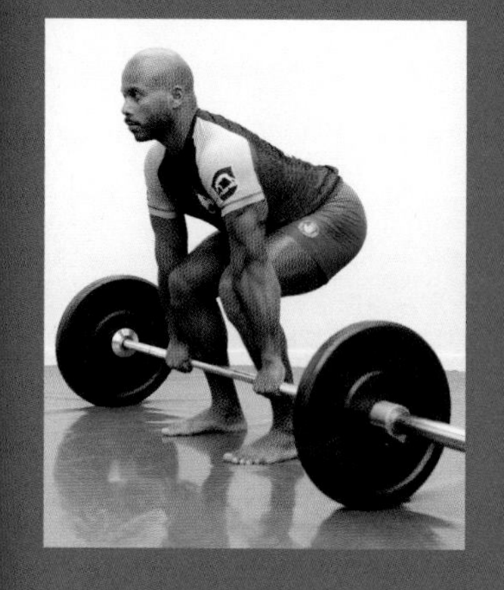

2. SHRUG

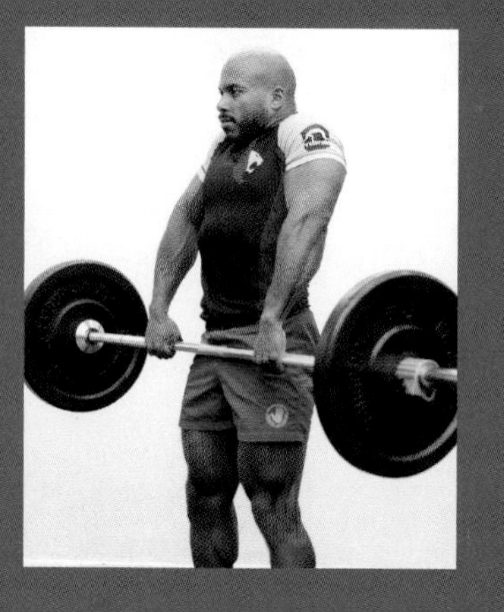

3. CLEAN

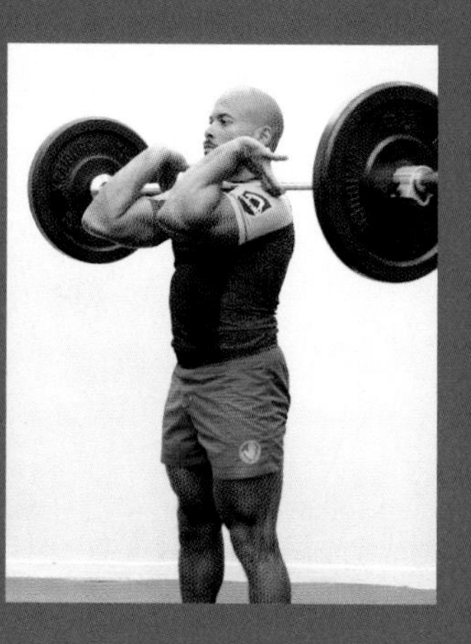

4. PUSH JERK

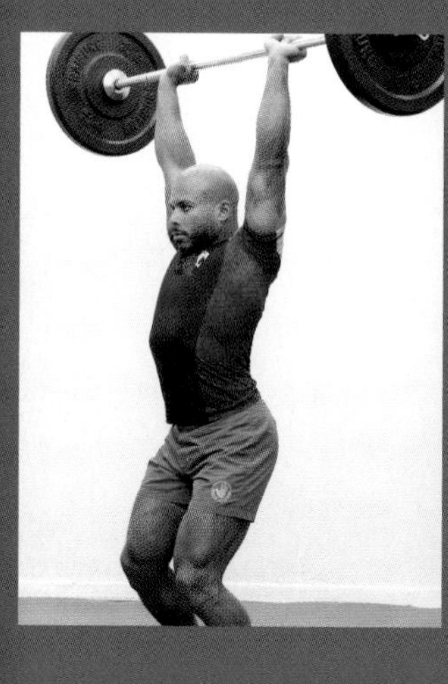

5. HIGH PULL

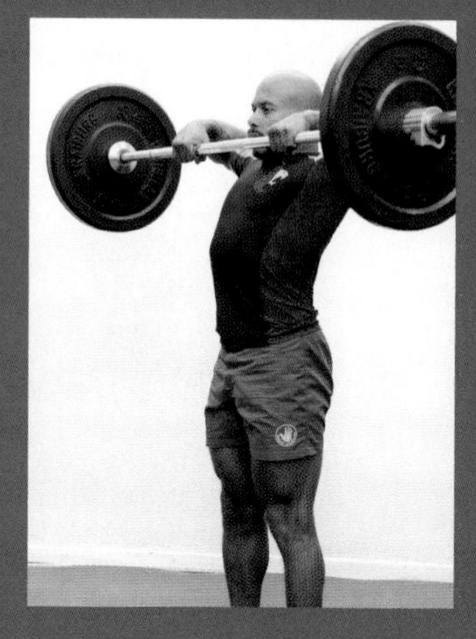

6. BENT-OVER ROW

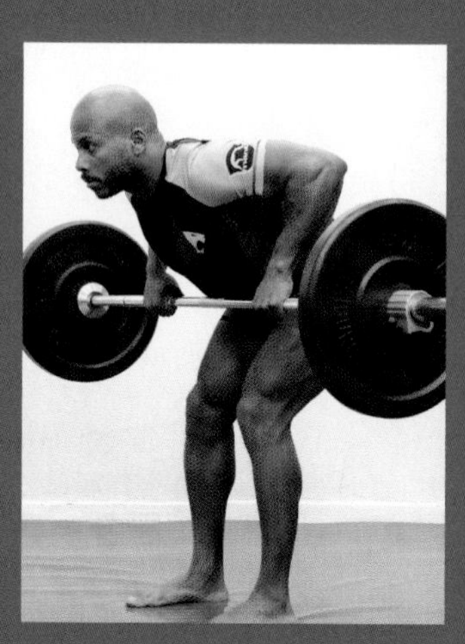

7. JUMP SQUAT

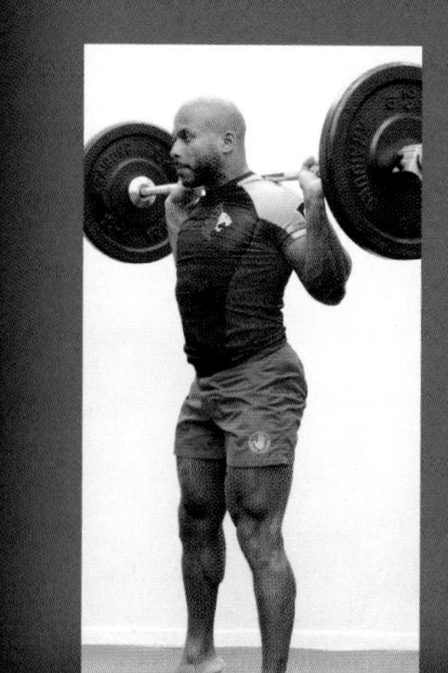

8. GOOD MORNING

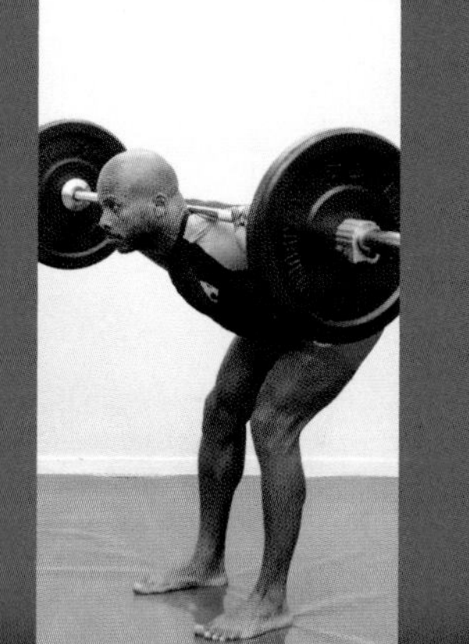

9. TRICEP EXTENSION

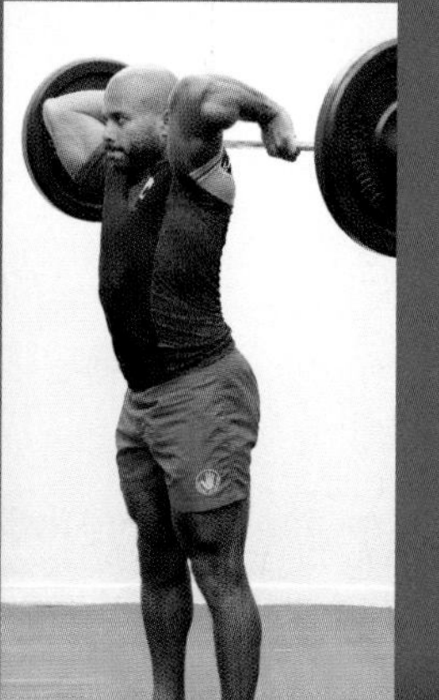

10. BICEP CURL

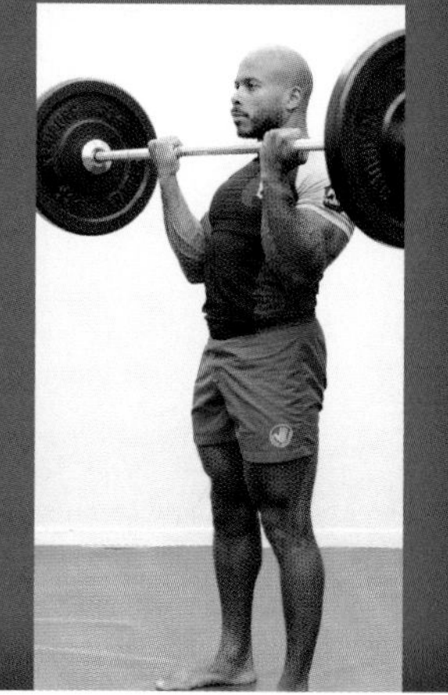

LOWER-BODY DUMBBELL COMPLEX CHEATSHEET

1. DEADLIFT

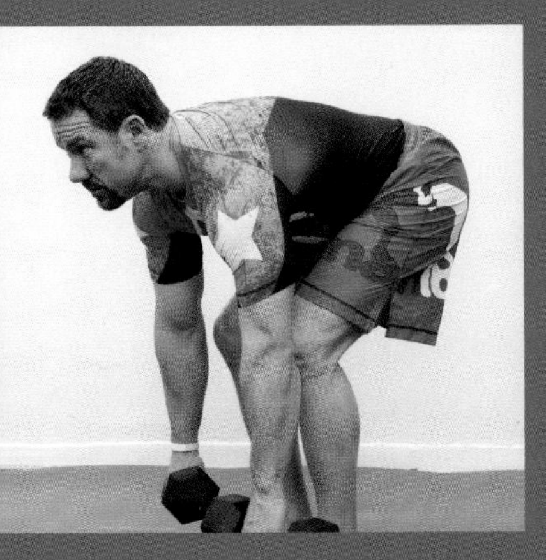

4. SNATCH

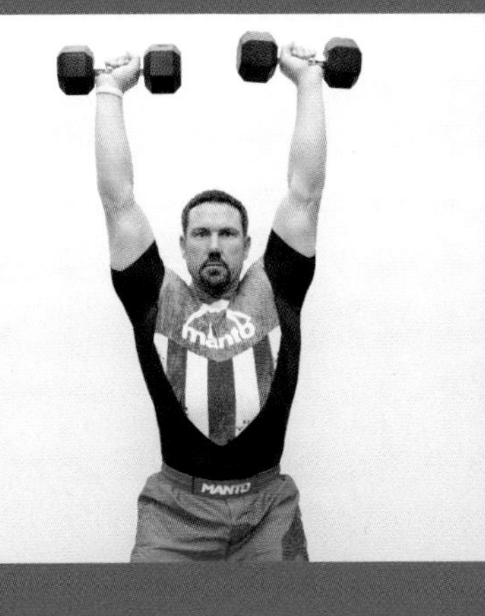

2. HAMMER CURL

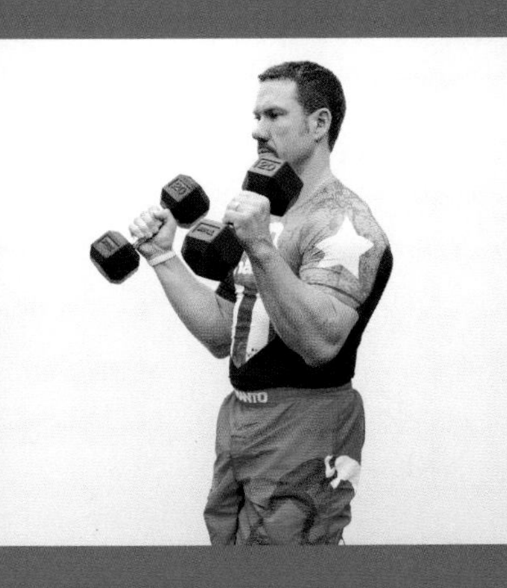

5. SQUAT

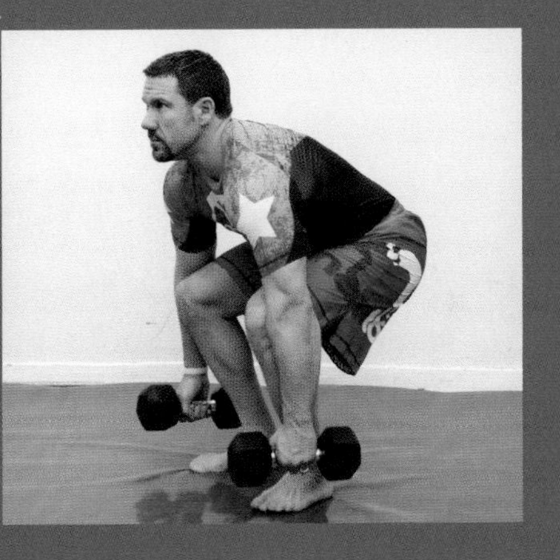

3. BENT-OVER ROW

6. LUNGE

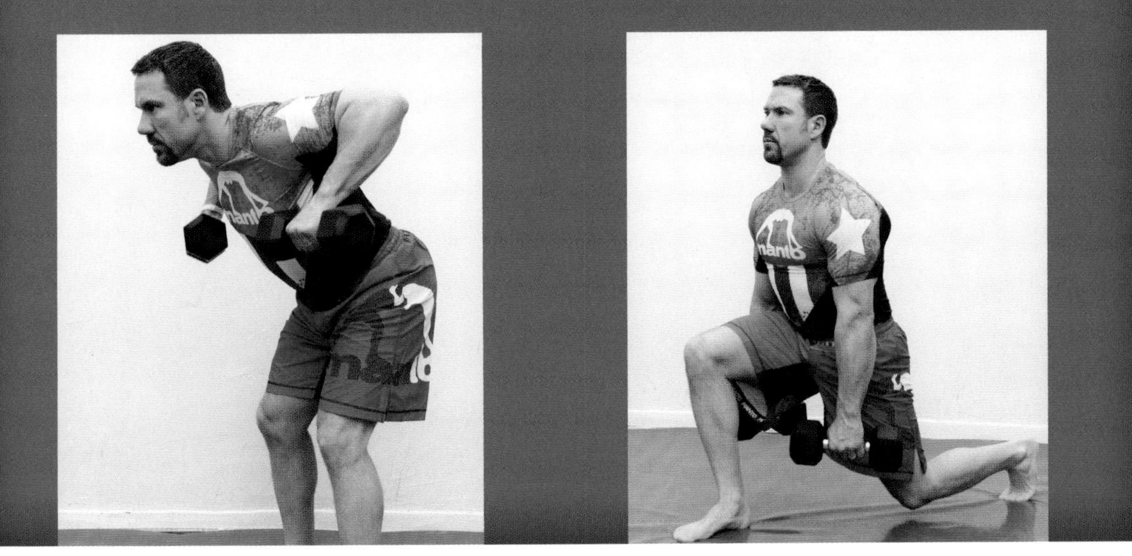

SINGLE DUMBBELL COMPLEX CHEATSHEET

1. SINGLE-ARM ROW

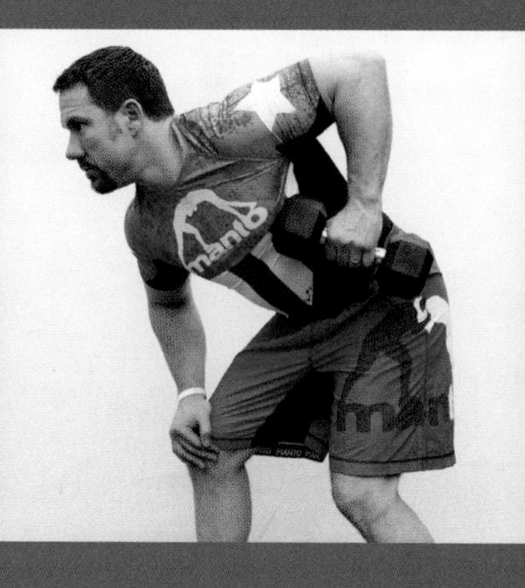

2. LUNGE ON SHOULDER:

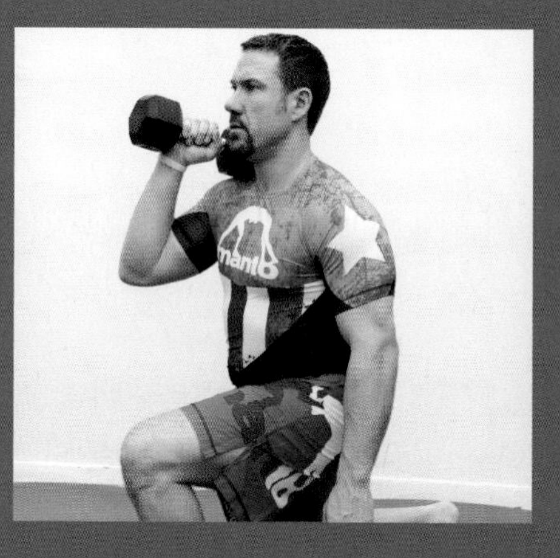

3. SNATCH

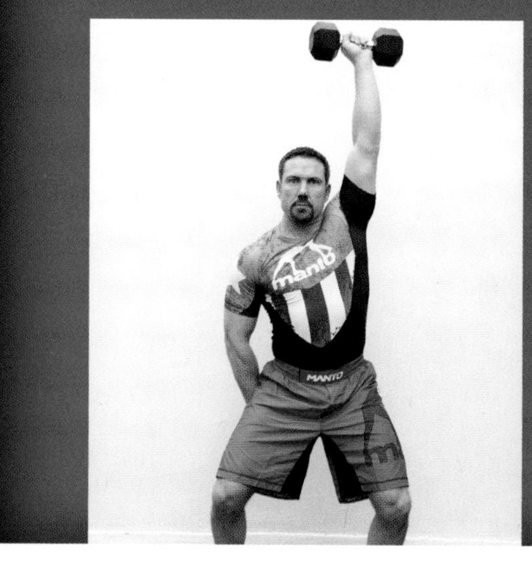

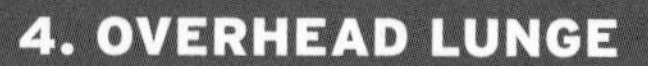

4. OVERHEAD LUNGE

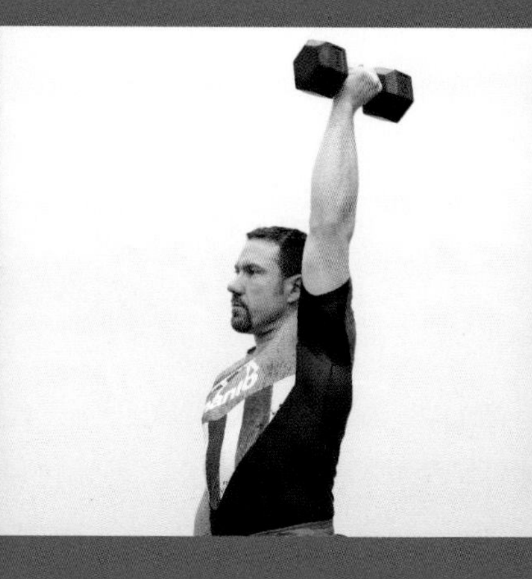

5. DUMBBELL SWING

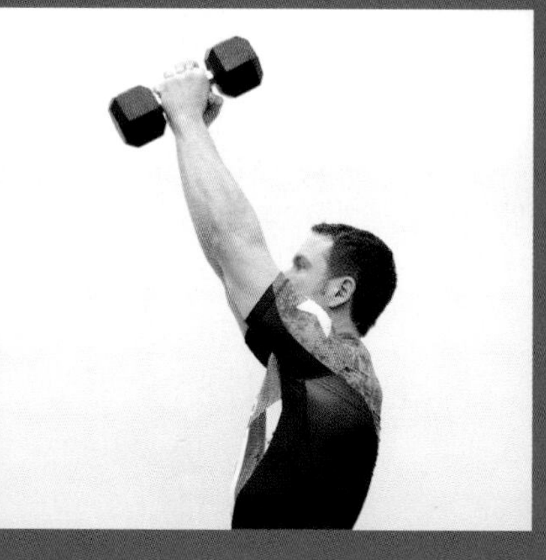

6. SIDE LUNGE

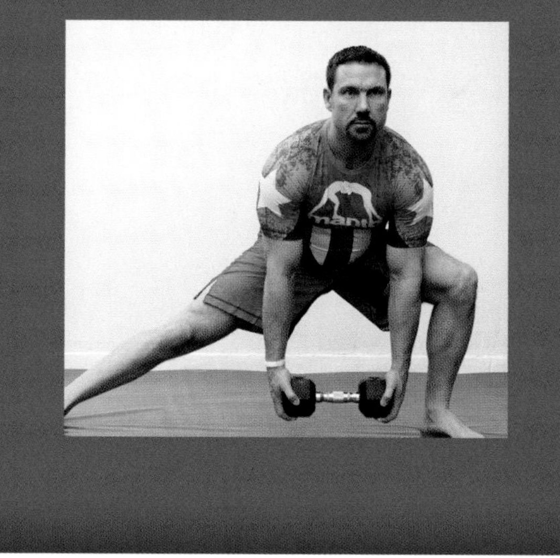

KETTLEBELL COMPLEX 5 CHEATSHEET

1. SQUAT

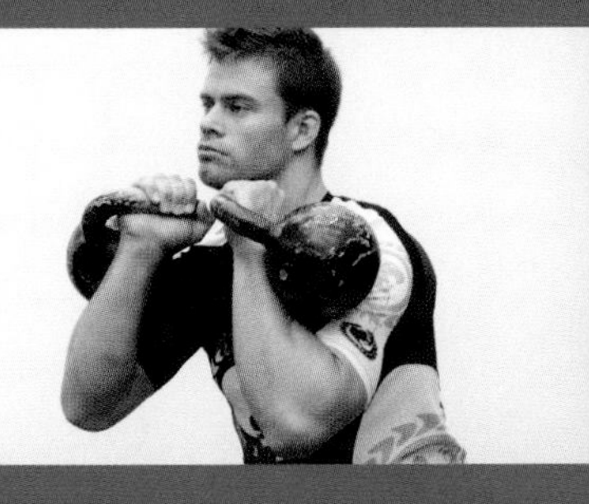

2. HUGH PULL

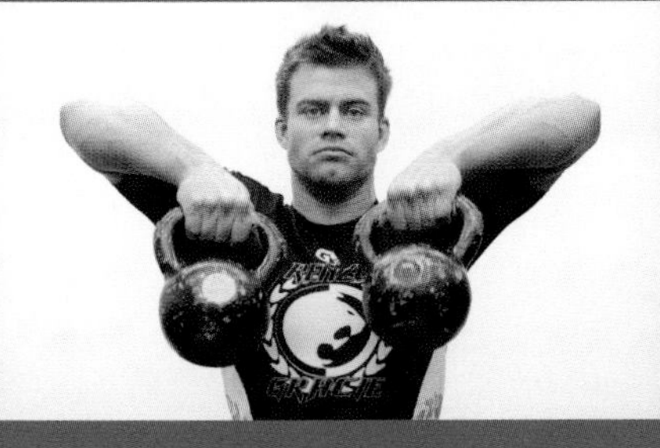

3. BENT-OVER ROW

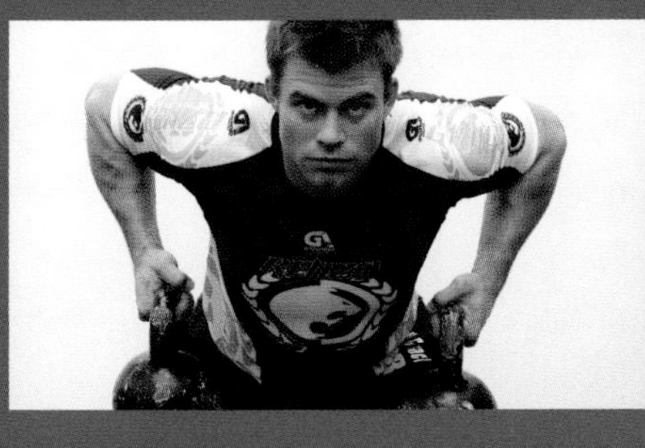

4. DEADLIFT

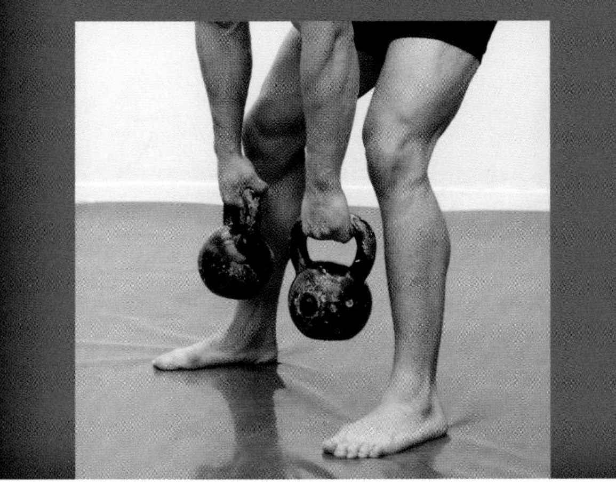

5. LUNGE

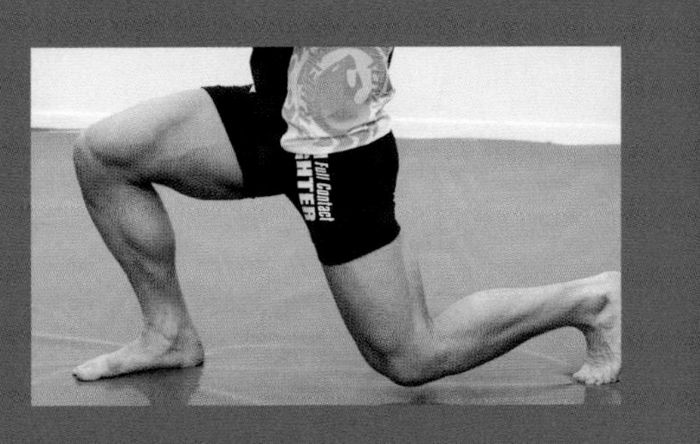

6. GOOD MORNING

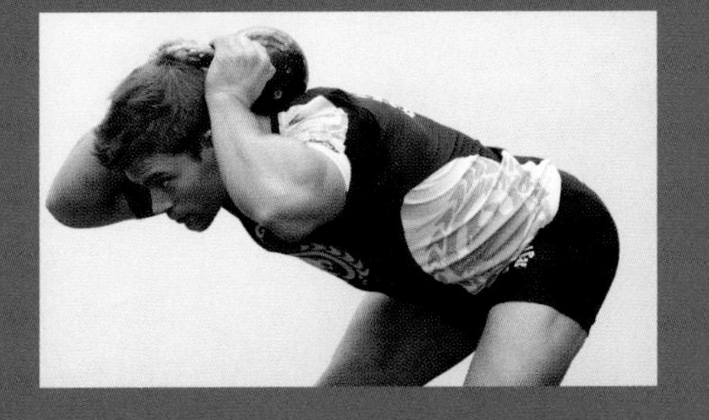

7. SIDE LUNGE

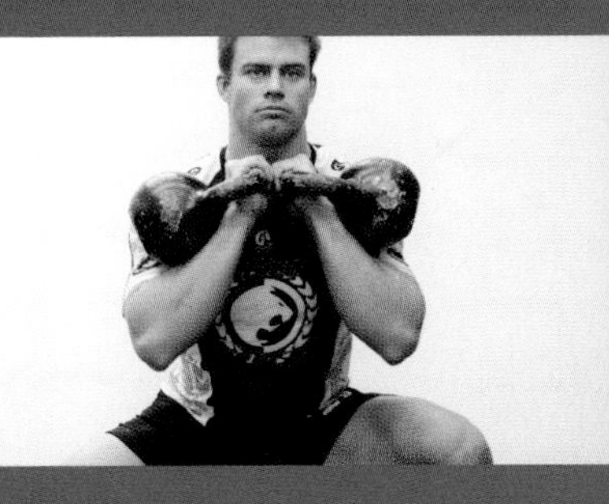

8. SWING TO ROW

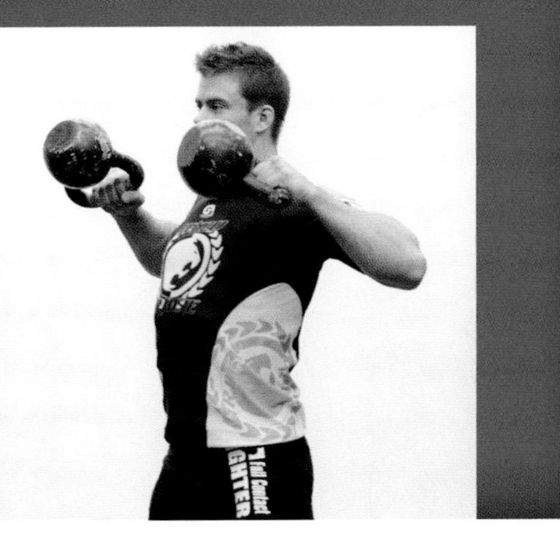

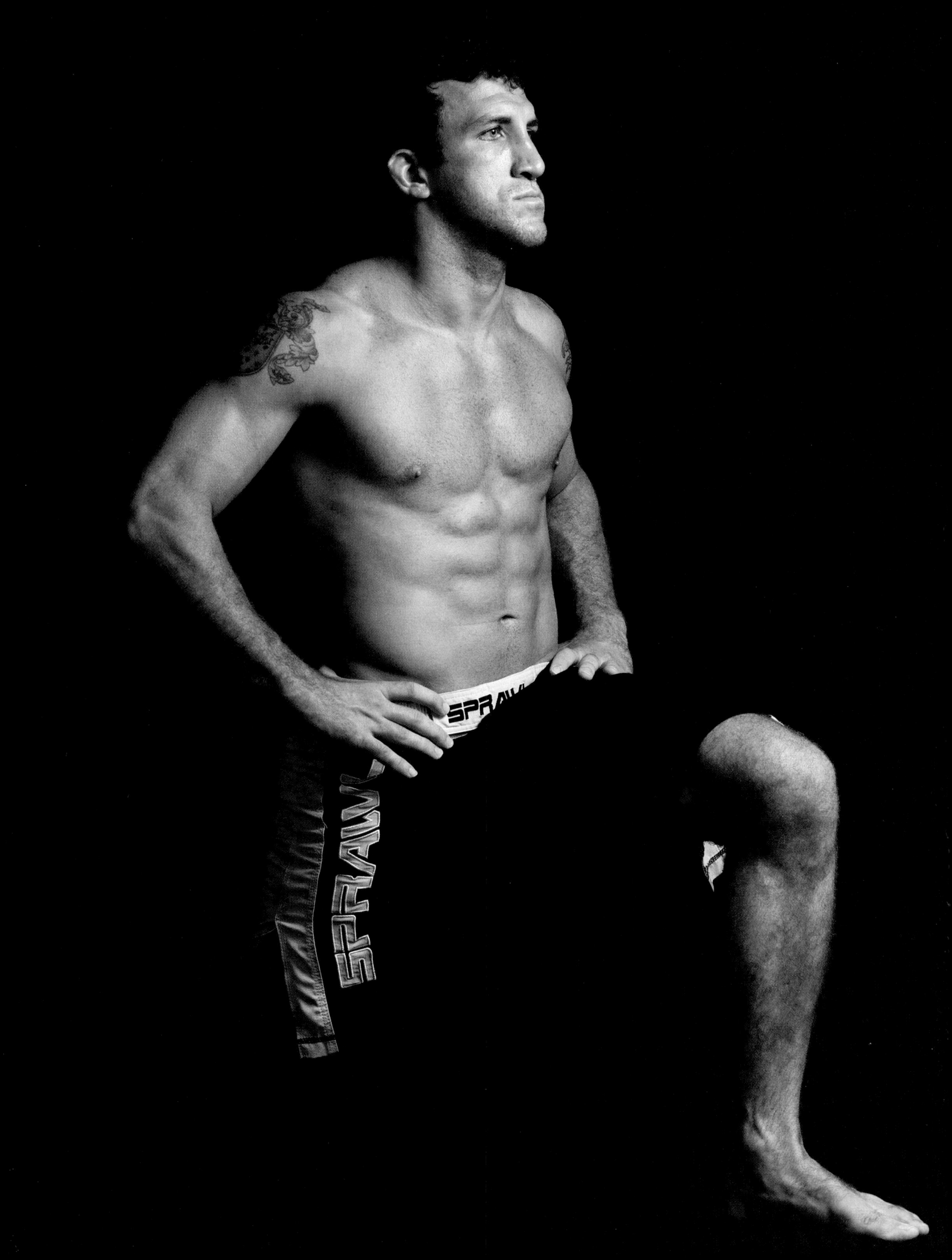
SPRAW
SPRAWL

11

BODY WEIGHT CIRCUITS

Today, much of the fitness industry is driven by new products, but before you worry about using weights or equipment, it is important to master the most important piece of equipment: your body. In the TFW system, relative body strength is the most important physical characteristic to possess. For instance, you cannot have great endurance if you are weak for your weight since it will take too much energy to move around. Without relative strength, you will lack speed and power of movement as well. So, relative strength, which I also refer to as "pound-for-pound" strength, is the characteristic you should be constantly attempting to improve through your training. An ultimate example of this type of strength can be seen by watching Olympic-level gymnasts compete using their bodies.

In my book *Ultimate Warrior Workouts*, I delivered a number of body weight challenges that have become very popular worldwide. All but one of these challenges involved performing a single body weight exercise for as many repetitions as possible in a set period of time. This chapter will focus instead on the use of multiple body weight activities combined in a circuit format to develop both relative strength and cardiovascular capacity.

Some of the circuits contain a prescribed number of repetitions that have to be performed in the best time possible, while others require performing as many repetitions as possible in the prescribed time. Using the element of time in these ways forces you to give your best effort.

TABATAS

One form of body weight circuit that we will use in this chapter is known as a tabata. The tabata, like many forms of training out there today, is something that has morphed from its original form as a result of being sensationalized over the Internet. To explain where this style of training came from, we need to look no farther than the name. Izumi Tabata was a researcher looking for forms of training that could produce excellent results in very short periods of time. As he studied different training methods in the mid-1990s, he discovered that when test subjects (elite-level speed skaters) pedaled at all-out maximum intensity on a resistance cycle for 20 seconds followed by 10 seconds of rest for eight total sets, they produced excellent results in terms of fat loss and cardiac benefit. In fact, he discovered that in only one set of this 4-minute circuit, he was able to produce better results in shorter periods of time than through other forms of training that required more time to complete.

The publication of the results, and the speed of the Internet, created a wave of interest in Tabata's study. Since not everyone had access to a resistance bike, "tabatas" began to refer to any exercise at any intensity for eight total sets of 20 seconds' work with 10 seconds' rest. Before long, some people began using variations, such as 15 seconds on, 5 off, so the tabata has lost a lot of its original meaning.

SAMPLE TABATAS

In the Training for Warriors system, we stick to the original 20 seconds on and 10 off and use only complex exercises at maximal intensity. Because of this approach, there are only a few ways that you can affect the expenditure of the tabata: through exercises selected, speed of movement, weight of the exercises (intensity), number of repetitions, number of total circuits, and total time of the circuit.

To perform each of the following five different tabatas, you need to perform an exercise for 20 seconds and then rest for 10 seconds before starting the next 20 seconds of exercise. This is to be repeated for a total of eight sets, which will take 4 minutes to complete. As you will see, some of the tabatas involve only one exercise, some involve two exercises, and another involves four. If the tabata has only one exercise, repeat that for all eight sets. If the tabata involves two exercises, alternate each exercise four times for all eight sets. If the tabata involves four exercises, perform all four and then repeat to complete the eight total sets.

A. THE CLIMBER

1. MOUNTAIN CLIMBER

Begin in the pushup position with the back straight. Bring one foot up inside the hands while keeping the hips low. Alternate feet to complete the exercise.

1

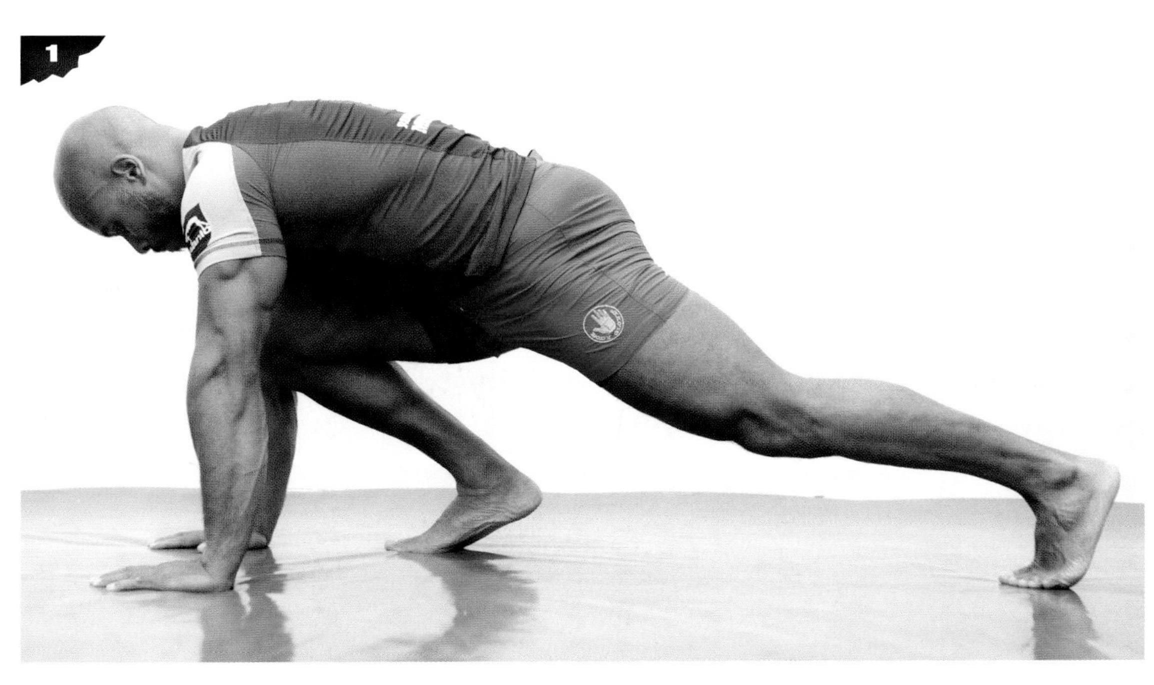

2

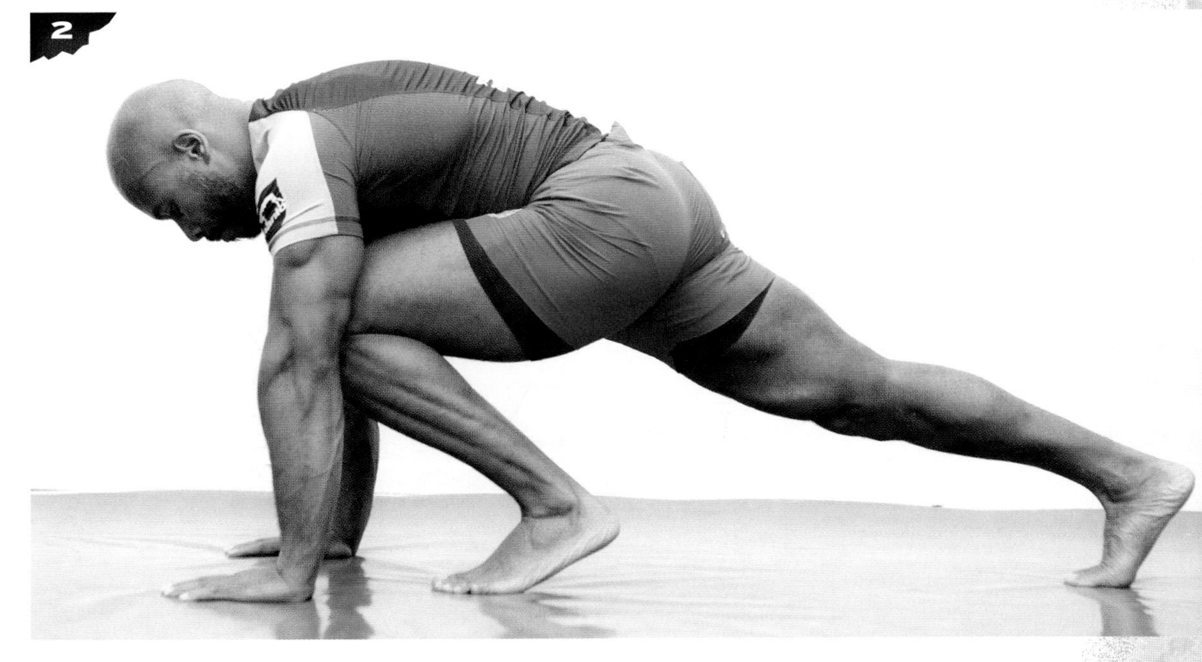

2. SINGLE-LEG MOUNTAIN CLIMBER

Begin in the pushup position with only one foot on the ground. Hop the foot up in between the hands. Return the foot to the original position and repeat.

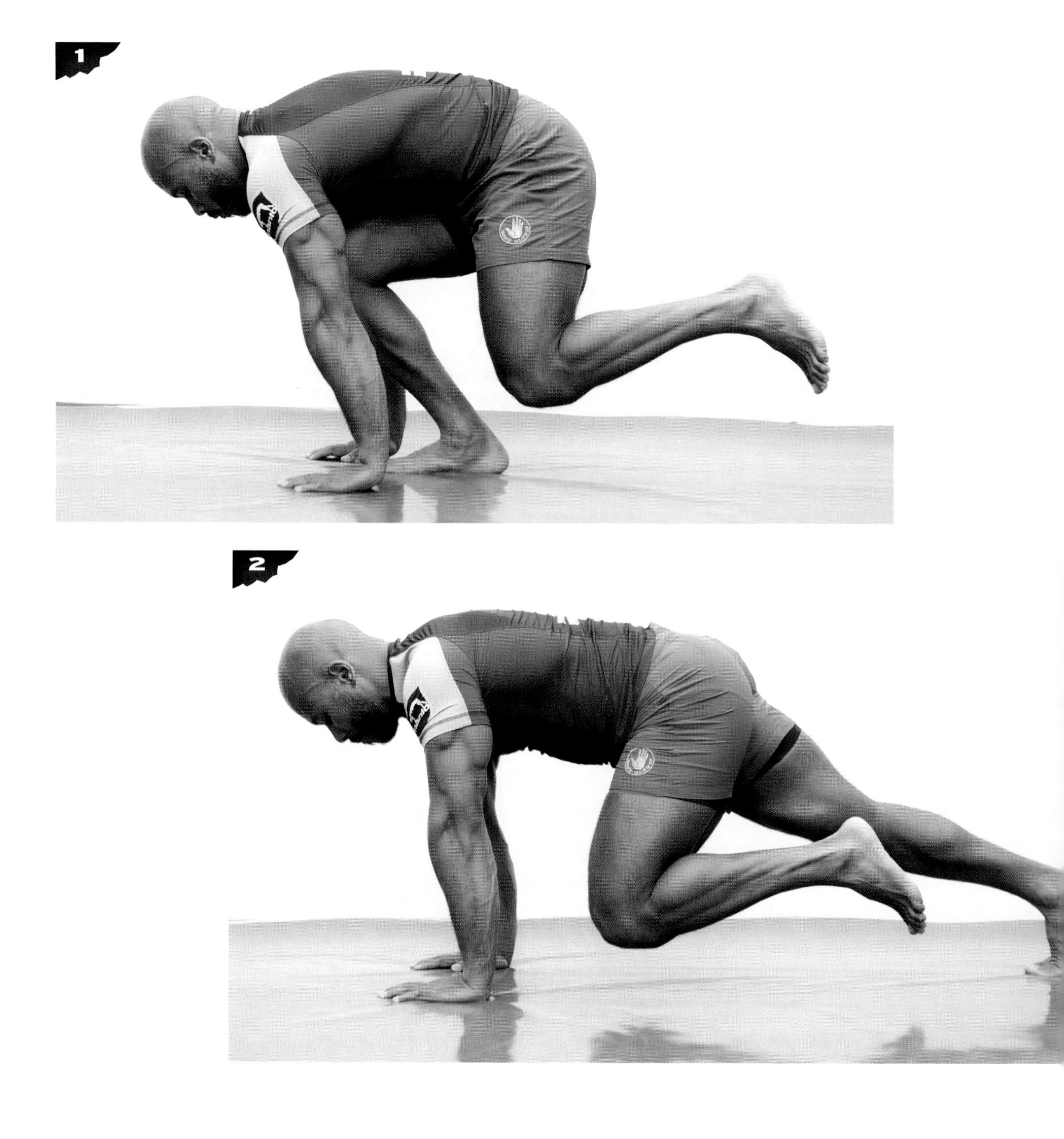

3. GROINER

Begin in the pushup position with the back straight. Bring one foot up outside the hand while keeping the hips low. Alternate the feet to complete the exercise.

1

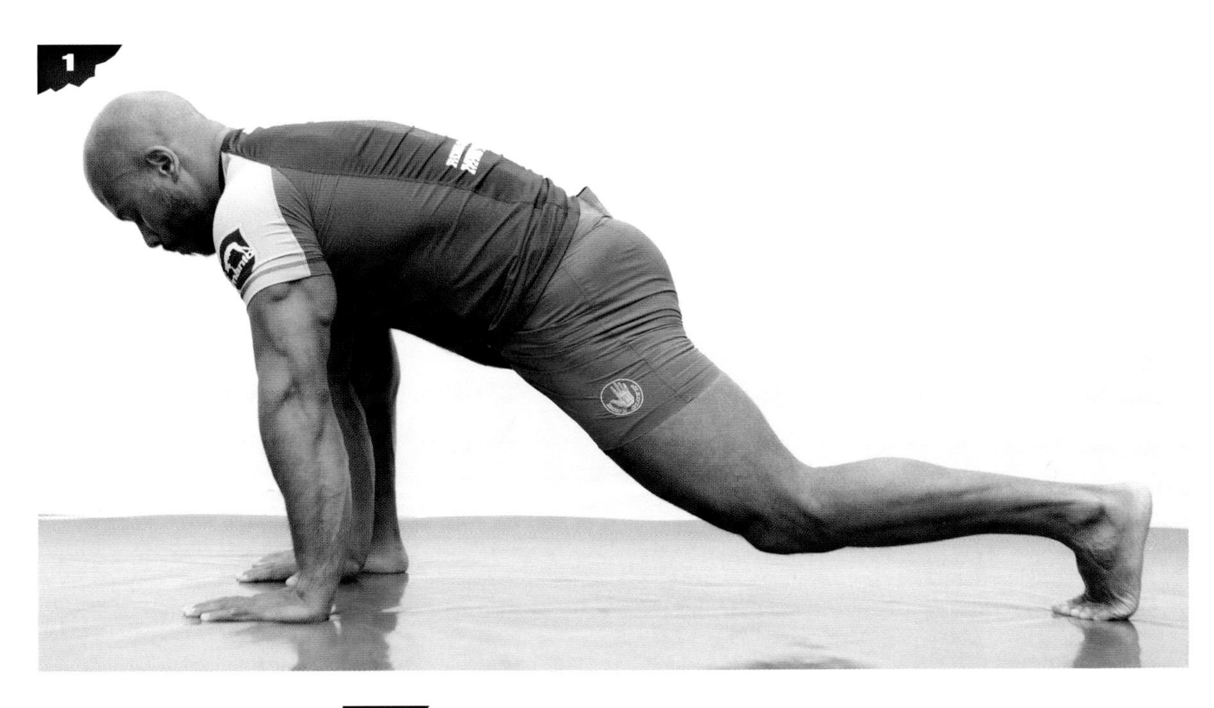

2

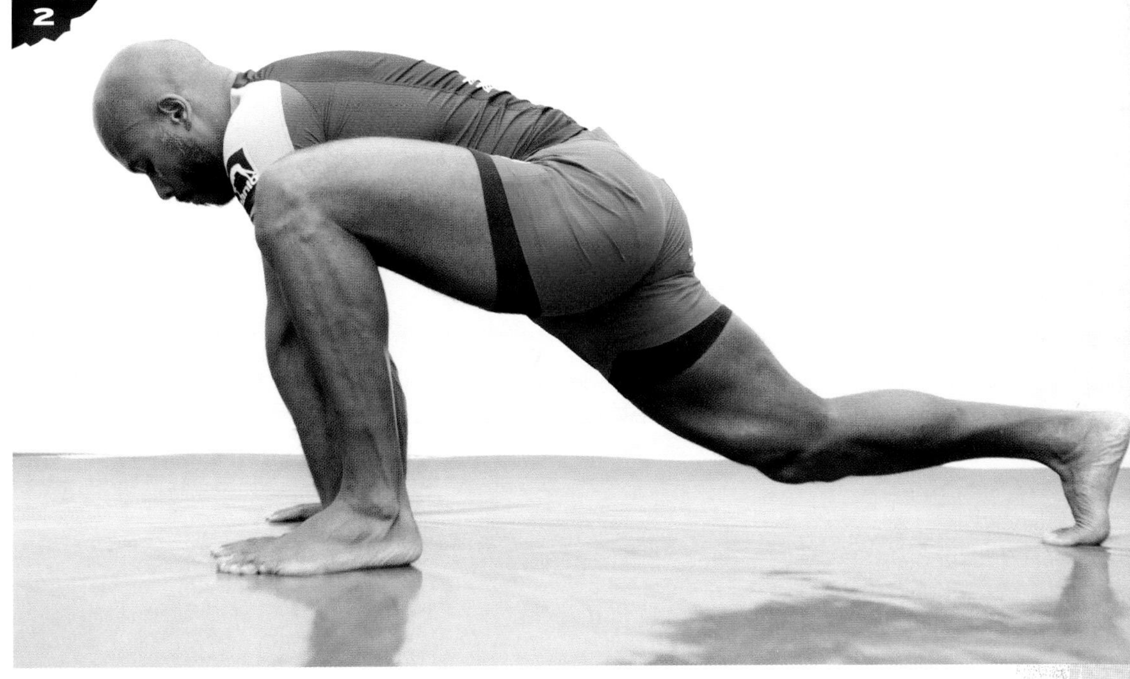

4. DOUBLE-LEG HOP-UPS

Begin in the pushup position. Jump both feet up in between the hands. Return the feet to the original position and repeat.

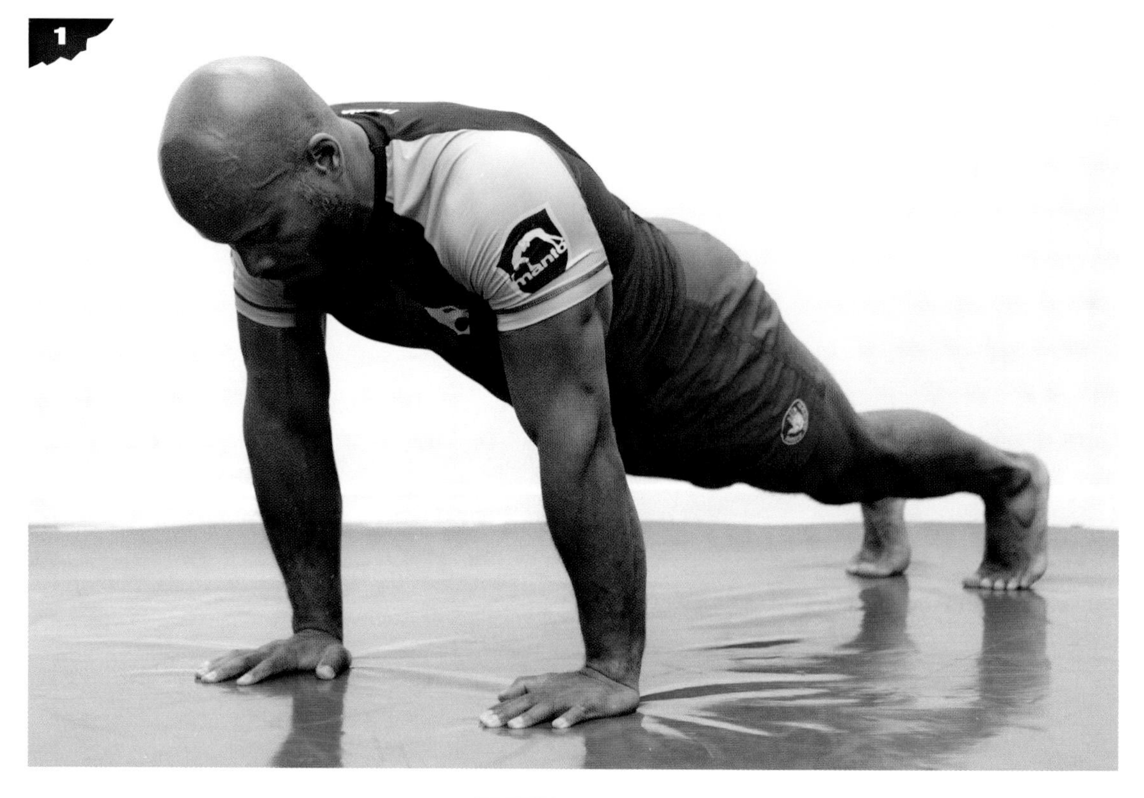

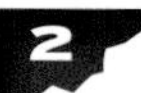

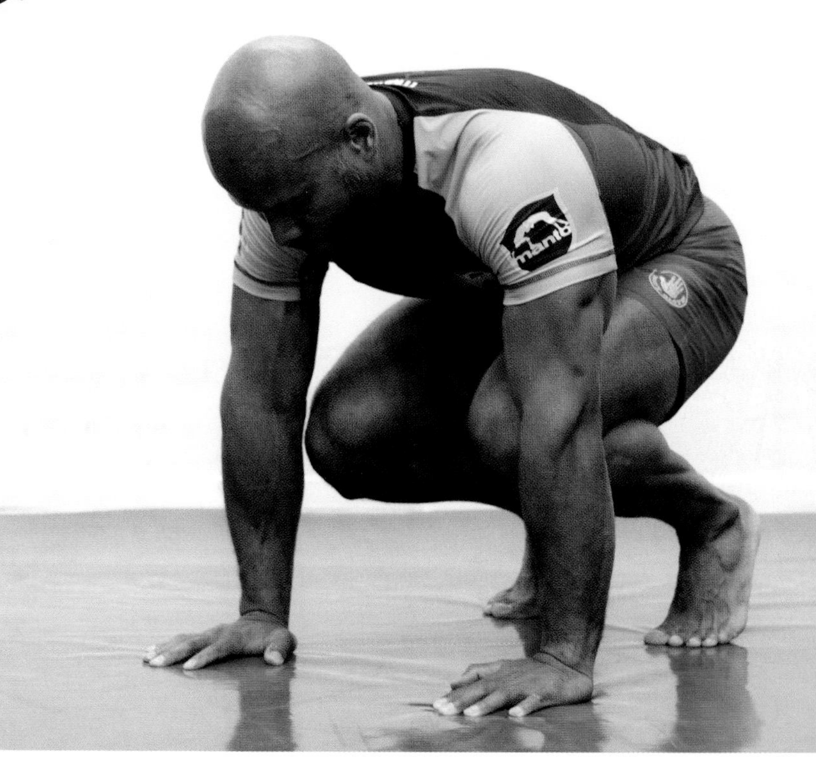

B. THE LUNGER

1. SIDE LUNGE

Begin standing with the hands out front and the elbows tucked at the sides. Step out to one side and lower the hips. Press back up and repeat on the other side.

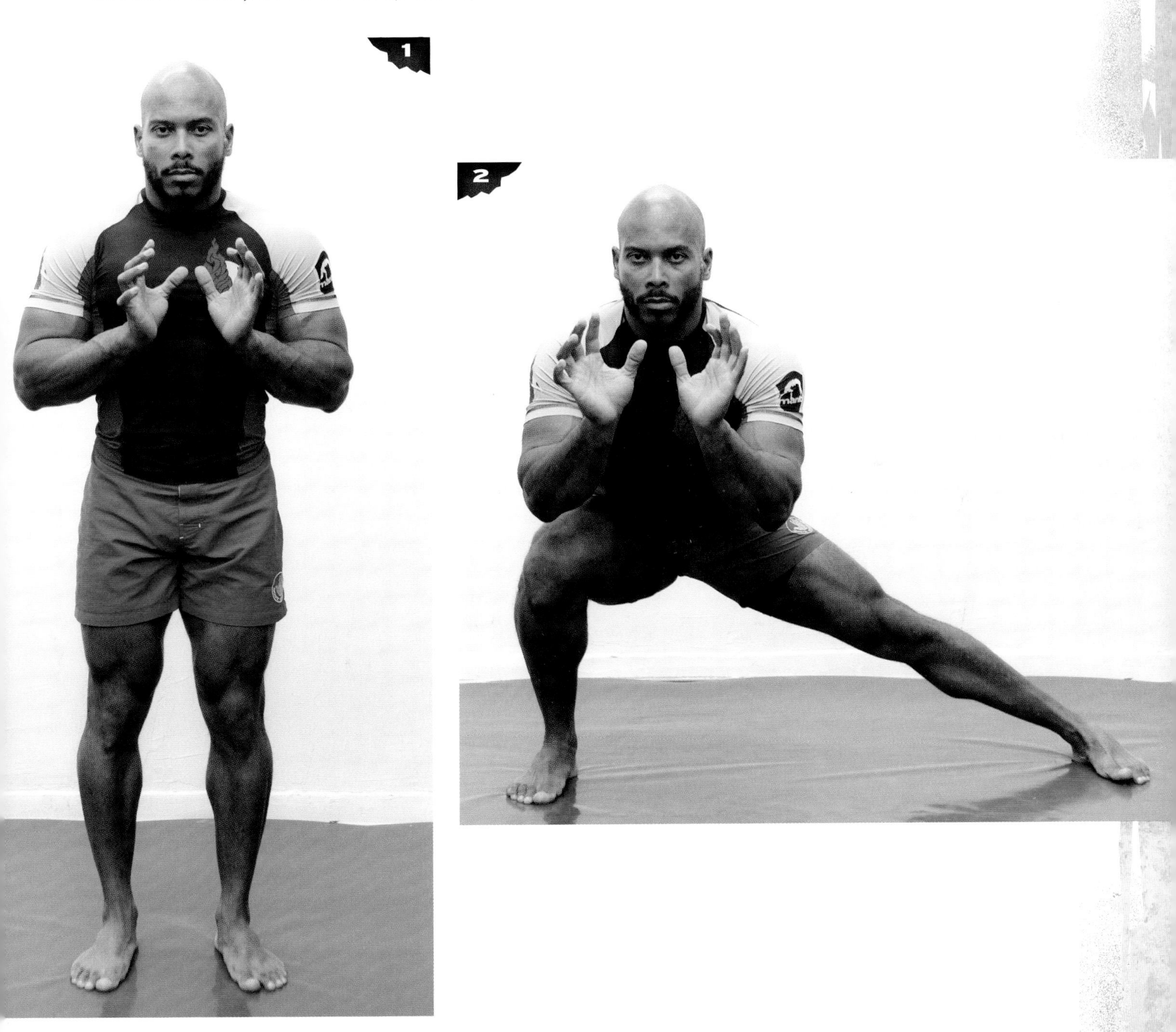

2. FRONT LUNGE

Begin standing with the hands up and elbows tucked at the sides. Step forward and drop the back knee almost to the ground. Press back up with the lead leg and repeat on the opposite side.

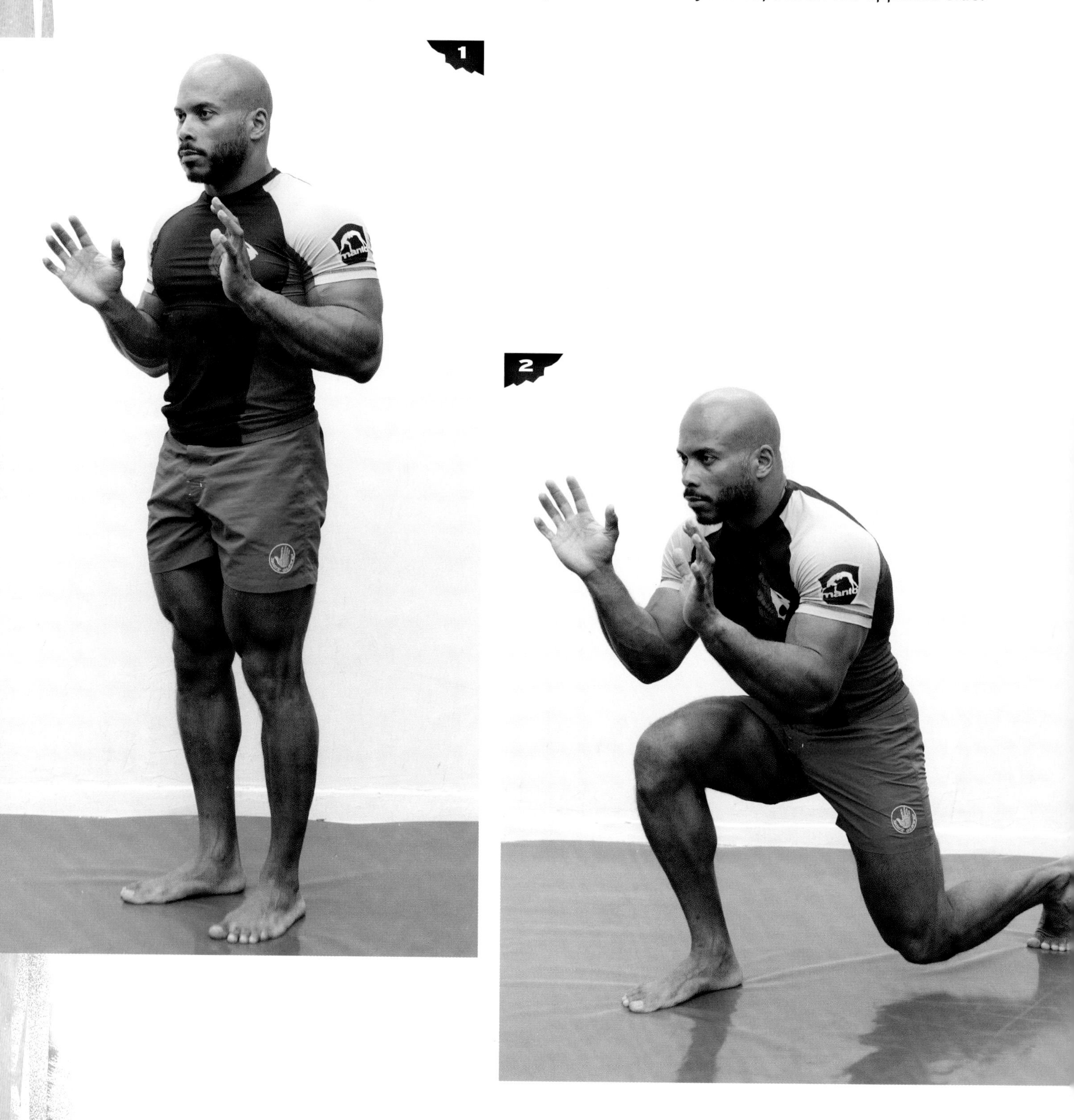

C. THE SQUATTER

1. HINDU SQUAT

Begin standing with the hands at the sides. Drop down, lifting the heels off the ground and raising the hands out in front of the body. Extend the legs and stand back to the original position.

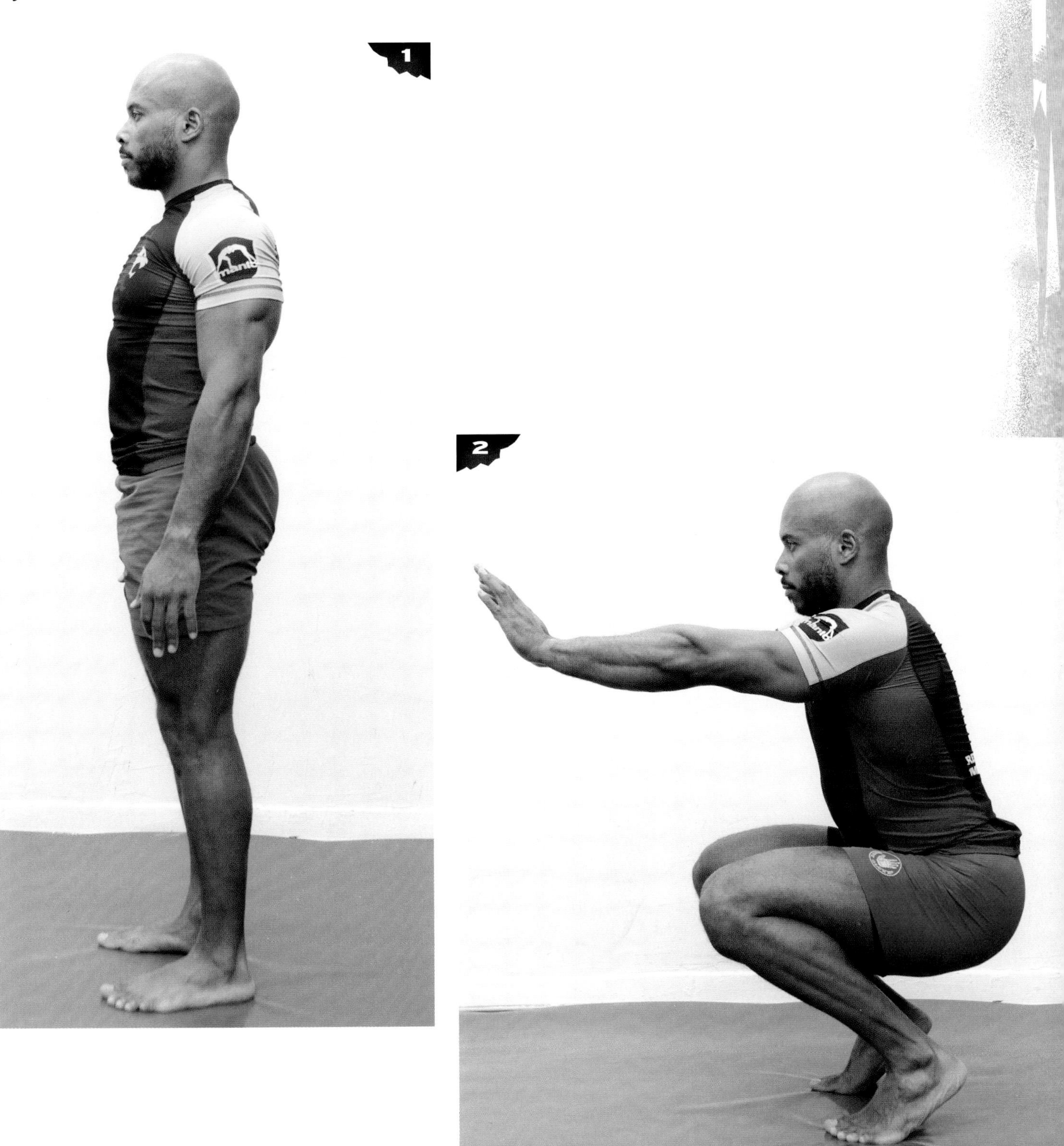

D. THE JUMPER

1. JUMP SQUAT

Start standing with the knees bent and the hands out front. Swing the arms and jump into the air as high as possible. Land under control and quickly jump again.

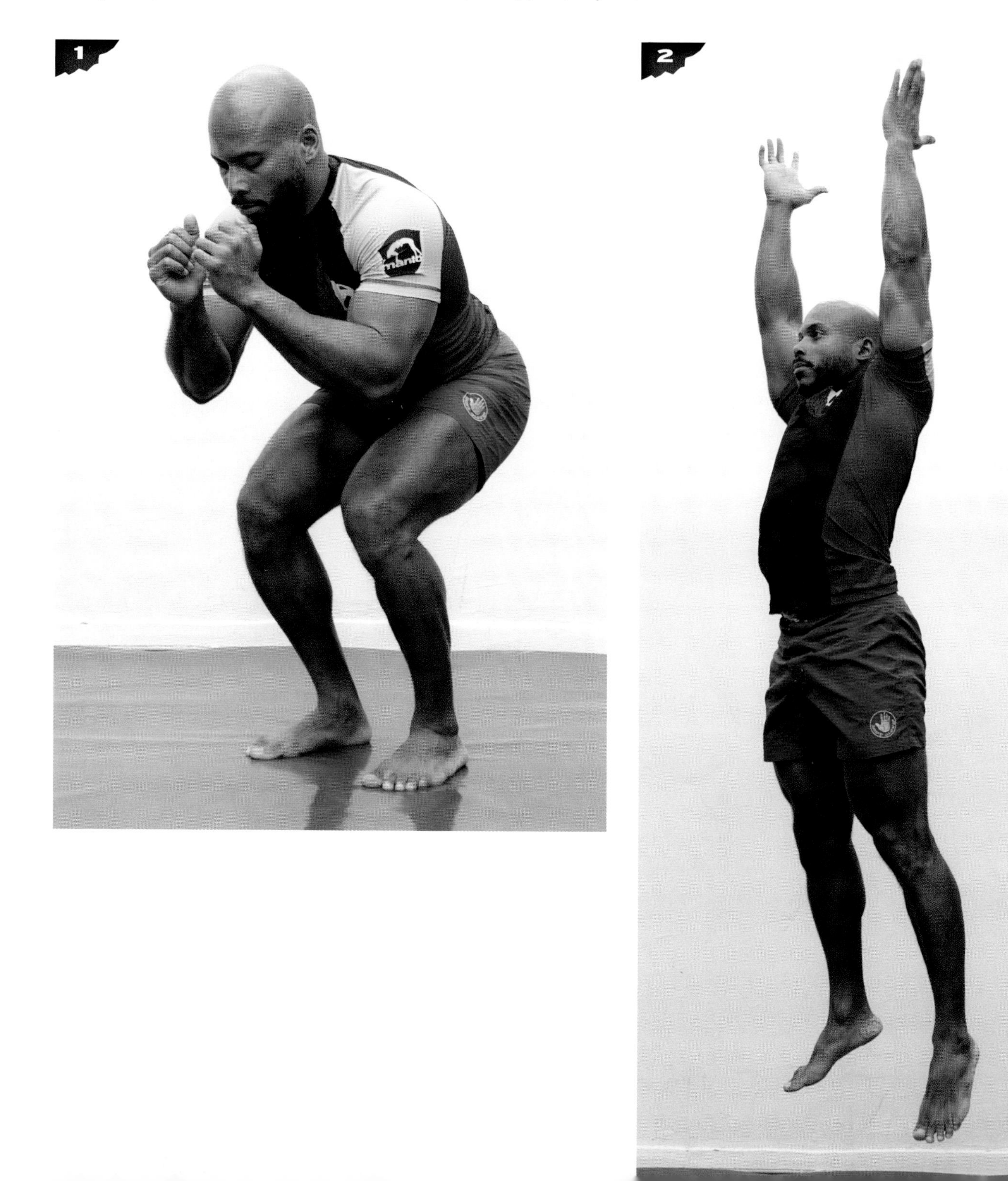

E. THE BURPER

1. BURPEE

Begin standing. Drop down and place the hands on the floor. Kick the feet back to the pushup position and then return the feet toward the hands and stand back up.

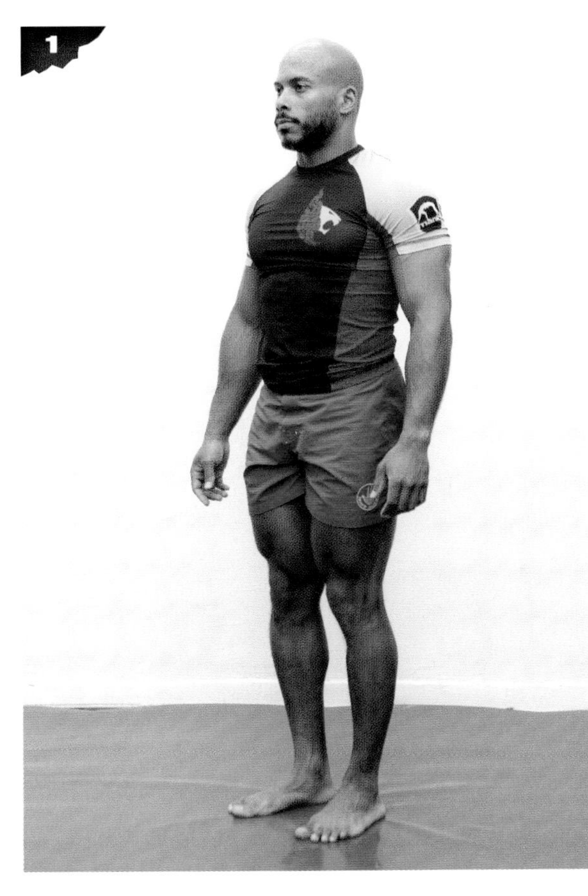

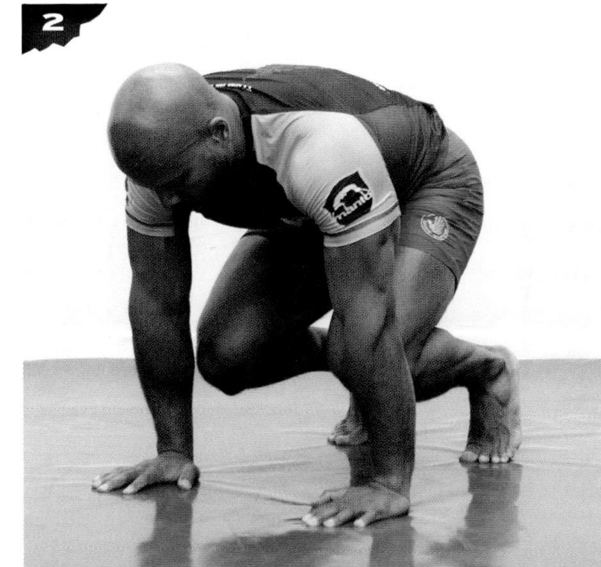

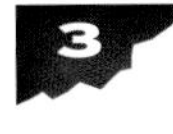

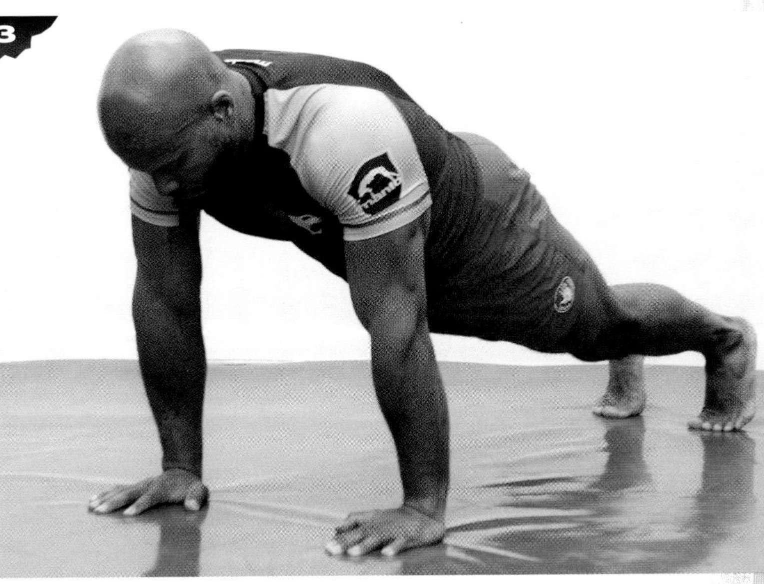

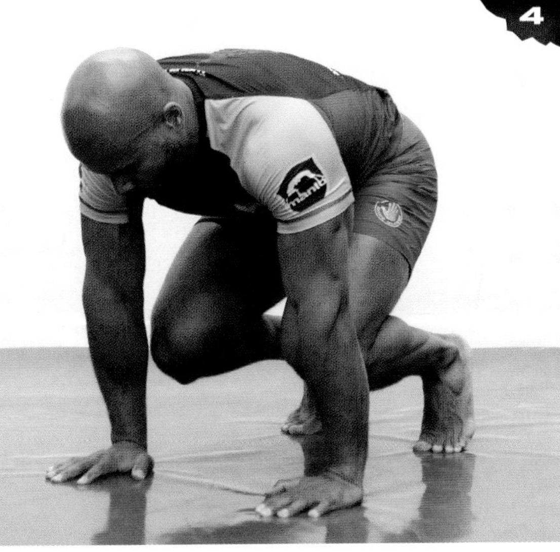

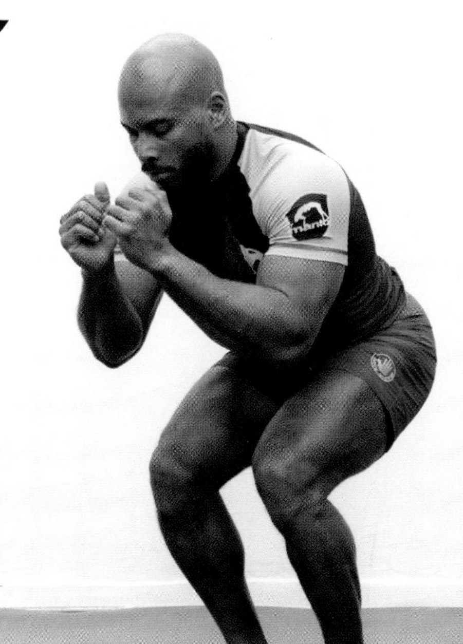

F. BODY WEIGHT CIRCUITS: 80 REPS

Perform the following circuit for 20 reps of each exercise. Record the best time for each circuit.

1. BODY SQUAT

Begin standing with the fingers interlocked behind the head. Lower the torso by bending at the knees and hips. Extend the legs and return to the original position.

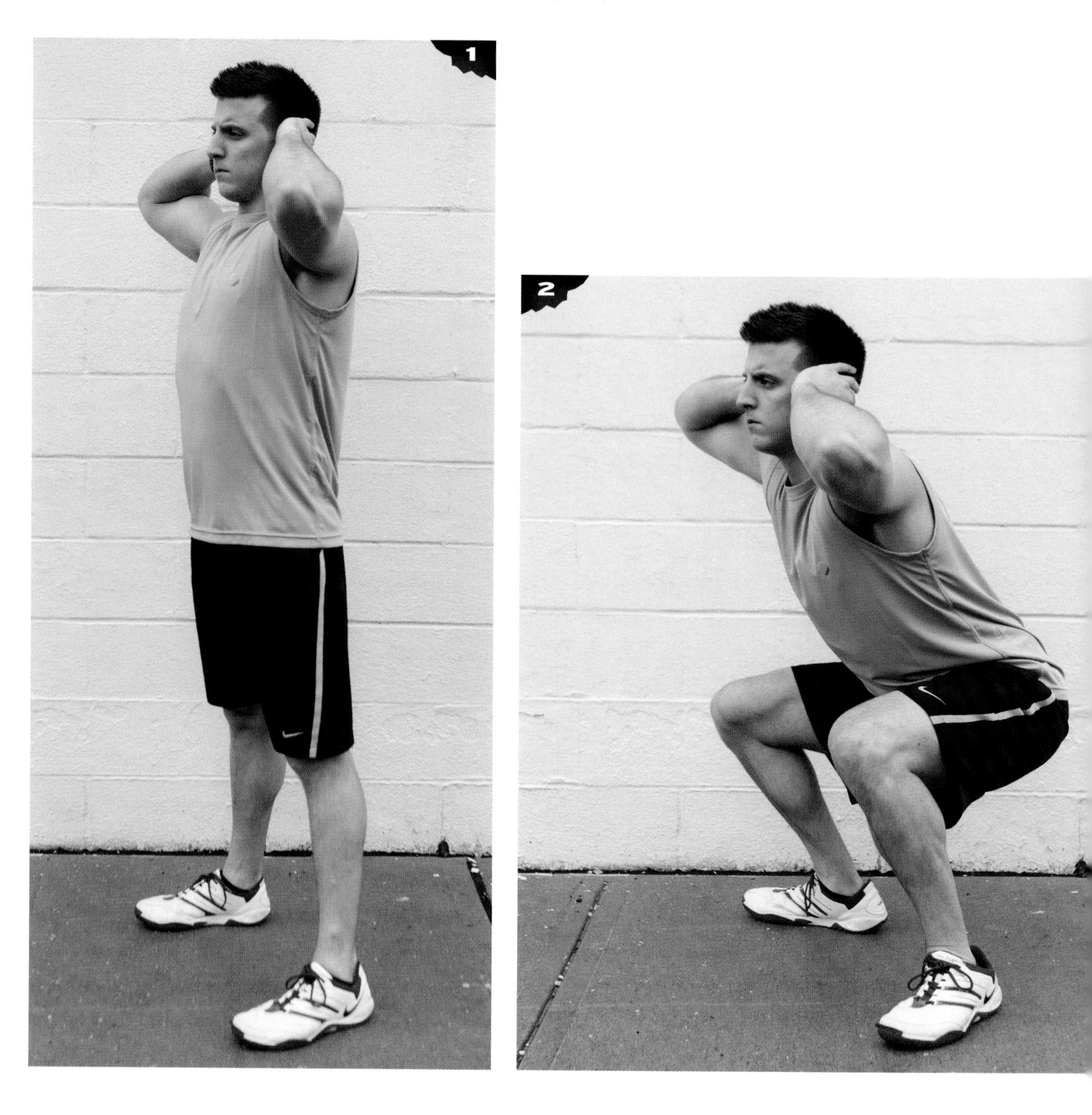

2. WIDE-OUTS

Begin in the half-squat position with the hands out front and the feet together. Without changing the height of the head, jump the feet out to the side and return them to the original position as quickly as possible.

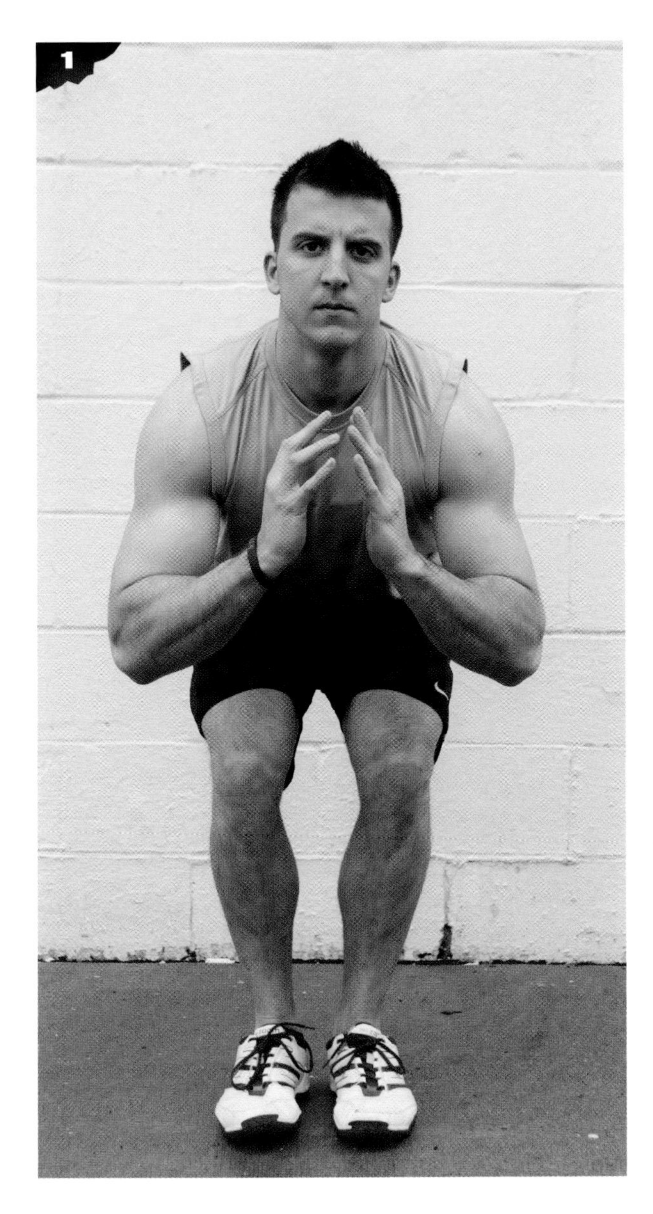

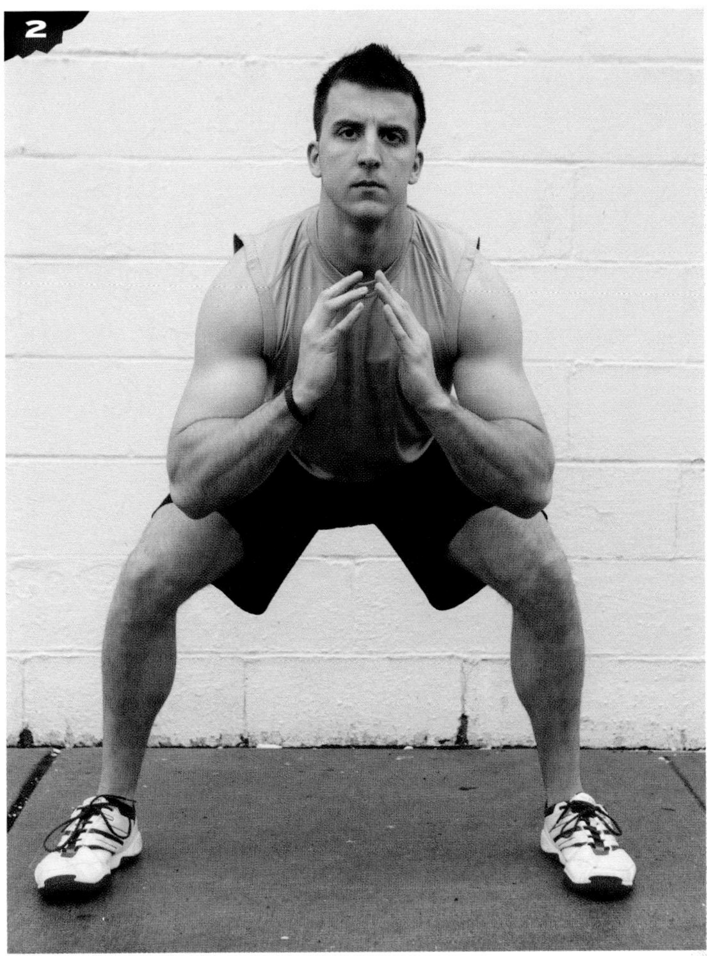

3. JUDO PUSHUP

Start in a pushup position with the hips held high, feet apart, and head facing down. Bend at the elbows and lower the head and chest to the ground. Bring the head upward while keeping the hips close to the ground. Press the hips back up to the original position as you drop the head.

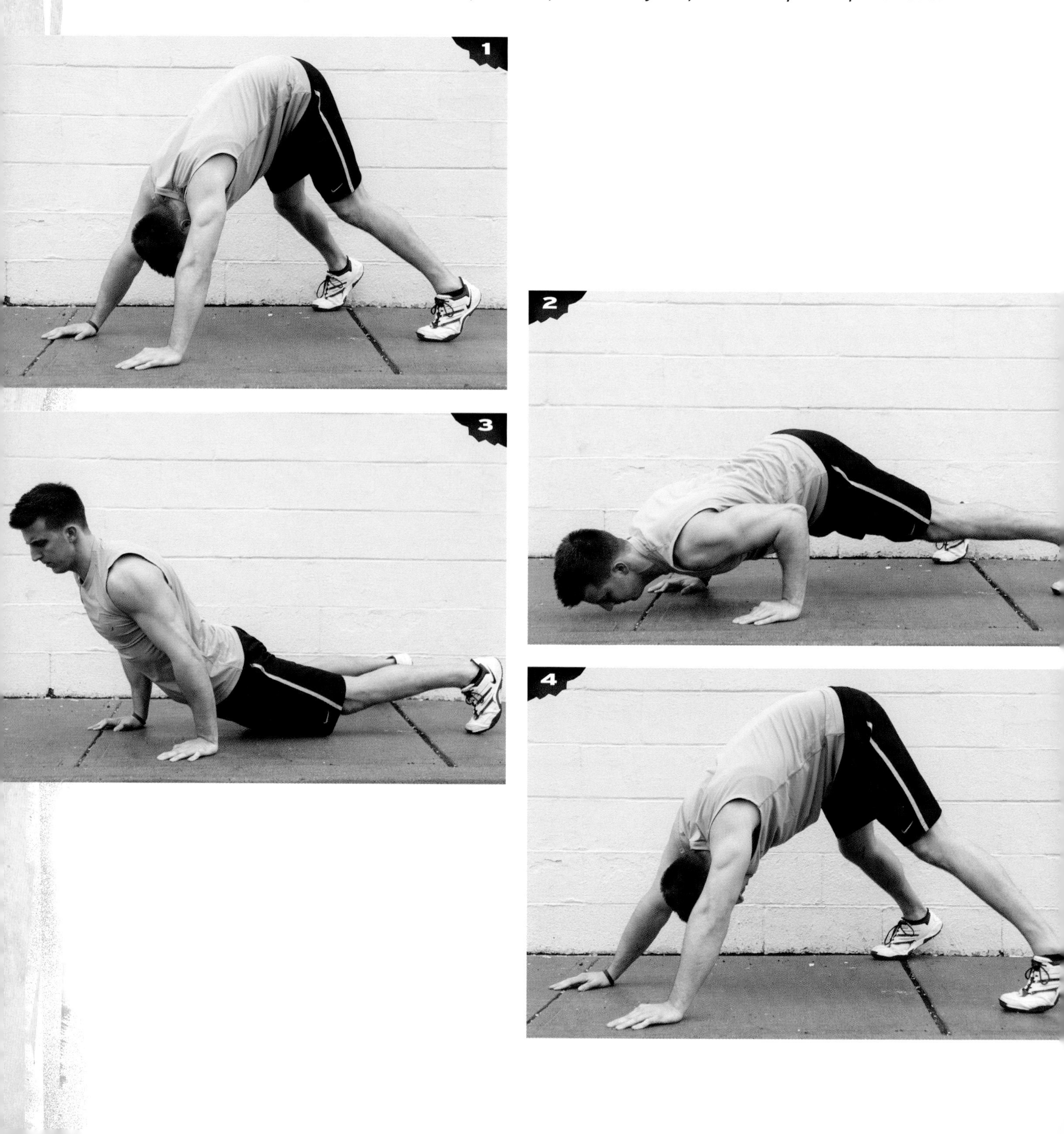

4. SPRINTER SIT-UP

Begin on the back with the legs straight and the elbows at the sides. As you sit up, bring one knee up and the opposite elbow forward while the other elbow fires backward. Lower back down to the original position.

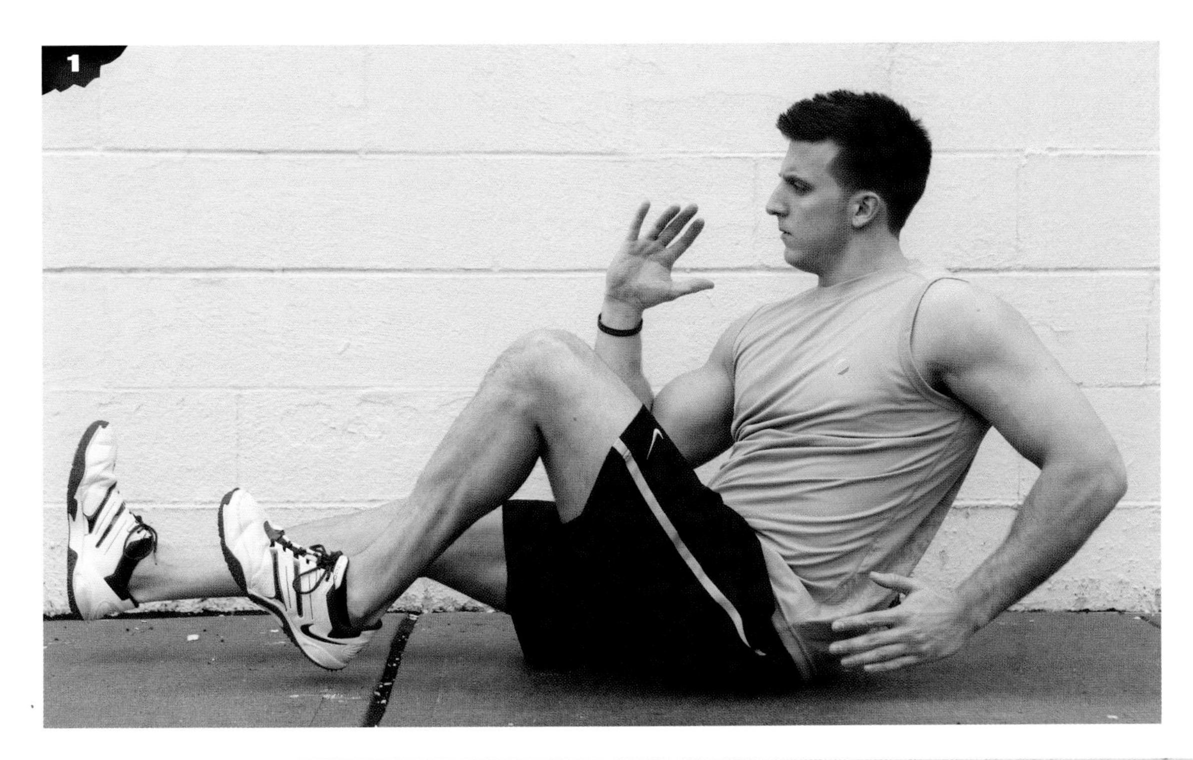

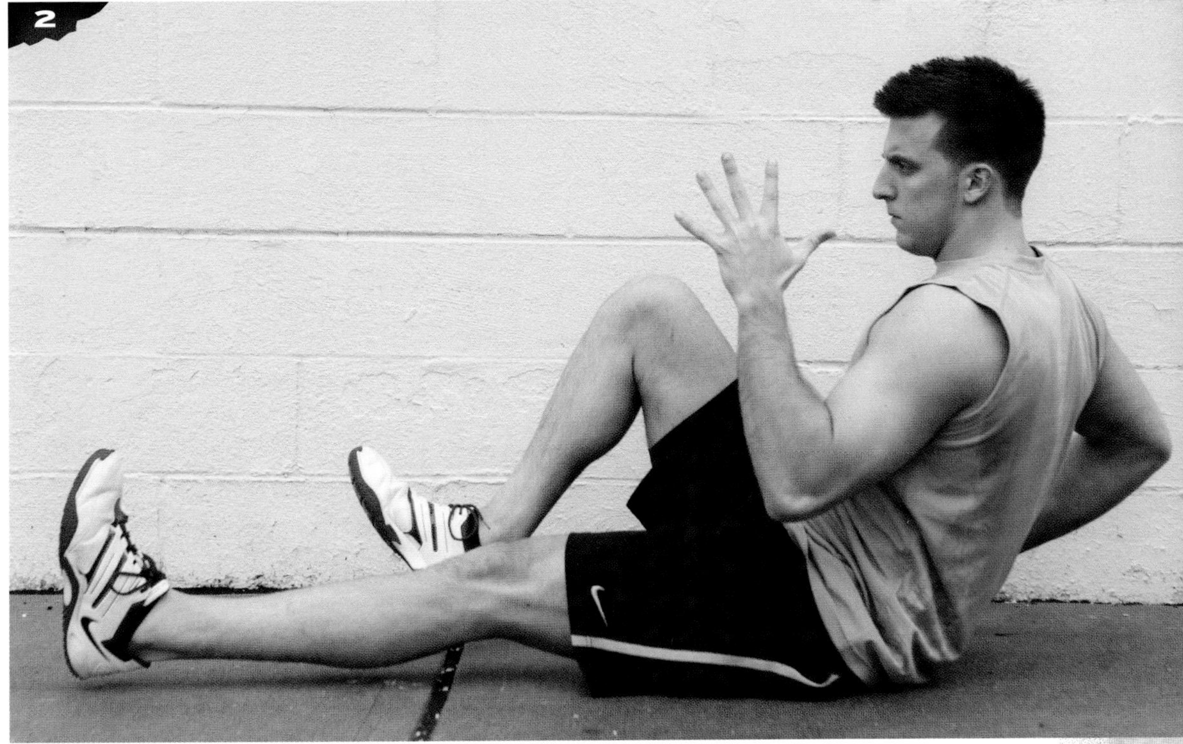

G. BODY WEIGHT CIRCUITS: 75 REPS

Perform the following circuit for 25 reps of each exercise. Record the best time for each circuit.

1. PUSHUP

Begin supporting the body on the hands and feet with the feet together and hands at shoulder width on the ground. Lower the chest to the ground while keeping the elbows close to the sides. Extend at the elbows to return to the original position.

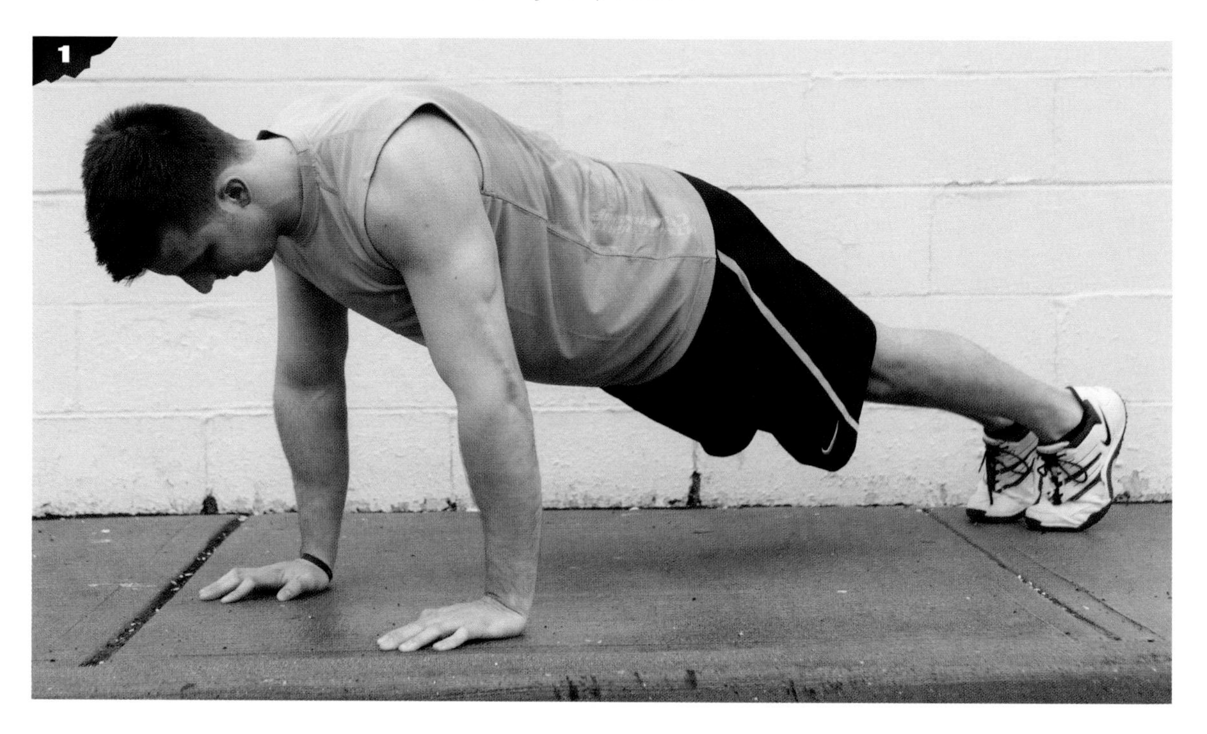

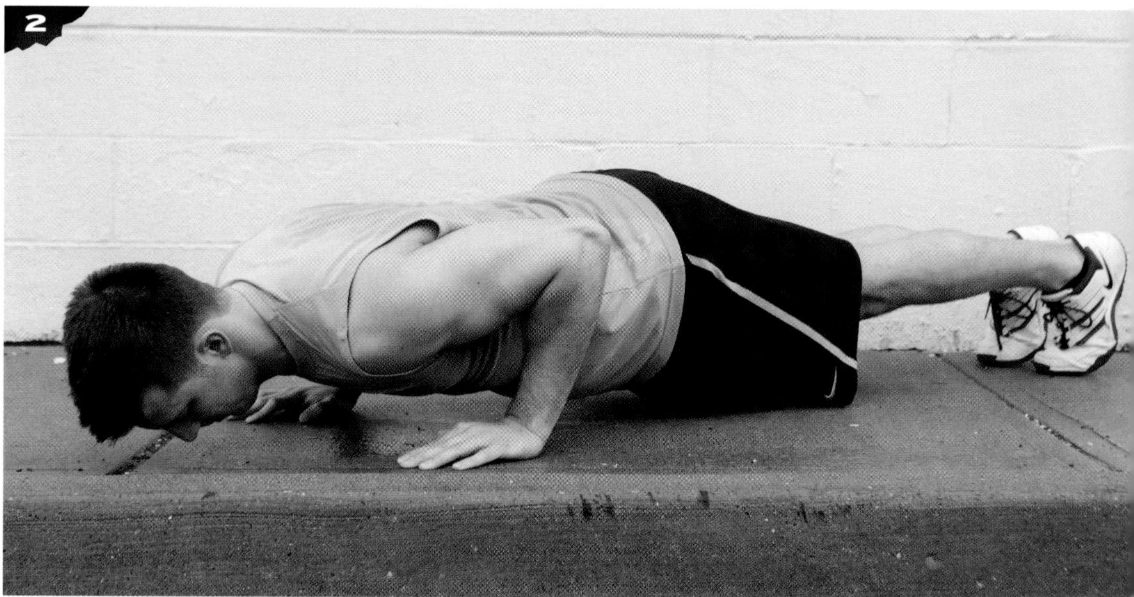

2. MOUNTAIN CLIMBER

Begin in the pushup position with the back straight. Bring one foot up inside the hands while keeping the hips low. Alternate feet to complete the exercise.

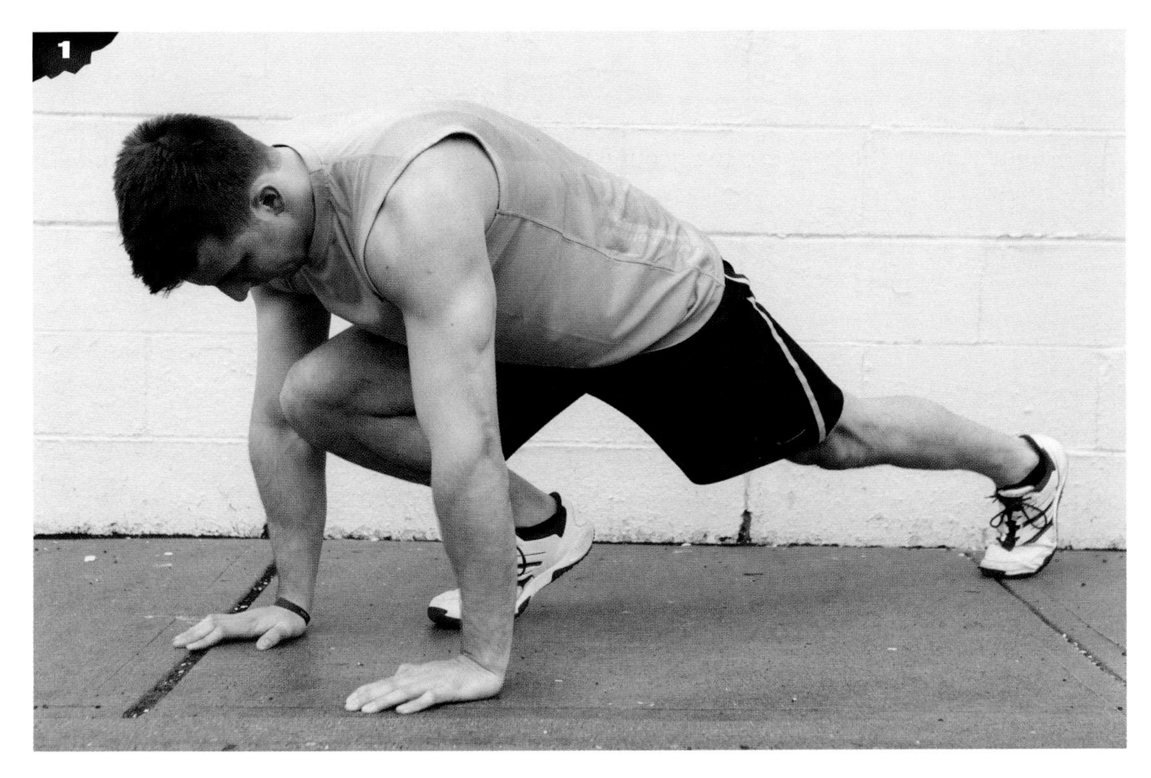

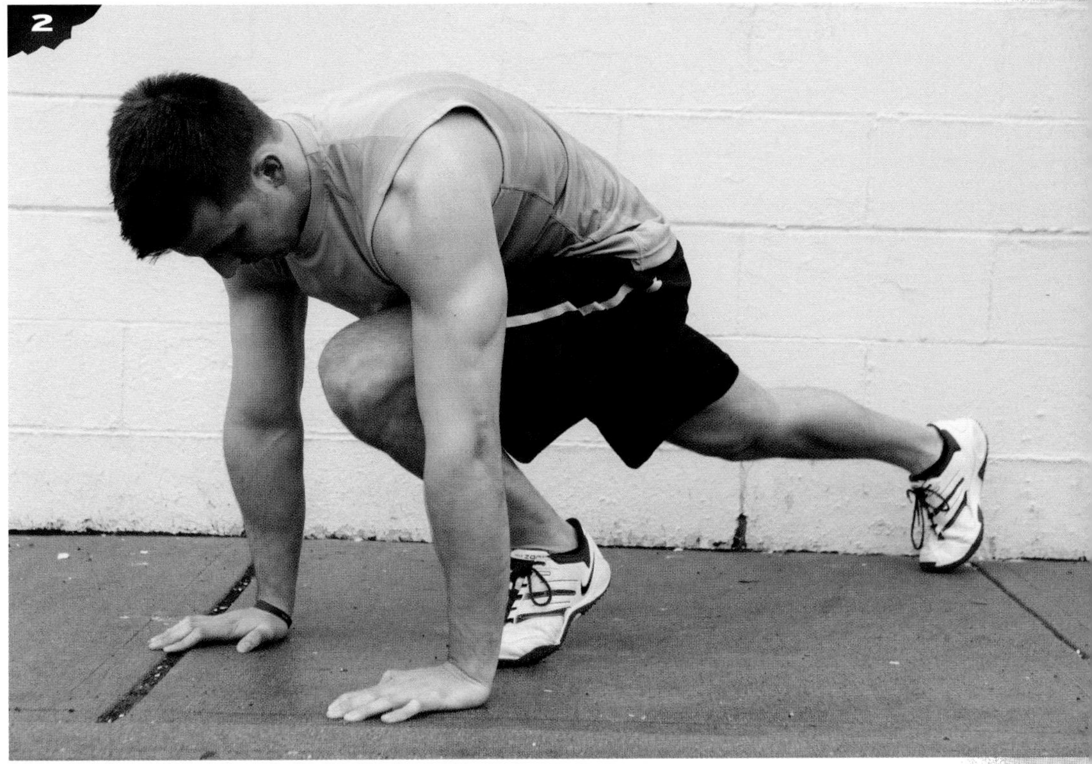

3. KNEE GRAB

Begin lying on the back with the knees straight and the hands held at the chin. Simultaneously bring the torso and knees up, and grab onto the ankles. Lower back down to the original position under control.

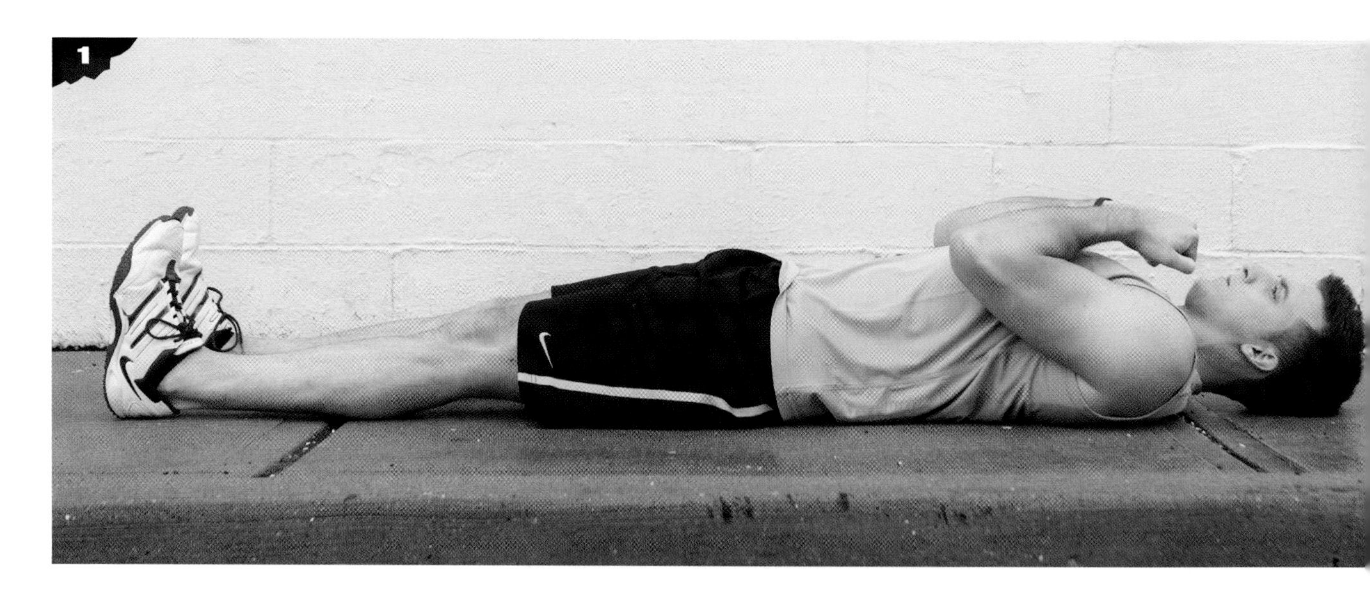

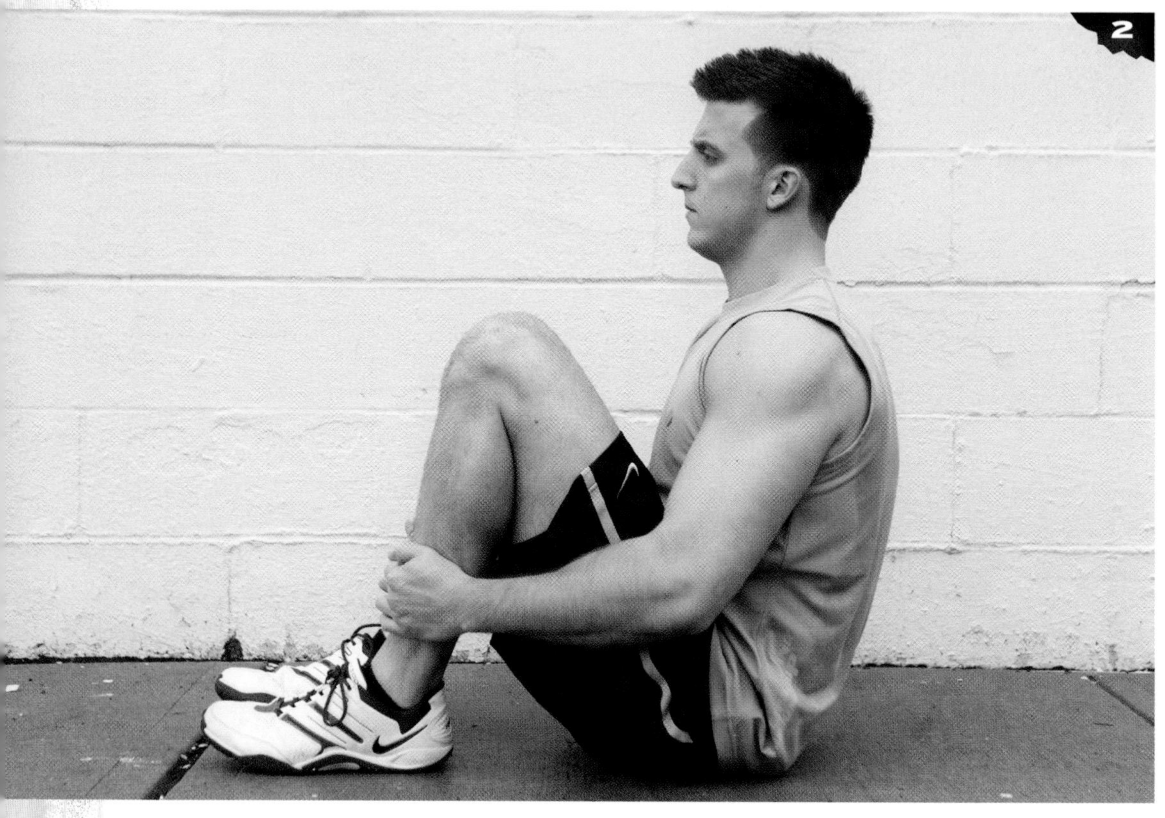

H. BODY WEIGHT CIRCUITS: PLYOMETRIC PUSHUPS

Perform the following circuit for 5 reps of each exercise. Record the best time for each circuit.

1. ONE-ARM-RAISE PUSHUP

Once you have lowered into the pushup position, extend at the elbows quickly and then, at the top of the motion, raise one straight arm overhead. Lower the hand back to the floor and then lower the body back down to the start position. Alternate arms on each rep.

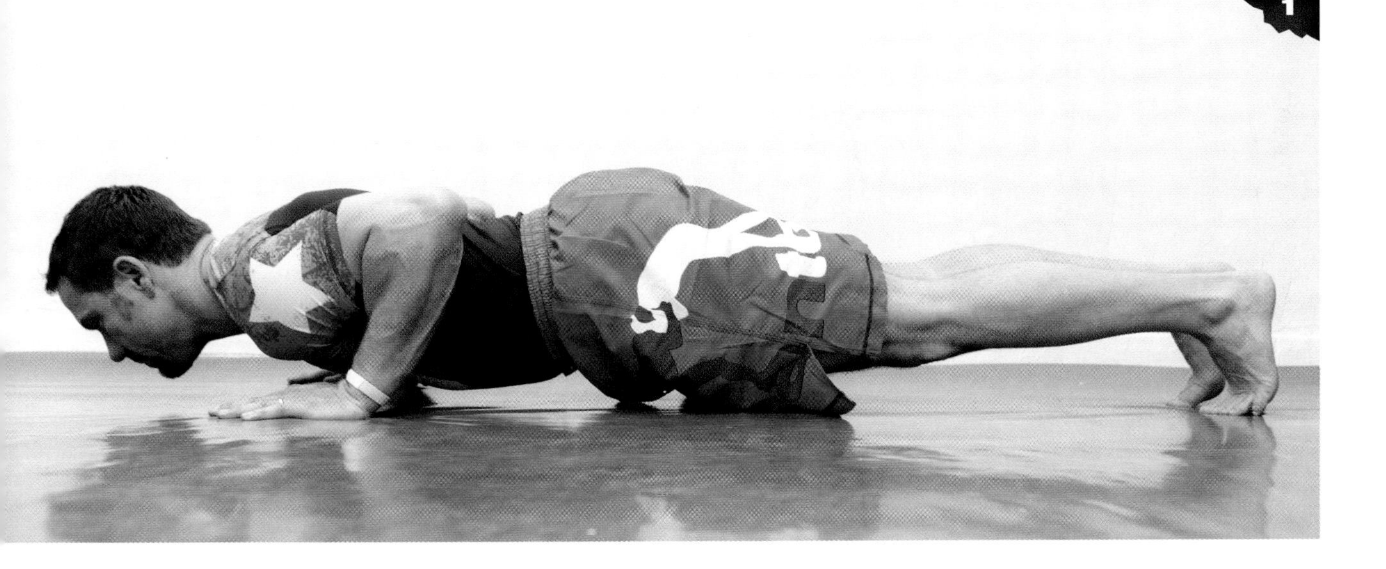

2. HANDS-OFF PUSHUP

Once you have lowered into the pushup position, extend at the elbows quickly so that the hands come off the floor at the top of the motion. Lower the hands back to the floor, and then lower the body back down for the next rep.

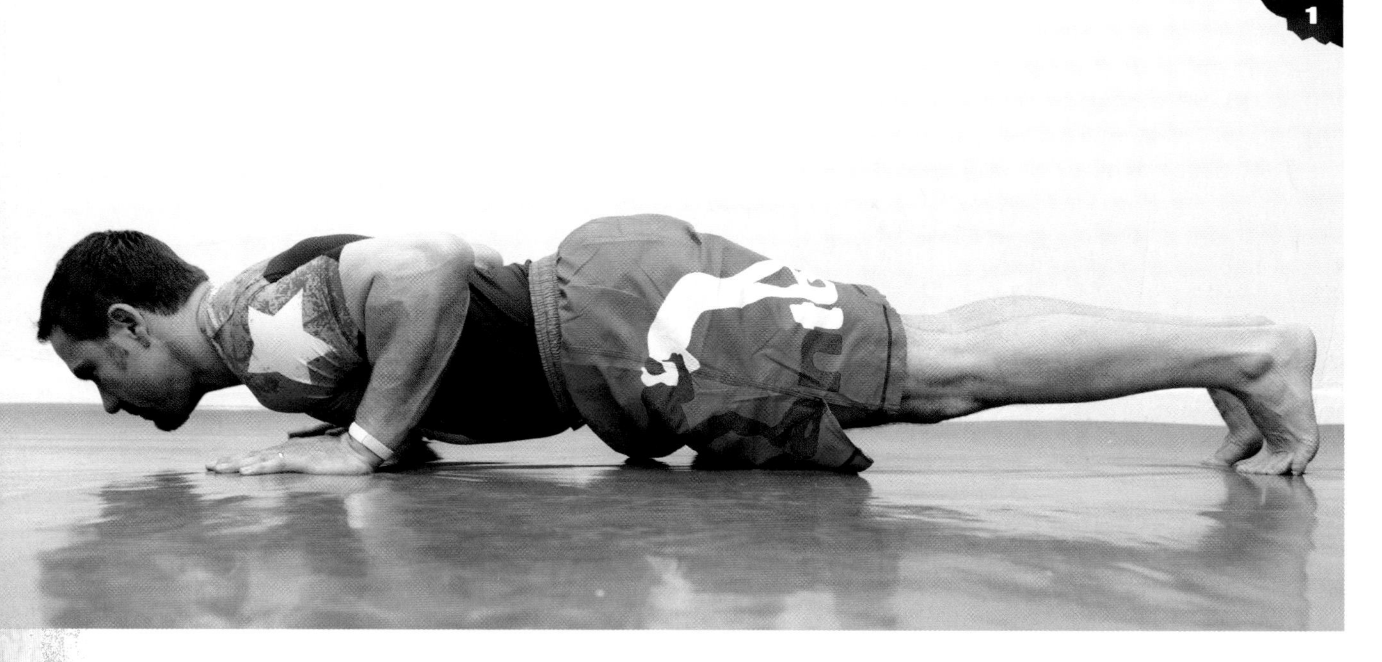

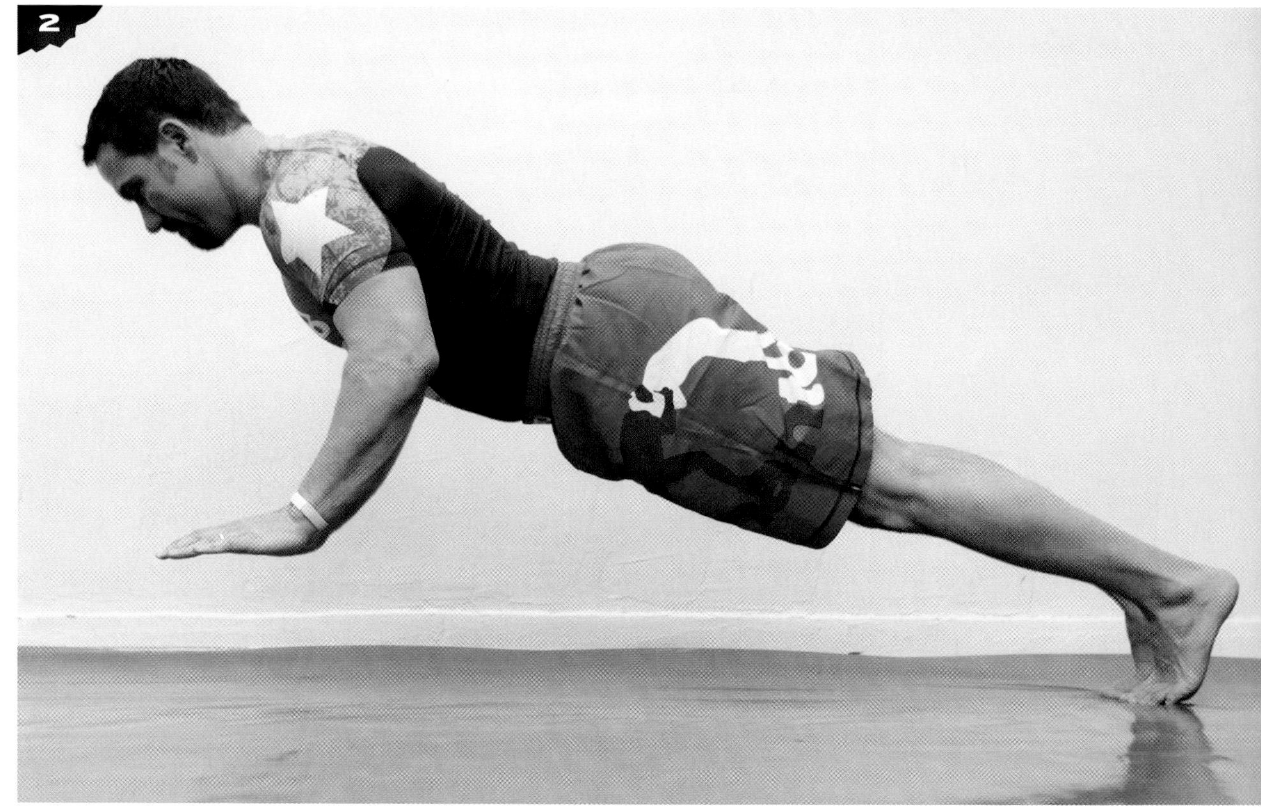

3. CLAPPING PUSHUP

Once you have lowered into the pushup position, extend at the elbows quickly so that the hands come off the floor at the top of the motion. Clap the hands together, lower the hands back to the floor and then lower the body back down for the next rep.

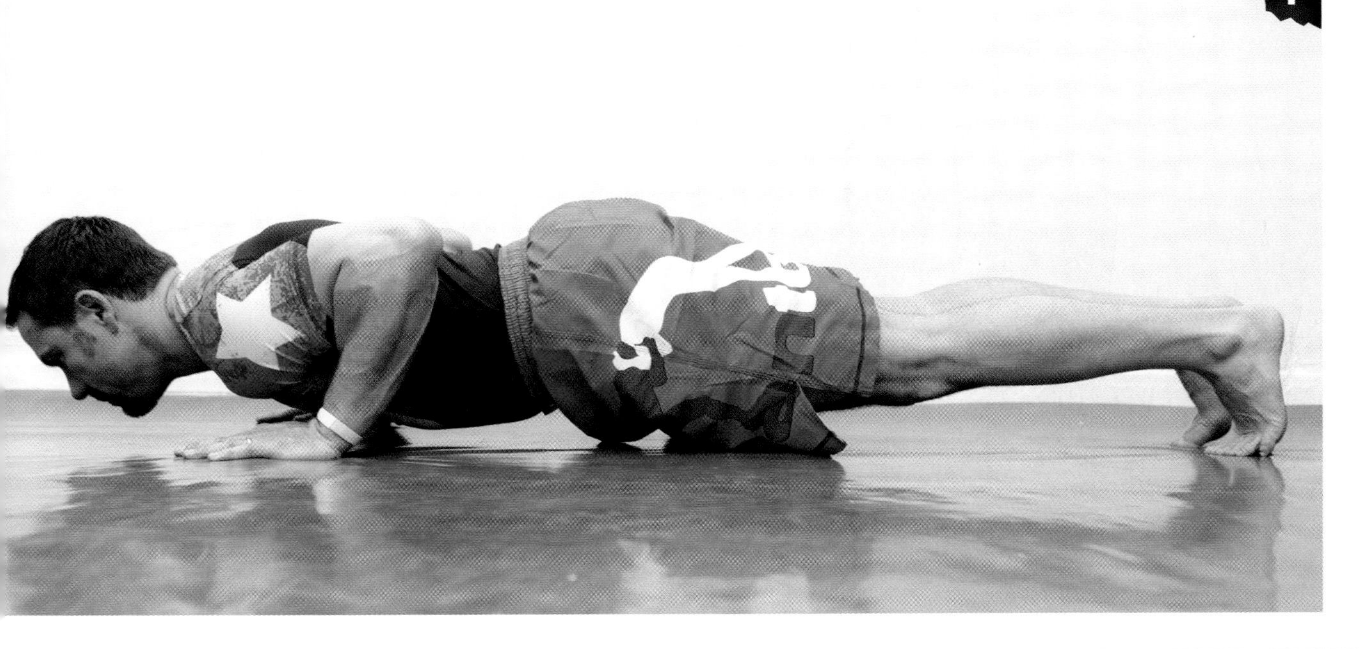

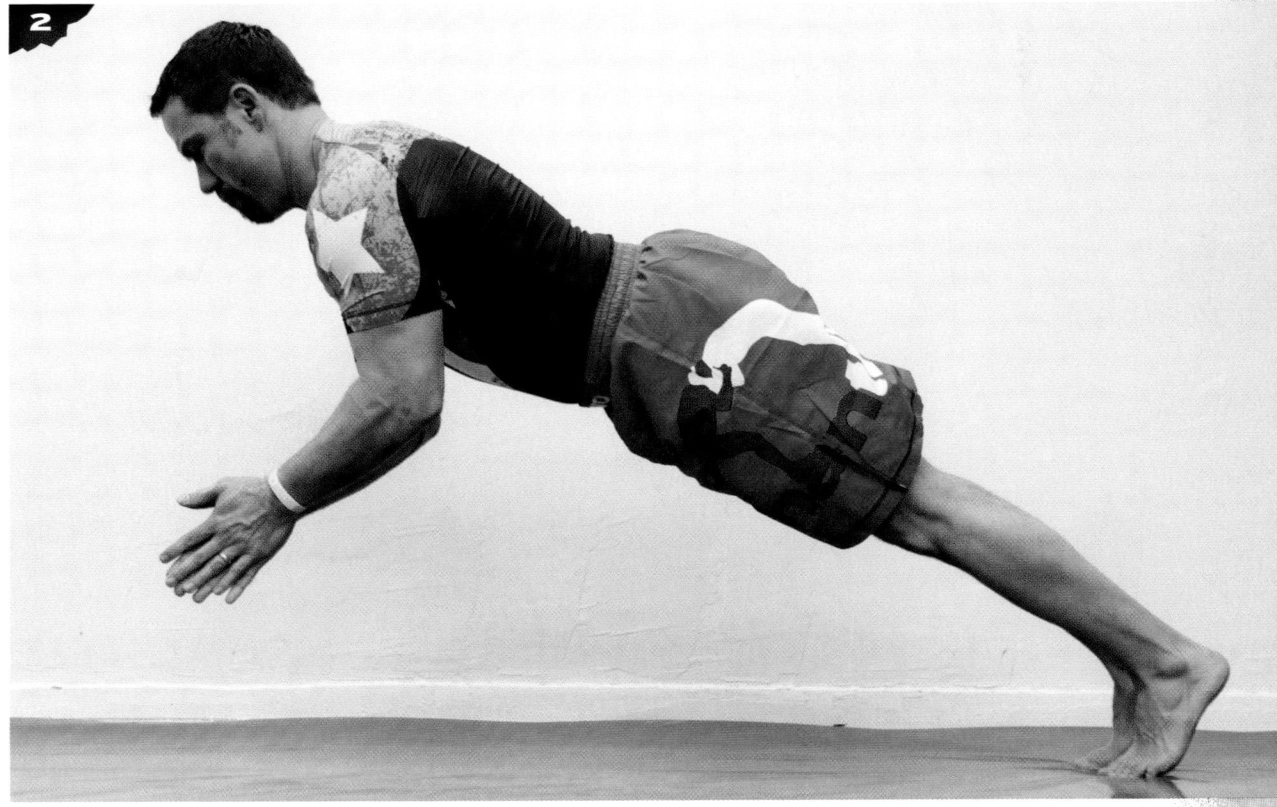

4. CHEST SLAP PUSHUP

Once you have lowered into the pushup position, extend at the elbows quickly so that the hands come off the floor at the top of the motion. Clap the hands against the chest, lower the hands back to the floor and then lower the body back down for the next rep.

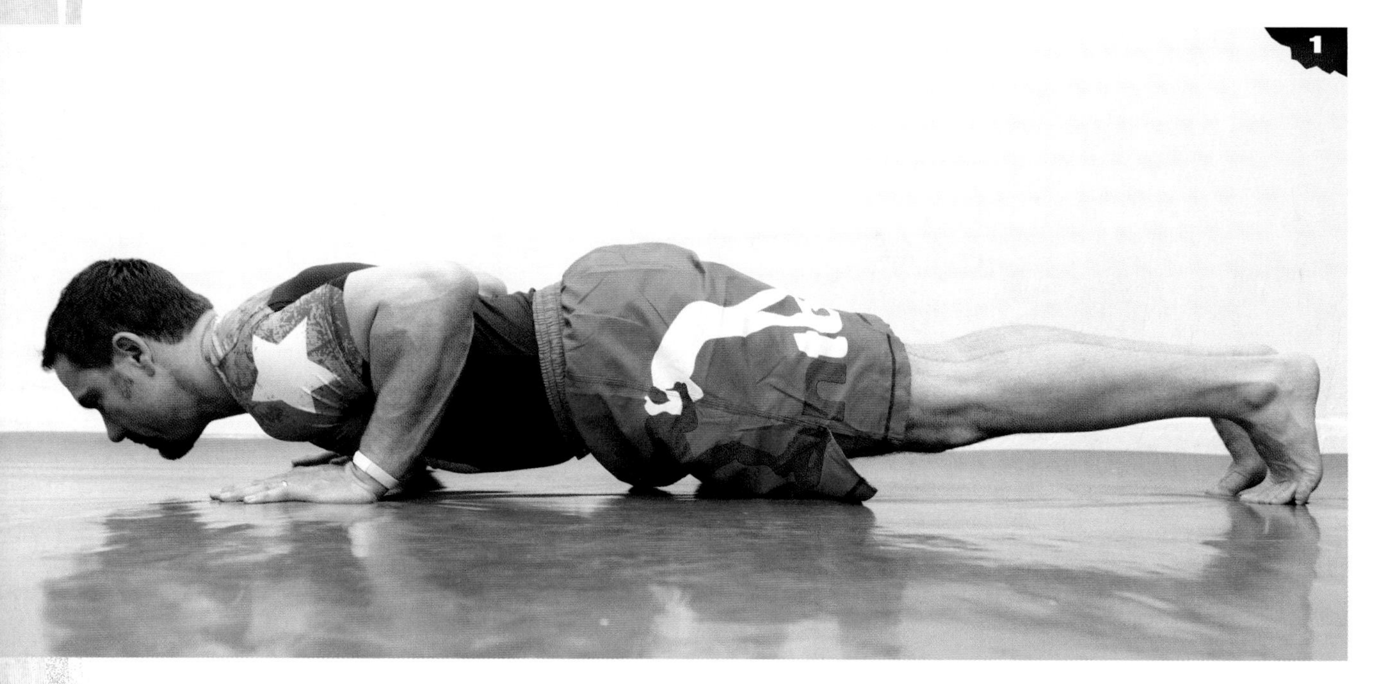

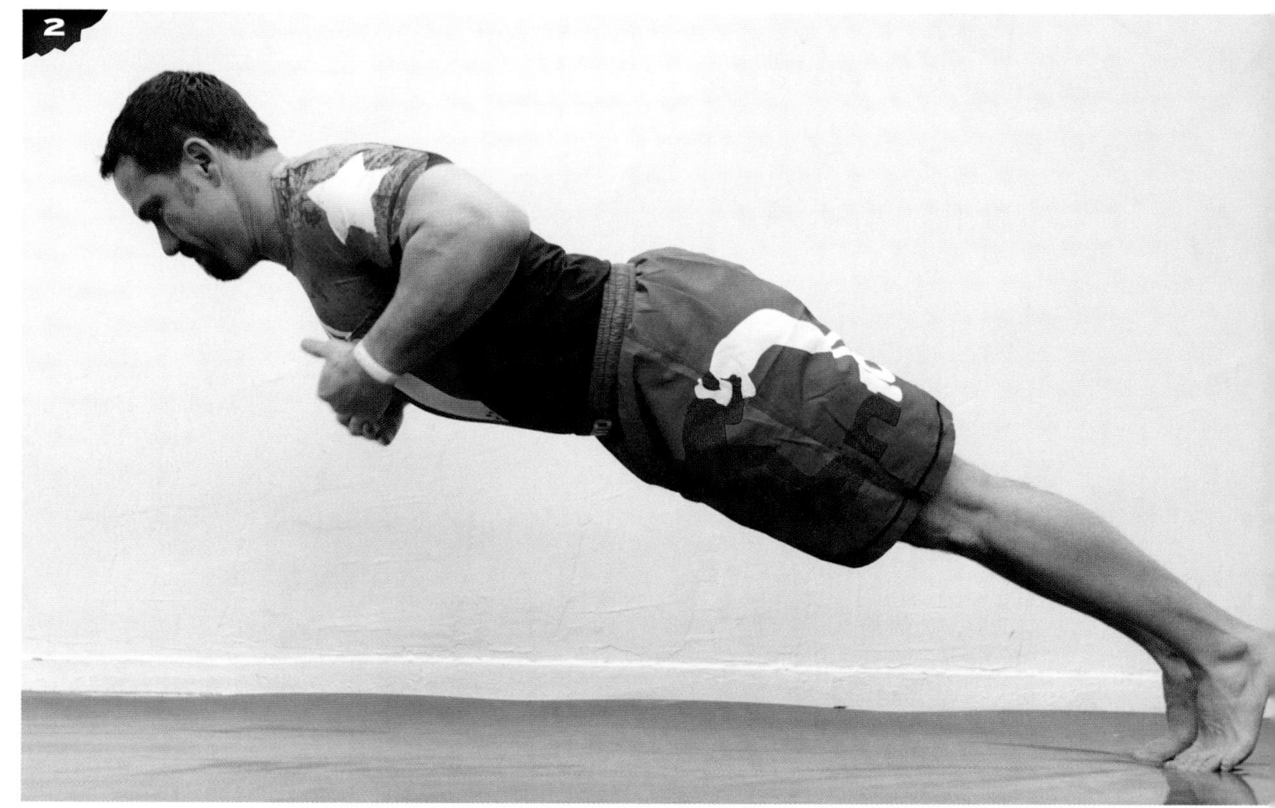

5. OVERHEAD-RAISE PUSHUP

Once you have lowered into the pushup position, extend at the elbows quickly and then at the top of the motion, raise both straight arms overhead. Lower the hands back to the floor and then lower the body back down for the next rep.

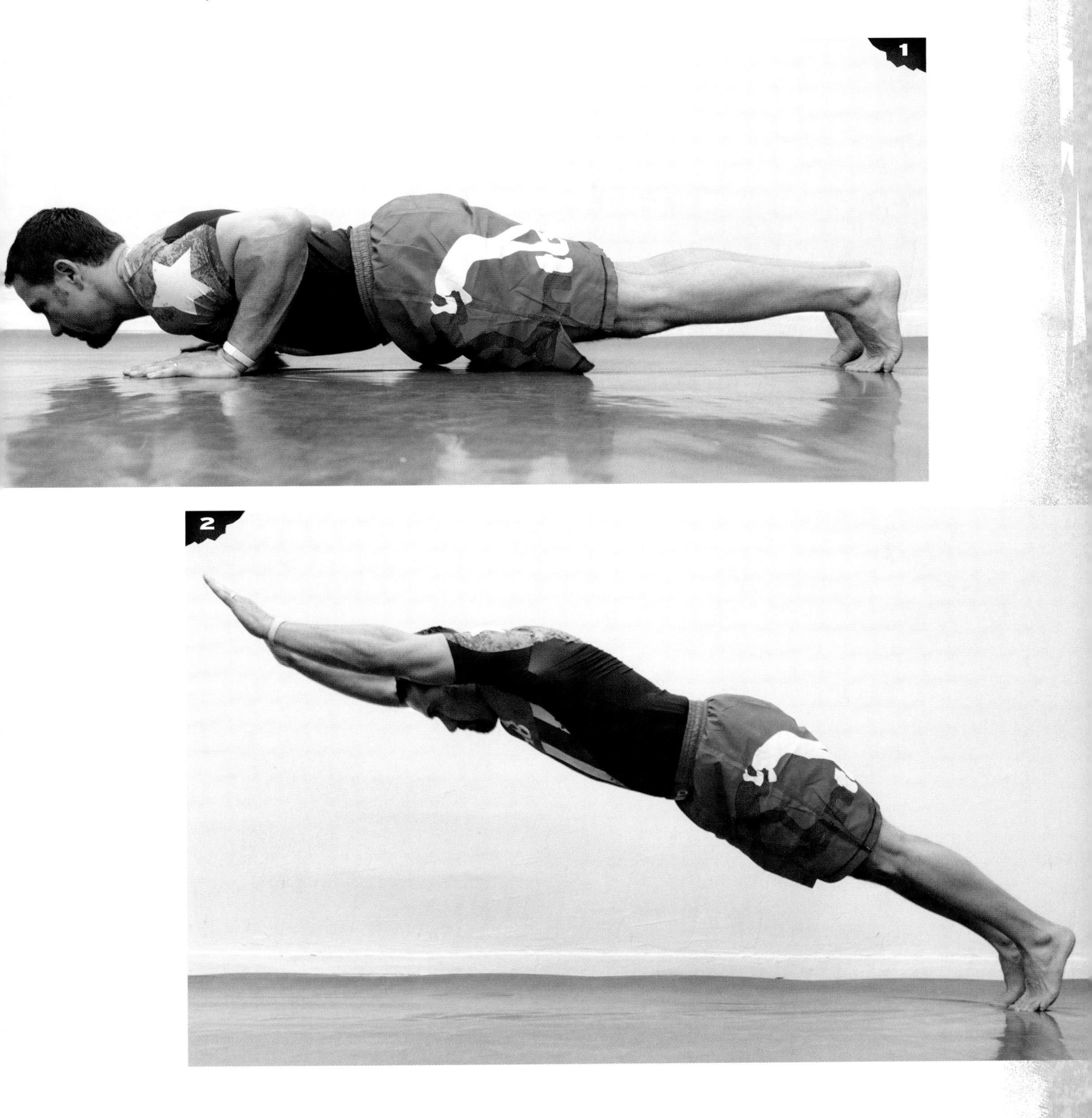

6. HIPS-SLAP PUSHUP

Once you have lowered into the pushup position, extend at the elbows quickly so that the hands both come off the floor at the top of the motion. Clap the hands against the thighs, then lower the hands back to the floor and then lower the body back down for the next rep.

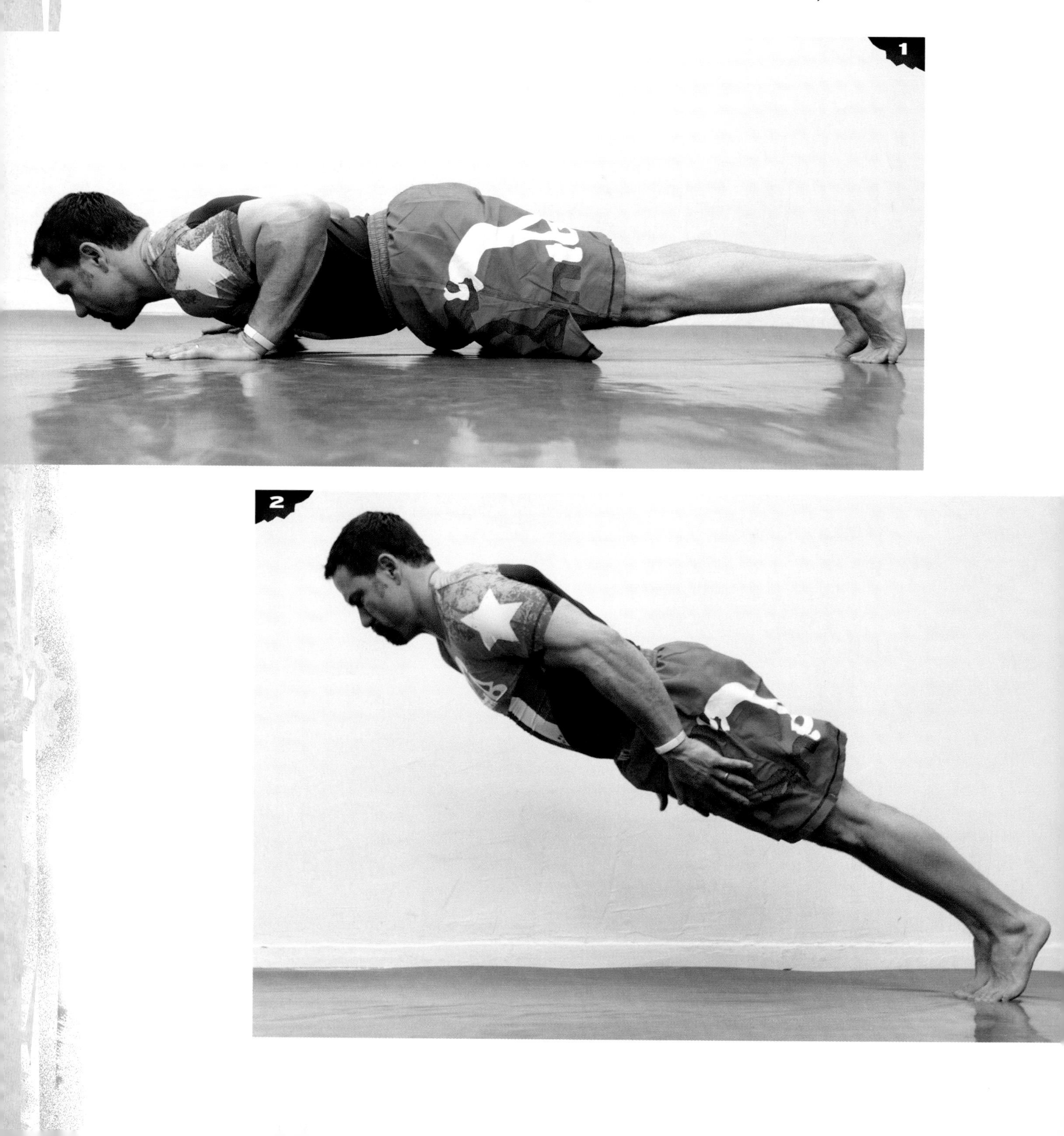

I. BODY WEIGHT CIRCUITS: FOUR-WAY LUNGE

Perform the following circuit for ten reps of each exercise. Record the best time for each circuit.

1. ALTERNATING FRONT LUNGE

Begin standing with the hands up and elbows tucked at the sides. Step forward and drop the back knee almost to the ground. Press back up with the lead leg and repeat on the opposite side.

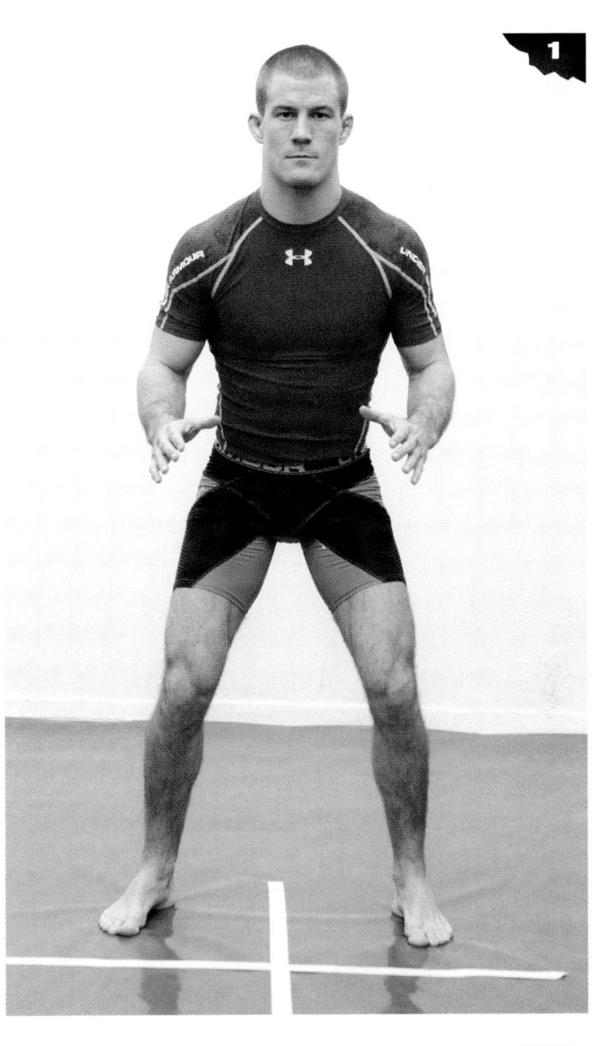

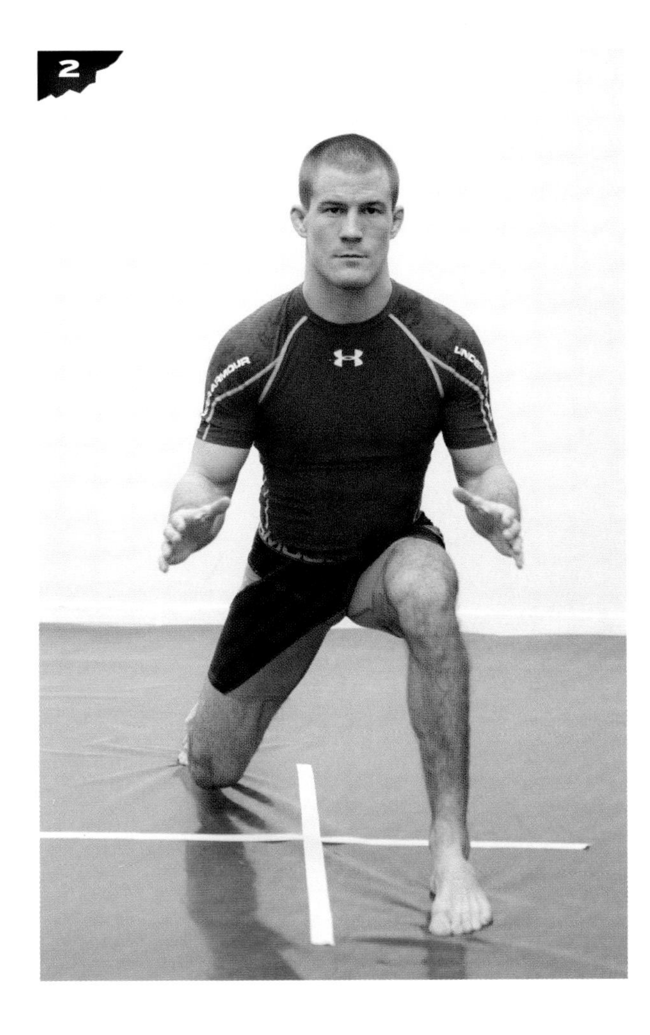

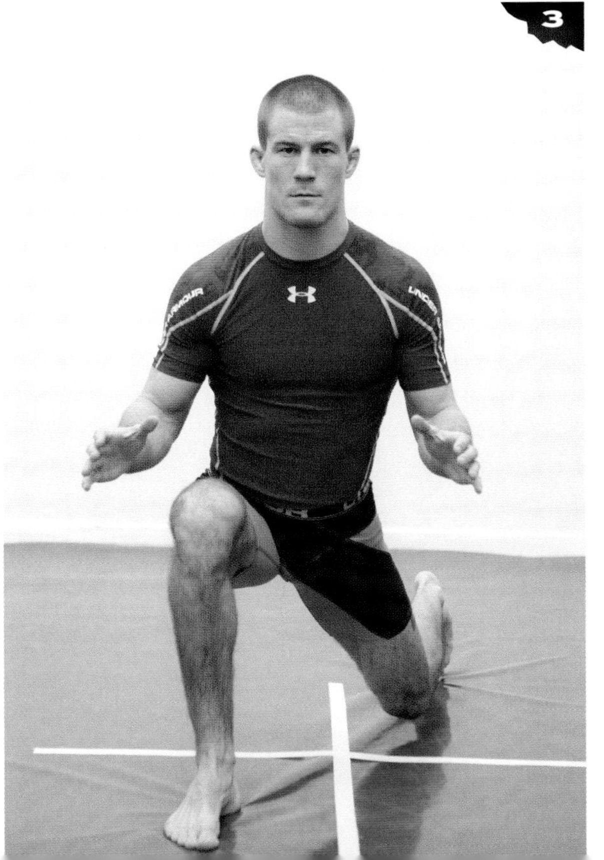

2. ALTERNATING SIDE LUNGE

Begin standing with the hands out front and the elbows tucked at the sides. Step out to one side and lower the hips. Press back up and repeat on the other side.

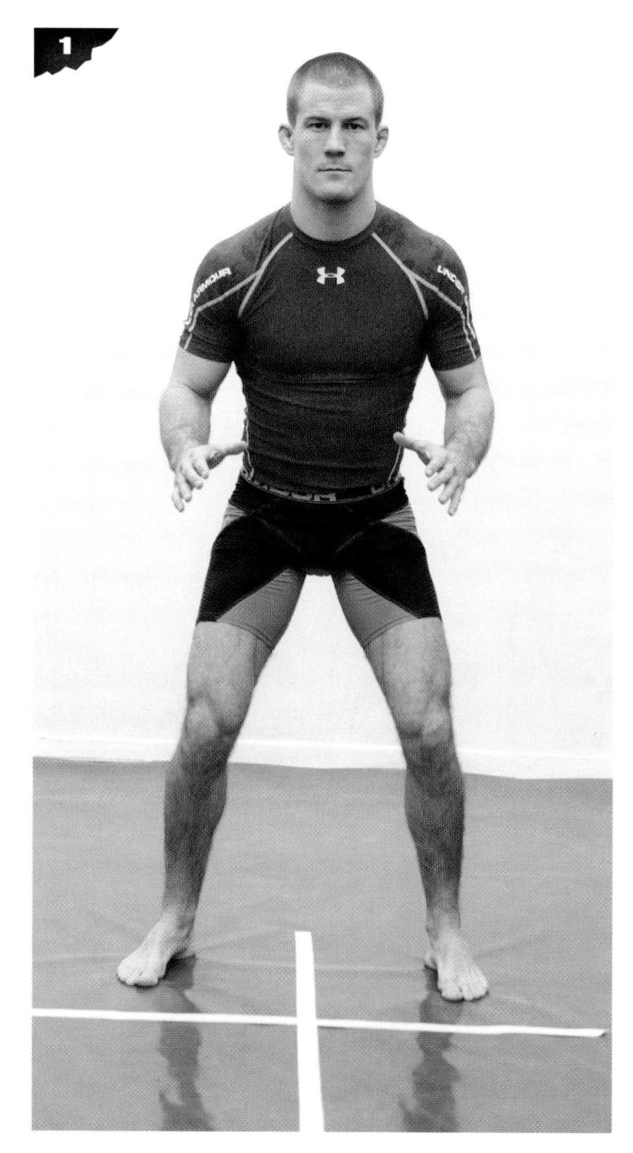

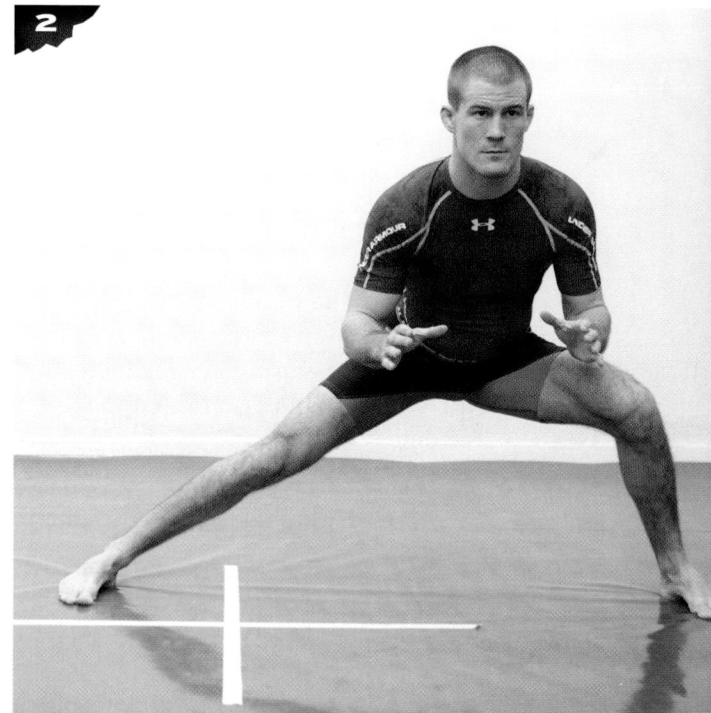

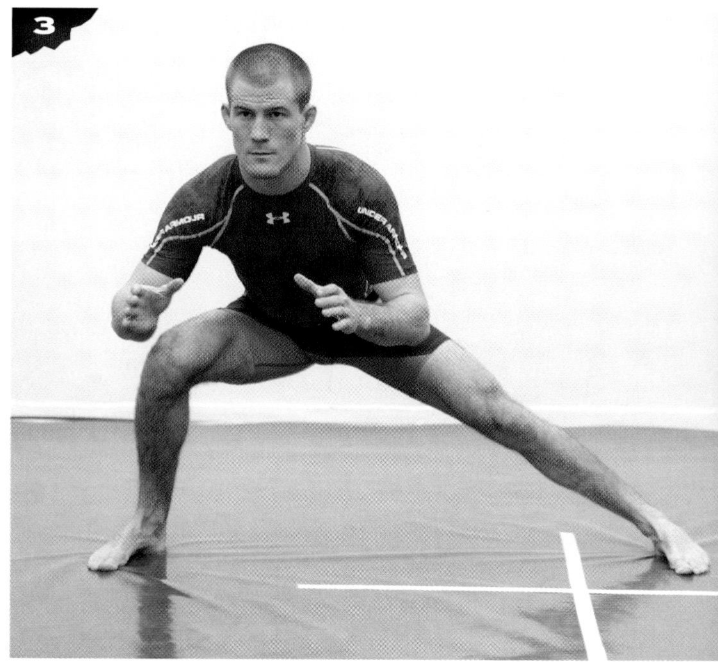

3. ALTERNATING REAR LUNGE

Begin standing with the hands out front and elbows tucked at the sides. Step back on an angle, opening the back hip as both hips drop and the front foot goes onto the heel. Press back up and repeat on the other side.

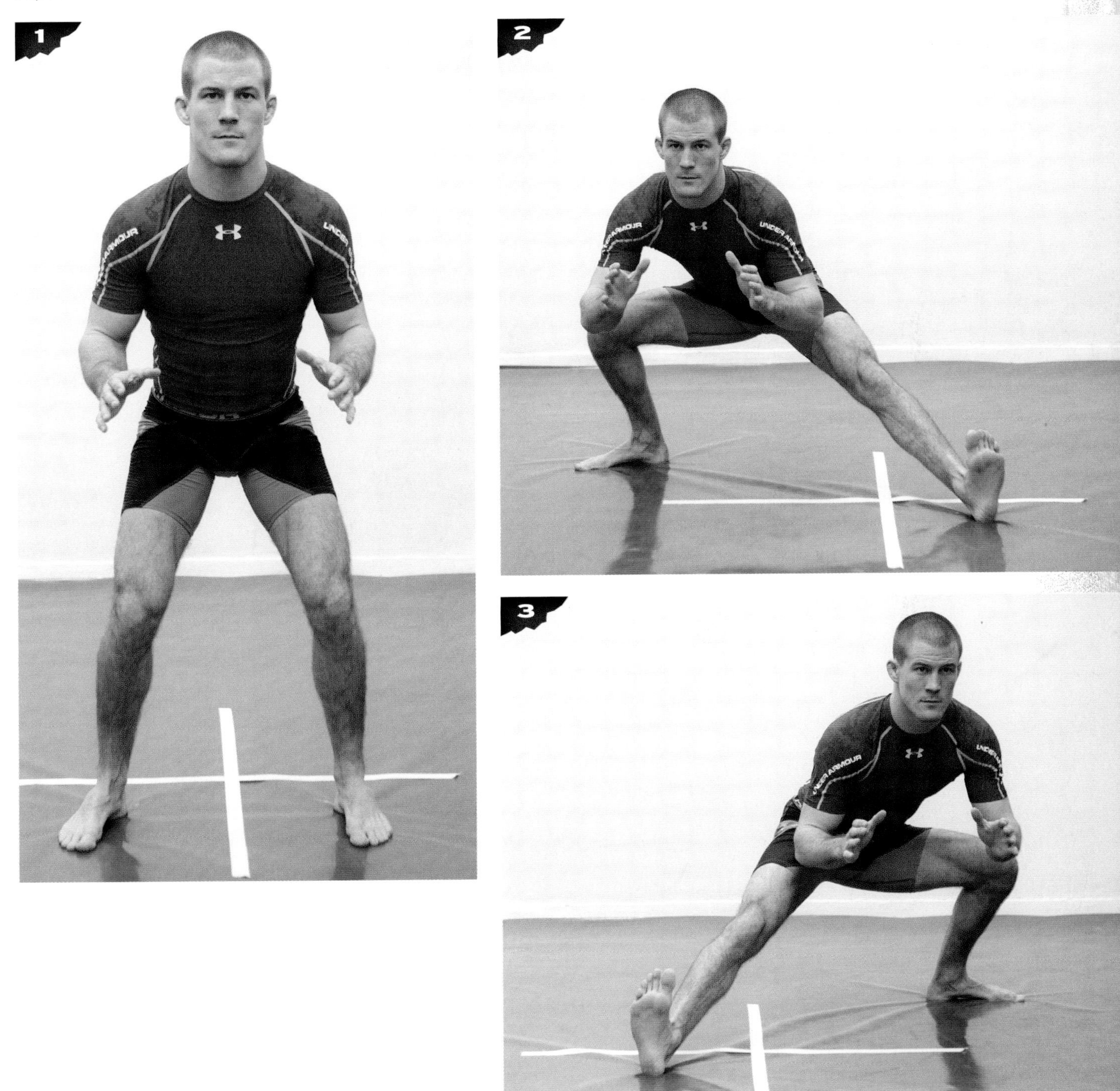

4. ALTERNATING CROSS-BACK LUNGE

Begin standing with the hands out front and the elbows tucked at the sides. Cross one foot back and behind the other as you drop your hips low to the ground. Step back up and repeat on the other side.

1

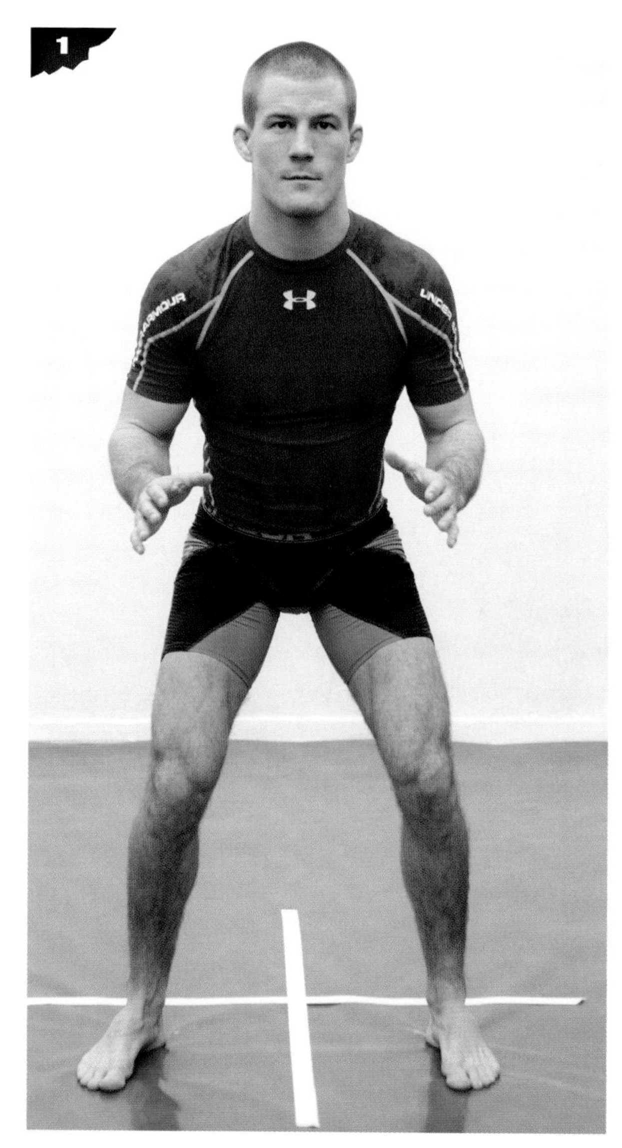

2

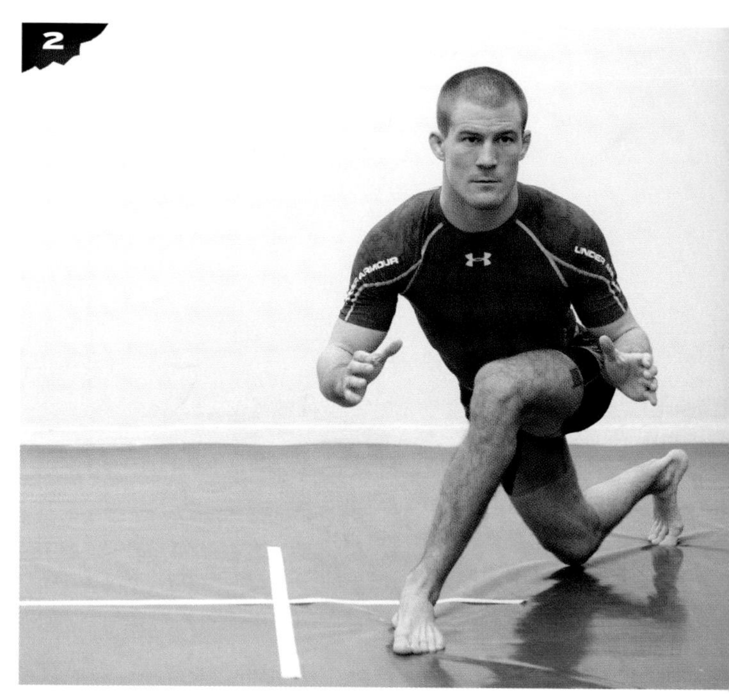

3

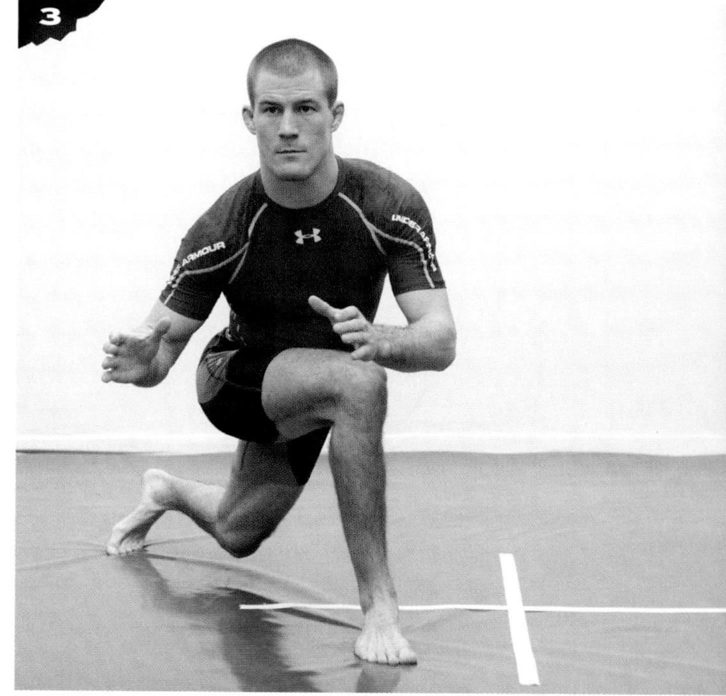

J. BODY WEIGHT CIRCUITS: ADVANCED PUSHUPS

Perform the following circuit for 10 reps of each exercise. Record the best time for each circuit.

1. PUSHUP

Begin supporting the body on the hands and feet with the feet together and hands at shoulder width on the ground. Lower the chest to the ground while keeping the elbows close to the sides. Extend at the elbows to return to the original position.

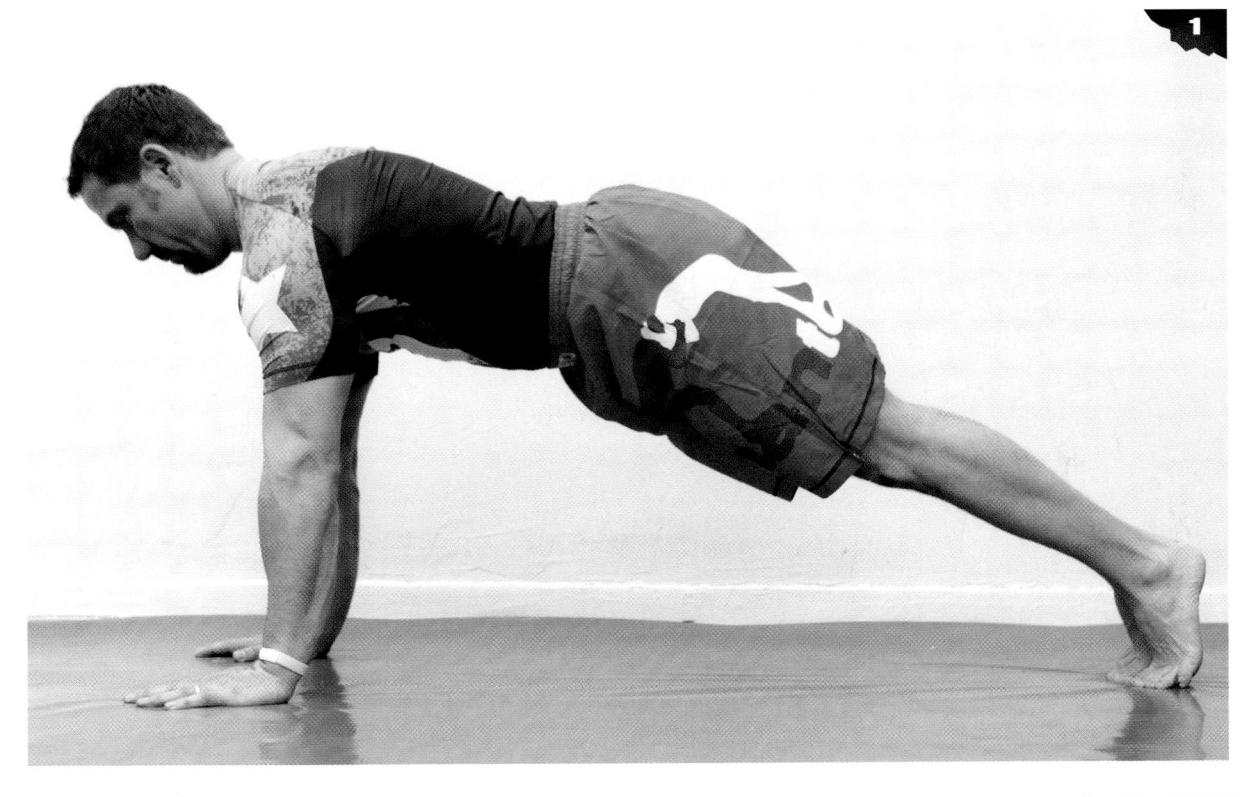

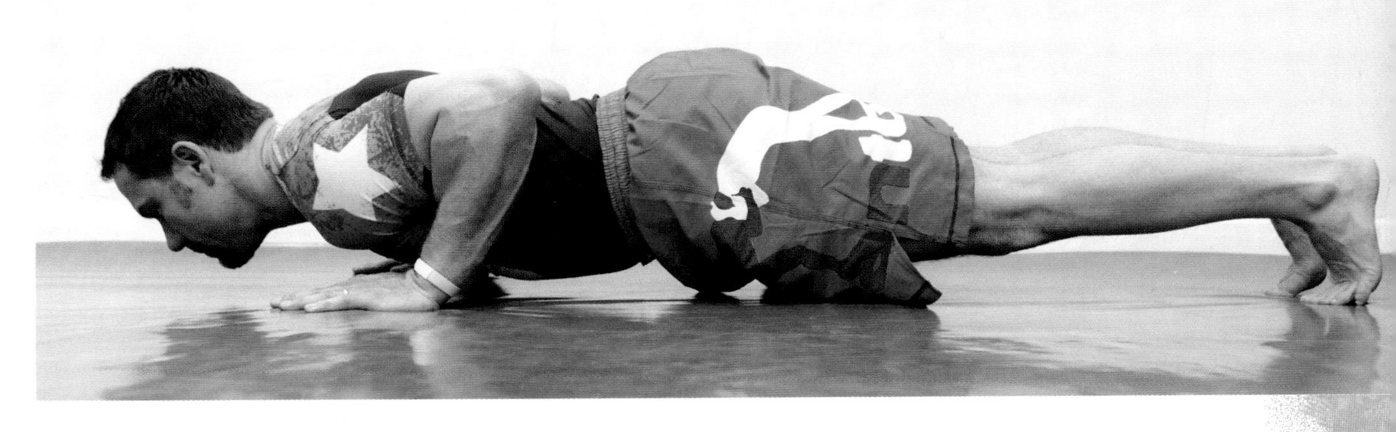

2. WARRIOR PUSHUP

Begin in the low pushup position and then extend at the elbows to reach the high position. Turn at the shoulders and reach one hand as high as possible toward the ceiling. Reverse the motion, replace the hand, and return to the start position. Alternate arms on each rep.

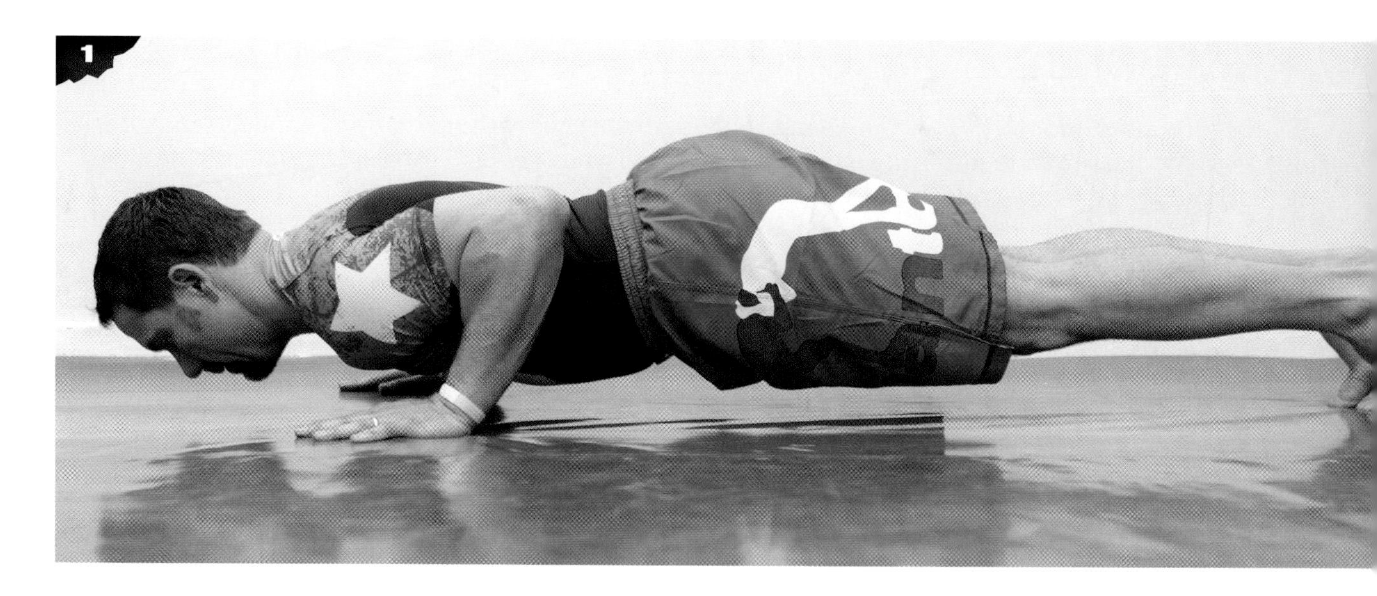

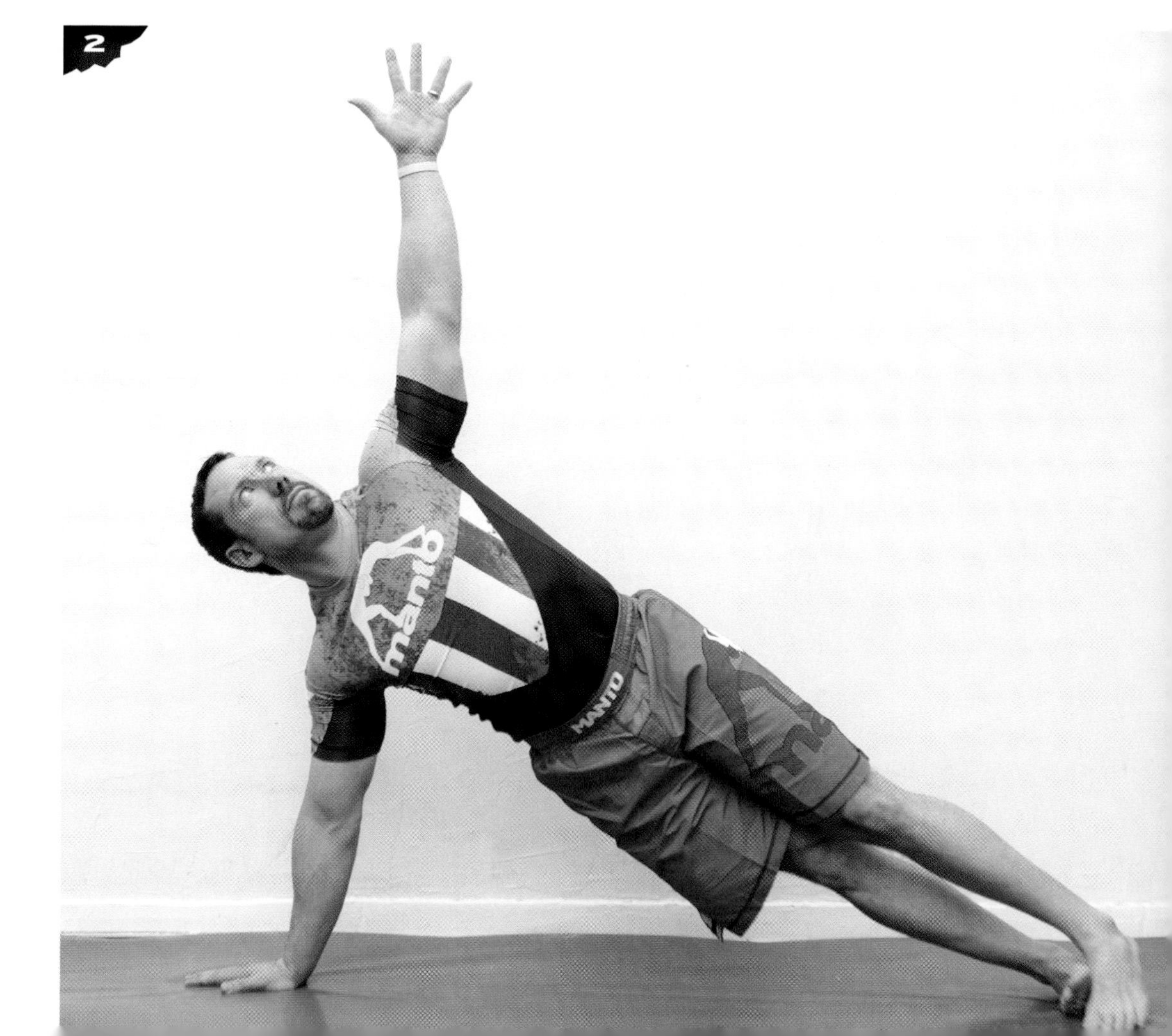

3. TOE-KICK PUSHUP

Begin in the low pushup position and extend the elbows to reach the high position. Turn at the shoulders and kick one foot under the body and as high as possible while touching that toe with the opposite hand. Lower that foot back to the original position.

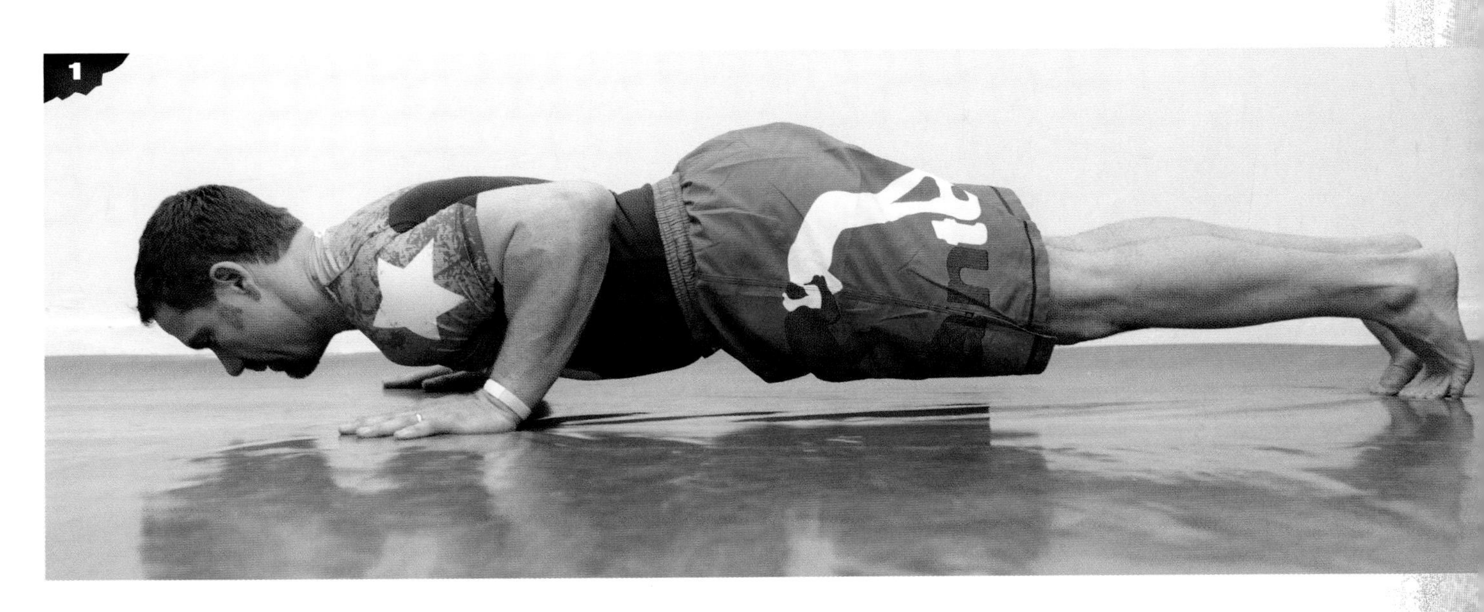

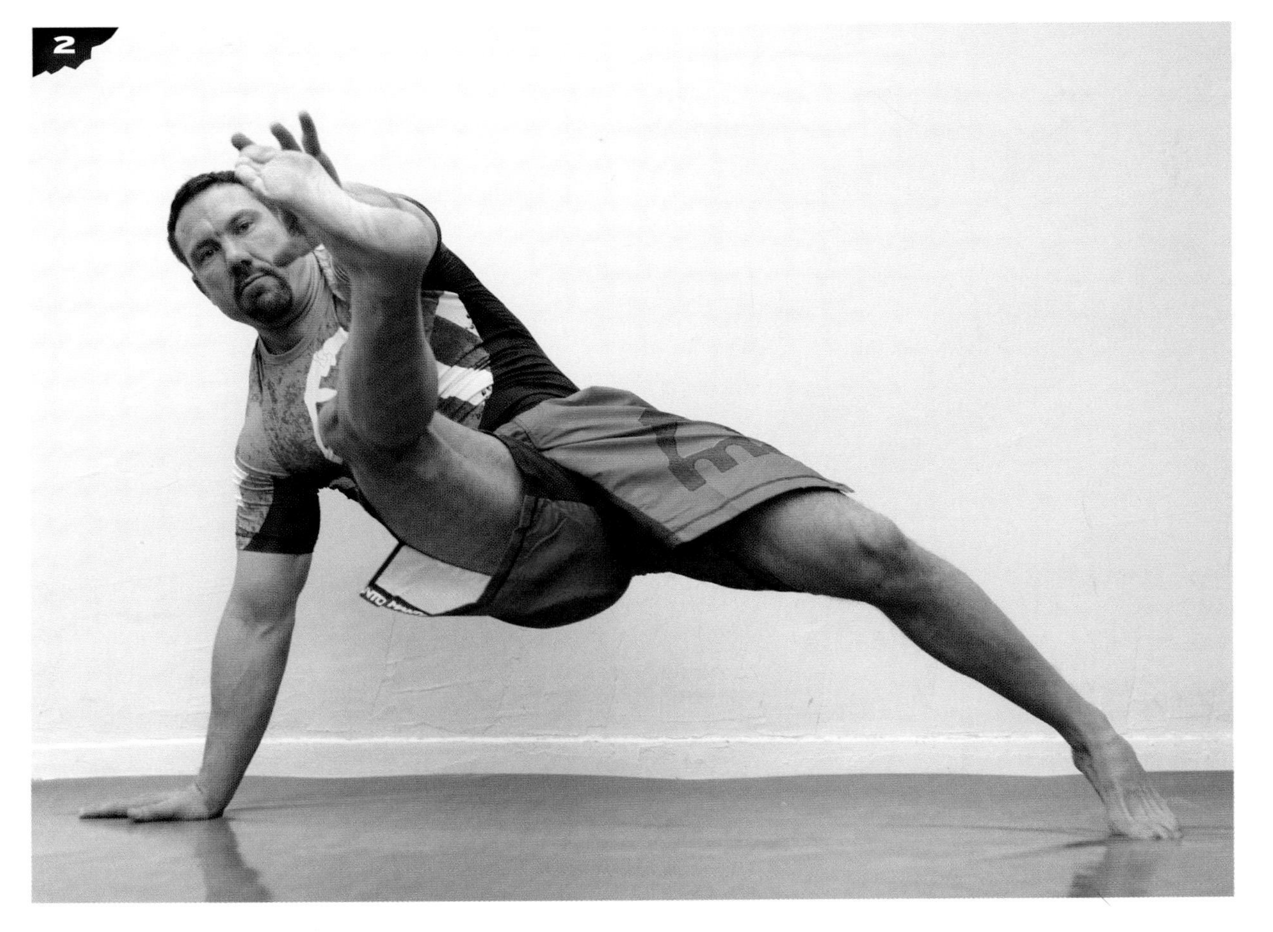

4. PIKE PRESS

Begin in the high pushup position. Lower the head and chest out as far in front of the hands as possible. Drag the forehead as close to the ground as possible while pressing the body backward and hips upward. Finish with the hips up, the head down, and the elbows extended.

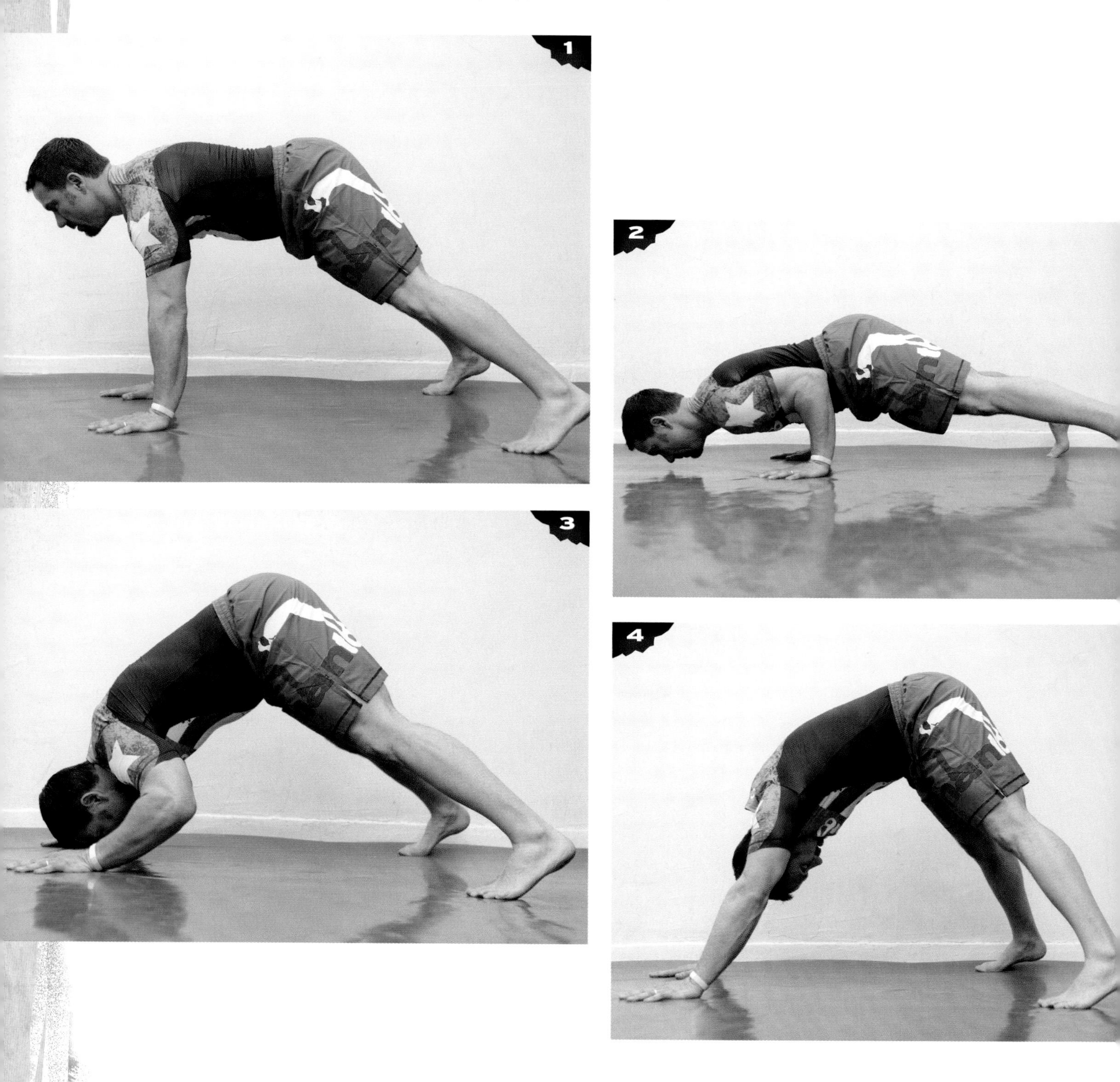

5. WALL PUSHUP

Begin in the high pushup position, using the hands to press the feet up into the wall. Lower the chest to the floor by bending at the elbows. Extend at the elbows and return to the original position.

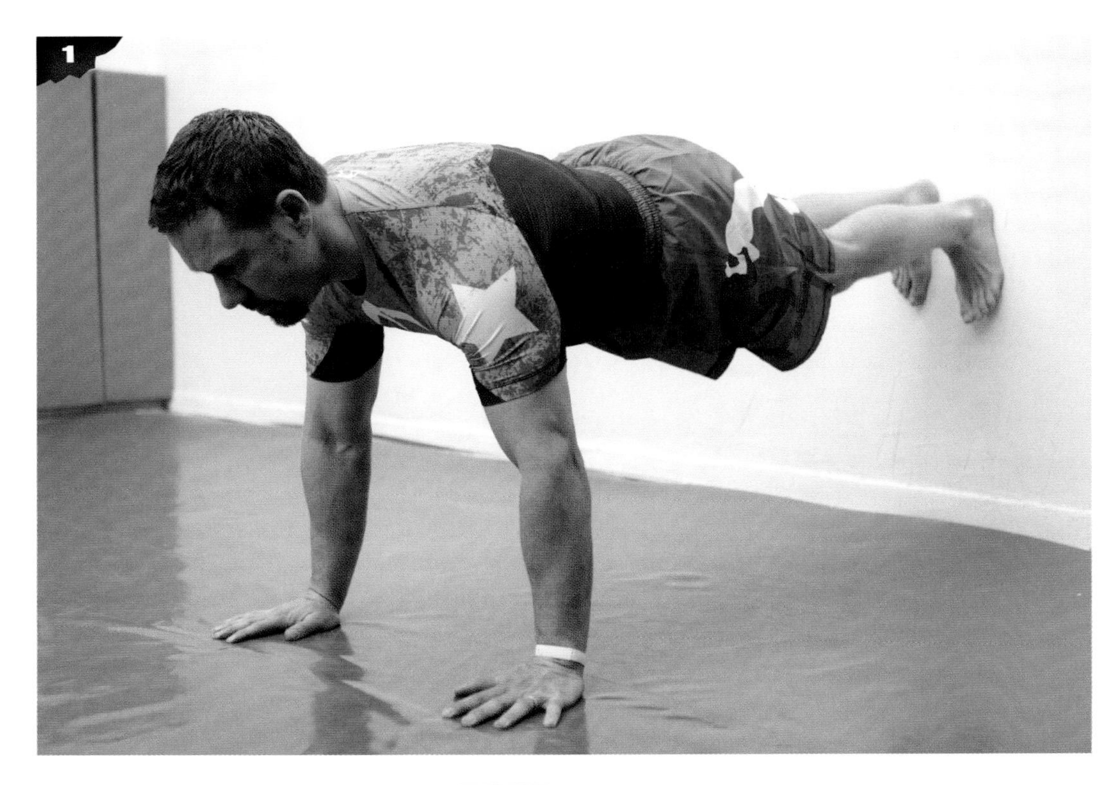

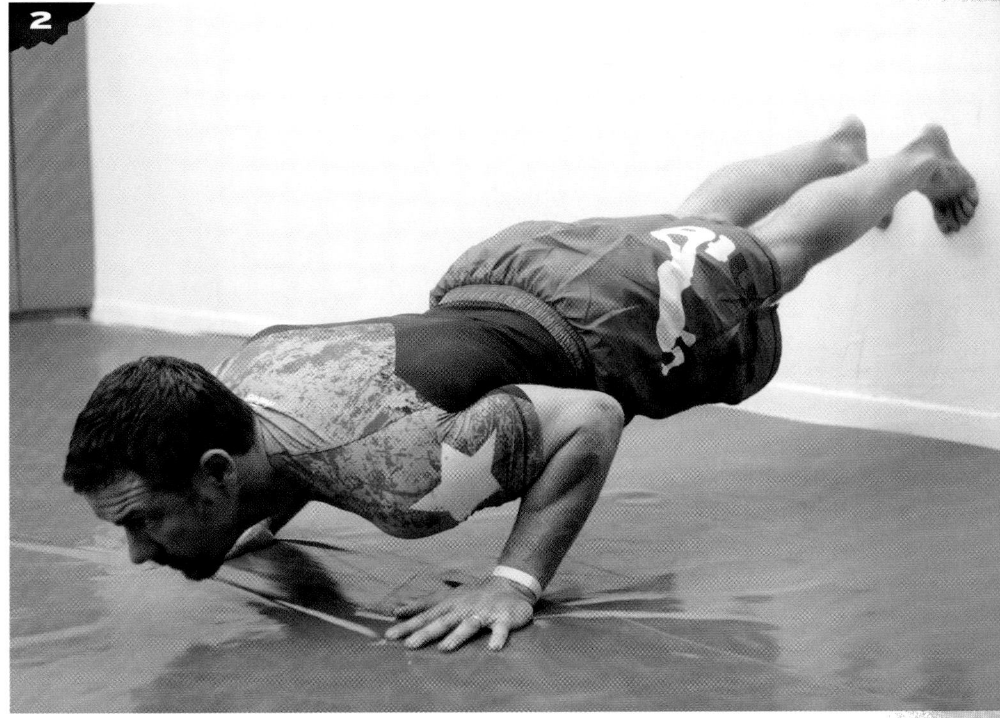

K. BODY WEIGHT CIRCUITS: THE TRAVELER'S WORKOUT

Over the last two years, I spent more than 100 days out of the country. In order to maintain my strength, size, and conditioning, in addition to eating well (which is always a challenge), I also needed to work out. Since many hotels of the world do not offer health clubs, I was forced to get creative with body weight training. Interestingly, not only did I find these workouts to be demanding, but I was pleasantly surprised to find that I actually gained strength in some areas when I returned to the weights! Whether on vacation or on a business trip, you can always find 15 minutes for a full body workout that is guaranteed to keep you fit and focused.

RULES OF THE WORKOUT

There are only three exercises and you have only 15 minutes. The goal is to perform as many reps of all three exercises as possible over that time. The exercises are to be performed in the following order:

BODY SQUAT

Stand with feet slightly wider than shoulder width and toes turned out slightly. Hands can be held behind the head or out in front of the body. Sit back while bending at the knees until thighs are parallel with the floor. Keep your weight on the heels with the feet remaining flat.

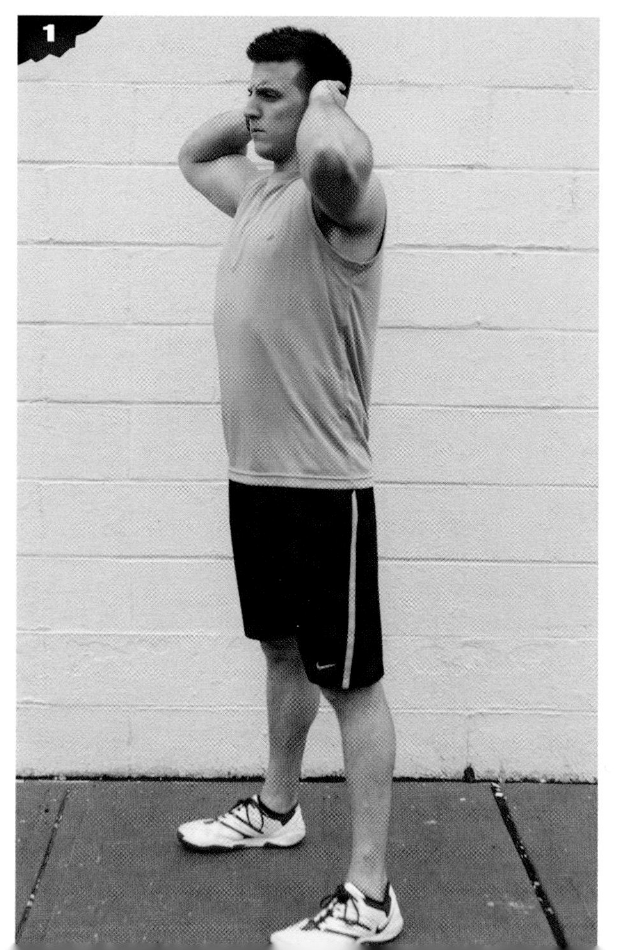

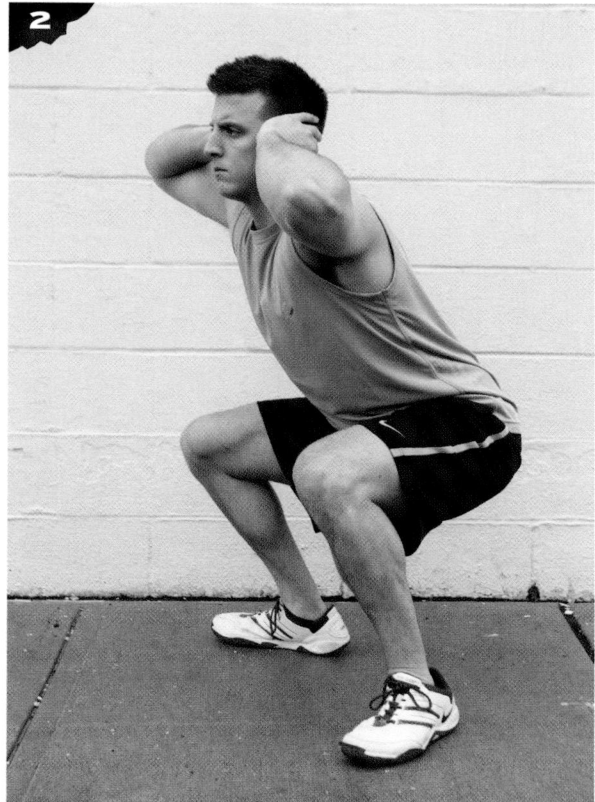

2. JUDO PUSHUPS

Begin in the pushup position with the feet wider than shoulder width and the butt held as high as possible. Bend at the elbows, bring the chest down to the ground and then push the hips through toward the hands as you raise your head (by extending the lower back). From this position, raise the hips and return to the start position.

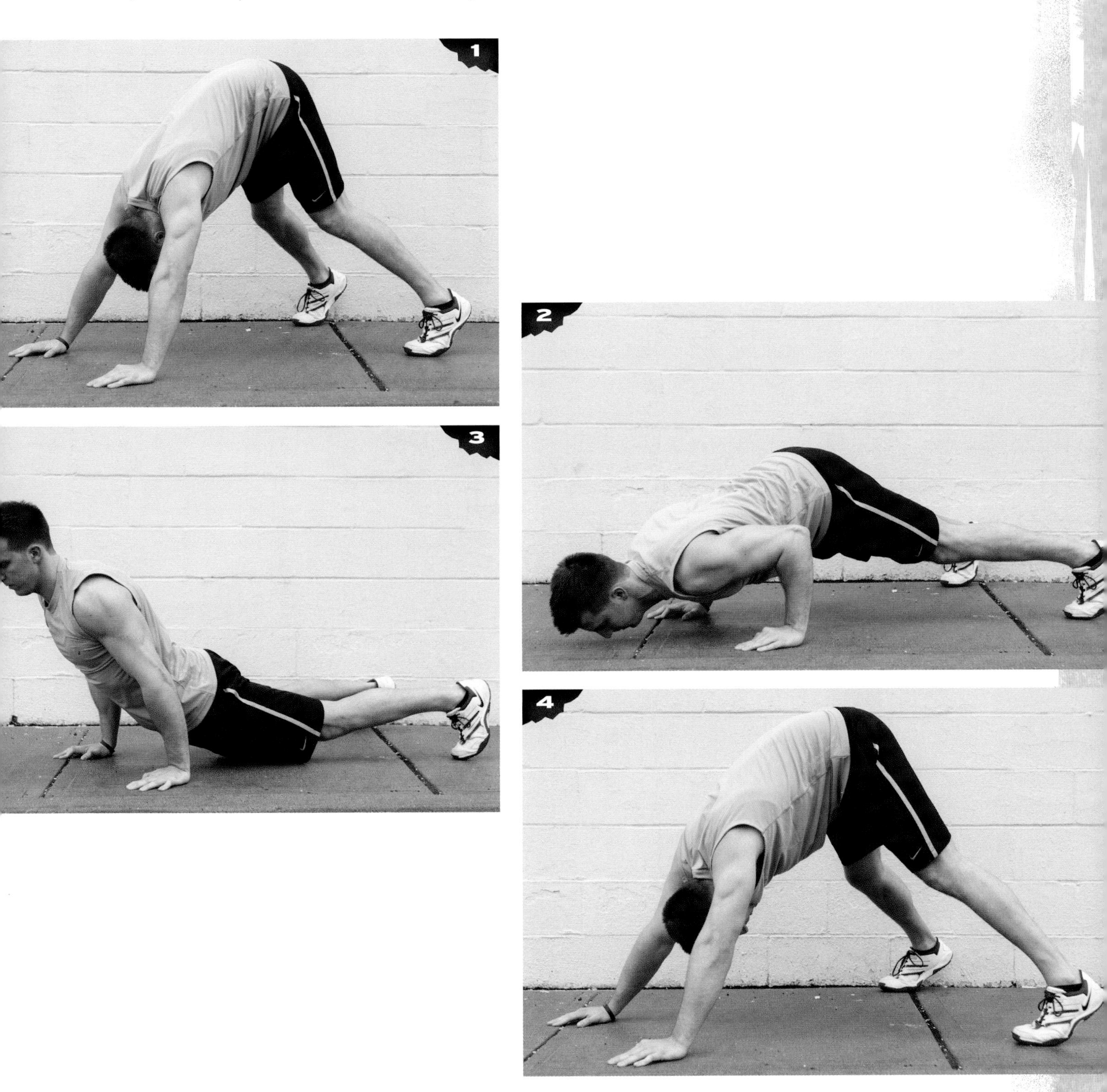

3. SPRINTER SIT-UPS

Begin on the back with the legs straight and the elbows held at 90 degrees at the sides. As you sit up, bring one knee up and the opposite elbow forward while the other arm fires backward. Lower back down under control to the start position and repeat on other side.

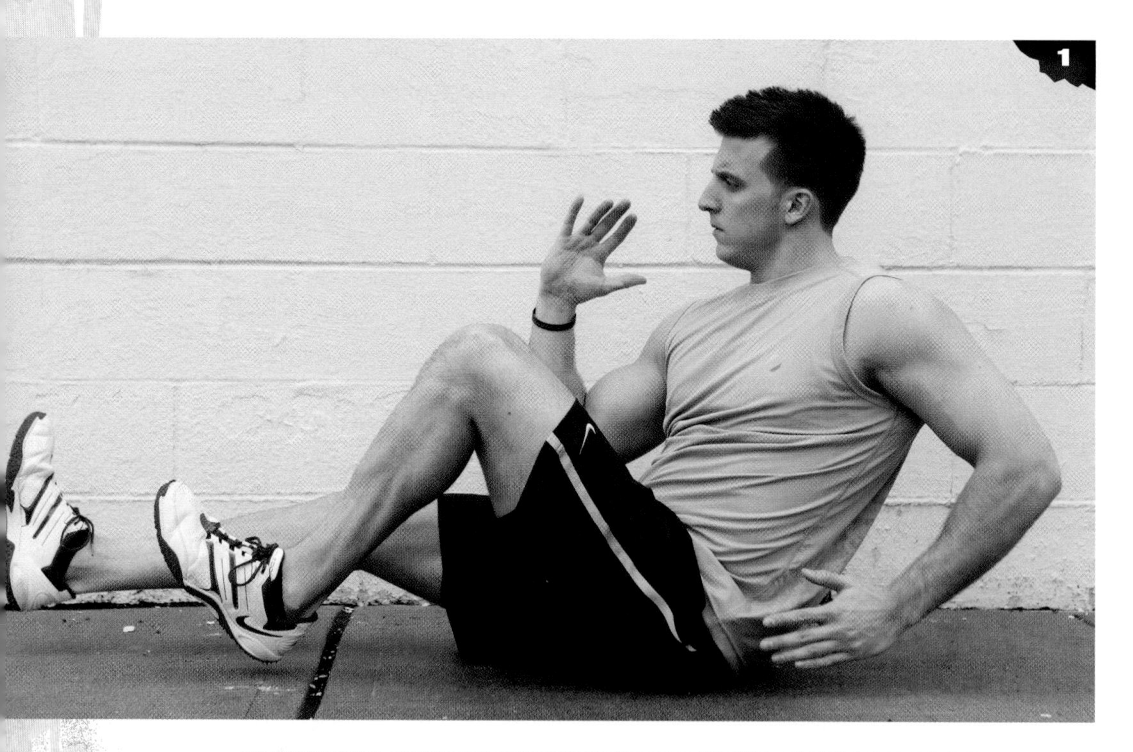

1

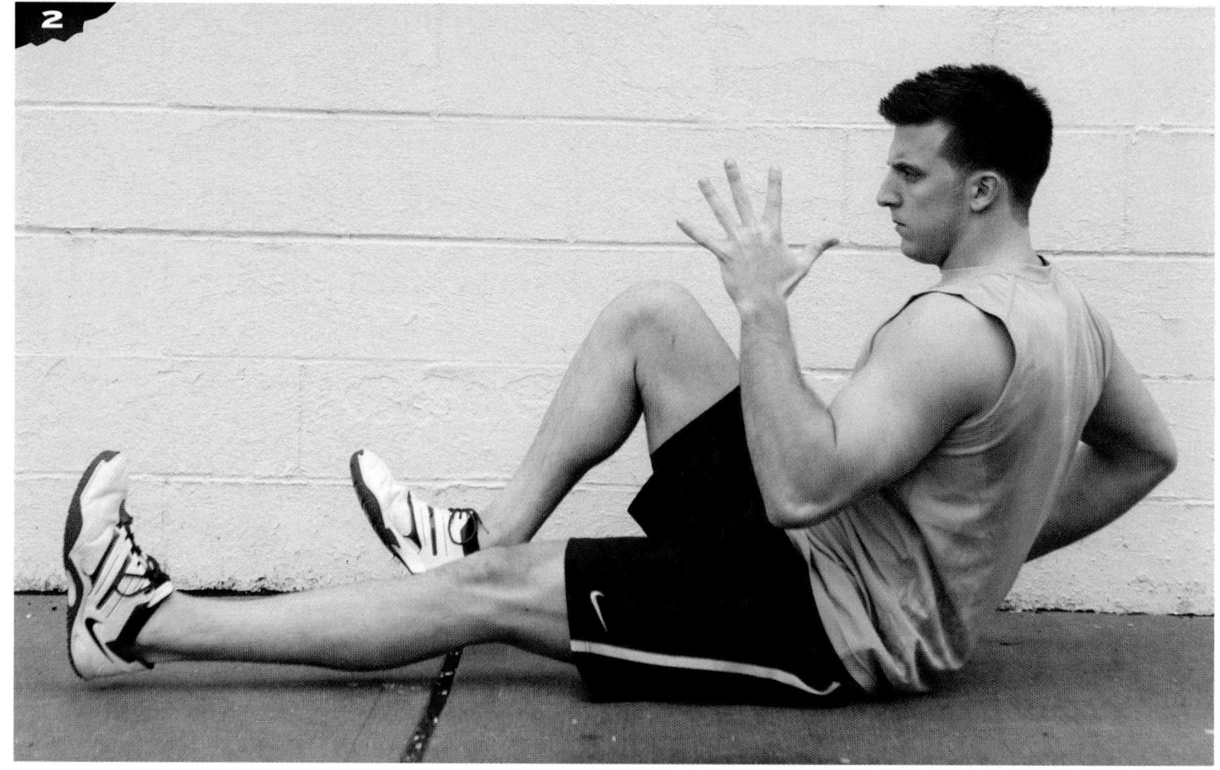

2

You choose how many reps per set to perform and the rest interval in between sets. For instance, I began with 10 reps of each exercise and tried to complete as many sets as possible in the 15 minutes. This would not only give me an easy calculation for the total reps of the workout, but also a number to improve upon on my next trip. Even if you get through only one circuit of all three exercises every 3 minutes, that would still be 50 reps of each for a total of 150 reps (and still leave time for a lot of rest, too)!

Once your body gets used to the workout, you can attack the exercises and shoot for a personal record on the road.

As you get more advanced, each set of the exercises can vary slightly in form for even more results. For instance, you can change the foot position for the squats, the direction of movement for the pushups, or the pattern of alternating sides with the sit-ups. This way, muscles are hit at different angles and the body is always kept both confused and stimulated.

80-REP CIRCUIT CHEATSHEET
1. BODY SQUAT
3. JUDO PUSHUP
2. WIDE-OUTS
4. SPRINTER SIT-UP

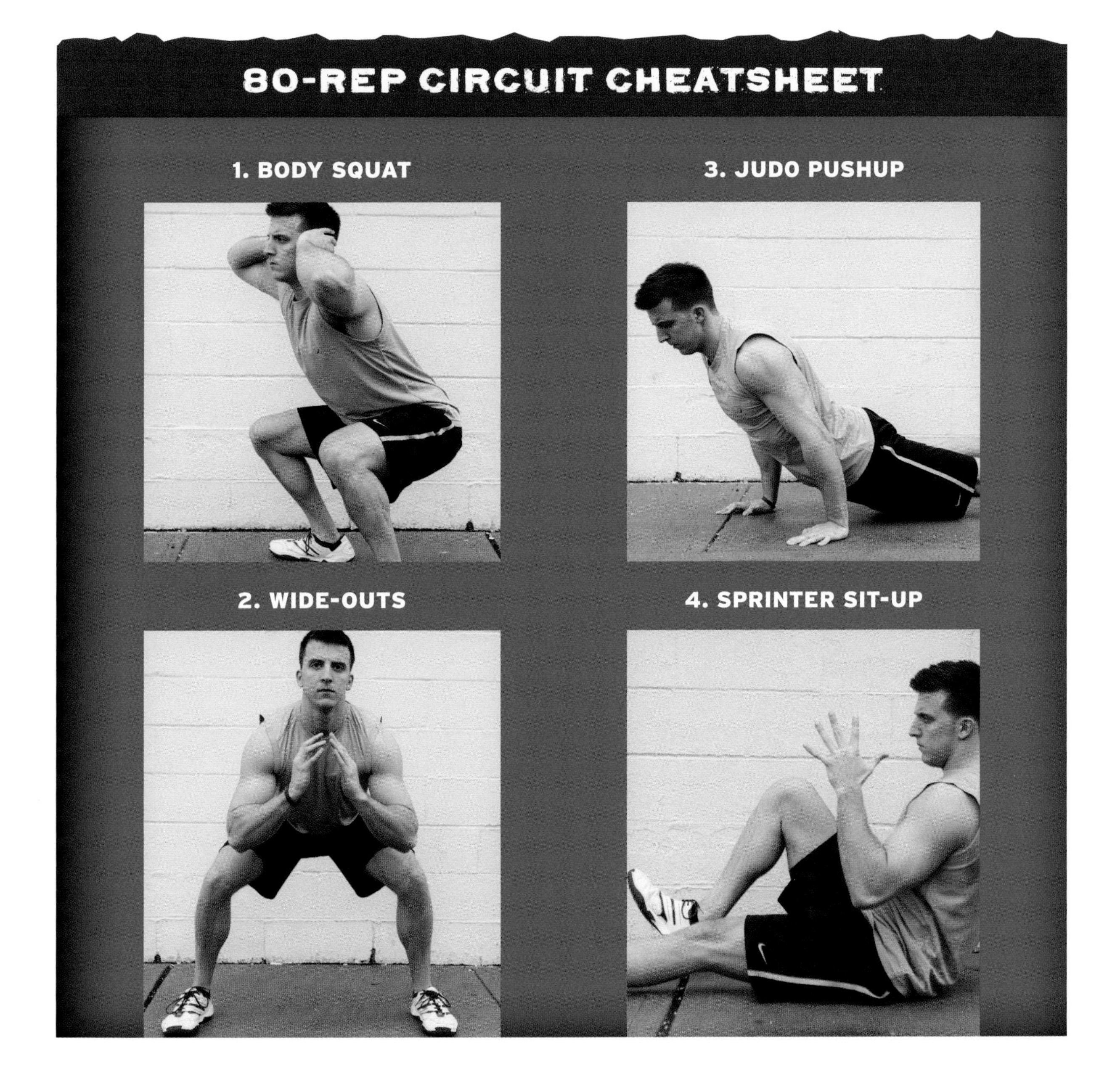

PLYOMETRIC PUSHUP CIRCUIT CHEATSHEET

1. ONE-ARM-RAISE PUSHUP

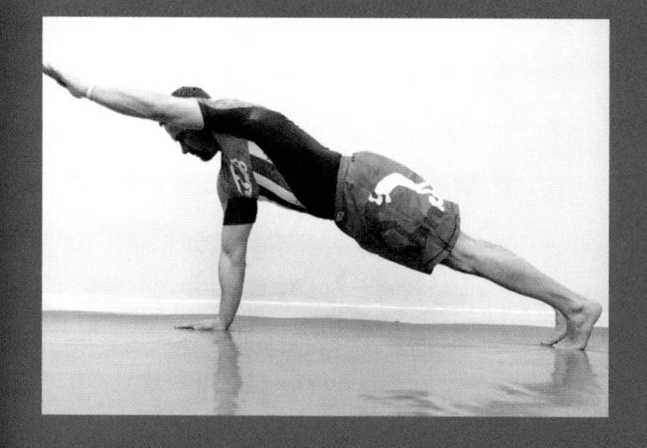

2. HANDS-OFF PUSHUP

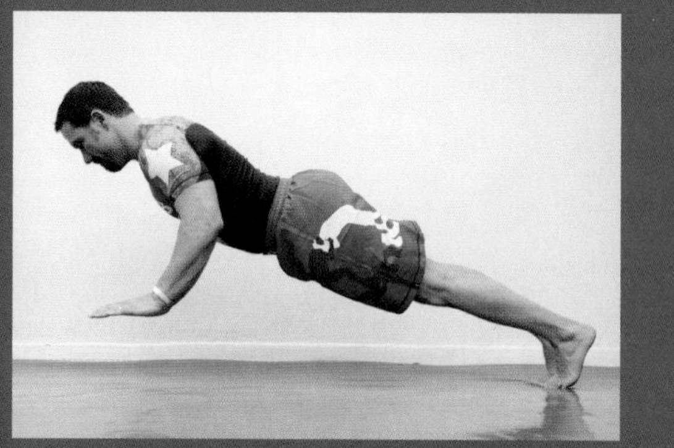

3. CLAPPING PUSHUP

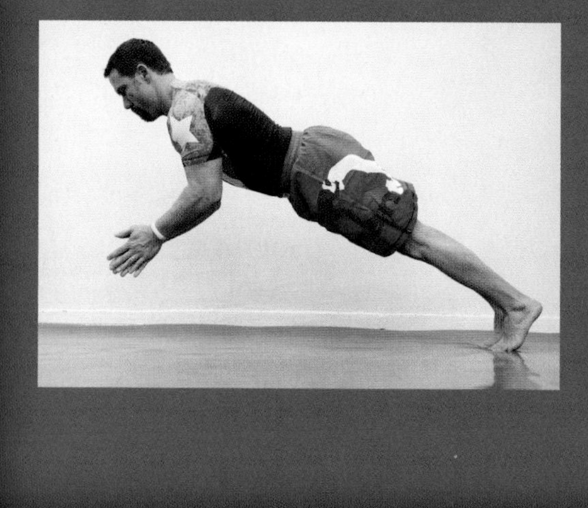

4. CHEST-SLAP PUSHUP

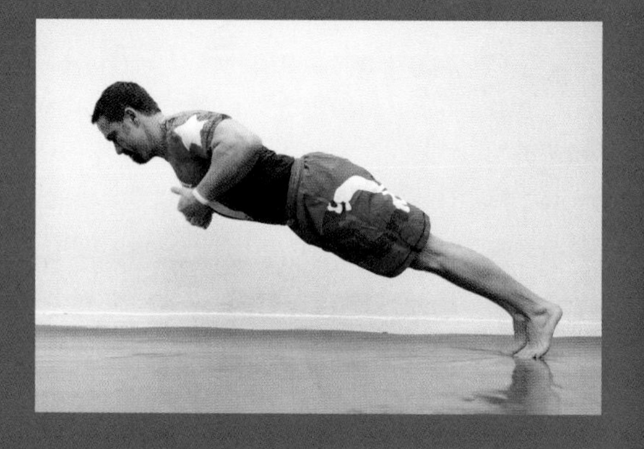

5. OVERHEAD-RAISE PUSHUP

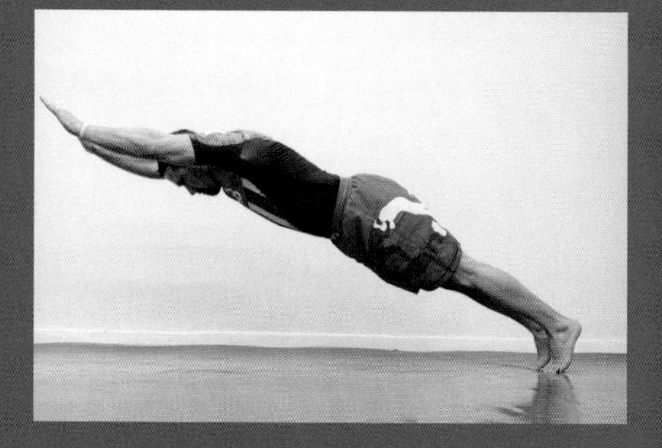

6. HIPS-SLAP PUSHUP

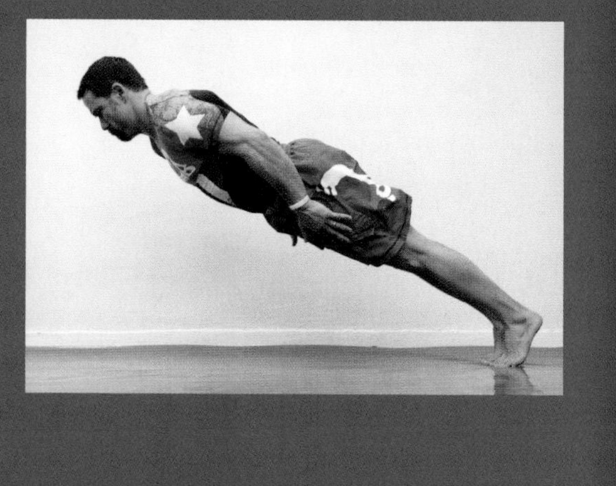

ADVANCED PUSHUP CIRCUIT CHEATSHEET

1. REGULAR PUSHUP

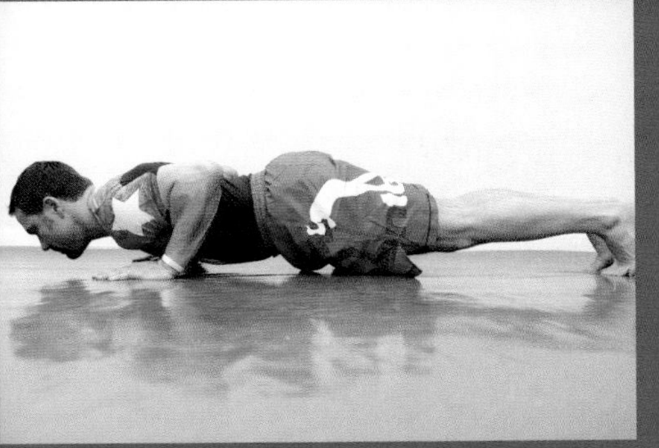

2. WARRIOR PUSHUP

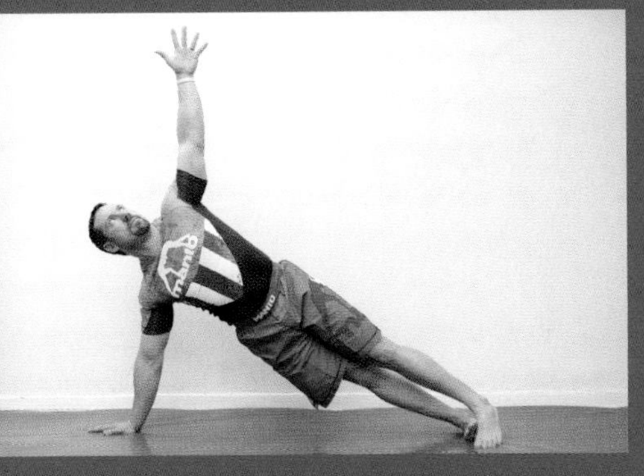

3. TOE-KICK PUSHUP

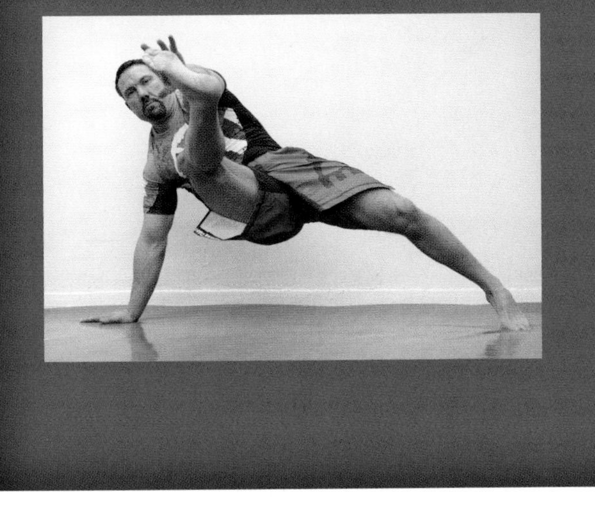

4. PIKE PRESS

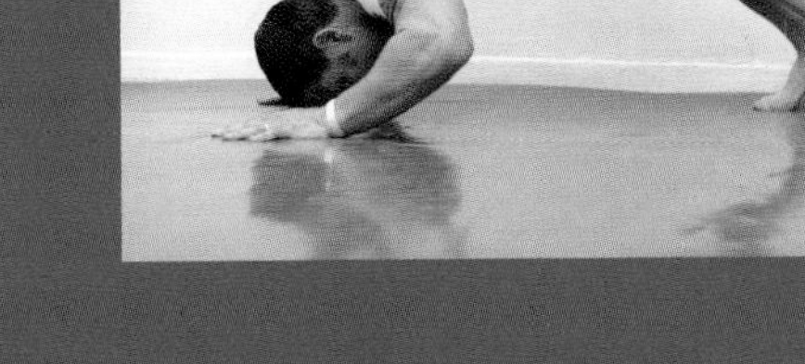

5. WALL PUSHUP

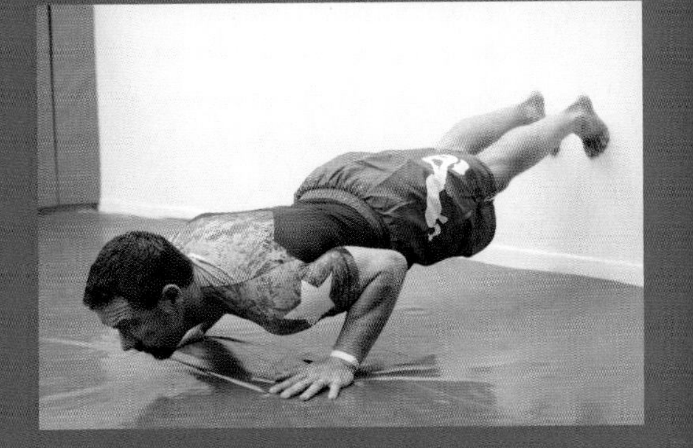

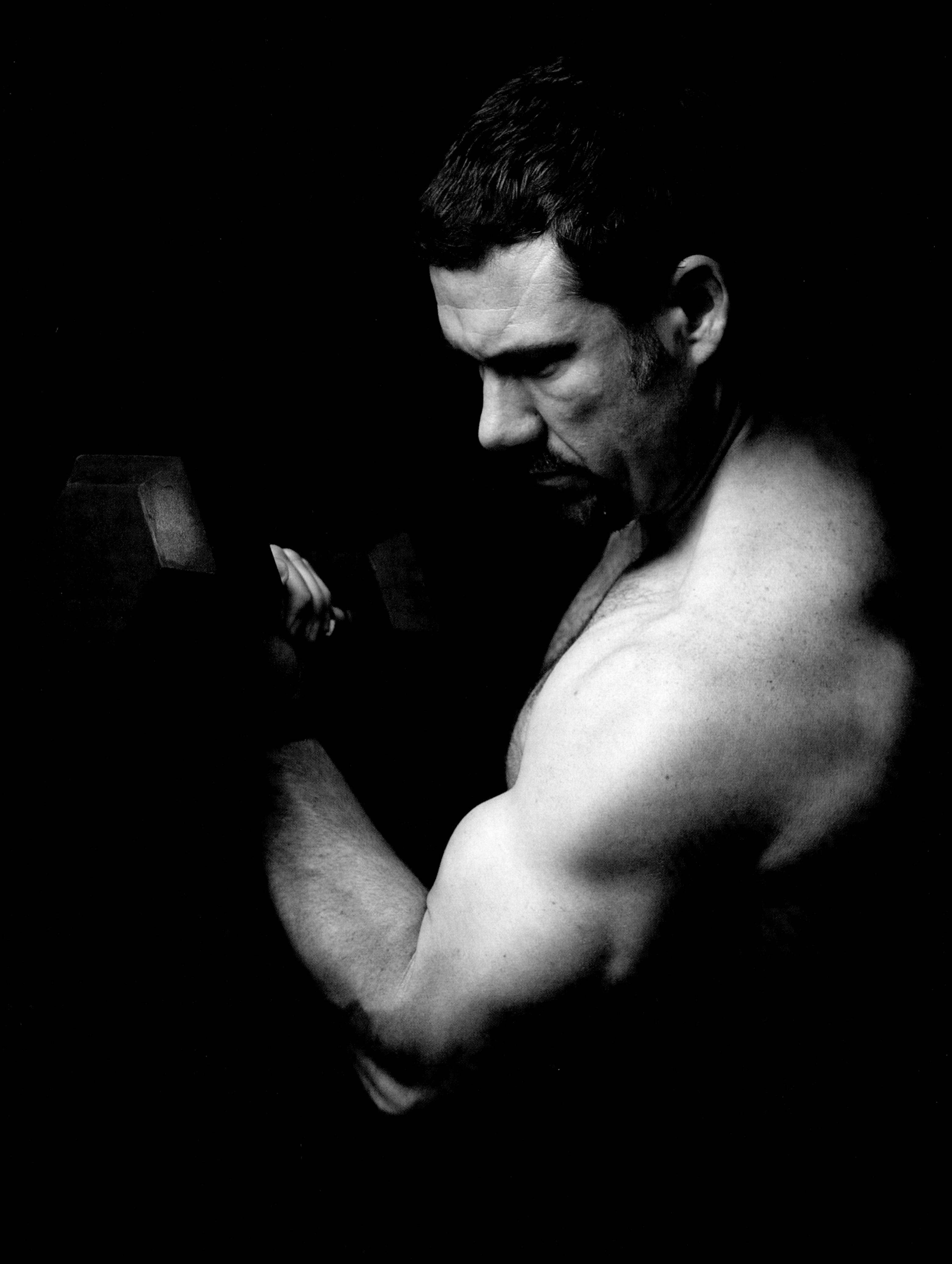

12

SPECIALTY STRENGTH CIRCUITS

Now that you have read the science of Cardio Training, you are aware that strength training can also produce losses in fat and gains in cardiovascular fitness. This is a revolutionary concept in terms of fitness and strength training. Over the last few decades, we have been convinced that hours of mind-numbing "cardio" work on a treadmill or bike was the most effective way to shed fat. Science (as well as the thousands of well-muscled and fit athletes) demonstrates that this is an archaic way of thinking. This fact should give you the confidence to leave the elliptical trainer for the weight room without the guilt that you still need hours of boredom to burn fat. In addition to some of the more popular ways that weights are used during Metabolic Training like the Hurricane Training, body weight circuits, and barbell complexes that were presented earlier in this book, there are a number of other TFW "specialty" circuits in which weights are used to simultaneously build muscular strength and cardiovascular fitness. Although these styles can be seen equally as mentally and physically challenging as the other training featured in *Warrior Cardio*, the main difference with the circuits contained in this chapter is that they utilize much heavier weights and resistances.

It could be argued that many of the circuits contained in this book are geared toward developing the cardiovascular system first and the muscular system second.

In the case of the circuits in this section, the opposite is true. These circuits are more geared toward strength and hypertrophy development, with the added benefits of fat loss and cardiovascular fitness that come along with them.

A. SADIV SETS

This workout is named after Rich Sadiv, my training partner and mentor. Sadiv is 47 years old with a 694.5-pound deadlift at 195 pounds, lifetime drug-free. To perform the Sadiv Sets, you must first have been training for a number of weeks in both the deadlift and the bench press before beginning with this style of training. (This is where the common sense comes in.)

1. DEADLIFT

Load a barbell with 60% of your deadlifting 1RM and set a timer for 12 minutes.

Perform as many single reps as possible in 12 minutes, shooting for a minimum of 20 reps. Each rep should be performed with maximal speed from the floor. Release the bar completely between reps, rest until you're ready, and repeat. Record your score.

Let's say you used 305 pounds and hit 20 reps in 12 minutes. It doesn't matter if you did it in 4 sets of 5, or 2 sets of 10. It's still 60% of your 1RM for 20 hard, fast reps, and that's a ton of muscle-building tension. Next week, get 21 reps.

Along with the muscles of your posterior chain, you will find your heart lift up with this one.

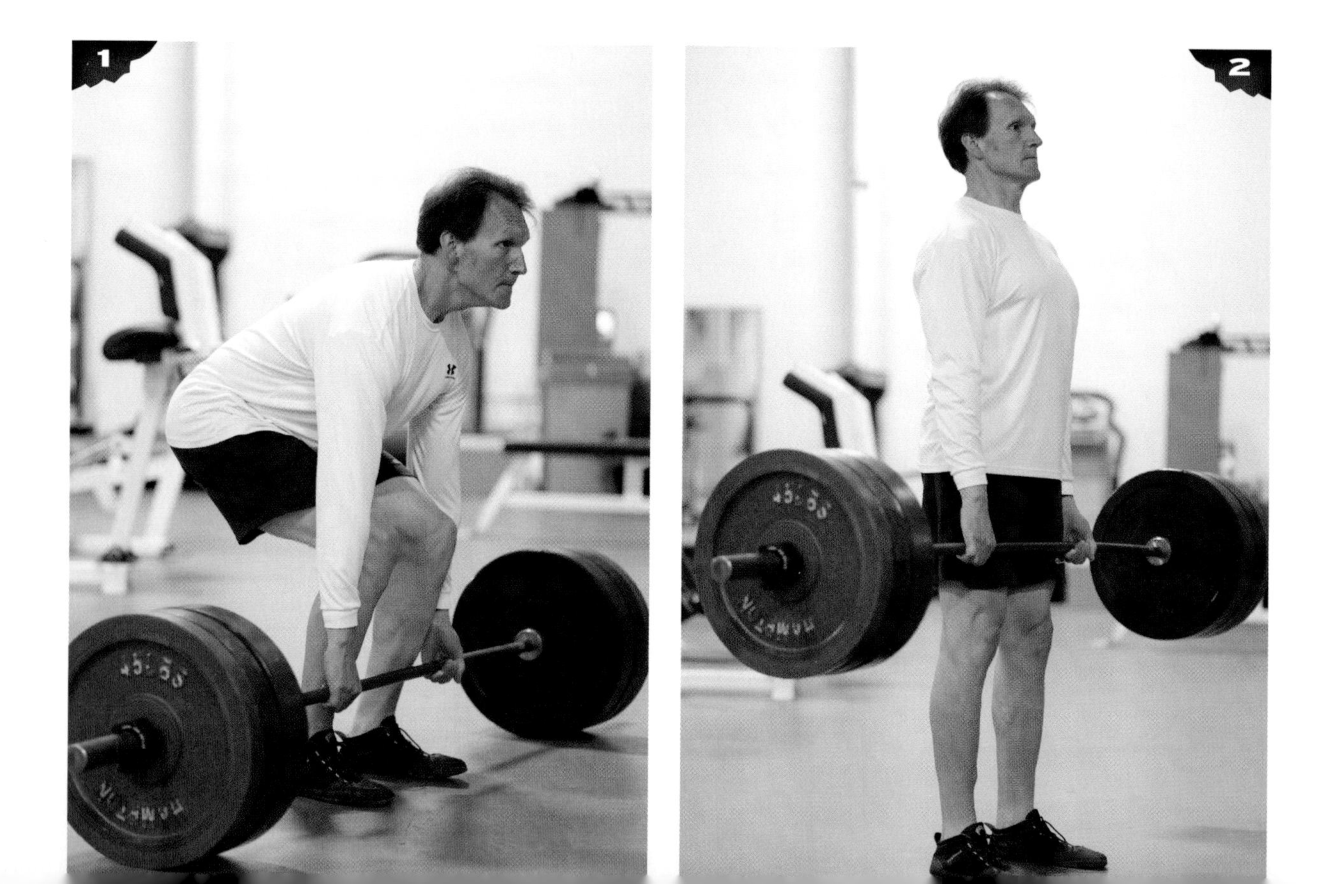

2. BENCH PRESS

You can do Sadiv Sets with bench presses as well—just raise the intensity to 90% and drop the timer to 10 minutes. This time, shoot for only 10 reps. Last week I hit 340 pounds for 10 reps in 10 minutes. This is a weight I can usually only get for a double, to do a weight for 2 reps. The result is 10 reps with a very high percentage of your 1RM. Can you say tension?

People commonly ask, why 60% for the deadlift and 90% for the bench? My answer comes down to the maximal weight that can be performed on each lift and the number of minimum reps required to attain. For instance, Sadiv has almost a 700-pound deadlift; 60% of that is 420 pounds. To be able to move fast and get the number of reps (20 minimum), we have found this to be a good percentage to use. Why 20 reps instead of 10? There is more muscle mass used in the deadlift, so we doubled the number of reps.

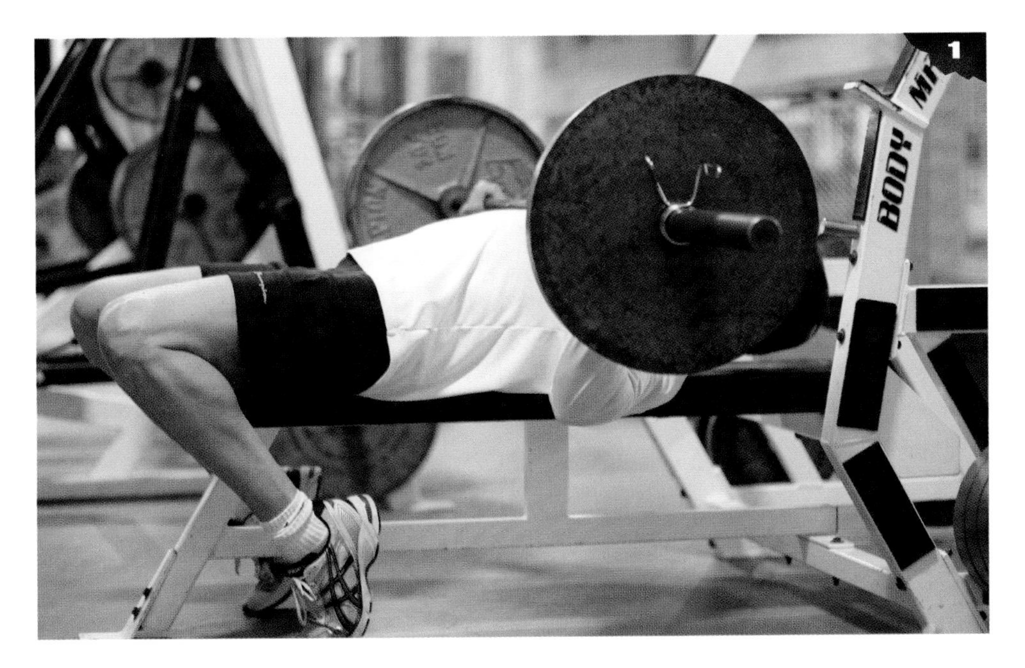

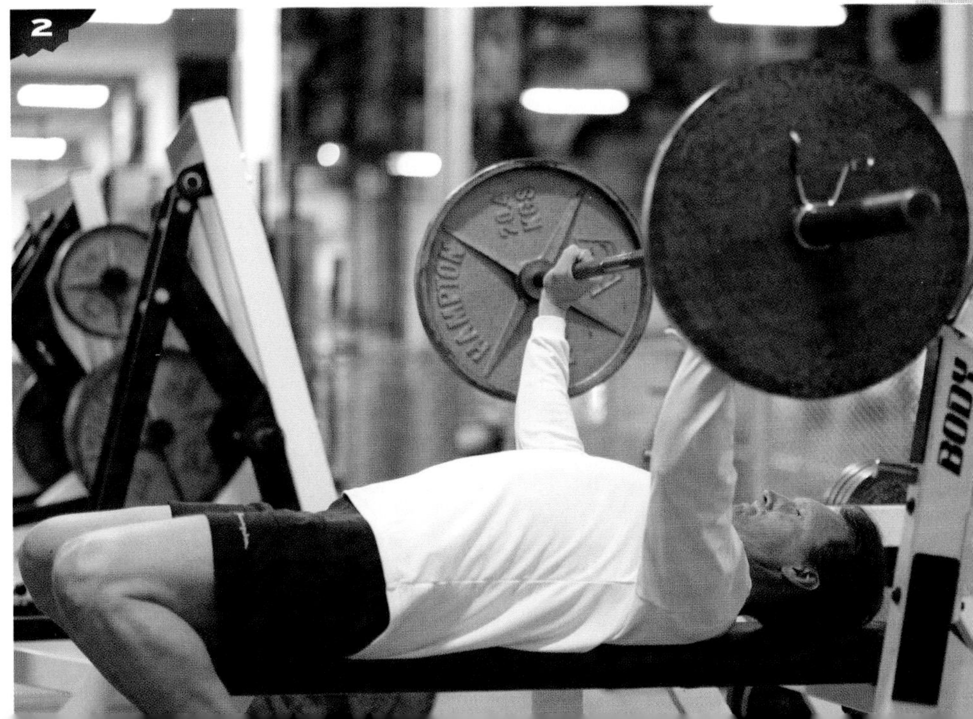

B. TERRIBLE 275'S

I believe that if you are doing more than about 6 reps, you are working cardio. Since fat loss and muscle gain are probably two of the most common desires of anyone in the gym, here is my version of cardio that will jack up both your arms and your heart.

If you weigh 200 pounds, put 275 pounds on a deadlifting bar, 275 on a flat bench press, and place a 75-pound dumbbell by the dip and chin-up station. Hit the bench for as many reps as possible. Rest 30 seconds and do the same with deadlifts, dips, and chins, and record your total number of reps. Rest 5 minutes and repeat for 1 or 2 more sets. Not only will you hit all the big muscles, you'll get a great workout done in less time with a cardiovascular benefit, too!

If 275 pounds is too much to begin with, regardless of what you weigh or where you're currently at for relative body strength, you can choose your own weight for the sets. You can do this at body weight or even begin by adding 5 or 10 pounds to body weight, and work up from there.

After a hard set of this, beware: the energy and noise of the set will make people around you nervous—if you look weary at the end of the set, make sure they don't call 911 by reminding them that this appearance of fatigue is often associated with something called exercise.

C. CHIN-UP SERIES

This is a circuit that I have been doing for years. This one has always led to pumped-up forearms and back muscles as well as a high heartbeat. There are two ways to use this circuit: One way is to find a number you can complete in each set without stopping. The other is to pick an individual start number, allow yourself rest during the set if necessary, and find your best time.

1. WIDE-GRIP PULLUP

Begin grabbing the bar with an overhand grip that is wider than shoulder width. Pull the chin over and the chest to the bar. Lower under control and repeat.

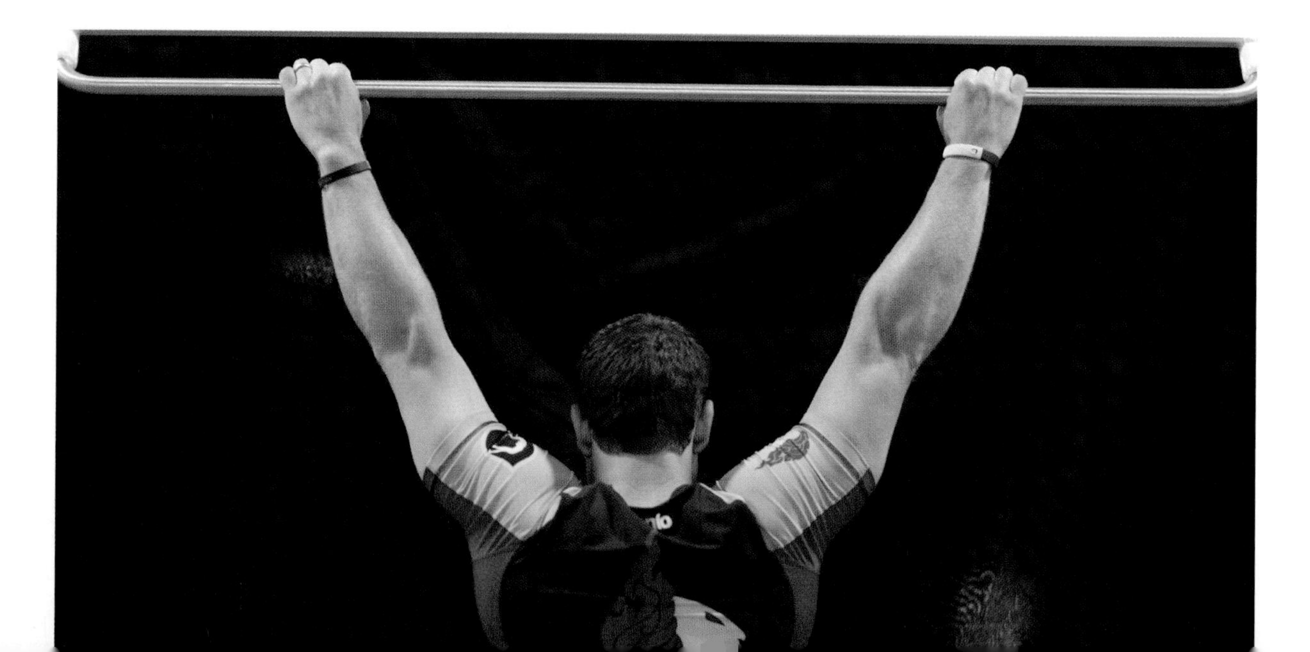

2. NEUTRAL-GRIP PULLUP

Begin grabbing the bar with a neutral grip (or on a handle, as shown) in which the palms face each other. Pull the chin up over one side of the bar. Lower under control and repeat on the other side.

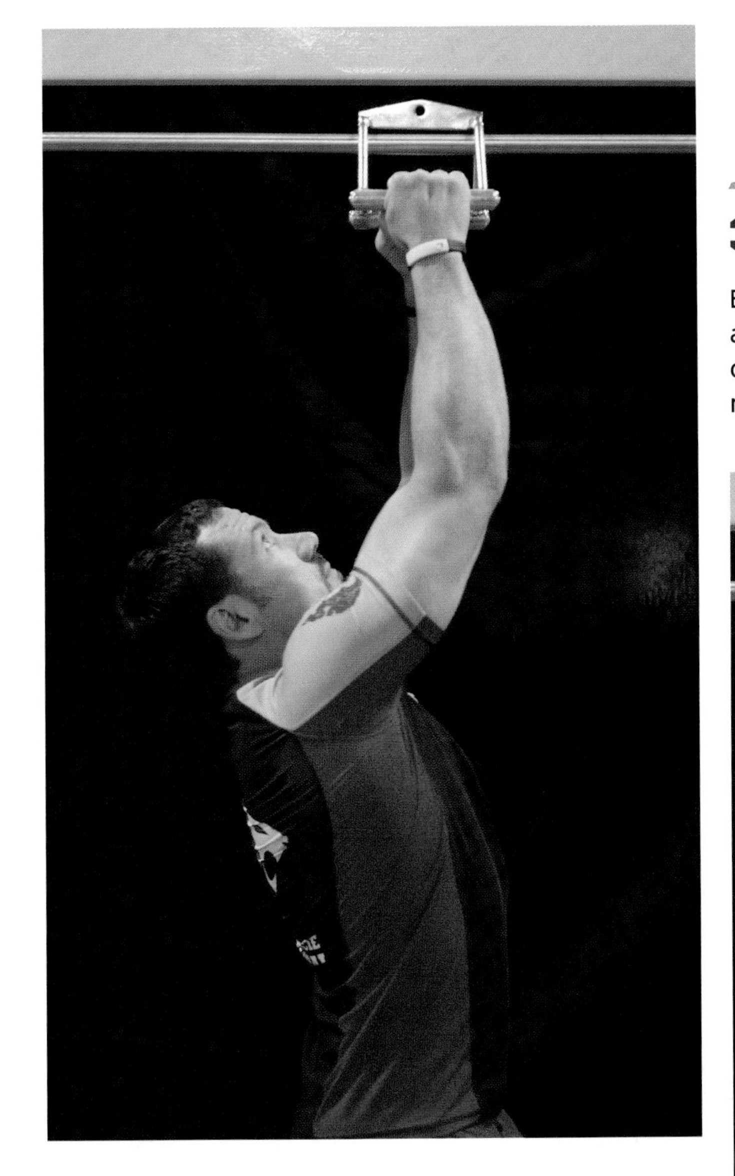

3. MIXED-GRIP PULLUP

Begin grabbing the bar with one palm forward and one backward. Pull the chin over and the chest to the bar. Lower under control and repeat.

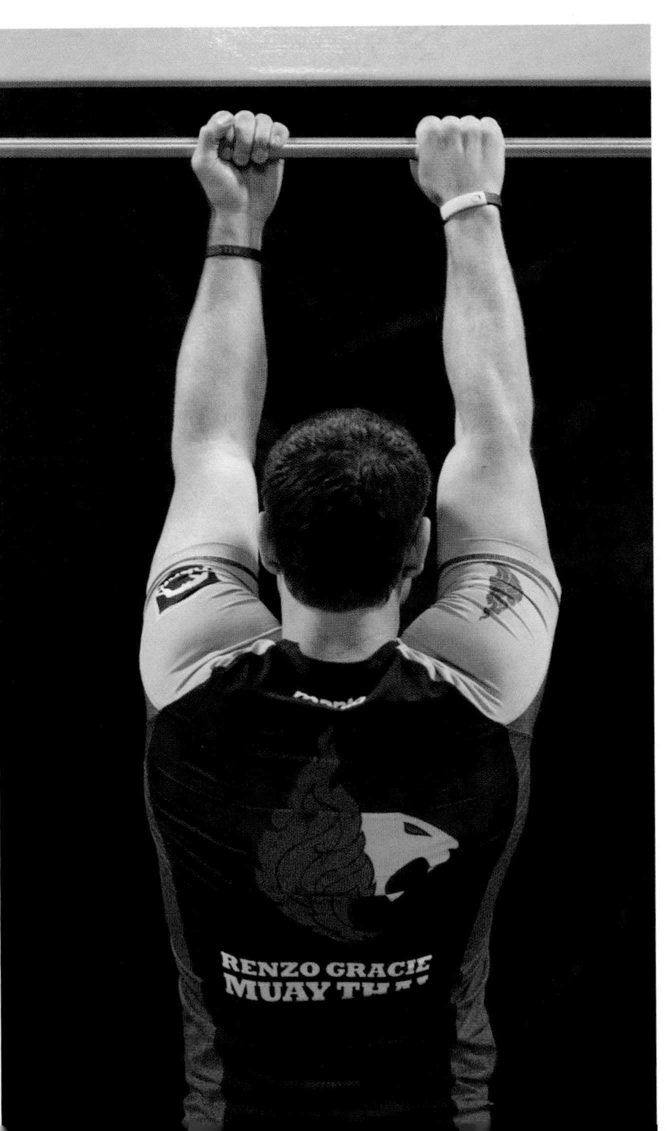

4. CHIN-UP

Begin grabbing the bar with both palms facing you. Pull the chin over and the chest up to the bar. Lower under control and repeat.

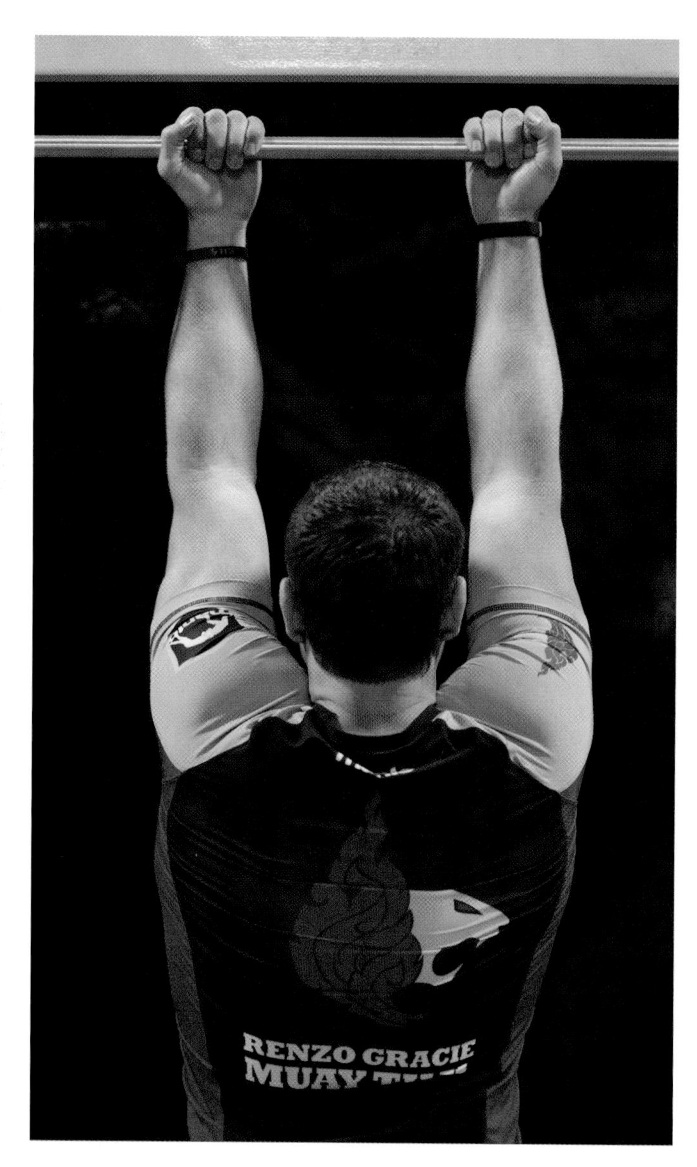

5. WRIST-GRIP CHIN-UP

Begin grabbing the bar with one hand, with the other hand holding onto the wrist. Pull the chin over and the chest up to the bar. Lower under control and repeat.

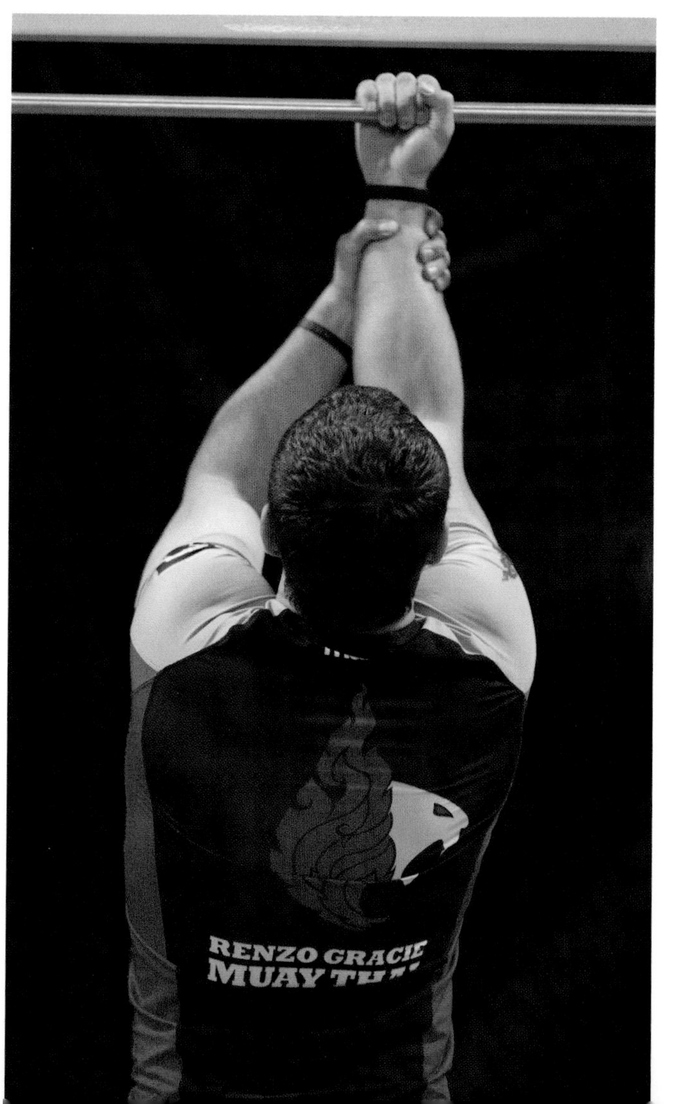

D. THE DOUBLER

The Doubler is an interesting strength circuit/challenge of TFW. To begin, select a start number for the first exercise (see repetition scheme on page 257). Once this is picked, you must complete double of the next exercise. Then you keep doubling the number for the next two exercises. There are two ways to use the Doubler: One way is to find a number you can complete without stopping. The other is to pick individual start numbers, allow yourself rest during the set if necessary, and find your best time.

1. BENCH PRESS WITH BODY WEIGHT

The bench should be loaded with a weight that matches your exact body weight. Begin lying on the back with the feet on the floor, gripping the bar with a shoulder-width grip. Take the weight off the rack and lower to the chest under control, keeping the elbows close to the body. Press the bar from the chest back up to full elbow extension.

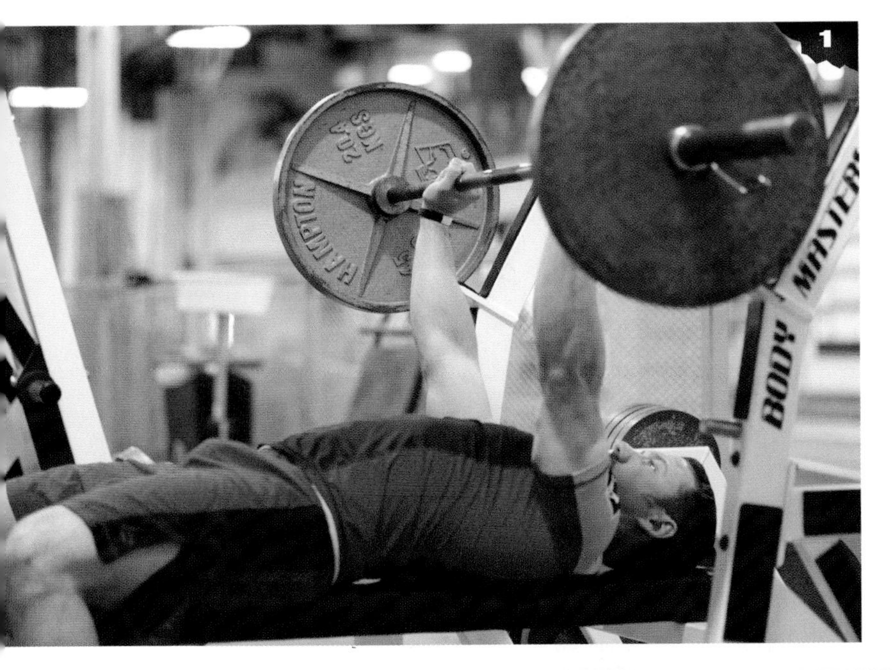

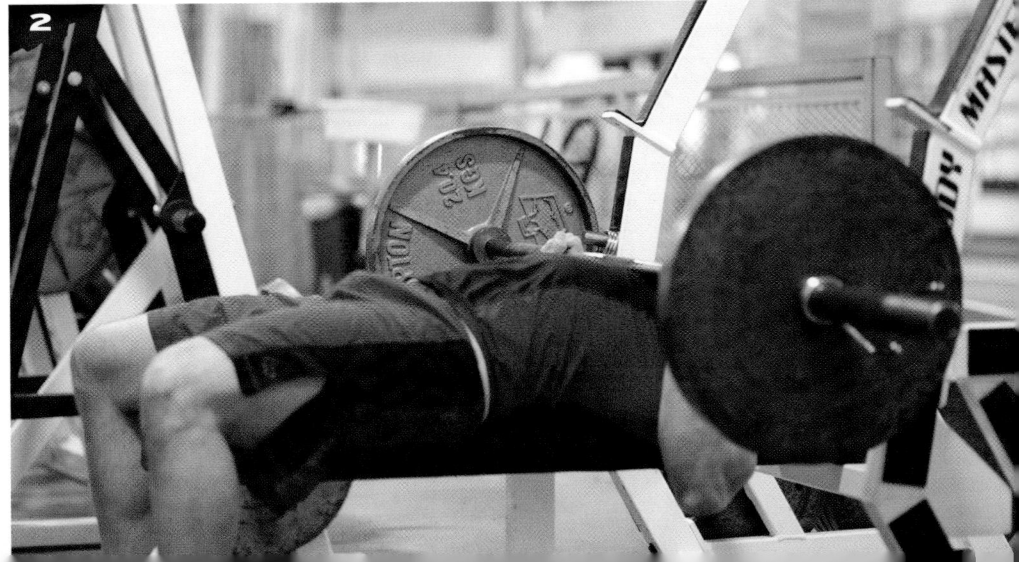

2. CHIN-UP

Begin grabbing the bar with both palms facing you. Pull the chin over and the chest up to the bar. Lower under control and repeat.

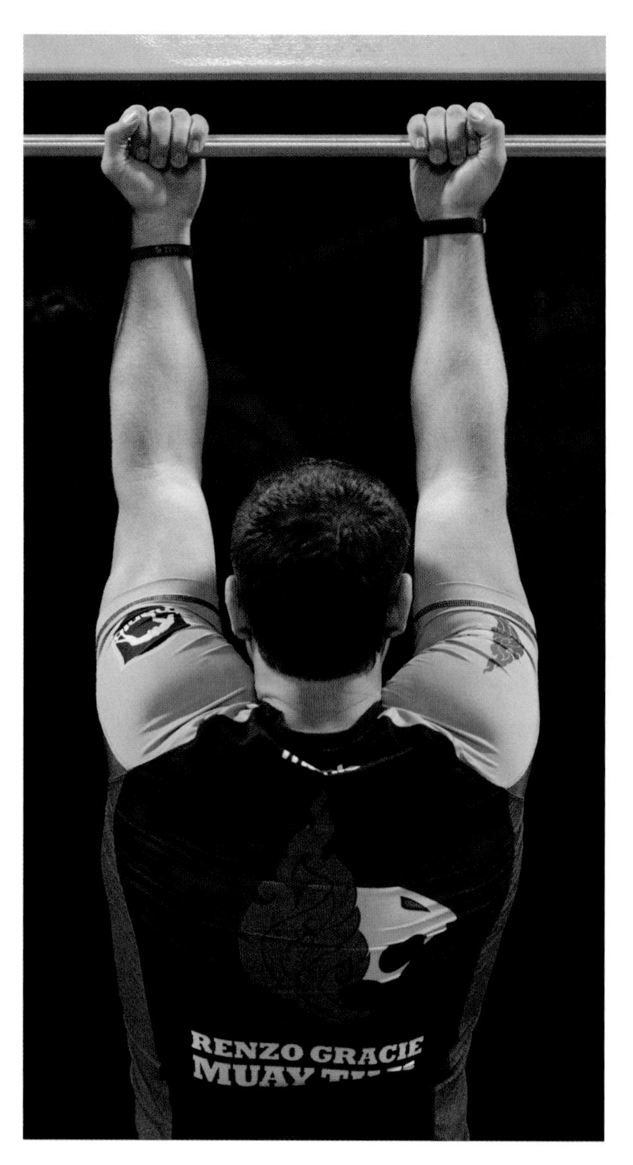

3. DIP

Begin in the first position with the elbows locked out. Lower past 90 degrees at the elbows. Extend the elbows to complete lockout.

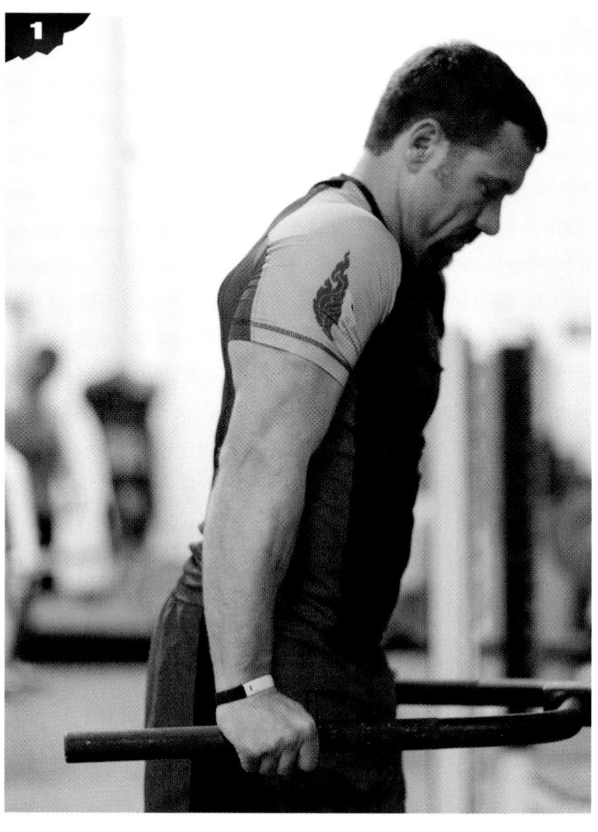

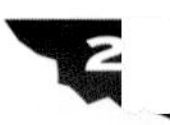

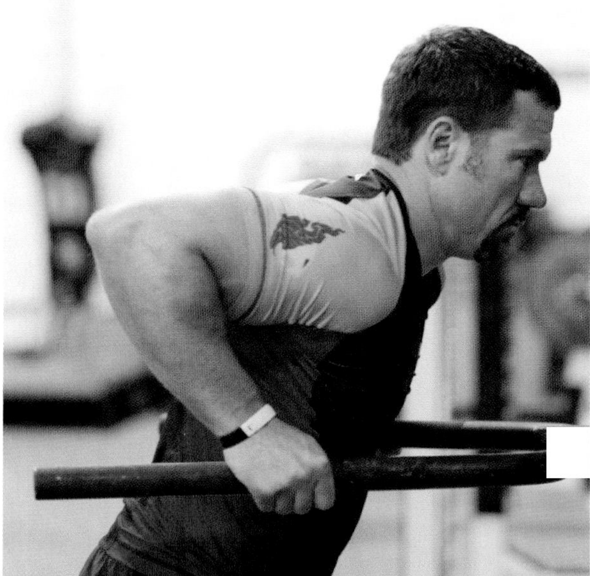

4. PUSHUP

Begin in the first position with the elbows extended and the hands at shoulder width. Lower the chest to the floor, keeping the elbows close to the body. Press through the floor and extend at the elbows to reach the start position.

Sample of "doubler" repetition schemes:

1, 2, 4, 8
2, 4, 8, 16
3, 6, 12, 24
4, 8, 16, 32
5, 10, 20, 40
6, 12, 24, 48
7, 14, 28, 56

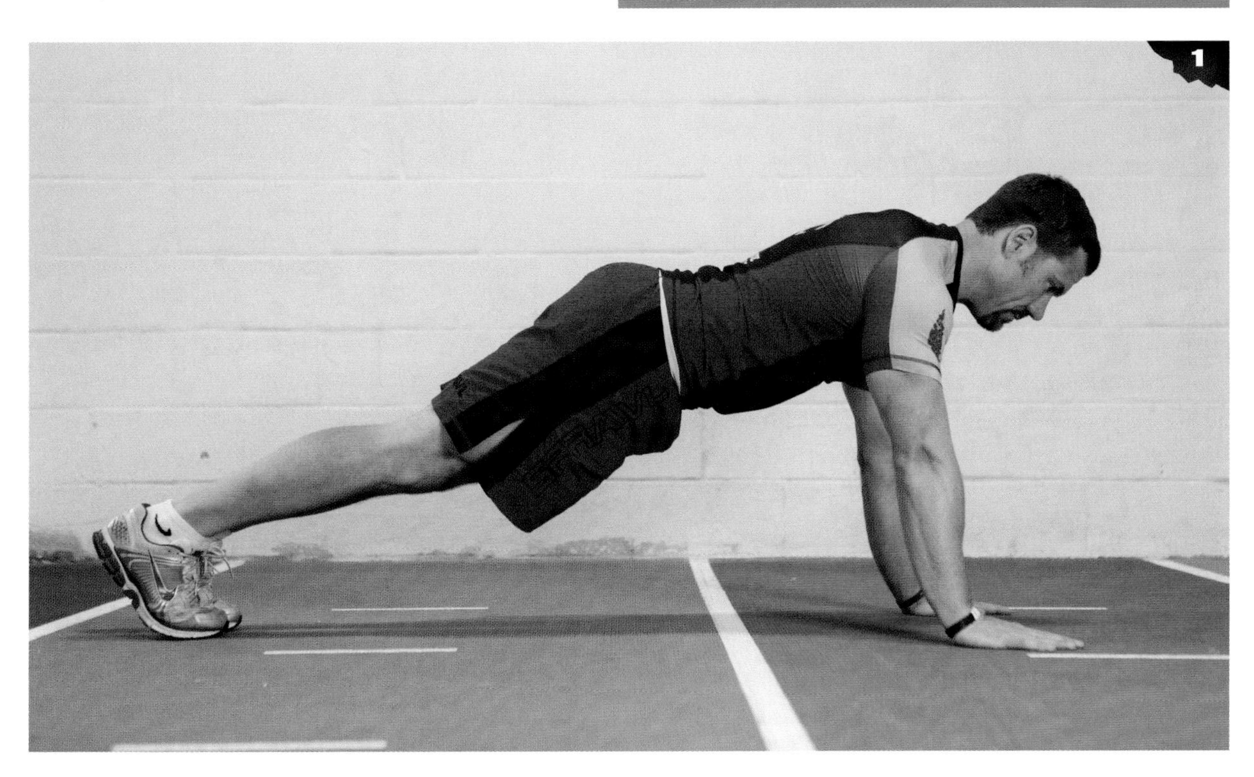

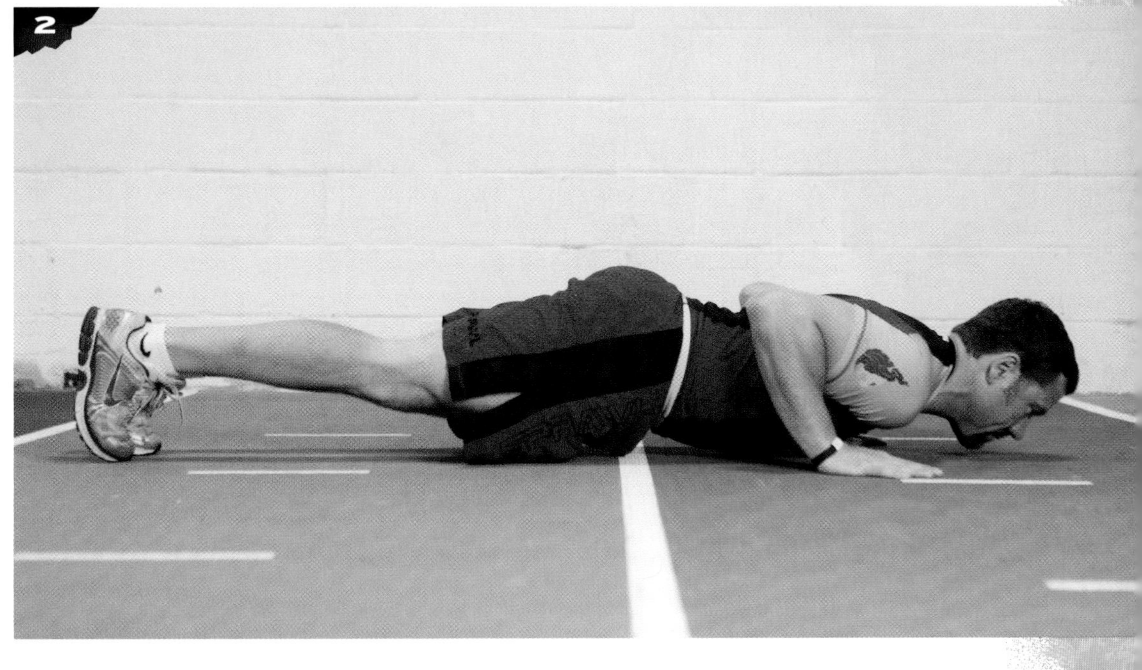

E. GAUNTLETS

In the TFW System, "running a gauntlet" is performed by choosing a certain number of exercises that can be alternated from one to another with the same weight and minimal time. You perform each of the exercises chosen for a certain number of repetitions, and then increase the weight for the next set with no rest in between gauntlets. I like dumbbells for the gauntlet, to challenge the nervous system even further with strength and stability. The sample gauntlet below is to be performed for 5 sets (increasing the weight 5 pounds per set) with six individual dumbbell exercises for 6 repetitions each. This can be performed in about 10 to 12 minutes. Talk about intense!

1. DUMBBELL BENCH PRESS

Begin lying on the back with the dumbbells on the chest as shown. Press the dumbbells up by extending the elbows and lower under control.

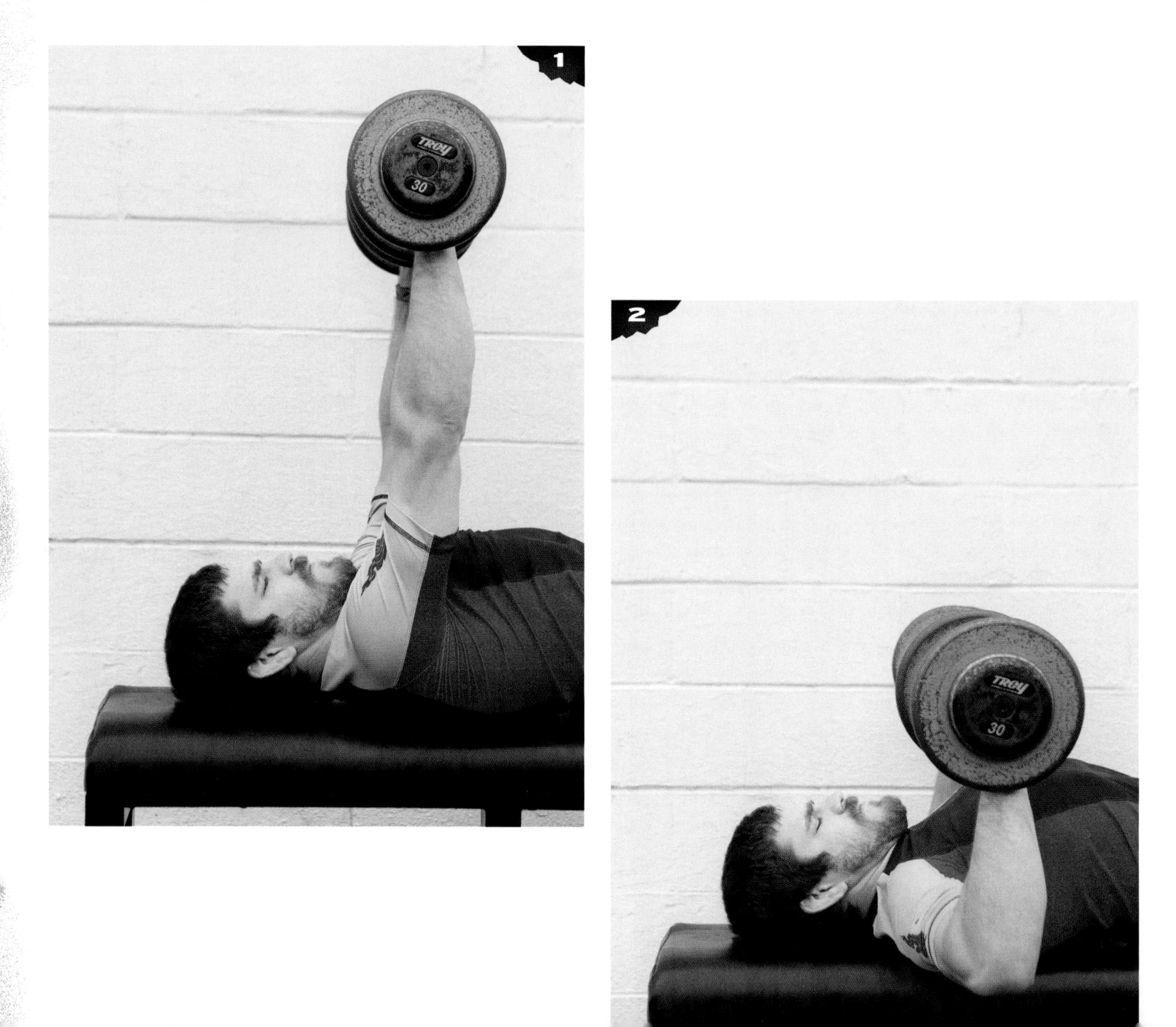

2. DUMBBELL CHEST FLYES

Begin with the arms extended and palms facing inward as shown. Turn the palms to face away from you as you lower the weight outward as shown.

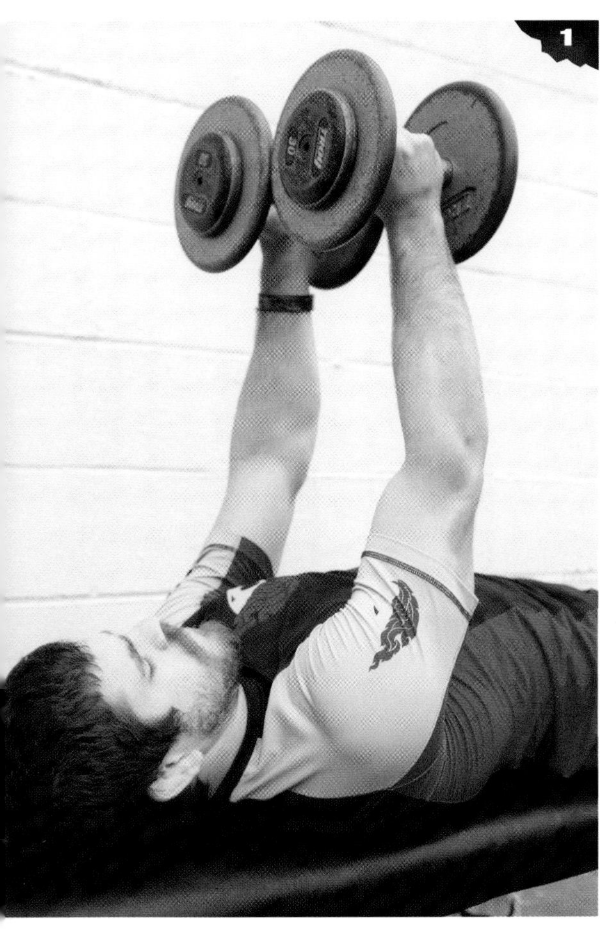

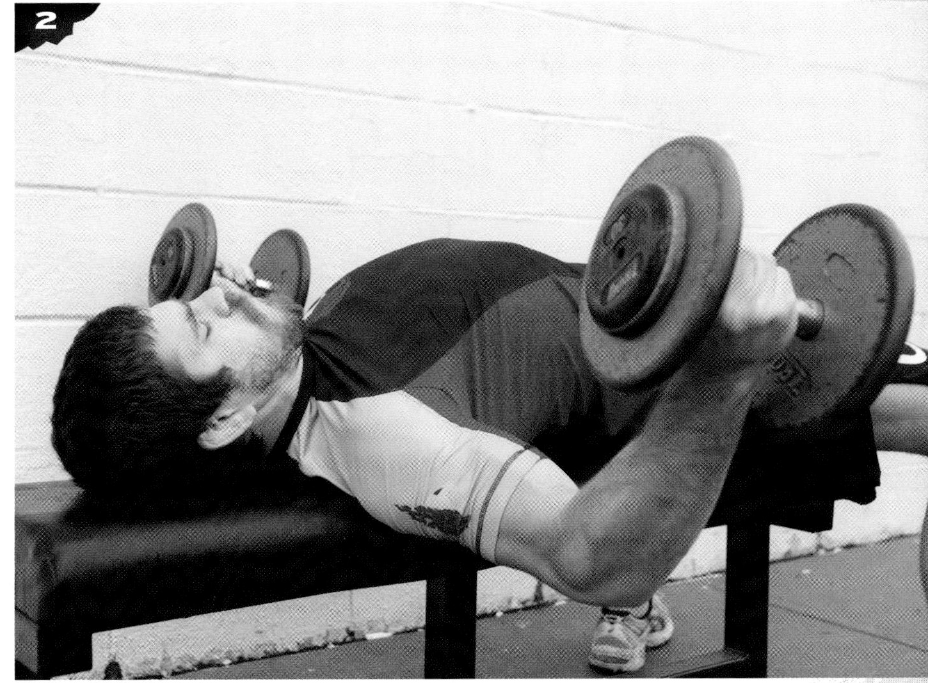

3. DUMBBELL ROLLING TRICEPS

Begin with the arms extended and palms facing inward. Bend at the elbow and lower the weight onto the shoulder. "Roll" the weight past the head and then return the weight quickly back to the original position.

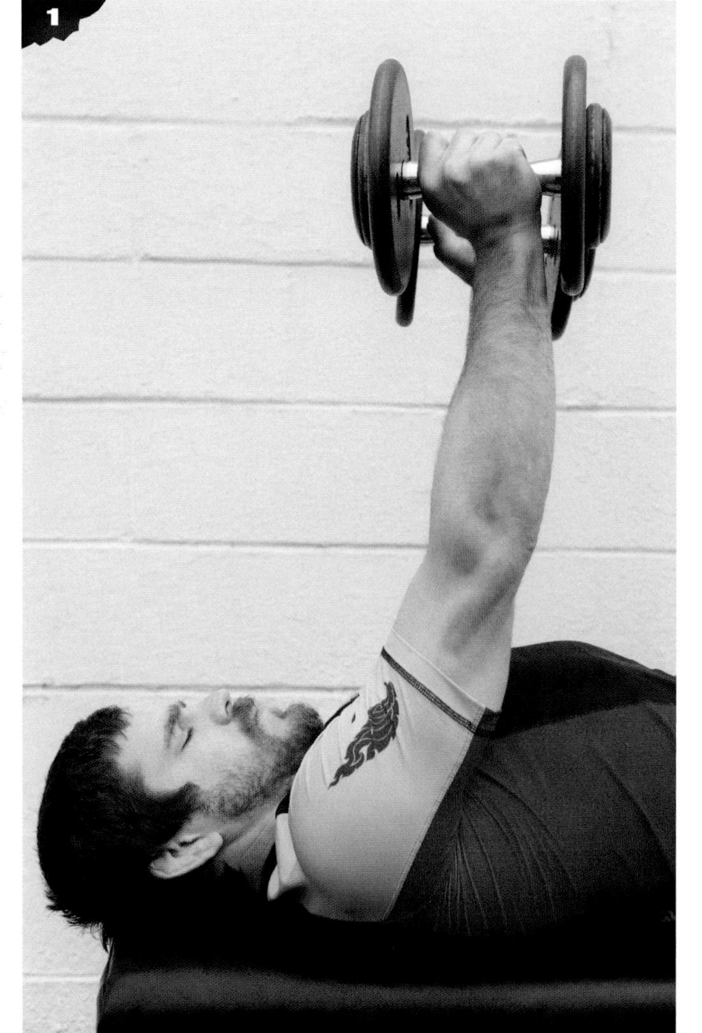

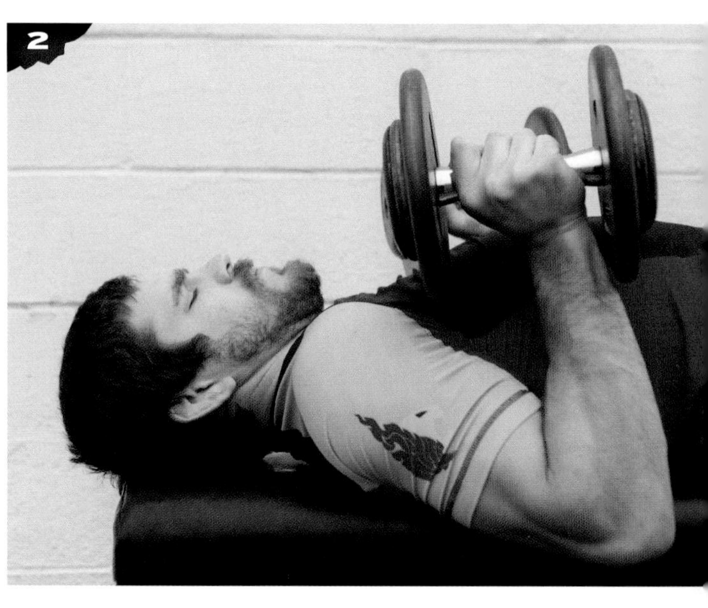

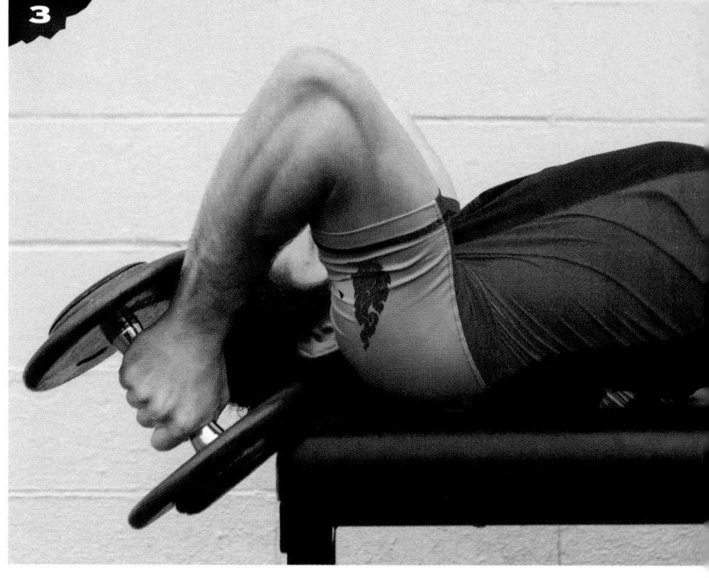

4. DUMBBELL BICEP CURLS

Stand and perform alternating curls with each arm, for six repetitions with each arm.

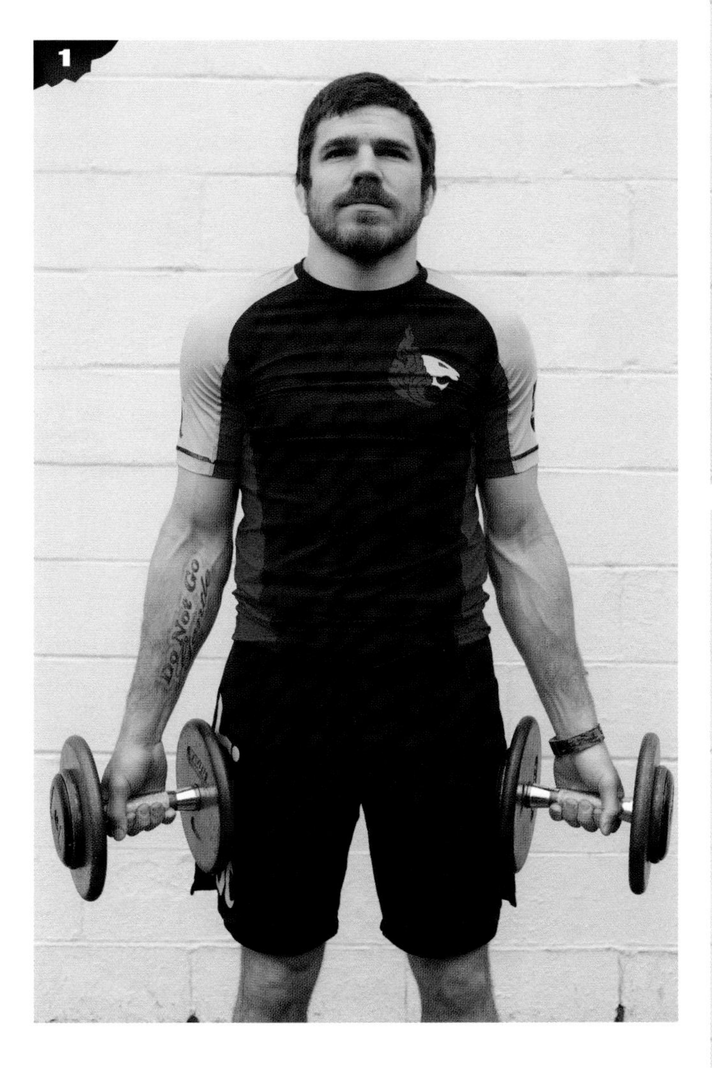

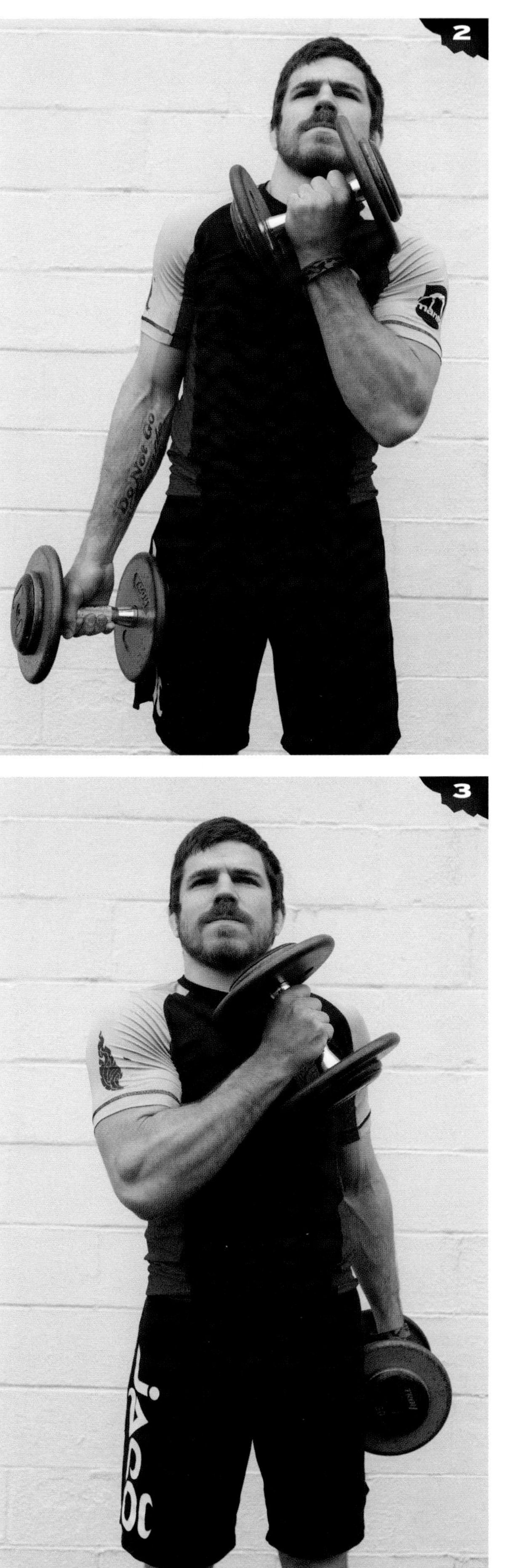

5. DUMBBELL SHOULDER PRESS

Stand and press the weight over the head as shown. Return the weight to shoulder height for the desired repetitions.

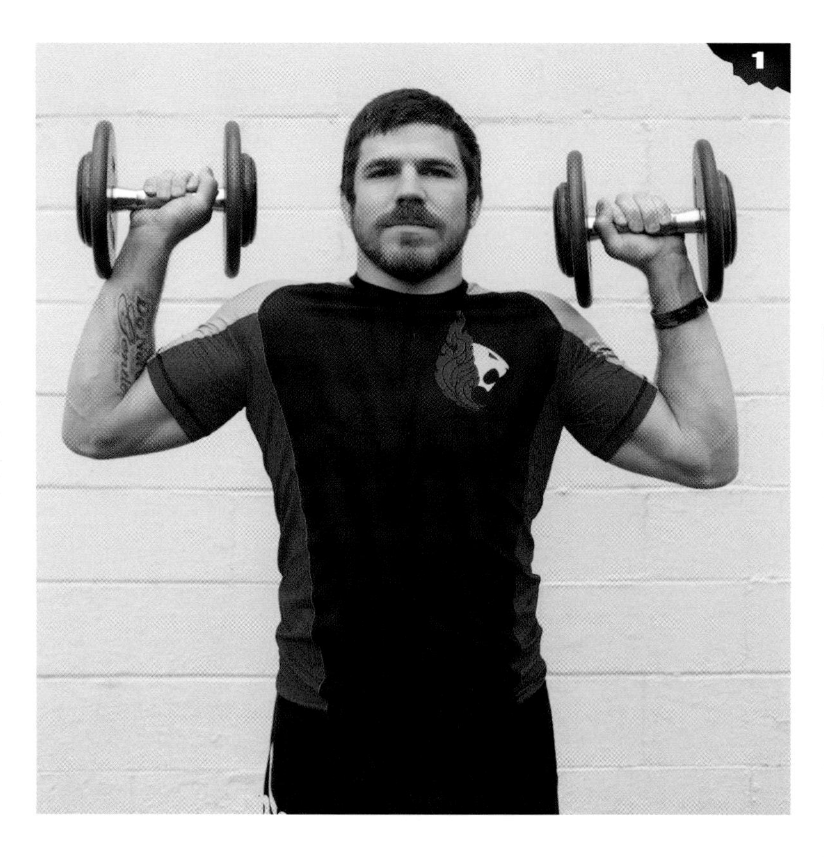

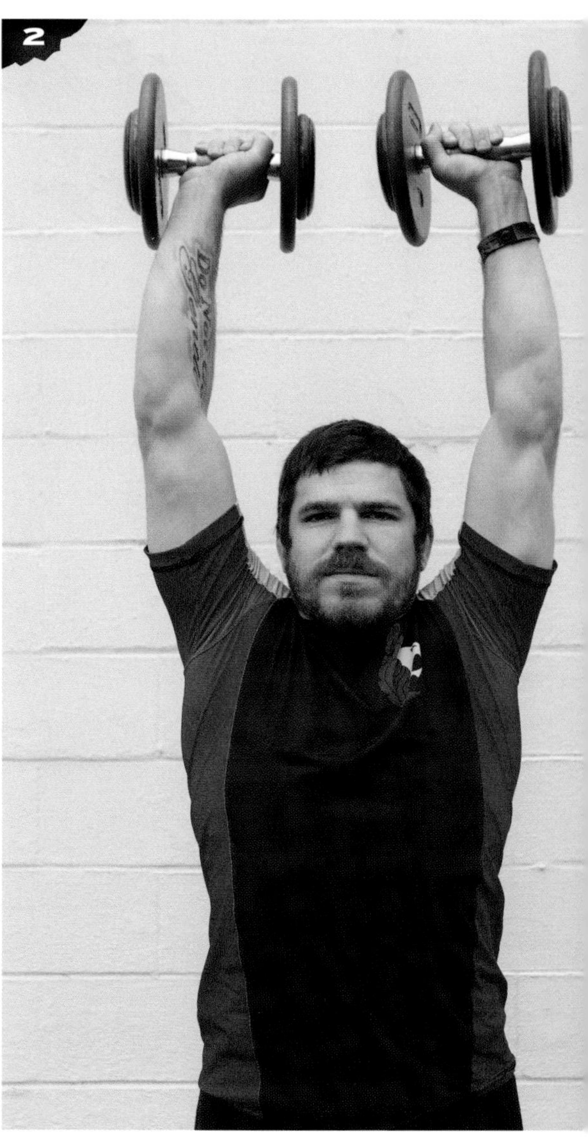

6. DUMBBELL SHRUGS

Let the weights hang at the sides with the elbows extended as shown. Raise the shoulders toward the ears. Lower and repeat for desired repetitions.

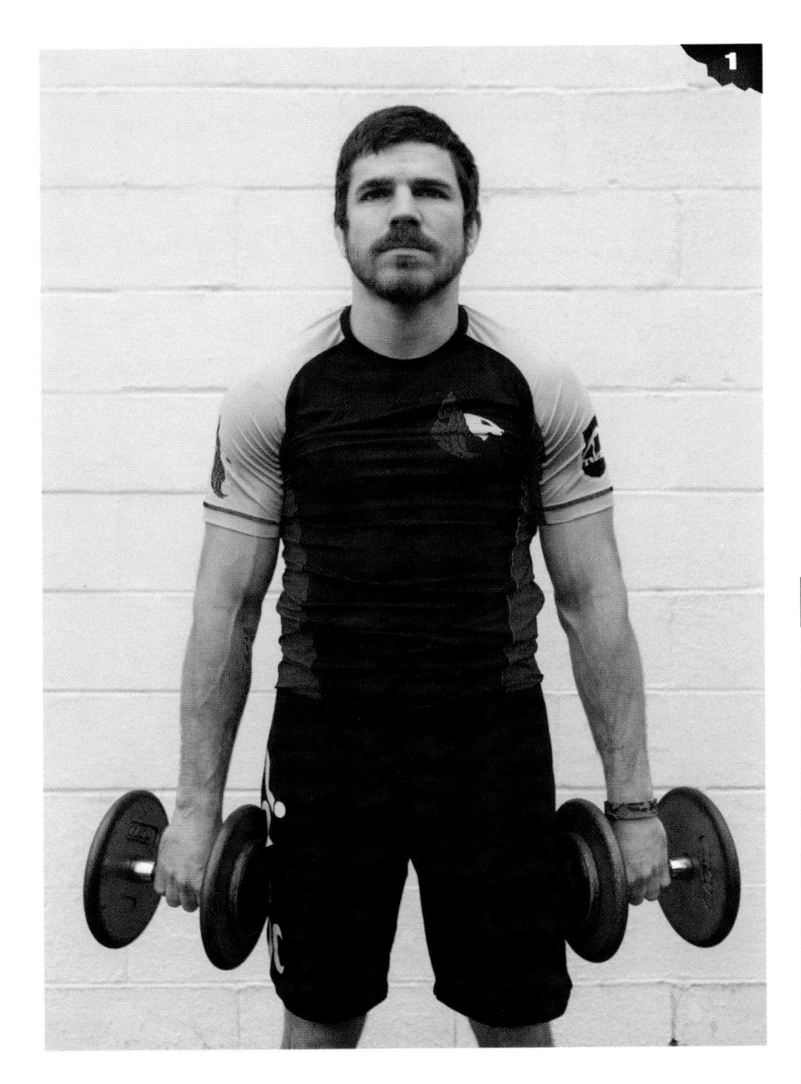

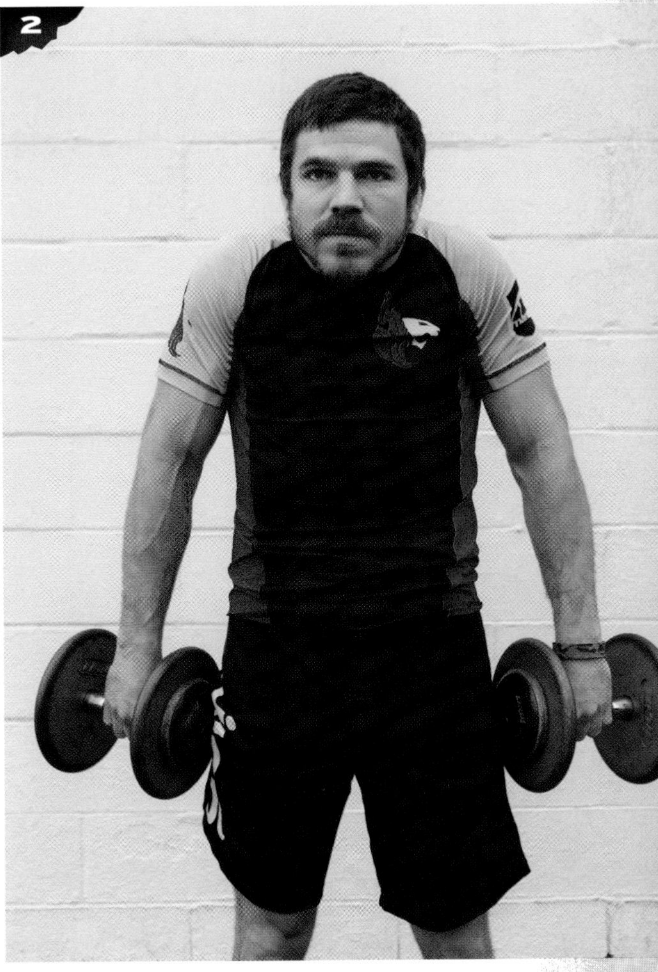

F. DUMBBELL SHOULDER CIRCUIT

This shoulder circuit is designed to develop the less often addressed muscles of the rotator cuff and the upper back. Each exercise is to be performed for 10 reps with light enough weight in order to complete the exercises without much rest in between.

1. LYING Y'S

Begin lying facedown on an incline bench with the palms facing each other. Lift the arms up overhead as if to form the letter Y.

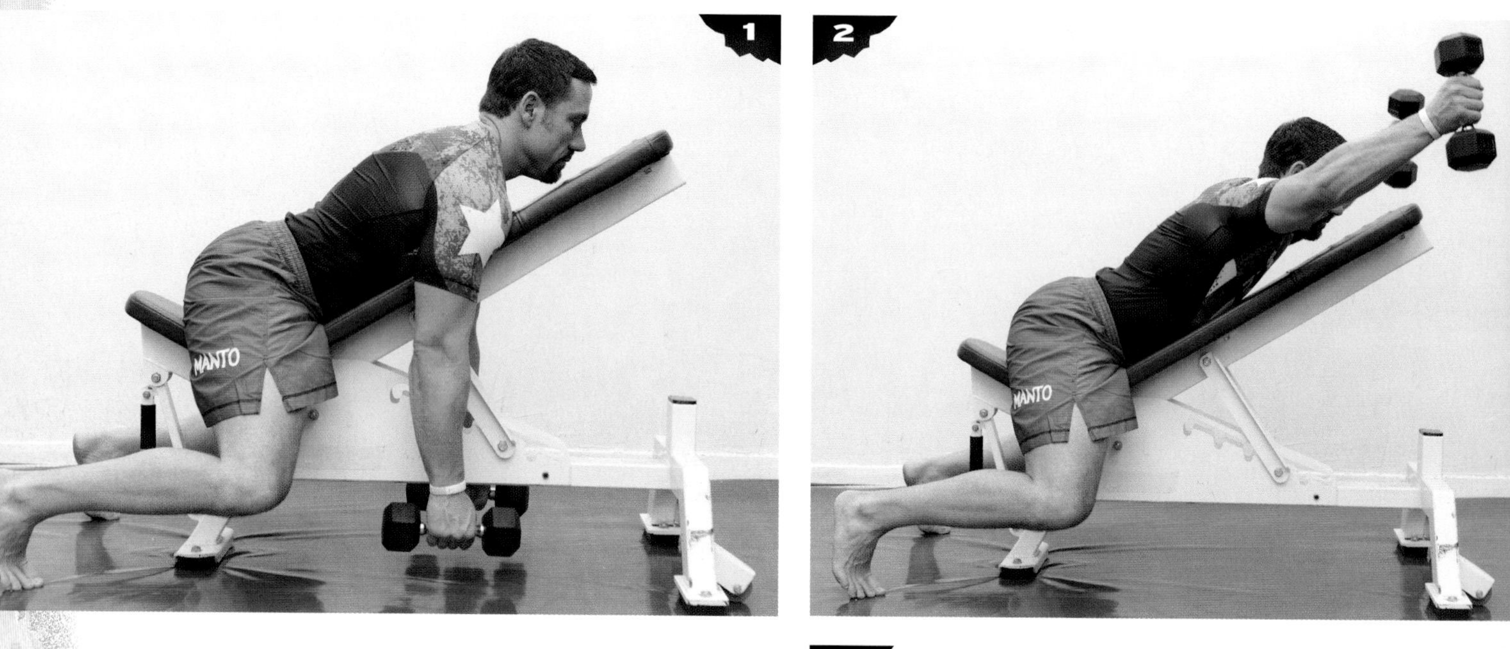

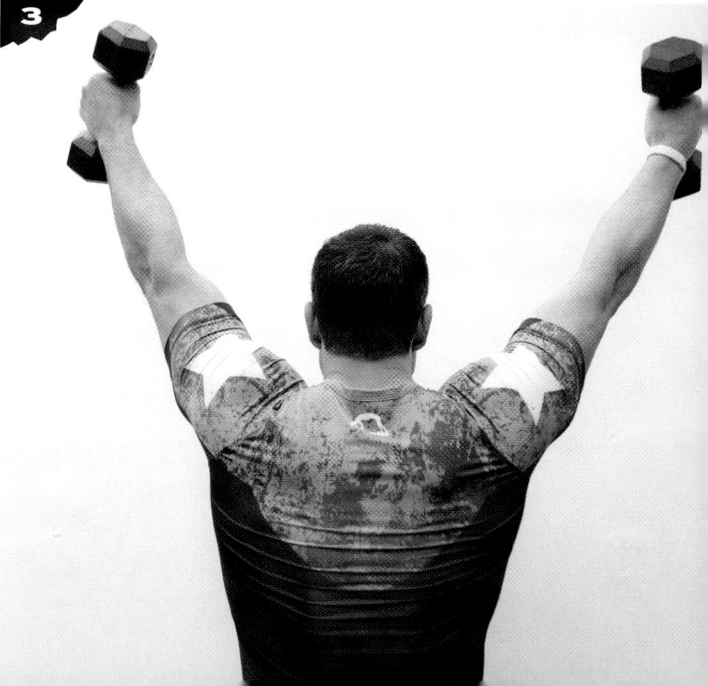

2. LYING U'S

Begin lying facedown on an incline bench with the palms facing each other. Bend at the elbows as you squeeze your shoulder blades together. Lift the elbows and externally rotate to bring the backs of the hands toward the ceiling as if to form the letter U.

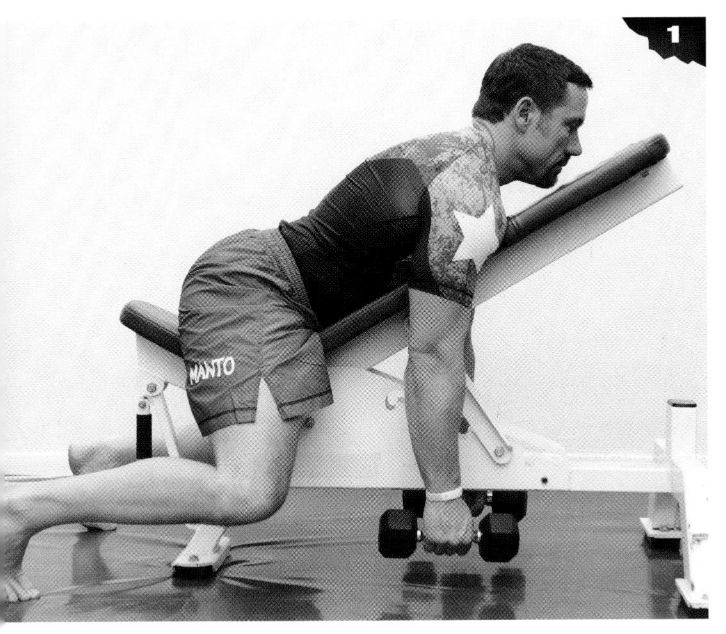

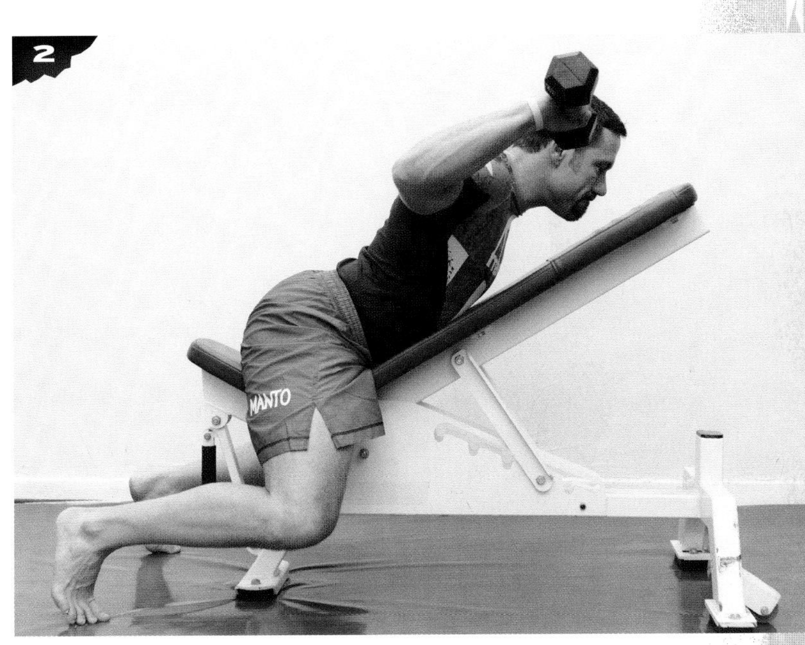

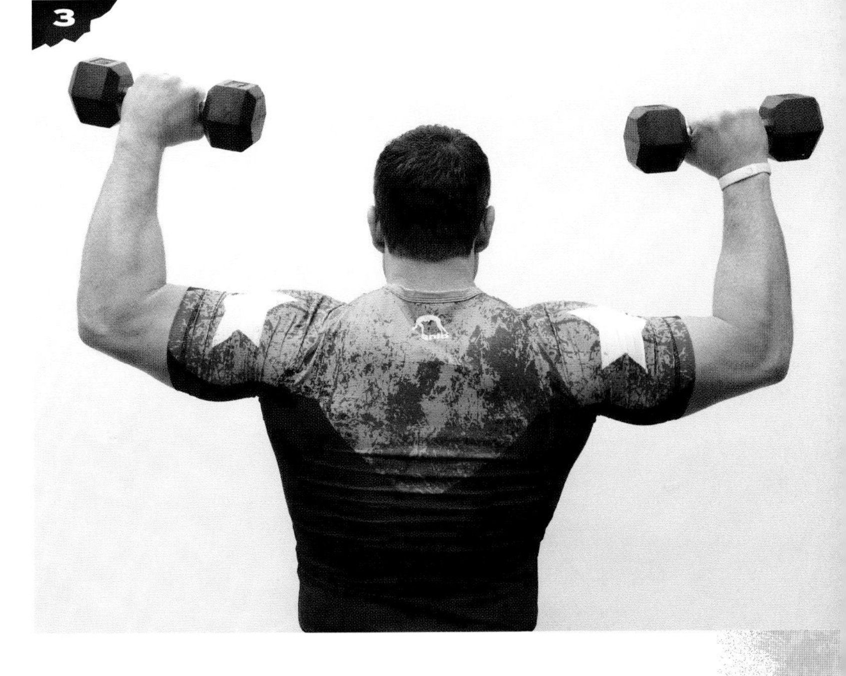

3. LYING T'S

Begin lying facedown on an incline bench with the palms facing each other. Lift the arms out directly to the sides as if to form the letter T.

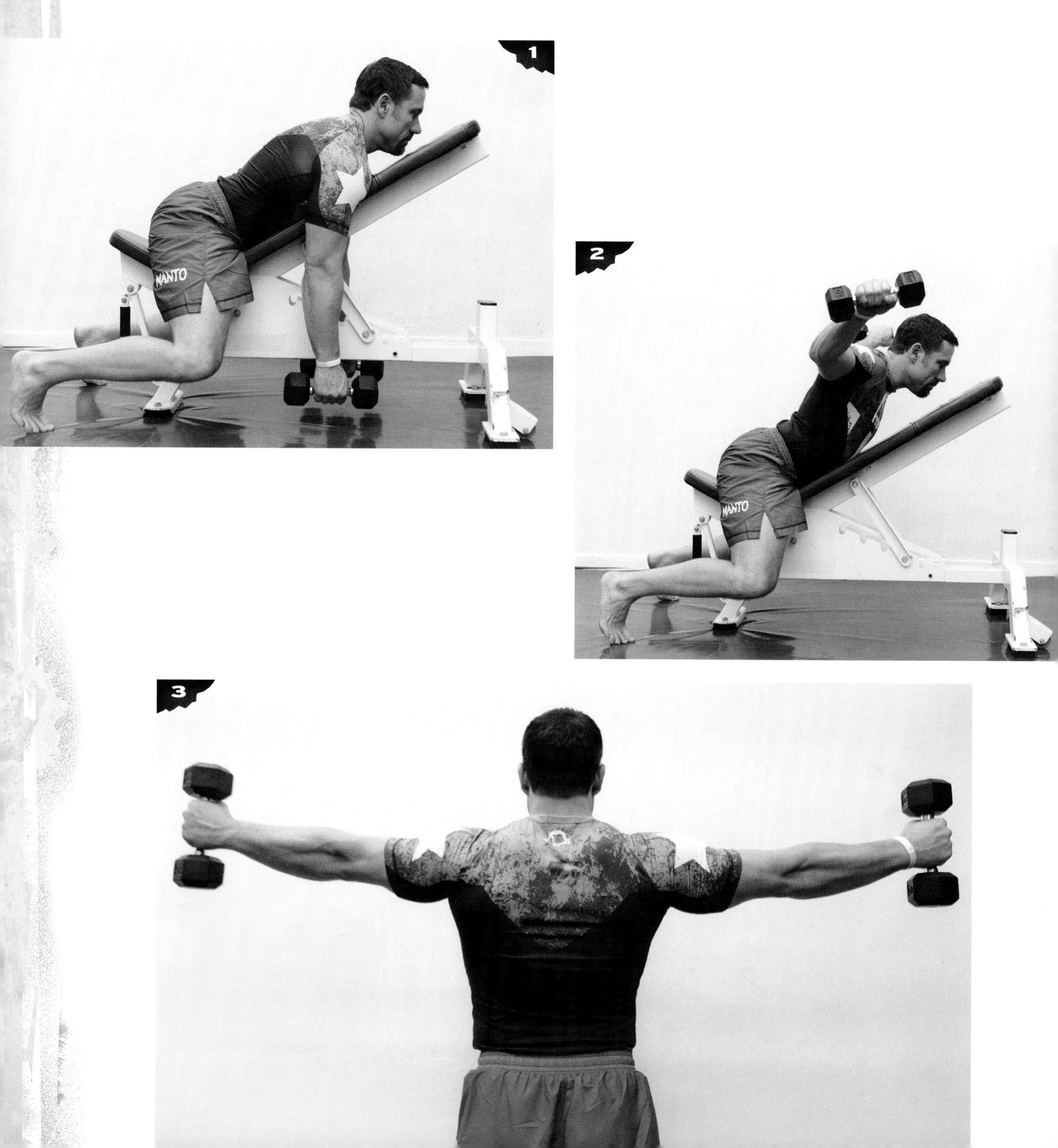

4. LYING W'S

Begin lying facedown on an incline bench with the palms facing each other. Bend at the elbows as you squeeze your shoulder blades together. Lift the elbows and externally rotate to bring the elbows to the sides and the backs of the hands toward the ceiling as if to form the letter W.

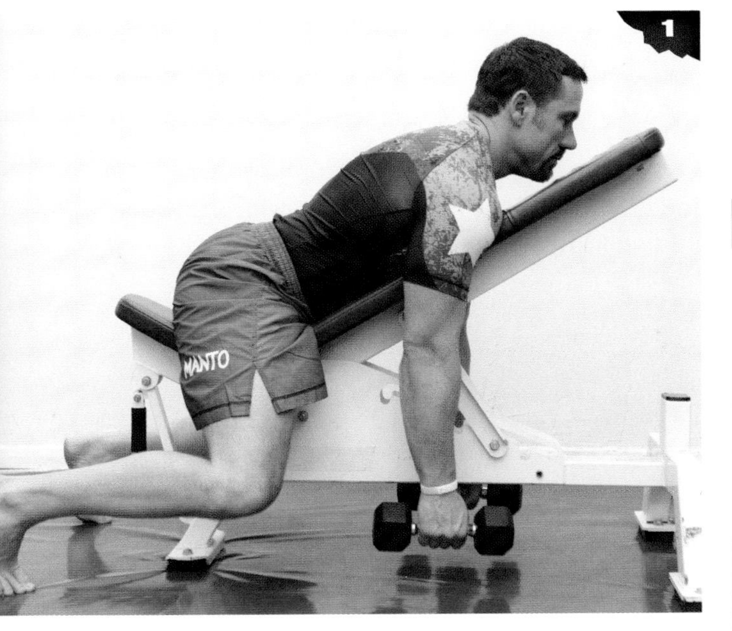

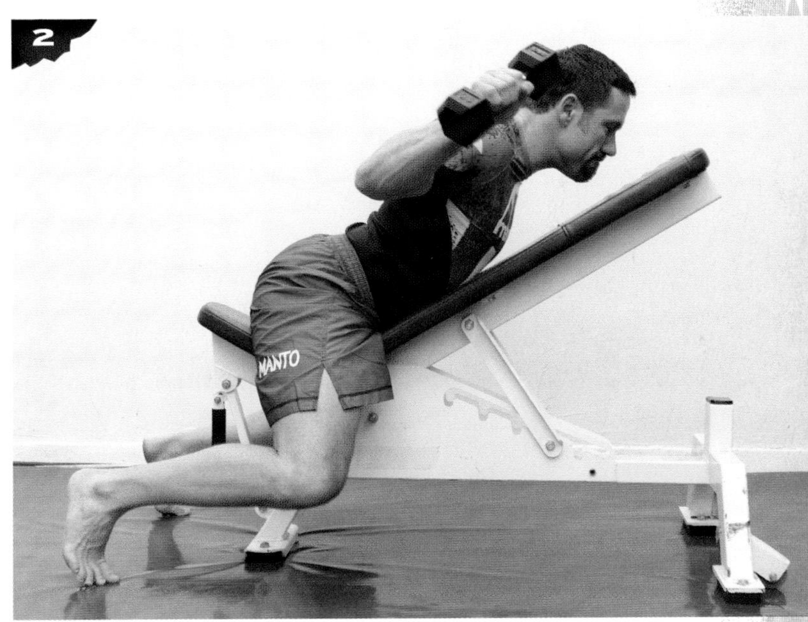

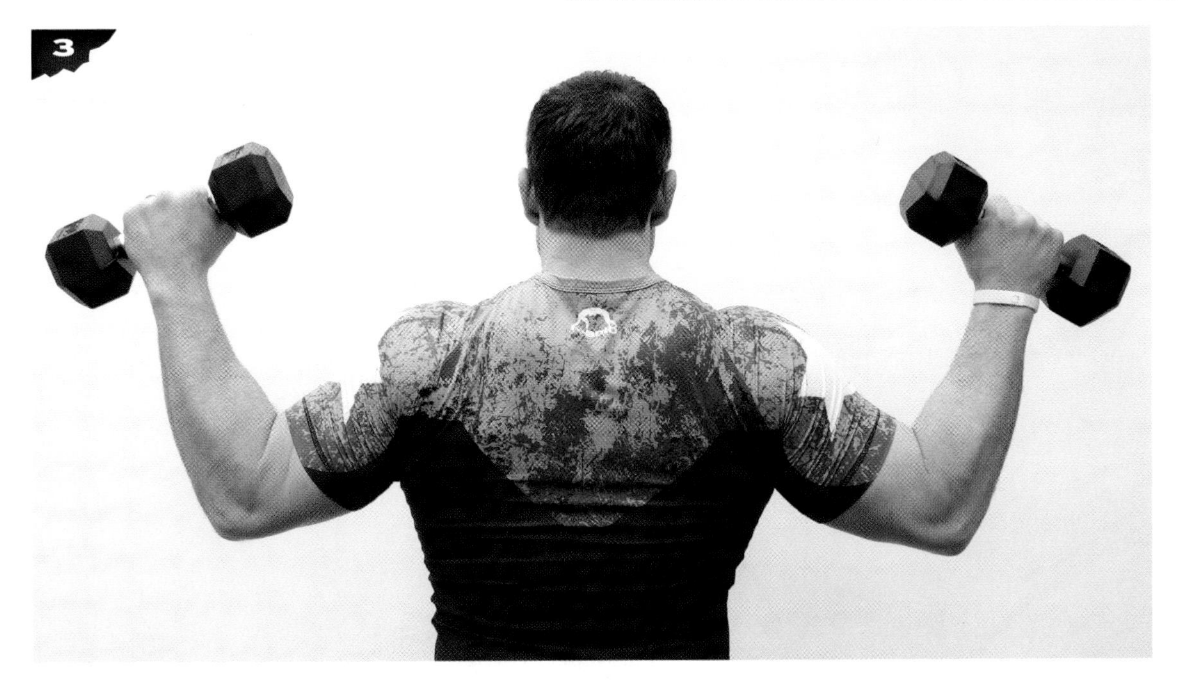

G. TFW 100-REP CHALLENGES

The TFW 100-Rep Challenges are physical tests in which a person attempts to complete 100 repetitions of a number of exercises linked together in a certain amount of time. The ultimate goal is to perform the 100 reps in less than 100 seconds. There is virtually an endless variety of tests. The following is a classic one used with our athletes, in which each exercise should be performed for 20 reps:

1. BAR PUSHUPS

Begin in the pushup position on the bar with the hands slightly wider than shoulder width. Lower the chest to the bar and then press back up by extending at the elbows.

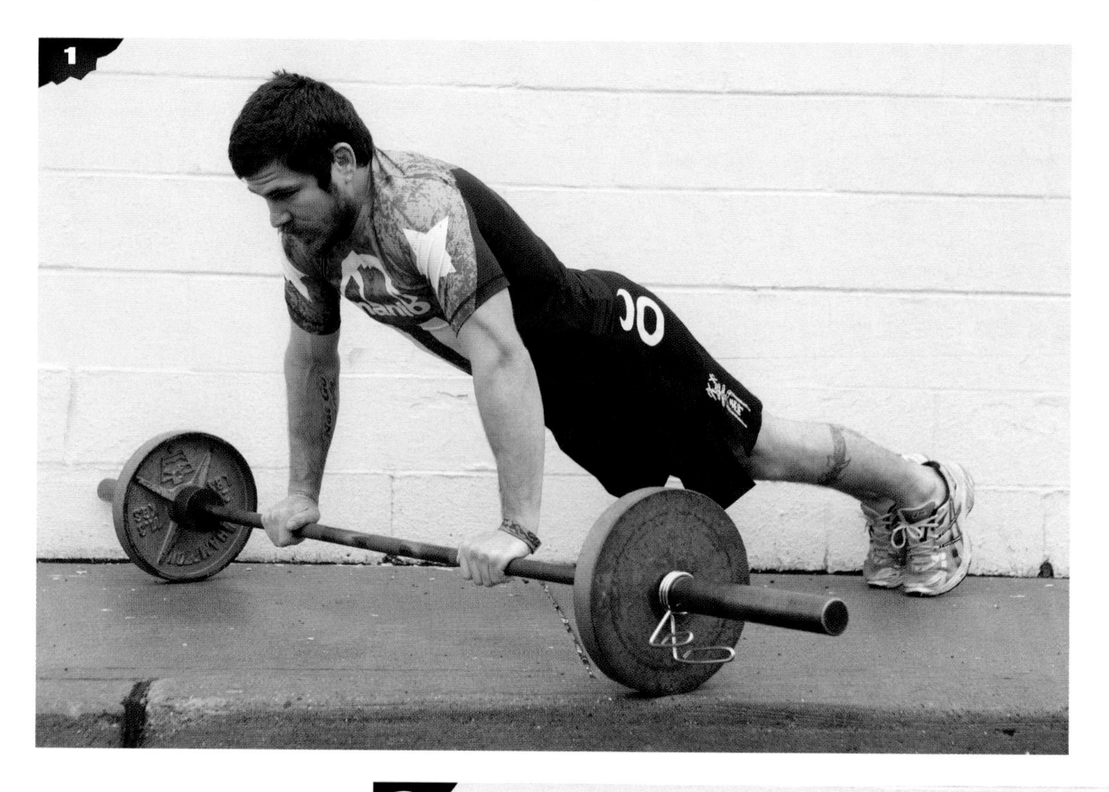

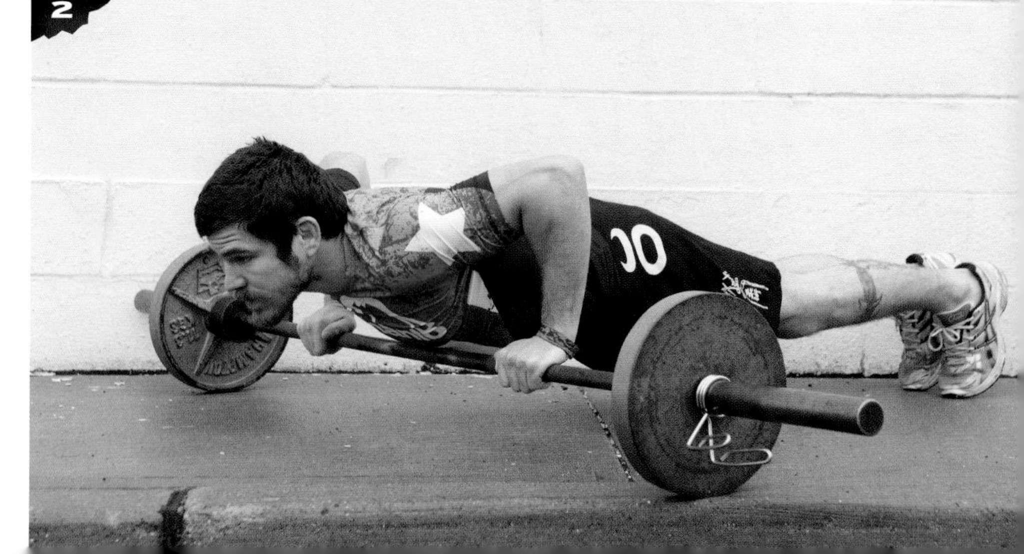

FULL-BODY HUNDRED CHALLENGE #1

2. DEADLIFT

Start by standing with the bar held with a shoulder-width grip at the height of the hips. While keeping the lower back flat and the knees slightly bent, bend forward at the waist so that the bar passes more than halfway down the shin. Extend at the lower back and return to the original position.

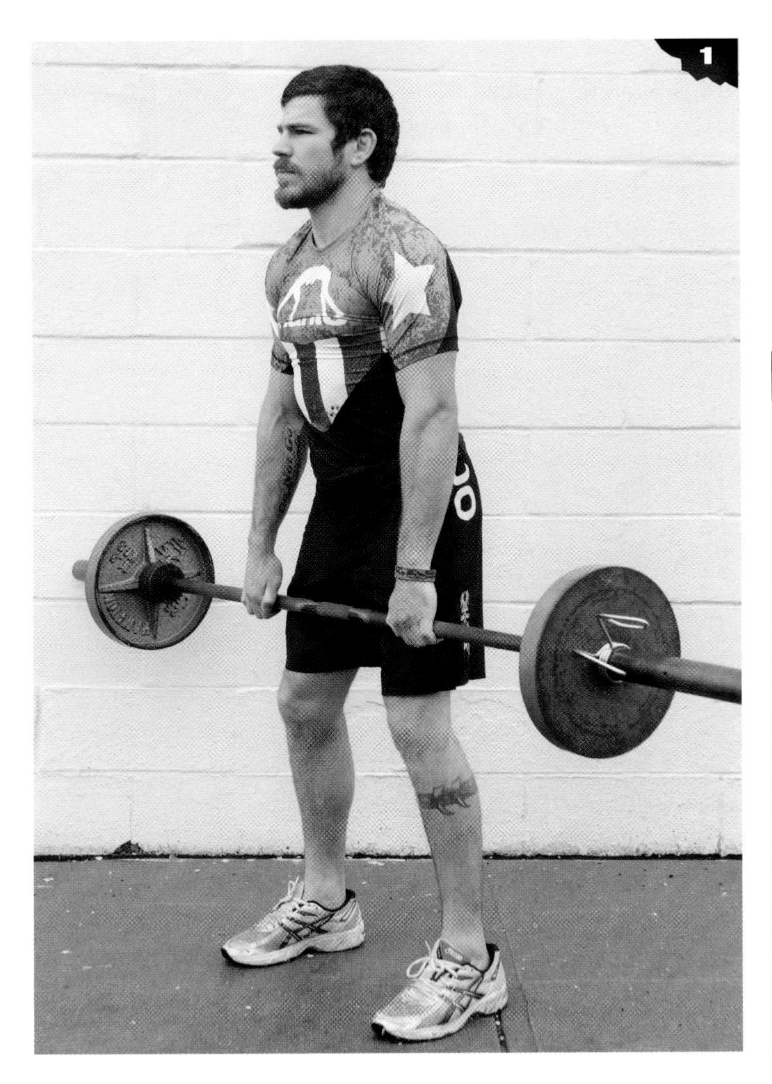

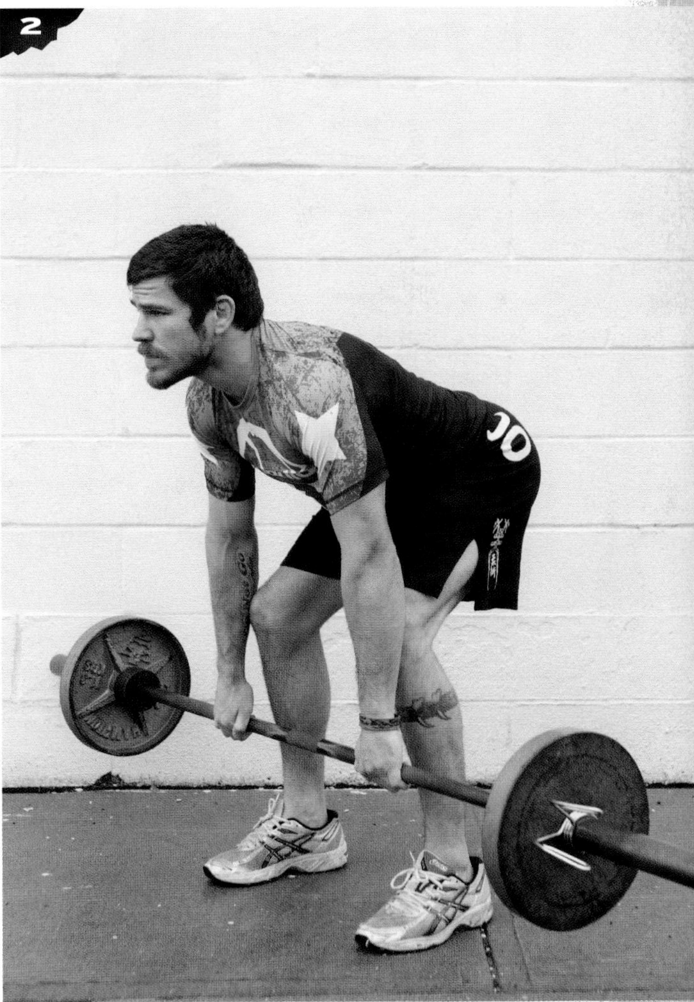

3. BENT-OVER ROW

Begin by leaning forward and holding the bar at knee height with a wider-than-shoulder-width grip. Pull the elbows back so that the bar touches the chest at nipple level. Lower to the original position and repeat.

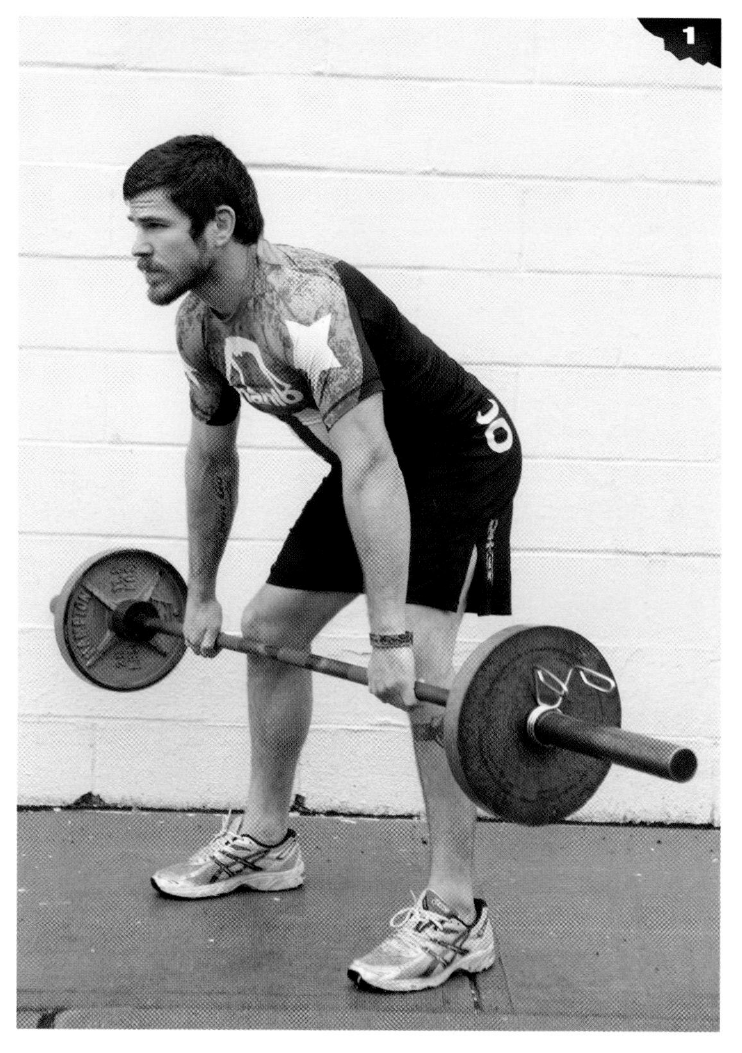

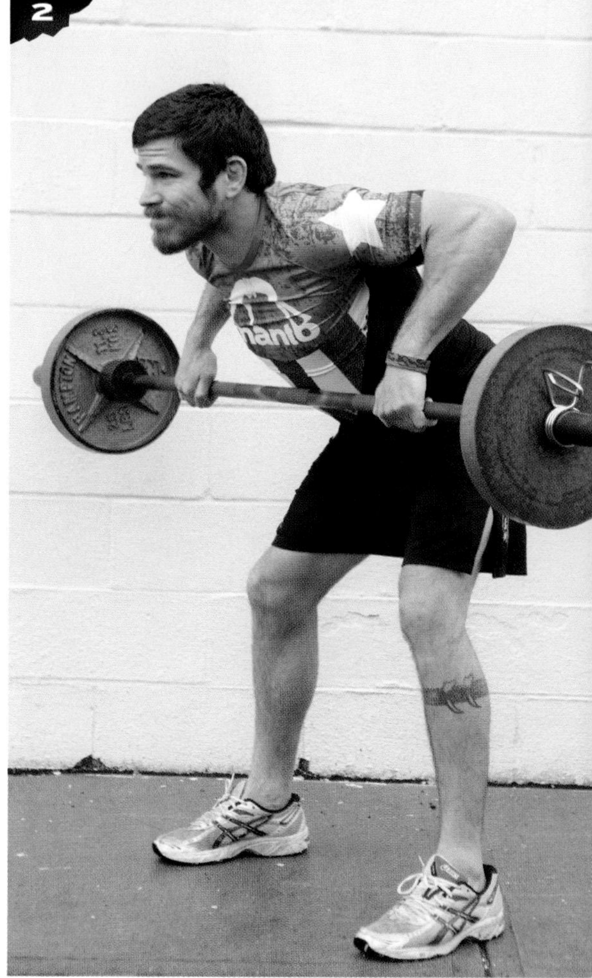

4. OVERHEAD PRESS

Hold the bar at chest height with a shoulder-width grip. Press the bar overhead by extending at the elbows. Lower the bar to the chest and repeat.

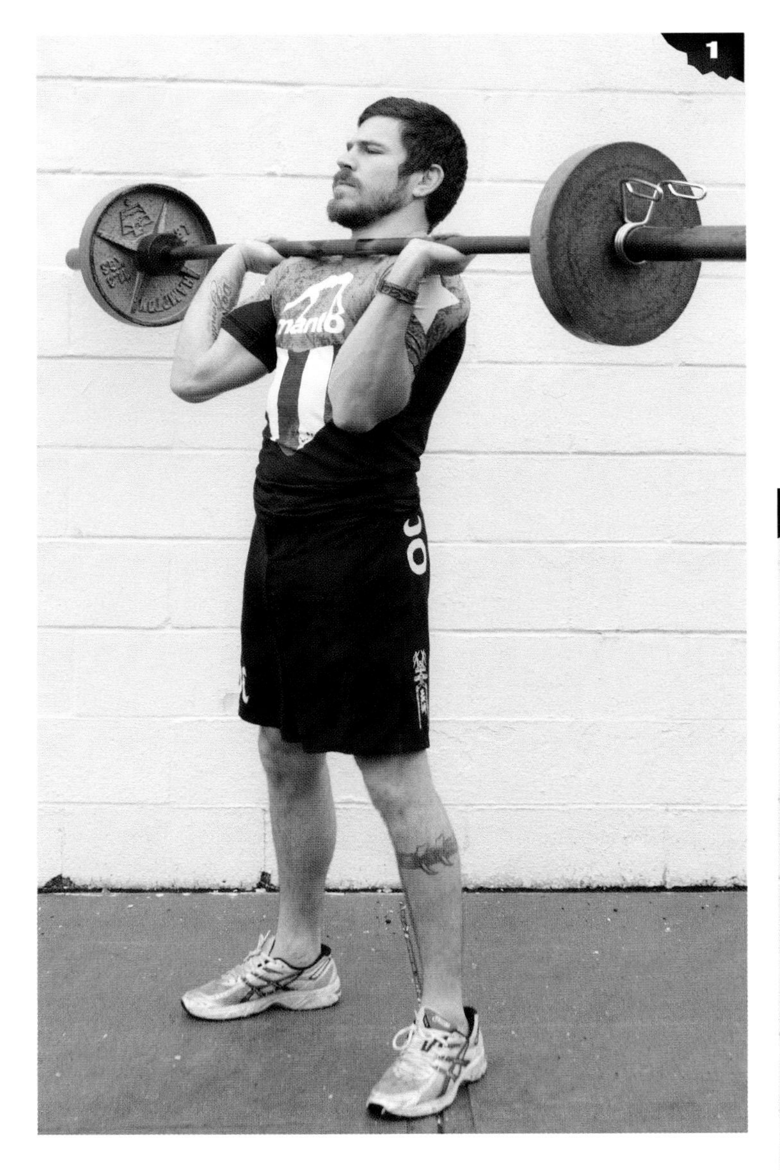

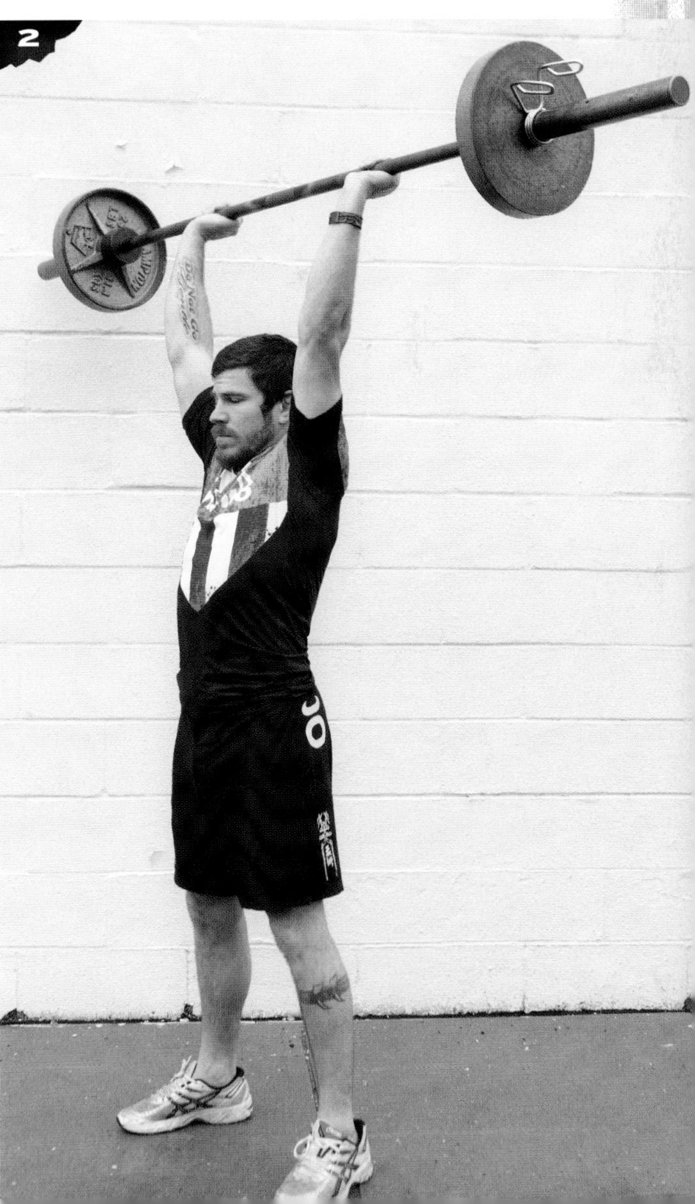

5. BACK SQUAT

Bring the bar overhead and place it behind the neck. Lower the hips to the parallel-squat position by bending at the knee. Press up by extending at the knees, hips, and lower back.

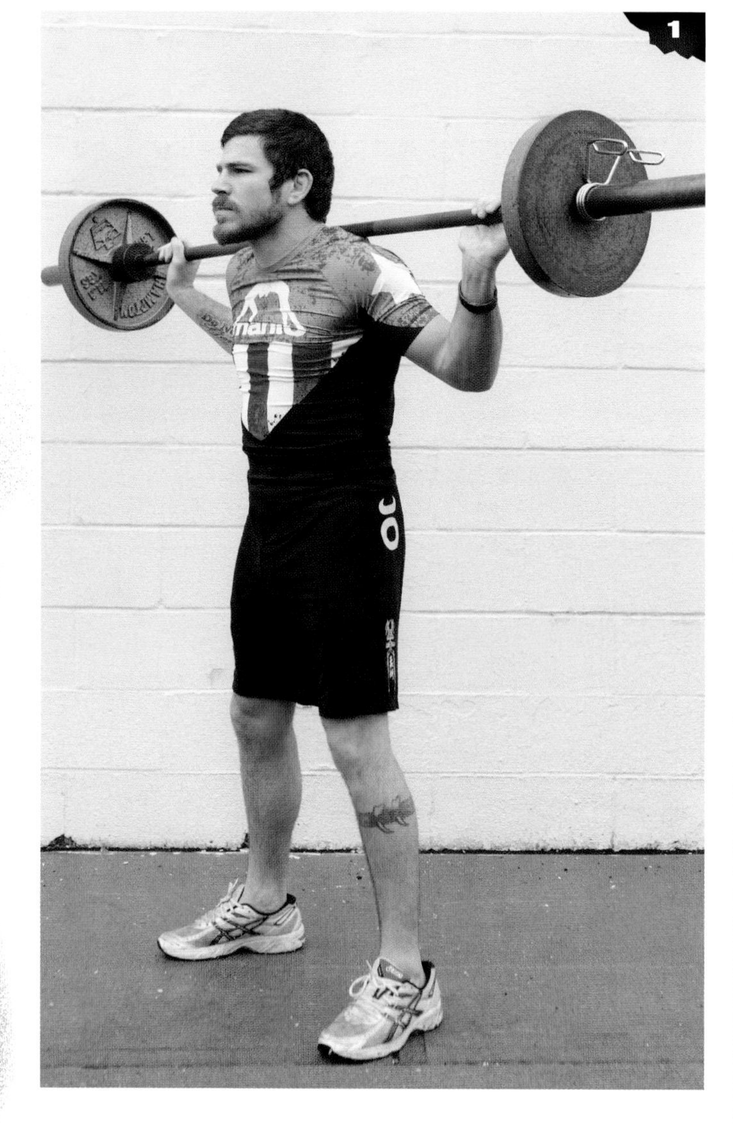

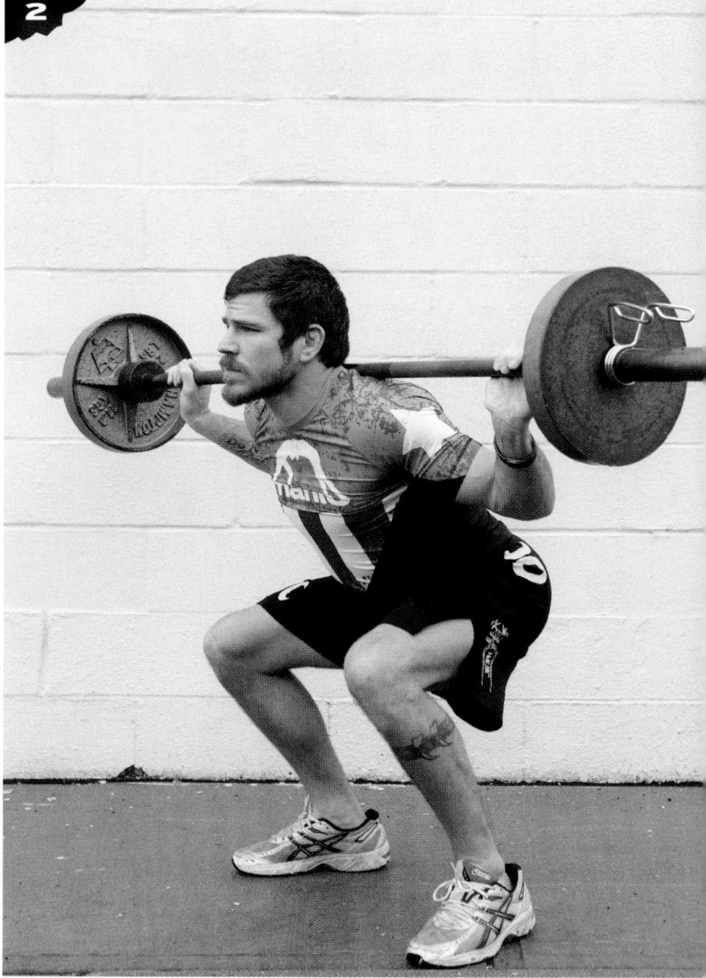

FULL-BODY HUNDRED CHALLENGE #2

To perform this challenge, perform 10 pushups and then immediately roll over and perform 10 knee grabs as quickly as possible. Perform 5 sets of each exercise for your best time.

1. PUSHUPS

Begin supporting the body on the hands and feet, with the feet together and hands at shoulder width on the ground. Lower the chest to the ground while keeping the elbows close to the sides. Extend at the elbows to return to the original position.

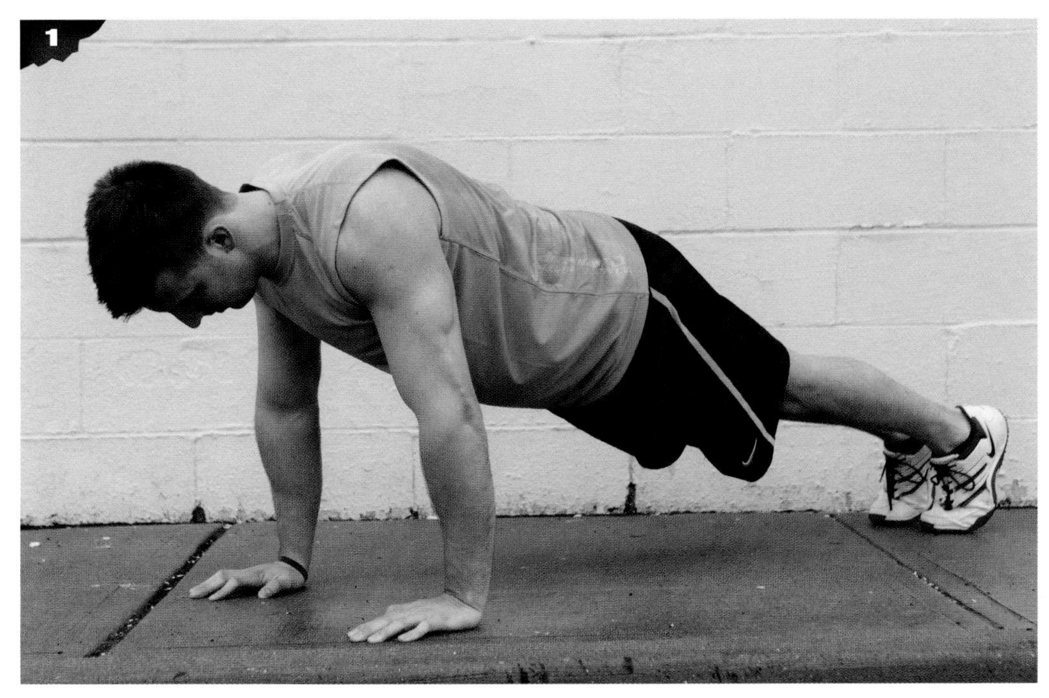

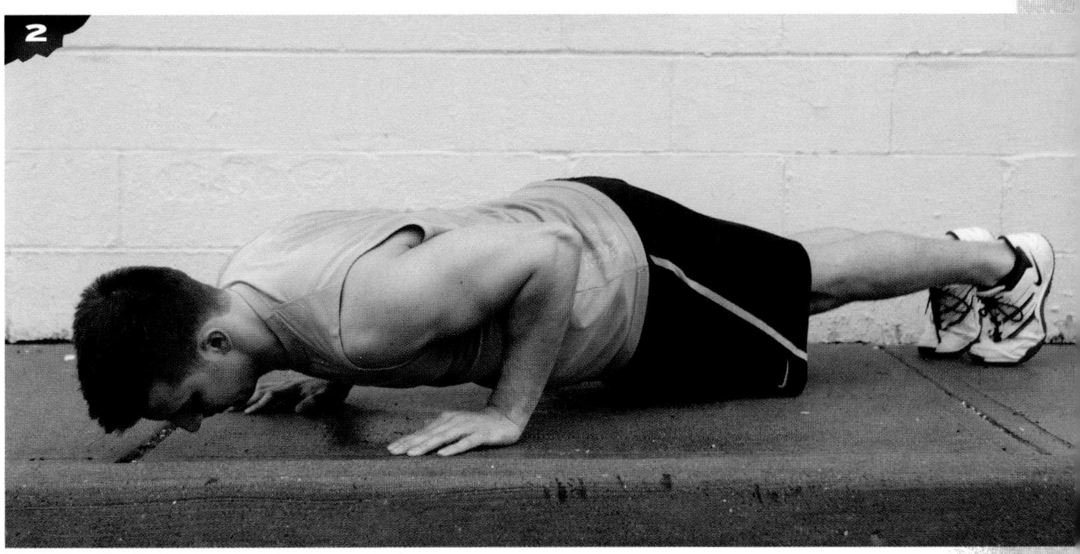

2. KNEE GRABS

Begin lying on the back with the knees straight and the hands held at the chin. Simultaneously bring the torso and knees up, and grab onto the ankles. Lower back down to the original position under control.

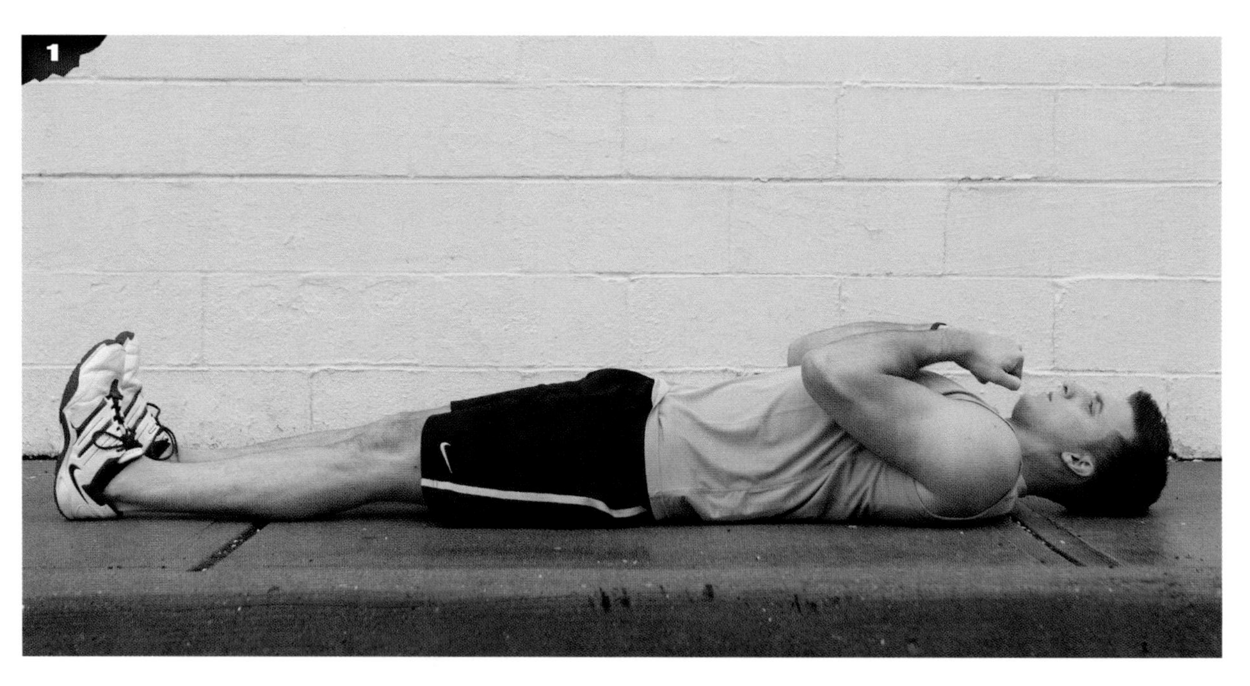

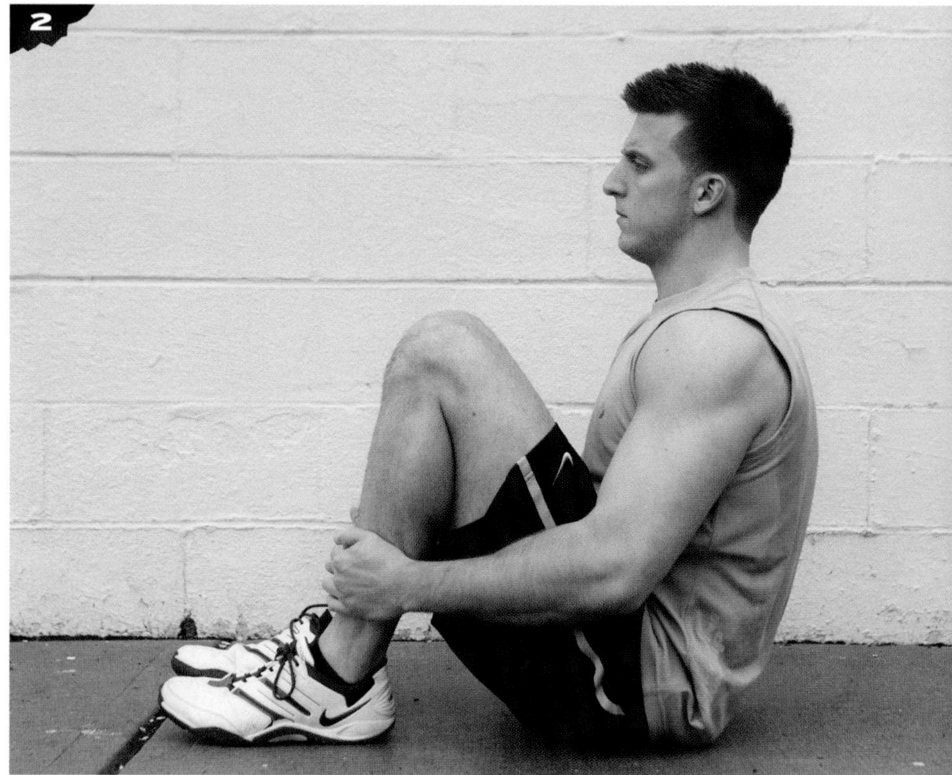

CHIN-UP SERIES CHEATSHEET

1. WIDE-GRIP PULLUP

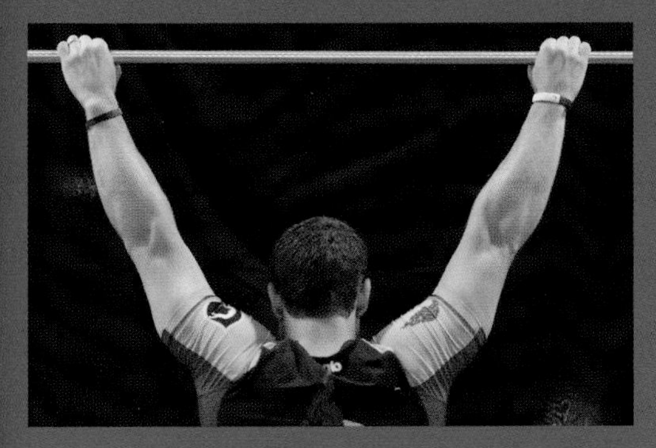

2. NEUTRAL-GRIP PULLUP

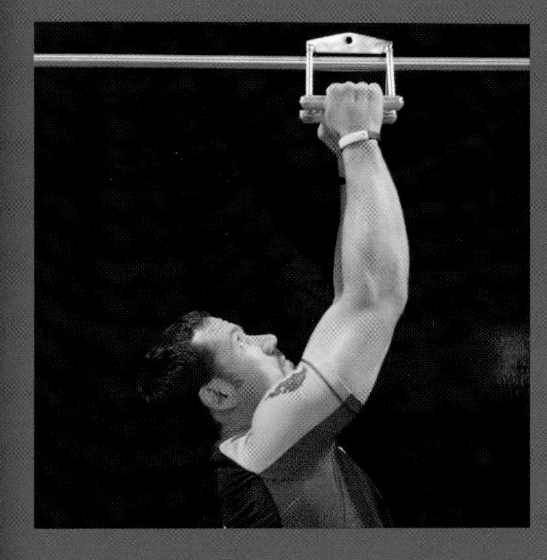

3. MIXED-GRIP PULLUP

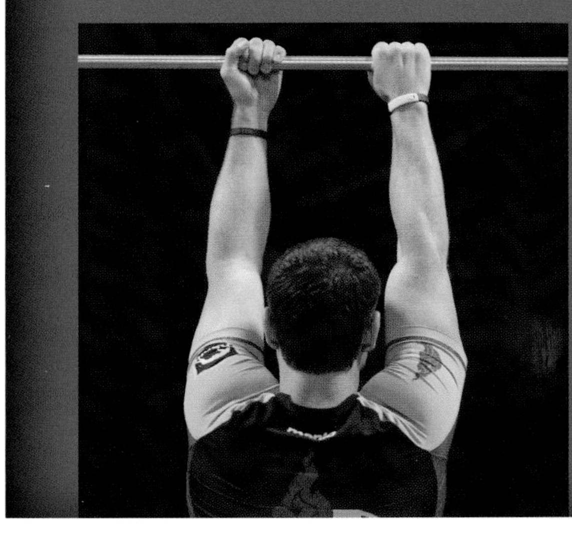

4. CHIN-UP

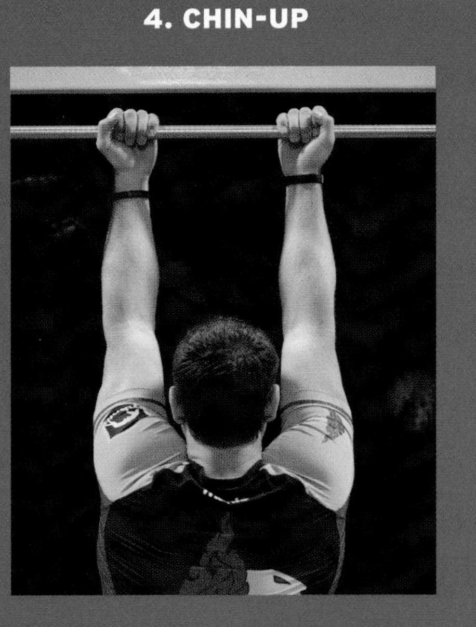

5. WRIST-GRIP CHIN-UP

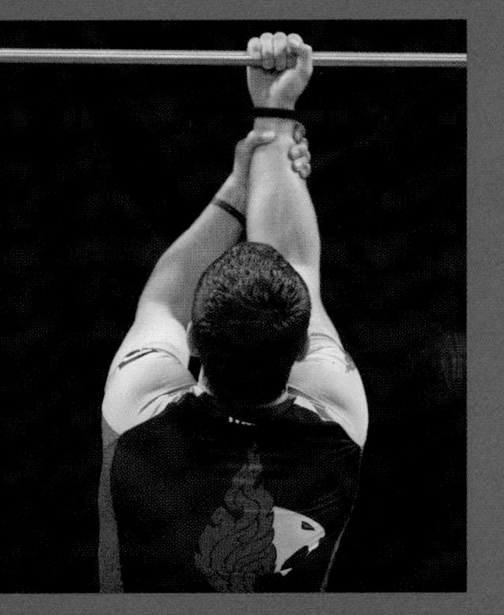

GAUNTLET CHEATSHEET

1. DUMBBELL BENCH PRESS

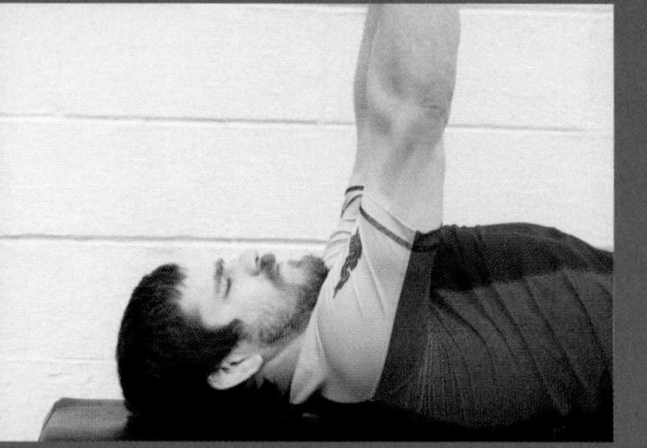

2. DUMBBELL CHEST FLYES

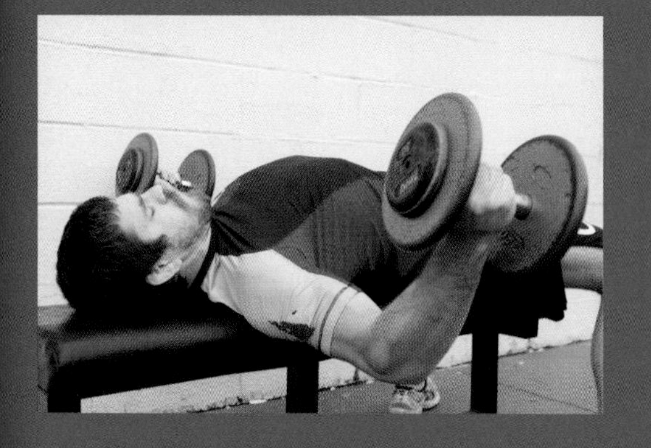

3. DUMBBELL ROLLING TRICEPS

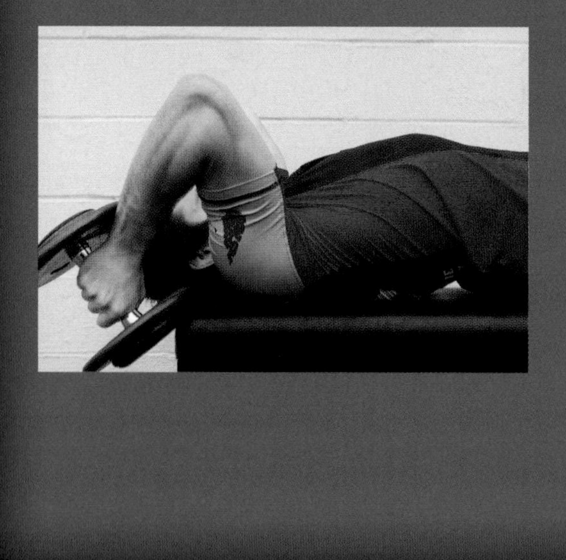

4. DUMBBELL BICEP CURLS

5. DUMBBELL SHOULDER PRESS

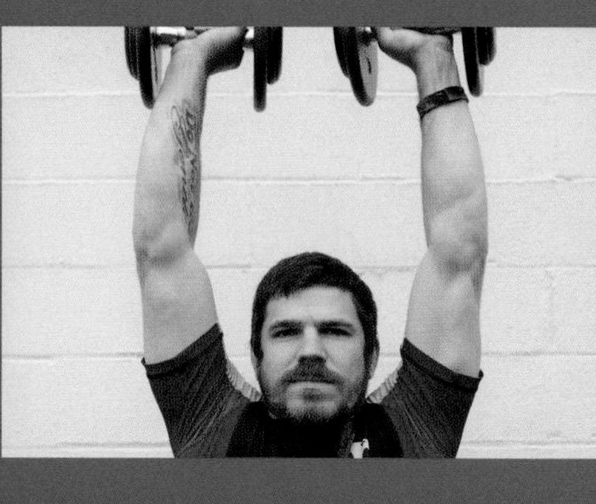

6. DUMBBELL SHRUGS

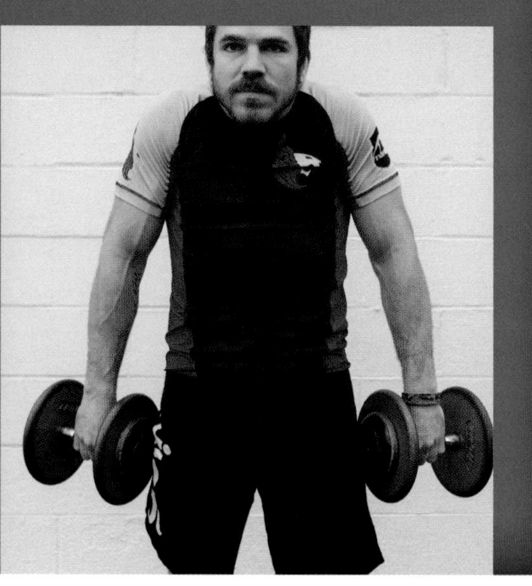

TFW 100-REP CHALLENGE CHEATSHEET

1. BAR PUSHUPS

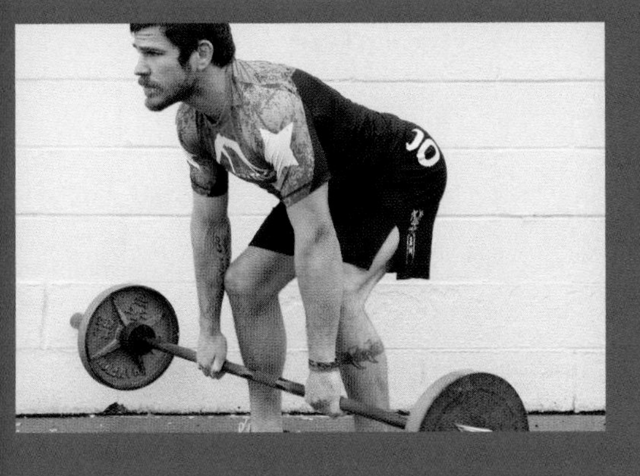

2. DEADLIFT

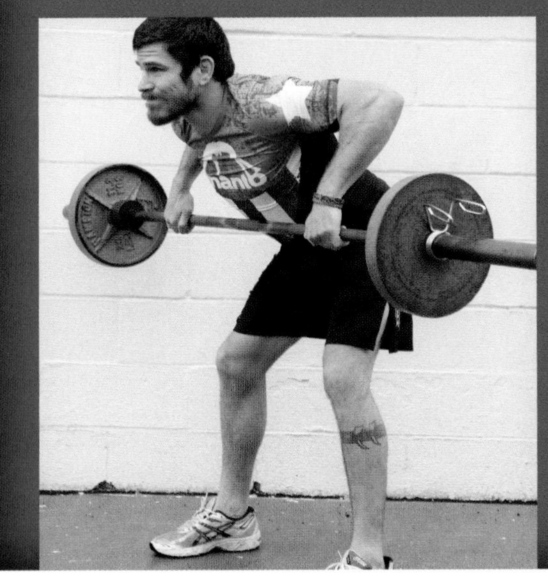

3. BENT-OVER ROW

4. OVERHEAD PRESS

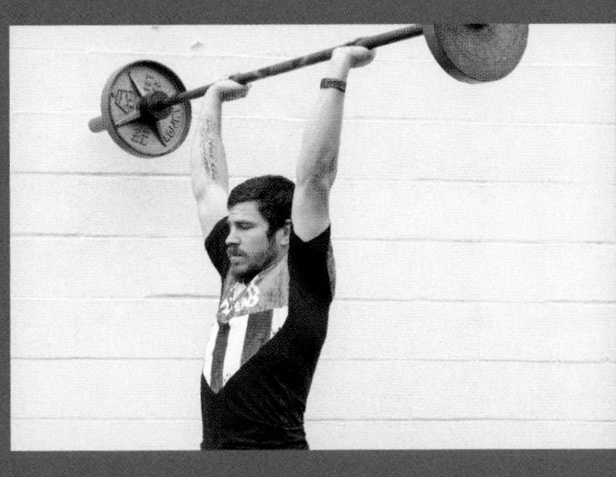

5. BACK SQUAT

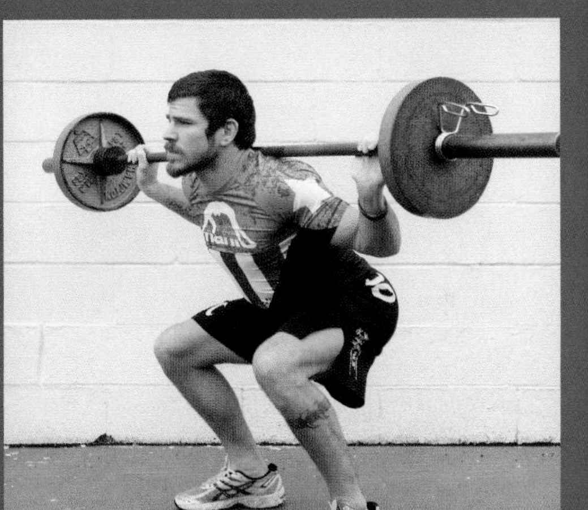

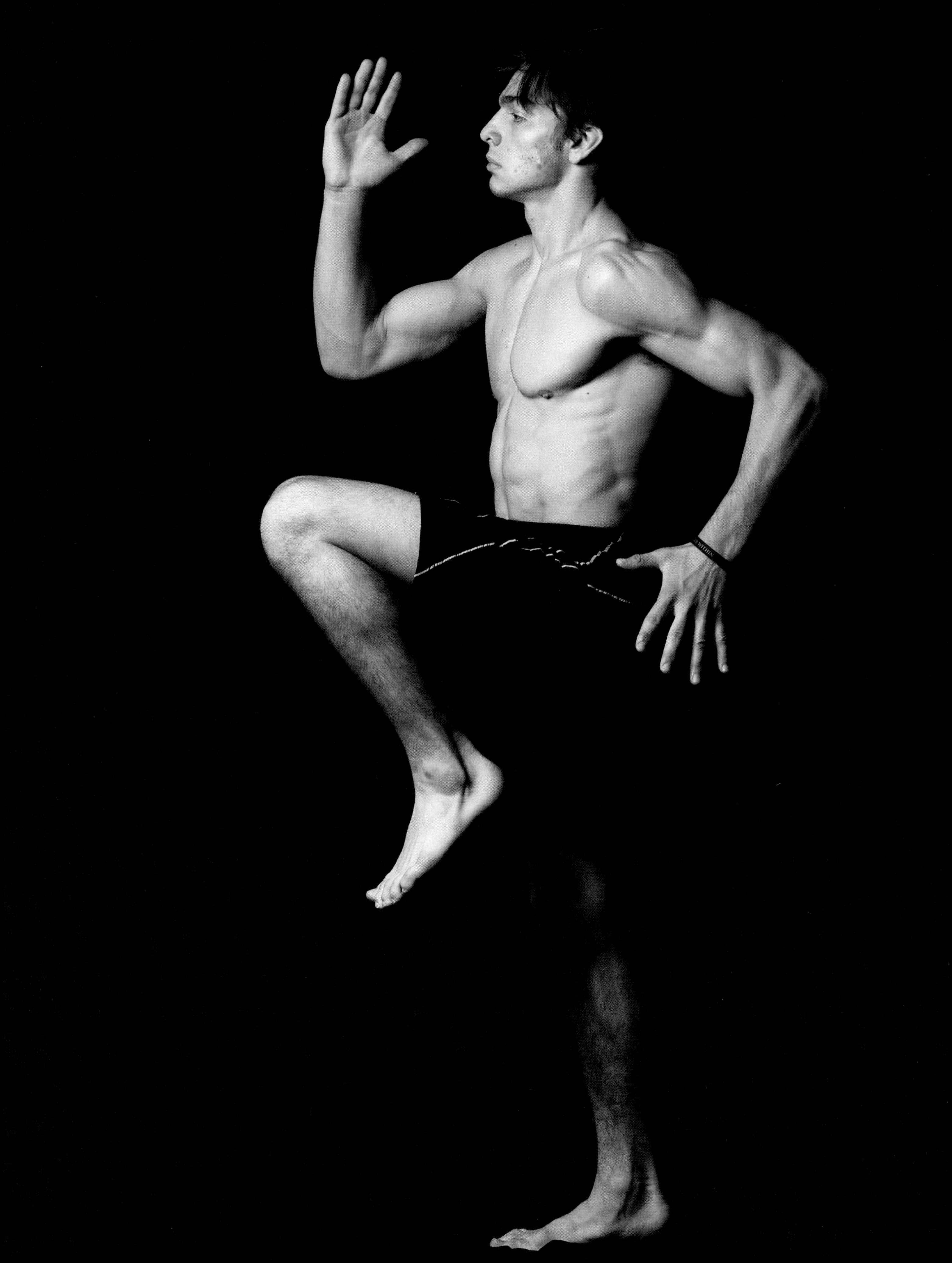

13

SPRINT TRAINING

Many people recognize that sprinting is an important athletic ability and may even incorporate some of this training into their workout routine. Most people, however, do not pay the same attention to form and technique with sprinting that they do with other sport motions or weight room exercises. This is a big problem, because poor sprinting form or technique can lead to decreased performance or potential injury.

I consider sprinting one of the greatest exercises that a person can perform. Sprinting involves almost every muscle in the body; it conditions the muscular, nervous, and energy systems; and its cyclical nature of work and recovery can help to prepare a warrior for battle. Due to the potential importance of this training, I am amazed when I see a sample training session covered on television that has athletes running with terrible form, in complete fatigue, on the wrong surfaces, and with little rhyme or reason. This improper training continues because they don't know what they don't know.

Here are five important TFW principles about sprint training that you may not know you don't know. If you internalize these principles and apply them to your training, your approach to sprinting will be forever changed.

1. SPRINTING IS A SKILL.

There is a best way to run. There is no use for sprinting with poor technique. Both arm and leg mechanics are critical, and body position is essential to assess. Sprint form is a motor program that requires as much technical work as learning any other motion in sport. In addition to technique, proper shoes, proper surface, and proper clothing all have an effect.

2. SPRINTING IS YEAR-ROUND.

Just as the farmer cannot rush his or her harvest, you cannot sprint for only a few weeks and expect to be prepared. Training should be a year-round thing, and that includes sprint work. If this is not consistent, injuries are bound to happen.

3. YOU MUST LEARN TO STOP BEFORE YOU START.

You must make sure that you are slowing down correctly after every sprint. Just as a Judo player must learn to fall safely before he can ever get thrown, a sprinter must learn to stop before he learns to run faster. Get low and use soft foot contacts during every deceleration. This will let the muscles absorb the force instead of the joints and ligaments.

4. INTENSITY MUST BE MONITORED.

Just as with weight lifting or other forms of training, you must monitor the intensity of the sprinting you perform. All too often, I see athletes sprint all-out every session. This is very detrimental to the nervous system and can wear the athlete out for other training. Make sure that you are using the appropriate intensity for that training day.

5. WORK-TO-REST RATIOS MUST BE MONITORED.

Sprinting involves coordination of most of the muscles of the body. When fatigue sets in, coordination, and hence technique, breaks down. The purpose of a sprint routine is to have a metabolic effect, not produce fatigue. Being tired may be a byproduct of this style of training, but it is not the goal. Ample recovery in between sets will insure good form and optimal results.

Note: If you are going to use sprinting as a form of metabolic training, you must ease into this style of training or shin splints and other issues like potential muscle pulls are sure to plague you. Give your body time to get ready for this style of training with a few easy weeks of lighter volume.

A. WARRIOR'S SPRINT CIRCUITS: TECHNIQUE

Now that you understand some principles behind sprint training, my goal is to deliver interval workouts that also get you to focus on technique, in order to avoid injury. These Warrior Cardio circuits will not only increase heart rate, but also force you to focus on sprinting correctly. I use these with all of my athletes successfully.

1. ARM ACTION DRILL

This exercise can be performed seated. Keep your elbow at a 90-degree angle and move the hands from the hip to the height of the chin. All the motion should take place at the shoulder joint. Do not cross the midline with the hands in front of the body.

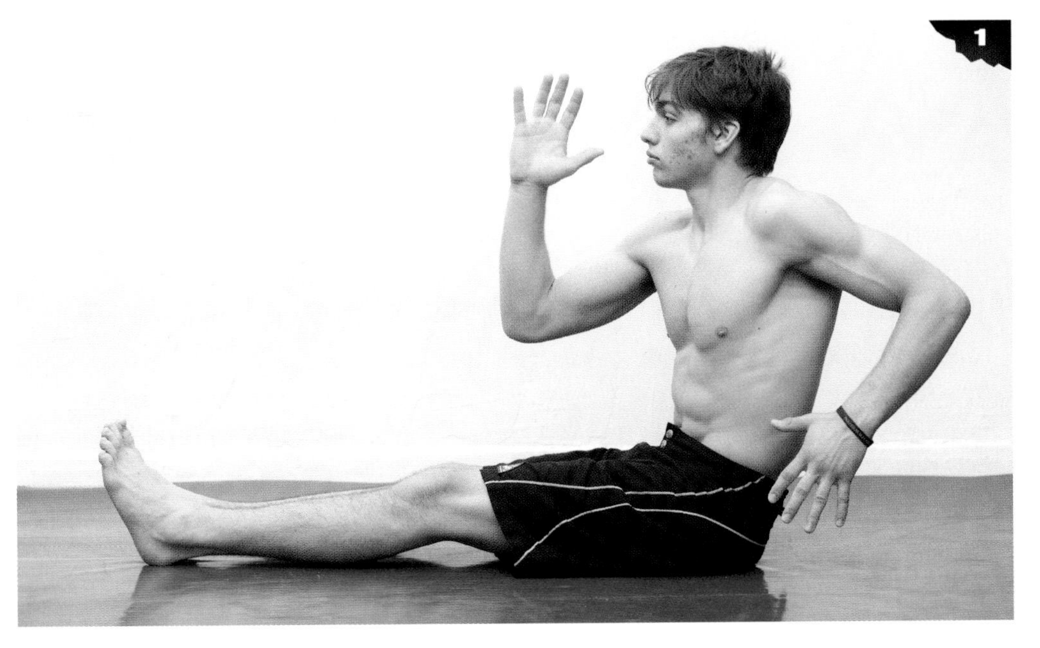

Perform this at slow, medium, and then full speed for 20 seconds each for 5 sets. Rest 1 minute between sets.

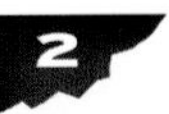

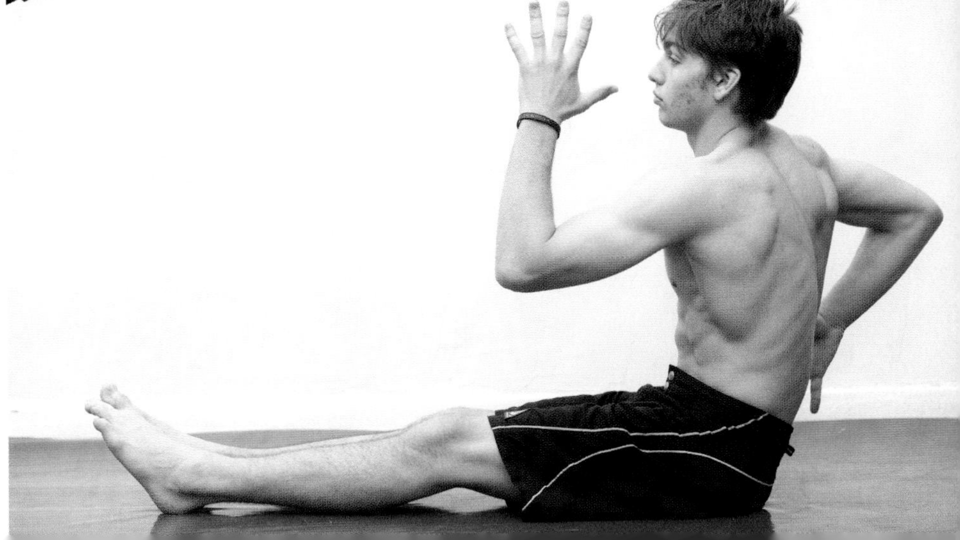

2. HIGH-KNEE FOLD DRILL

Once you have worked on the arm mechanics, the next piece of the puzzle is leg recovery. Leg recovery is critical to speed production and injury prevention. For the High-Knee Fold Drill, you are to run 5 yards with good arm form and high knees while concentrating on bringing the foot up under the butt as the knee and hip flex forward. The goal is to take as many steps as possible over the 5 yards. Then walk 5 more yards and repeat for 5 sets.

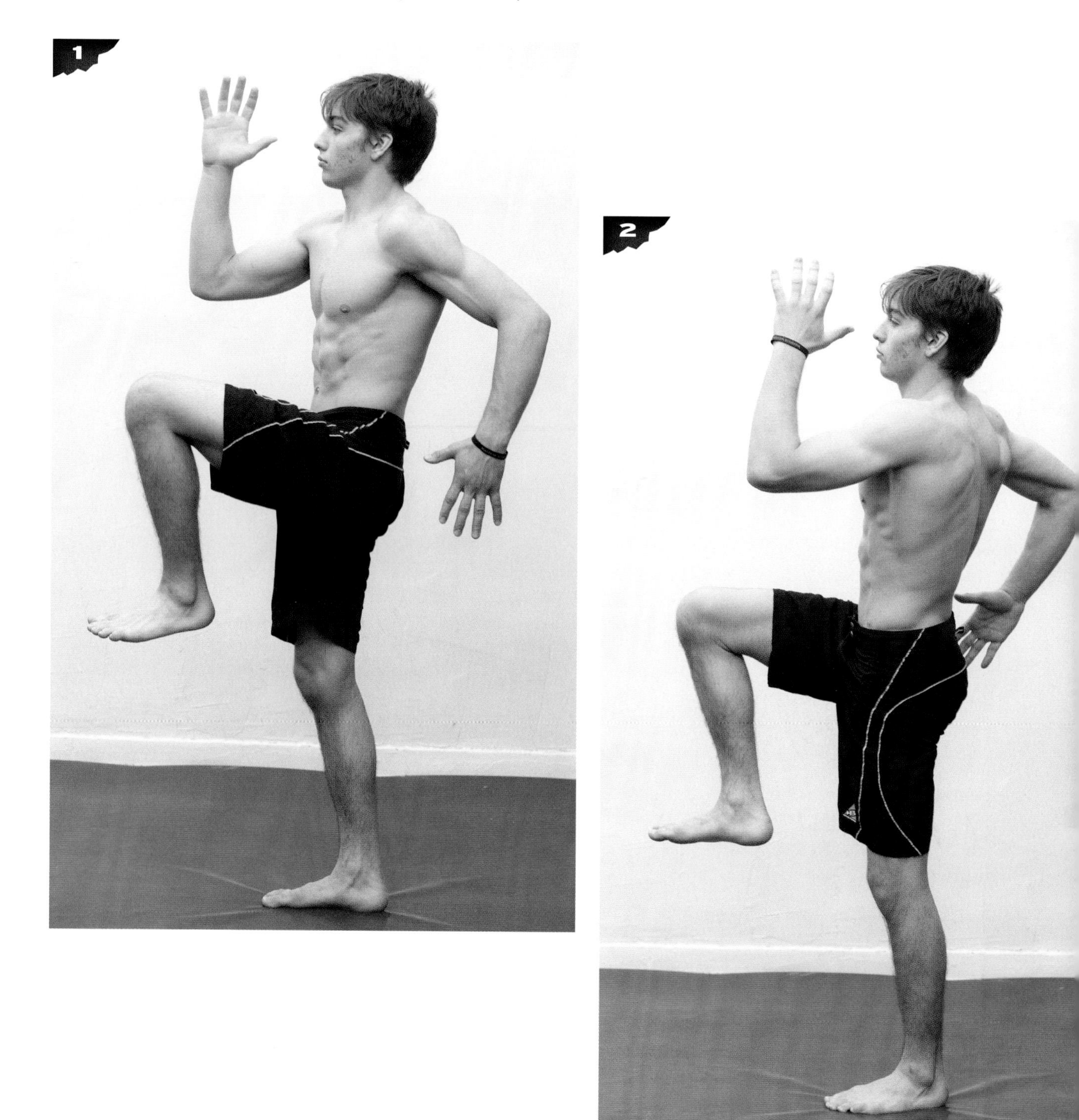

3. WALL DRIVE

The athlete leans into a wall at a 45-degree angle. The head is aligned with the body and one knee is up. Switch the leg positions explosively while pushing into the wall.

Perform this at a slow, medium, and then full speed for 20 seconds for 5 sets each.

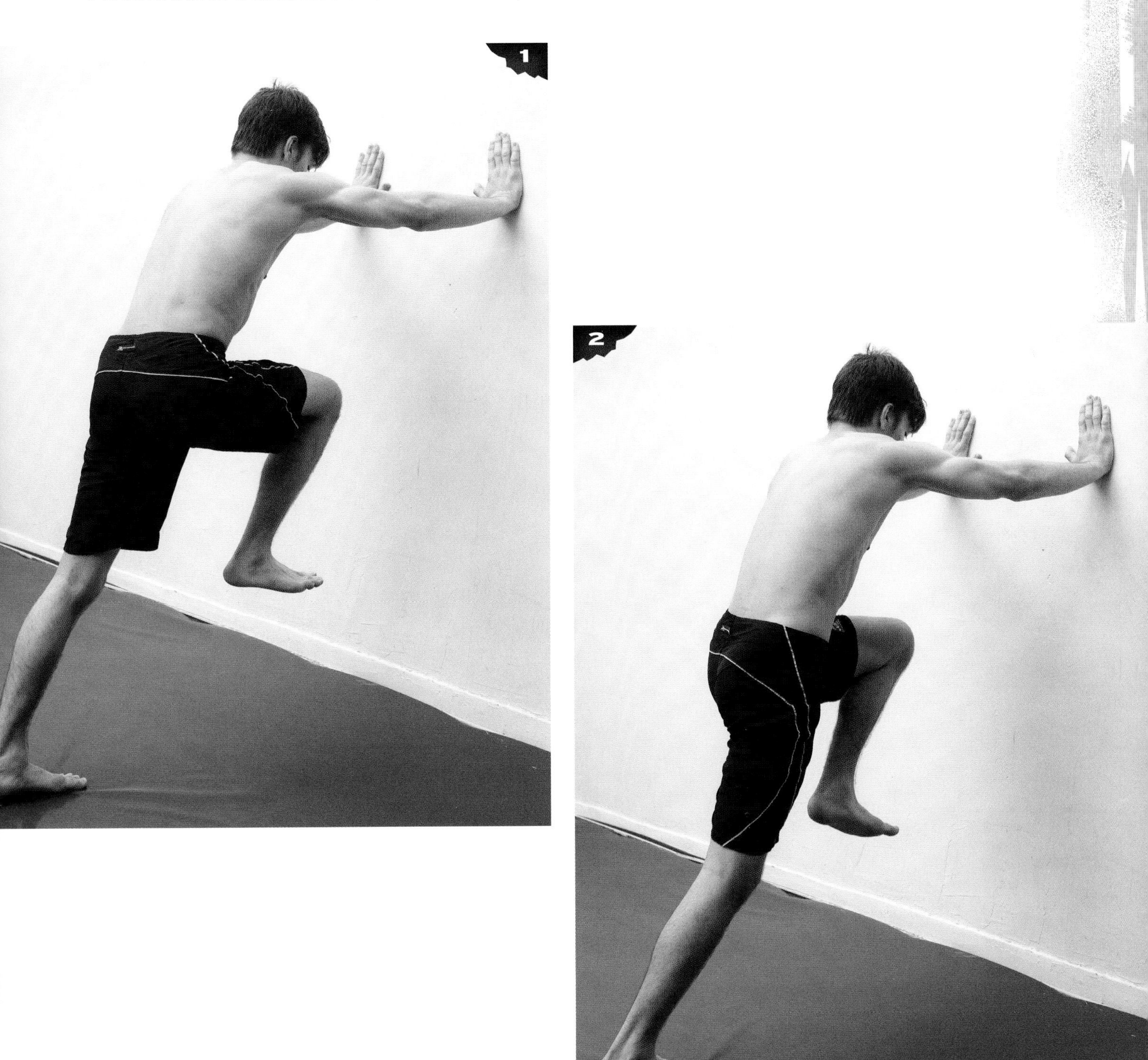

Once you have learned to perform these drills properly, you will be more aware of technique and better prepared to perform a sprint training workout. Although there is an endless variety of ways to utilize sprint training, here are the five most popular forms we use in the Training for Warriors system. Any of these metabolic sessions can be substituted in when you are completing the 12-Week Warrior Cardio Workout at the back of this book.

B. 20-METER SPRINTS

You should focus on staying low by leaning forward and taking long, powerful, "pushing" strides by driving the feet backward. Be aggressive with arm drive.

Perform 10 sprints at 90% to 100% intensity. Use 1 minute in between sprints as recovery.

C. 100-METER TEMPO RUNS

You should still drive out low and then at the 20- to 30-meter mark, run tall and focus on leg recovery and arm form.

Perform six sprints at 80% to 90% intensity while focusing on form and staying relaxed. Run 100 meters and then rest 2 minutes in between sprints.

D. "STRAIGHTS AND CURVES" TRACK CIRCUIT

If you have a track available, a great workout is ten 100-meter sprints at about 80% while walking the 100-meter curves for recovery. In this case, the recovery is shorter, with about a 1:3 work-to-rest ratio, so there is an increased metabolic demand.

E. 40-YARD DASHES

Another popular form of sprint training in TFW is sprinting ten to twelve 40-yard dashes and jogging the recovery.

When running the 40-yard dash, you should stay leaning forward and low for the first 15 to 20 yards and then run tall, focused on arm form and leg recovery, for the second half of the run.

You can time each individual set to determine the intensity at which you are working.

F. STADIUM STAIR RUNNING

If you have a nice set of stadium stairs nearby at either the local college or high school, they can be a great tool for your stamina training.

We like to create different patterns for running the stadiums to keep us fresh. A great way to run the stadiums is to run five separate 5-minute rounds. You can alternate the pace between running hard up the stairs and jogging the side and downward portions. The goal is to cover as much distance as possible. There are an infinite number of ways to use the stairs. The first step is getting out there and trying them out.

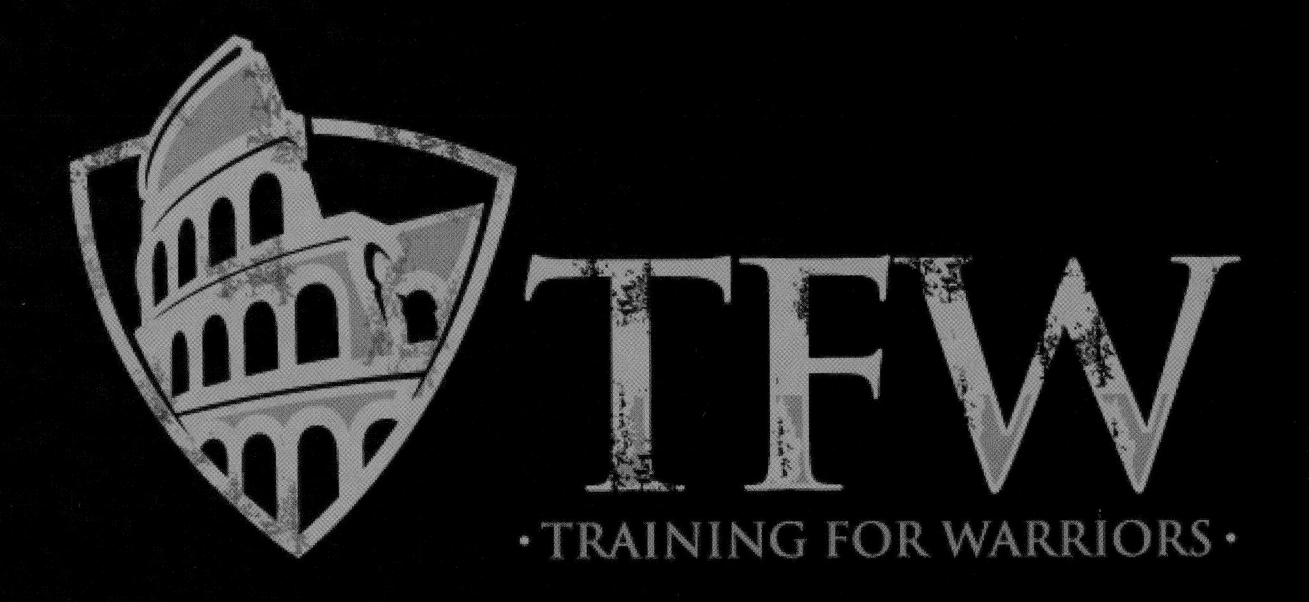
TFW
·TRAINING FOR WARRIORS·

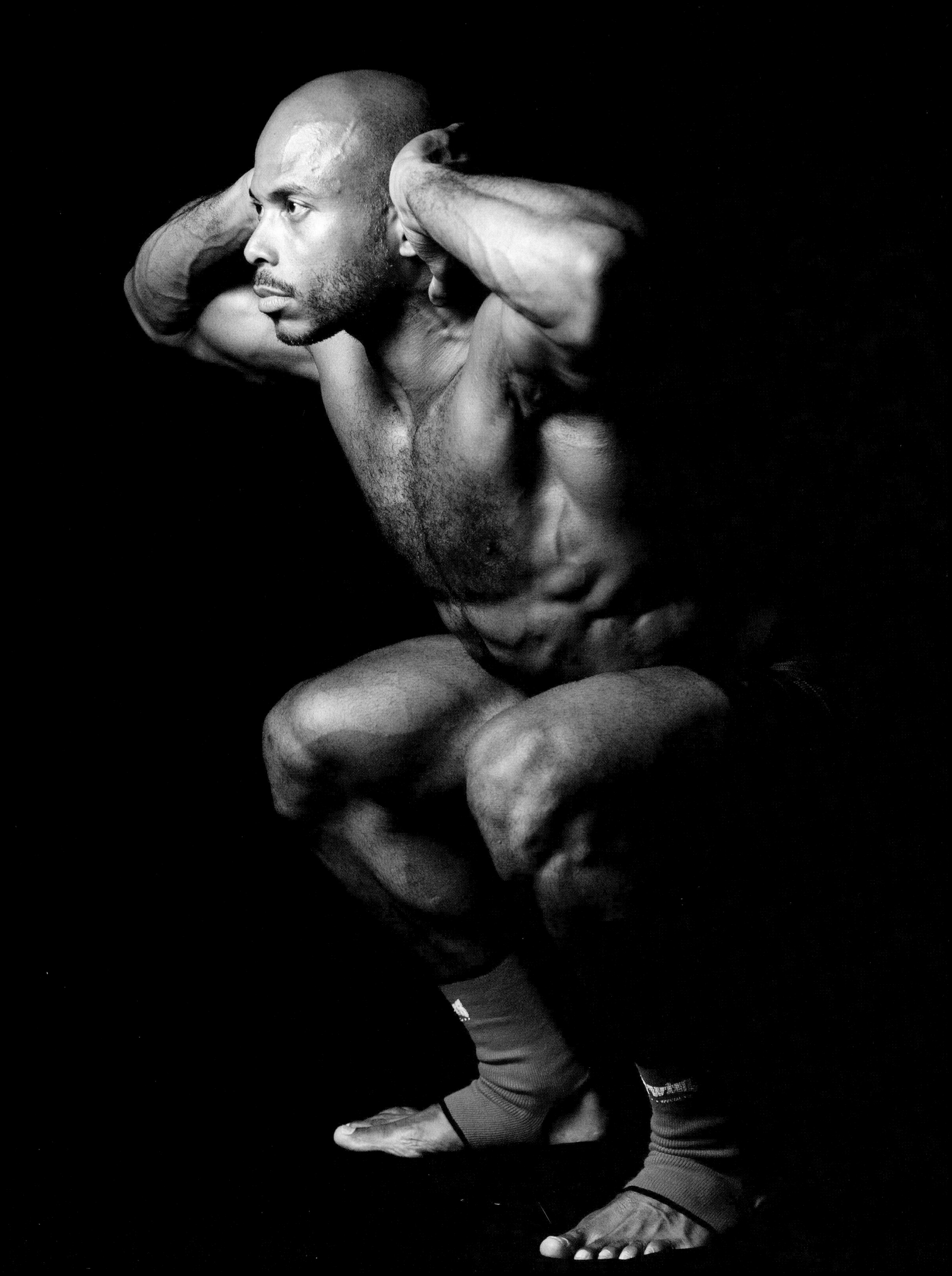

14

THE FINISHERS

In the TFW system, we use certain exercises and routines that are known as "finishers." These are exercises used to put an exclamation point at the end of a tough workout. The key to the finishers is that although they are demanding and challenge both the body and mind, they are relatively safe to perform, easy to control, and even as deeper fatigue sets in, form and technique do not drastically change.

The three finishers that are most commonly used in TFW are the Pulling Sled, the Prowler, and Plate Pushes. These exercises are similar in many ways, but their subtle differences are noticeable enough that they are considered different exercises.

One aspect that makes the finishers a good choice for the end of a workout is that they do not have much of an eccentric component (which means the muscles are not required to lengthen under tension during the exercise). When the eccentric component of an exercise is reduced, the muscles do not experience the damage that comes along with eccentric contractions of certain exercises like the squat, deadlift, bench press, and many other body weight exercises featured in this book. Because of the fact that this style can be less damaging, but still deliver a good workout, the sled can also be used as a recovery workout. Recovery training is featured in this chapter as well.

The challenge with the finishers is that the trainee is already in a fatigued state by the end of the workout. As a result, be cautious to monitor the total volume of work that was performed during the session. For instance, if you have already done three 5-minute circuits or five full bar complexes, even though you may feel like doing a lot more, your body may have already had enough. Over time, you will learn how much you can handle.

Finisher exercises can be performed for time, for distance, or for a number of repetitions while monitoring the work-to-rest ratio.

A. FINISHERS: SLED DRAGGING

One method for metabolic work using the sled is pulls for time. In this case, the sleds are weighted moderately, but the length of the entire circuit is quite long. Depending on the length of the upcoming fight or athletic endeavor, you will walk 50 yards forward, backward, sideways, bear crawling, and with duck walks while pulling moderate weight for the duration of the set. This could be anywhere from 3 to 20 minutes with no rest. This takes time to get used to, but in addition to the physical adaptations that take place, mental toughness is increased. The sample order of the drag series is as follows:

1. FORWARD DRAG

Begin with the back to the sled, holding the ropes in the hands. Take as big of a step forward as possible, staying on the balls of the feet while maintaining a 45-degree angle with the body.

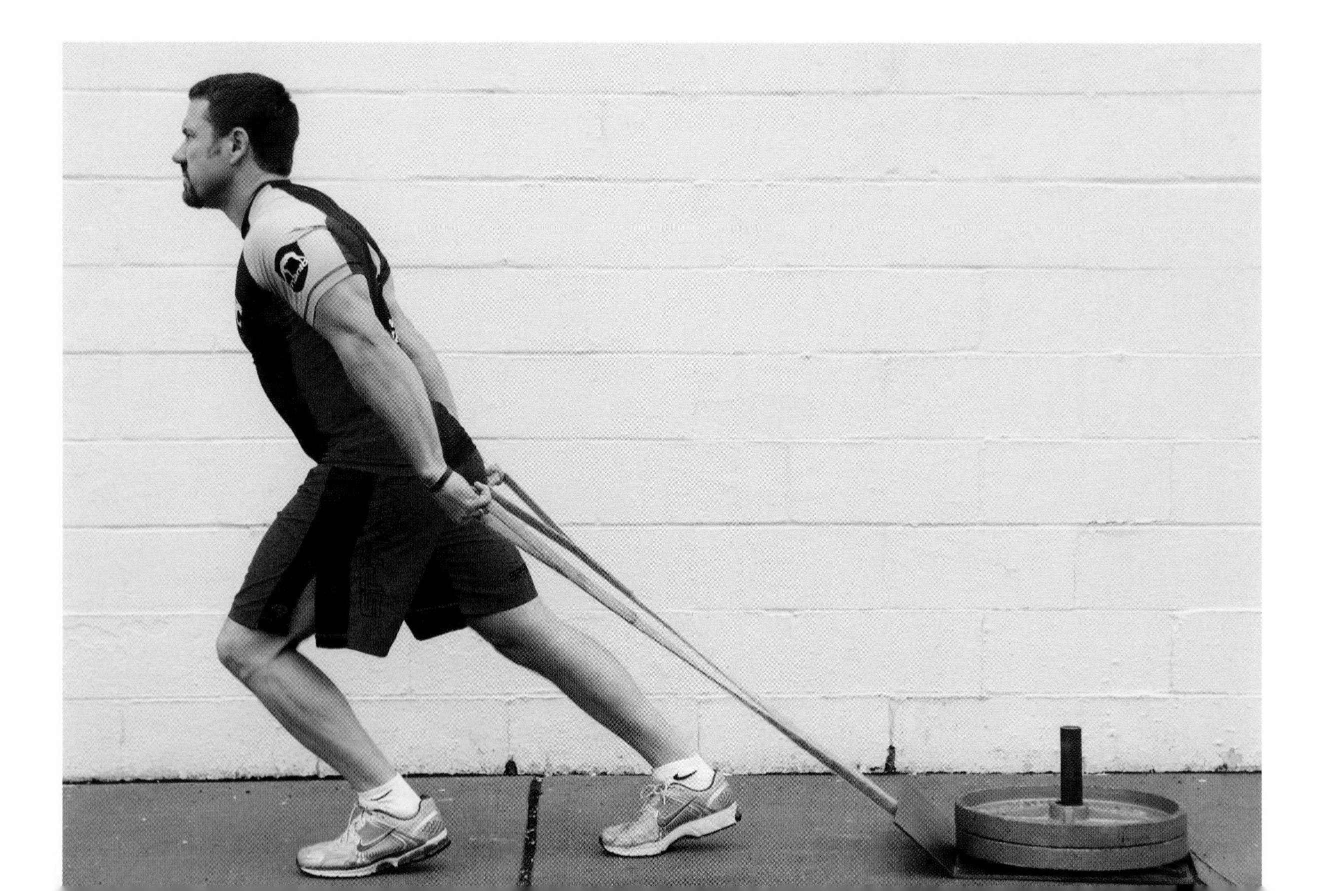

2. BACKWARD DRAG

Begin facing the sled, holding the ropes in the hands. Take small backward steps using a toe-to-heel relationship while leaning slightly backward.

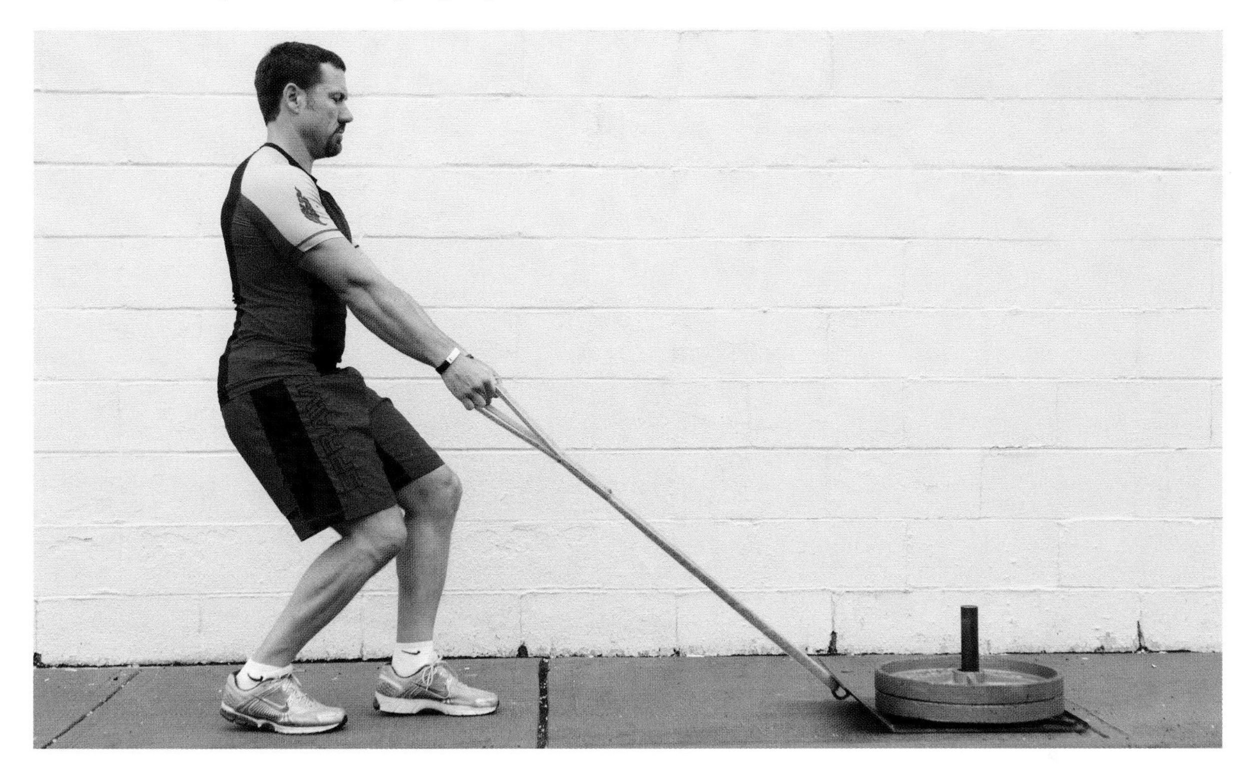

3. SIDEWAYS DRAG

Begin facing sideways to the sled with the ropes fastened around the waist. Take crossover steps while keeping the feet and hips facing perpendicular to the sled.

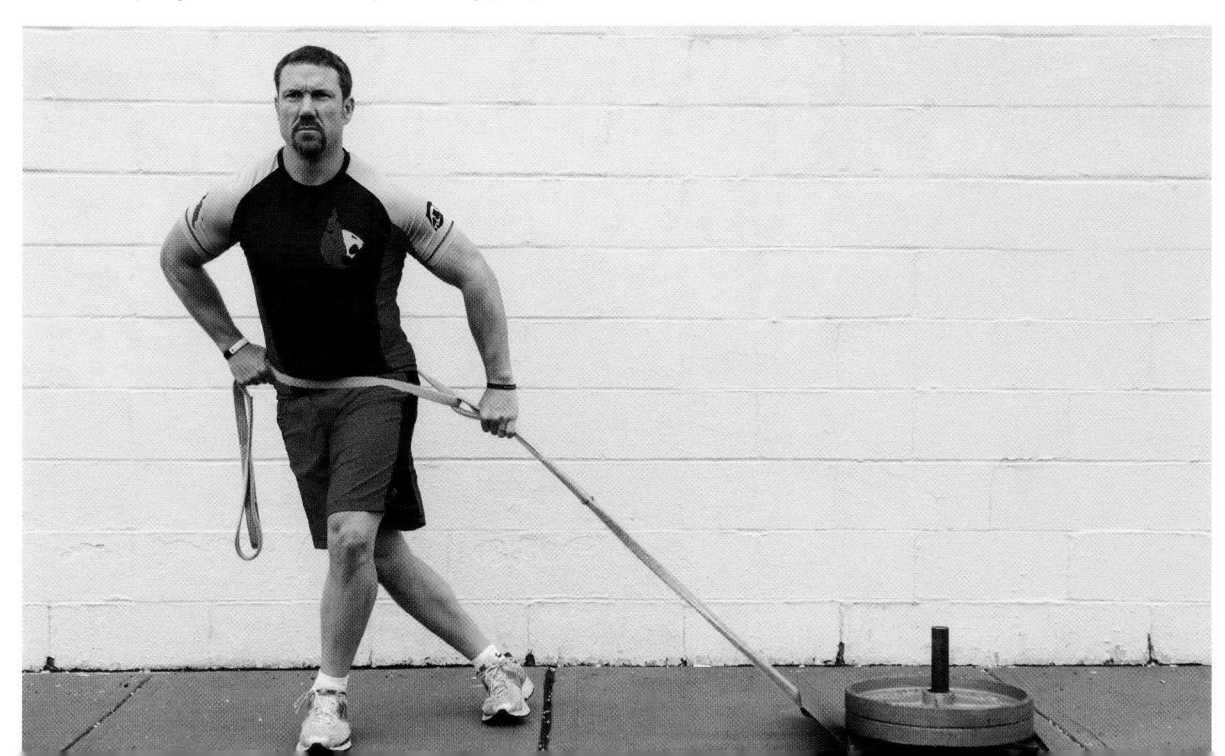

4. BEAR-CRAWL DRAG

Begin with your back to the sled, with your weight supported by the hands and feet and the ropes tied around the waist. Crawl forward to drag the sled.

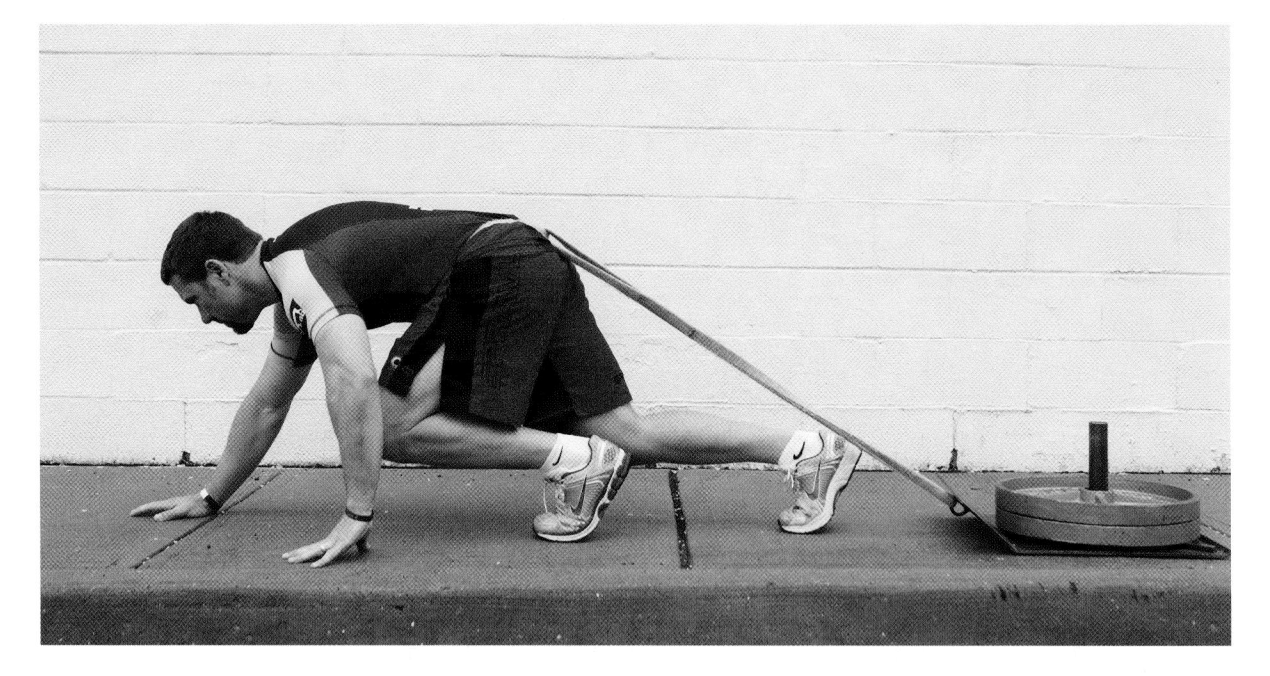

5. DUCK-WALK DRAG

Begin with your back to the sled, standing in a half-squat position with the hands holding the ropes in between the legs. While keeping the torso tall and the feet slightly wider than shoulder width, take steps forward.

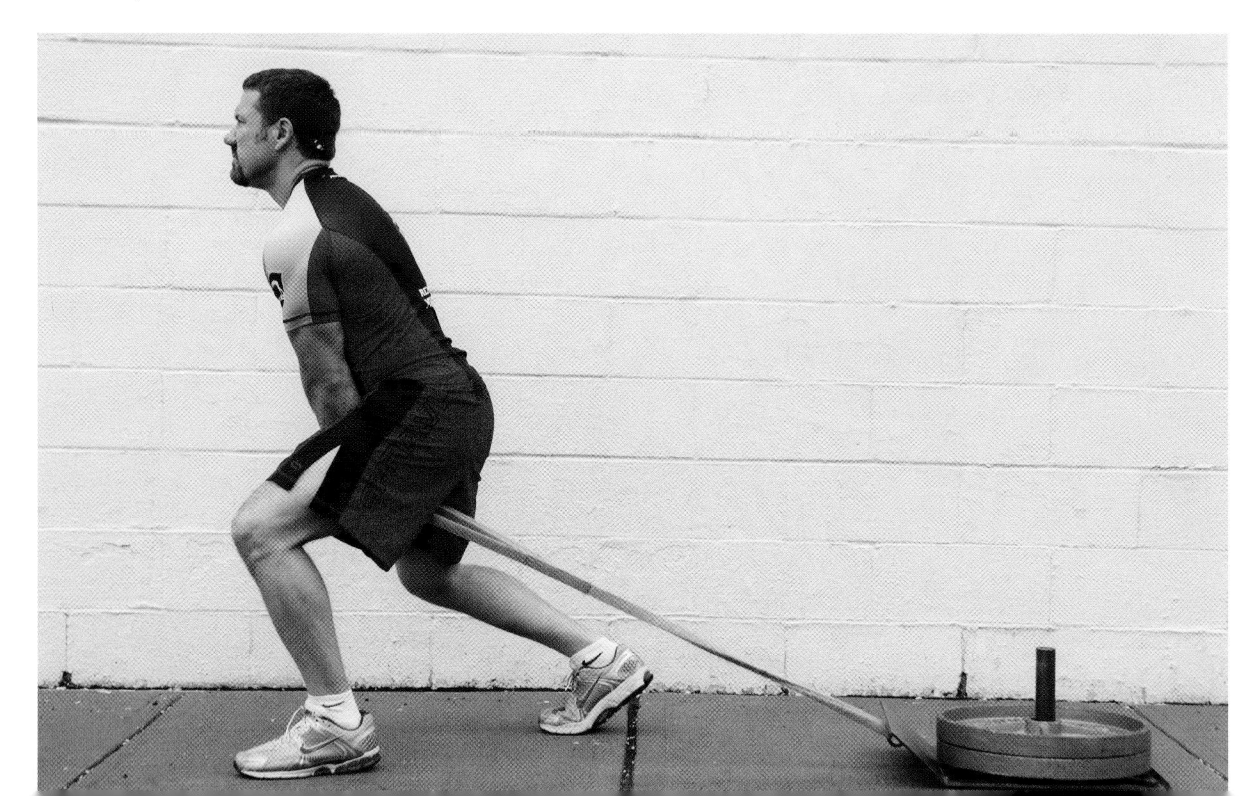

B. FINISHERS: PROWLER

The major difference between the sled and the Prowler is that this tool is used by pushing instead of pulling. This allows for more recruitment of the upper-body musculature in addition to the legs. The Prowler can be pushed for speed for sets of work and recovery or for distance and time. In the case of this finisher, the Prowler can be pushed 20 yards down with the high grip and back with the low grip for five total sets of each. These 200 yards can be covered quickly, but the demands on the body and mind are quite strenuous.

1. HIGH-GRIP PUSH

Begin with the hands on the high grips of the Prowler. Push into the sled and take as big a stride as possible, staying on the balls of the feet.

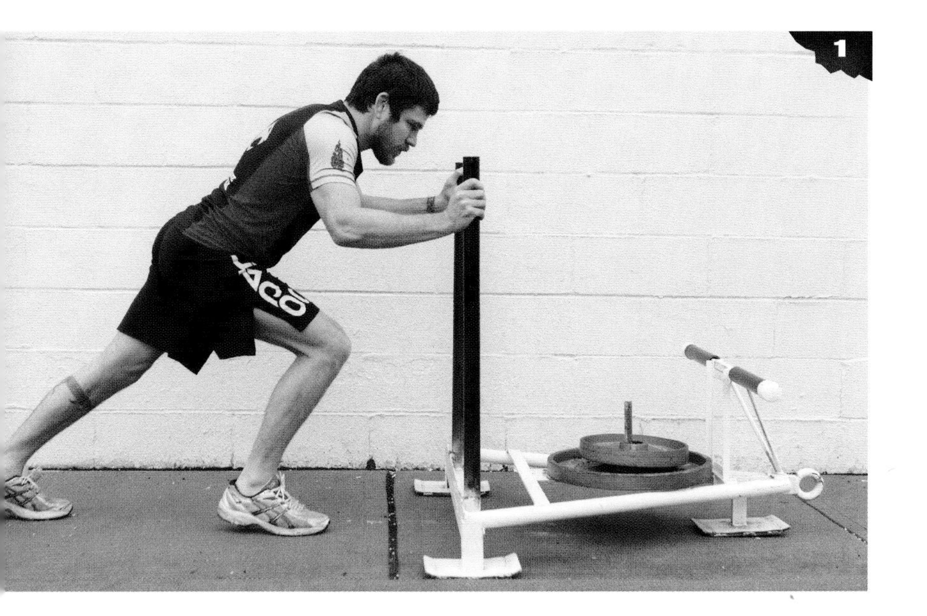

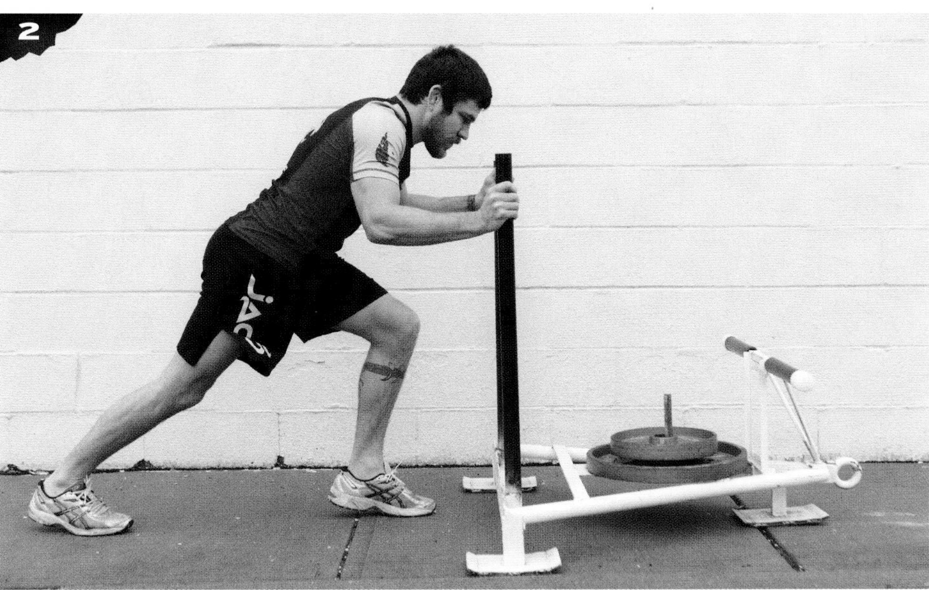

2. LOW-GRIP PUSH

Lean forward while keeping the core tight and place the hands on the low grips of the Prowler. Push into the sled and take as big a stride as possible, staying on the balls of the feet.

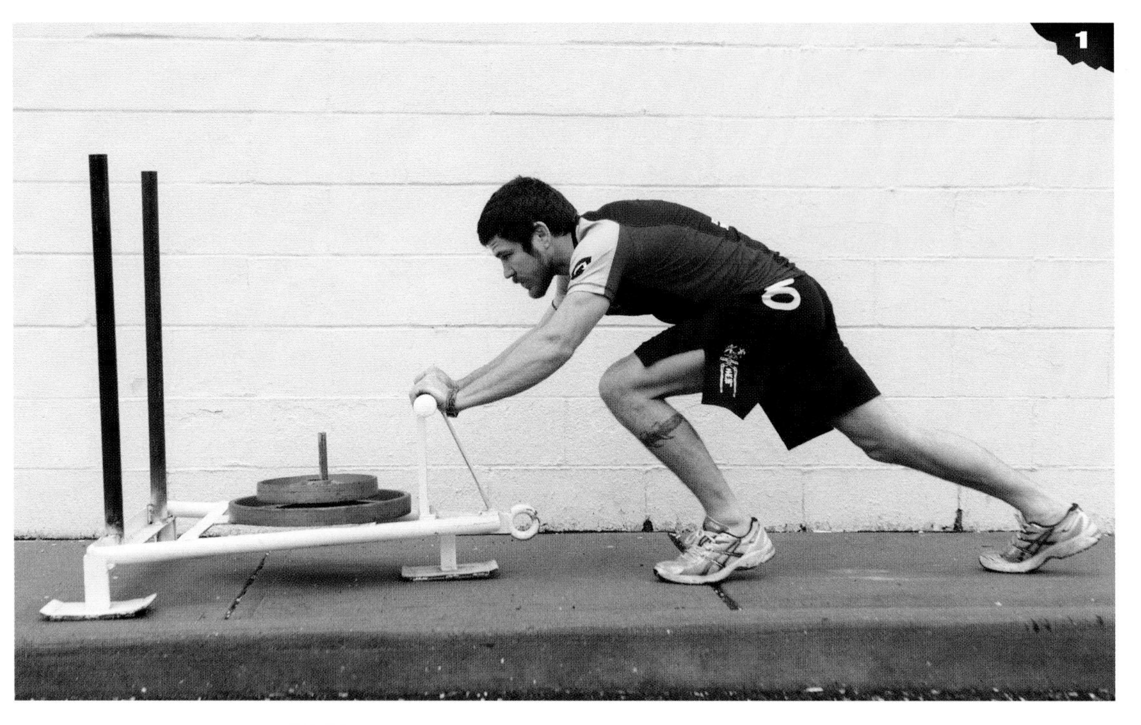

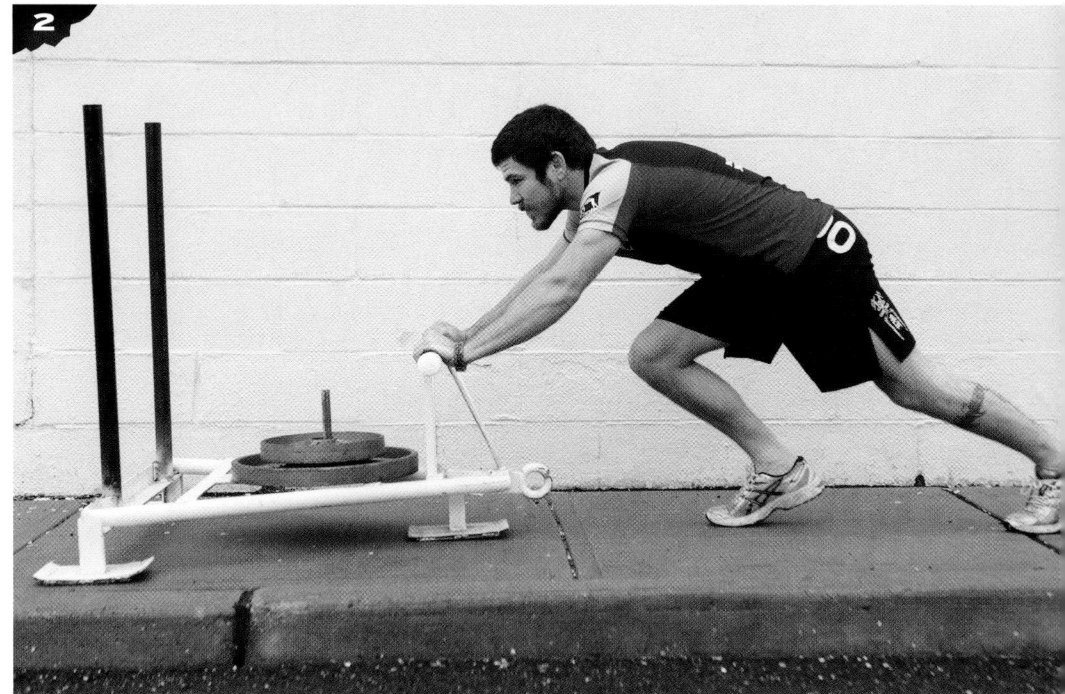

C. FINISHERS: PLATE PUSHES

Due to the plate's lack of height, this is perhaps the most demanding of the finishers. The Plate Push is very taxing for the legs (especially the quadriceps) and the shoulders. Since this finisher is difficult to perform, these pushes are performed as individual reps with greater rest periods in between than the previous two methods.

A sample Plate Push finisher workout would be to perform six 20-yard pushes down and back as fast as possible with 1 1/2 minutes' rest in between sets.

Begin with elbows extended and the hands on top of the plate on the ground. Push forward into the plate and take as big a stride as possible, staying on the balls of the feet.

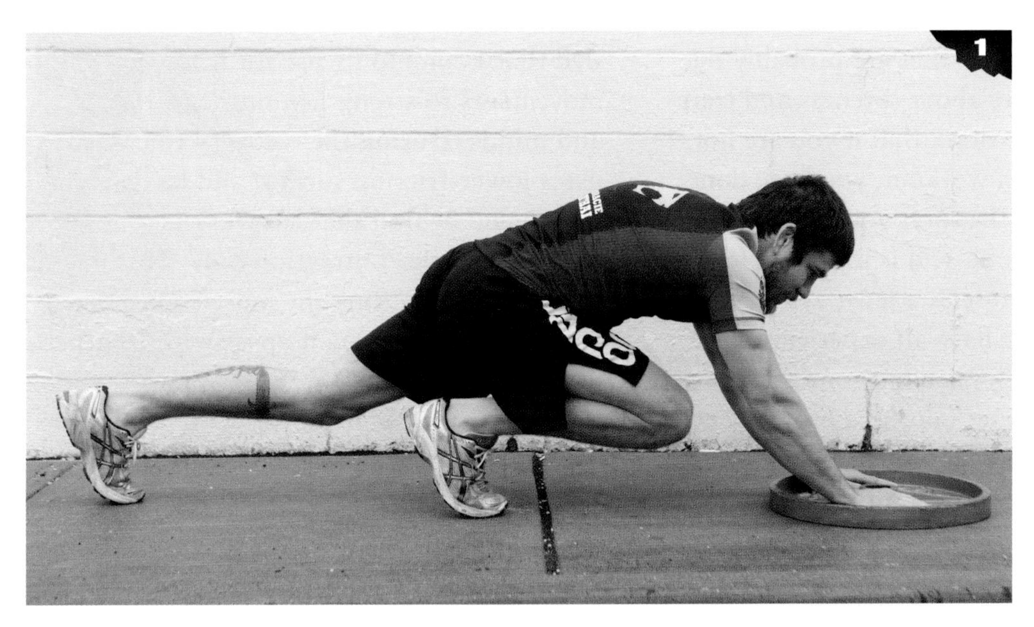

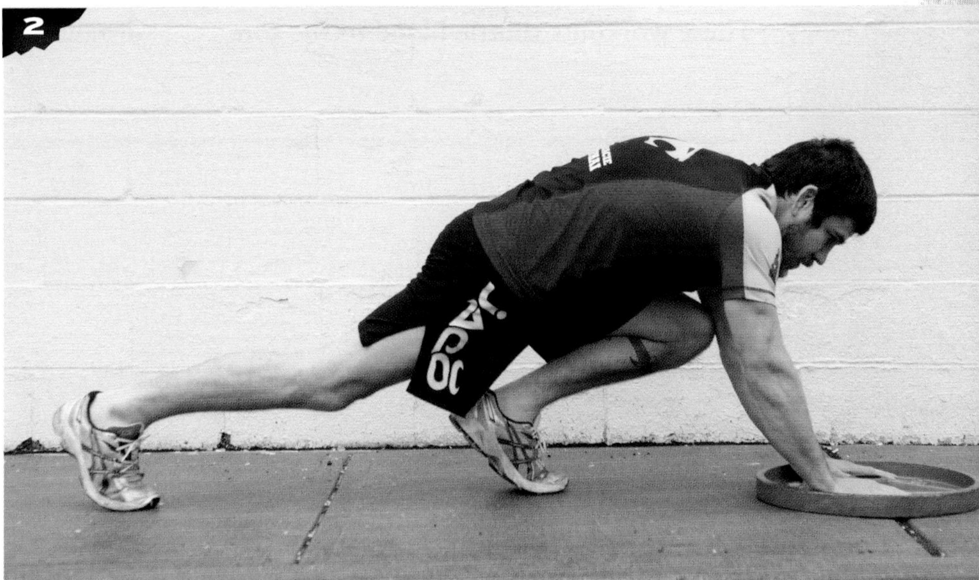

4. UPPER-BACK FLY

Begin facing the sled and start with arms out front, which is then turned into external rotation at the shoulder as the hands are brought up and palms turned to the sky.

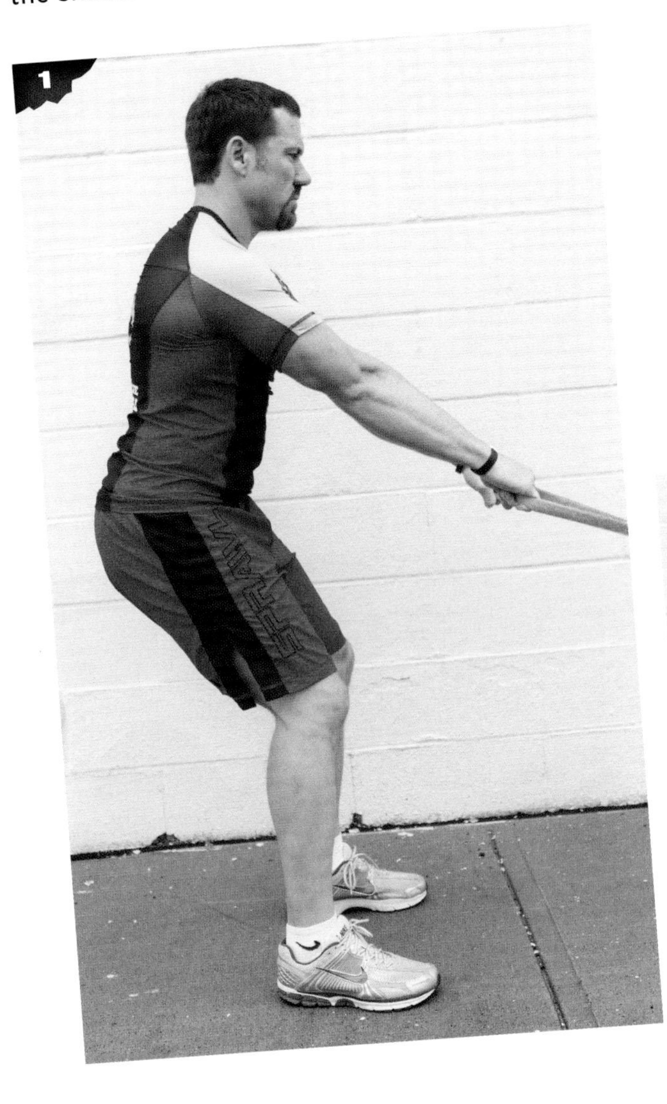

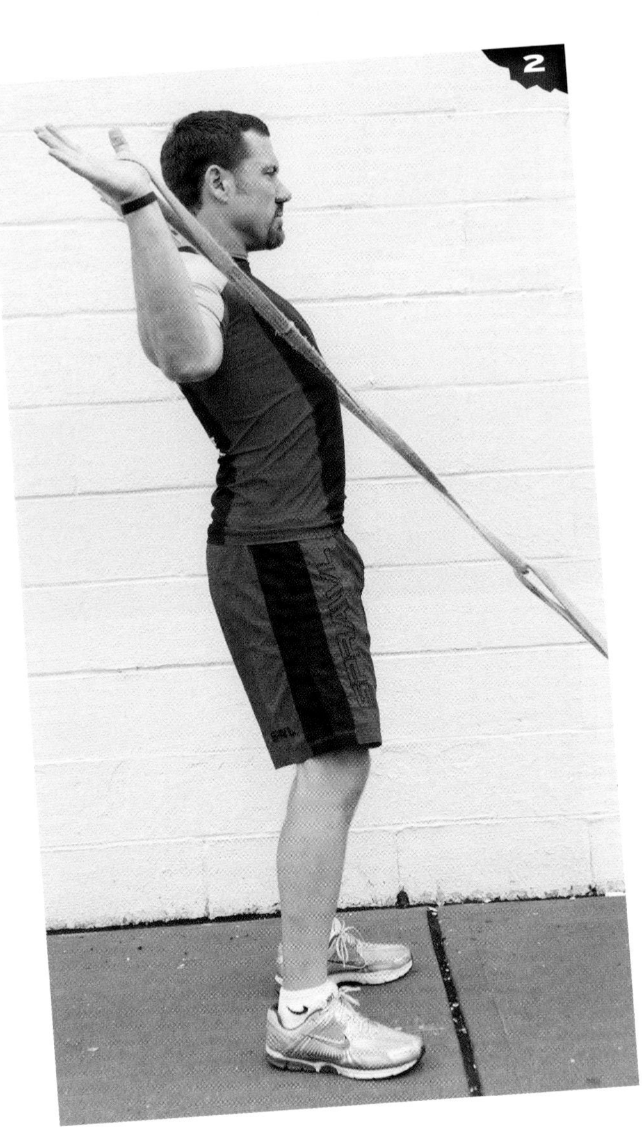

C. FINISHERS: PLATE PUSHES

Due to the plate's lack of height, this is perhaps the most demanding of the finishers. The Plate Push is very taxing for the legs (especially the quadriceps) and the shoulders. Since this finisher is difficult to perform, these pushes are performed as individual reps with greater rest periods in between than the previous two methods.

A sample Plate Push finisher workout would be to perform six 20-yard pushes down and back as fast as possible with 1 1/2 minutes' rest in between sets.

Begin with elbows extended and the hands on top of the plate on the ground. Push forward into the plate and take as big a stride as possible, staying on the balls of the feet.

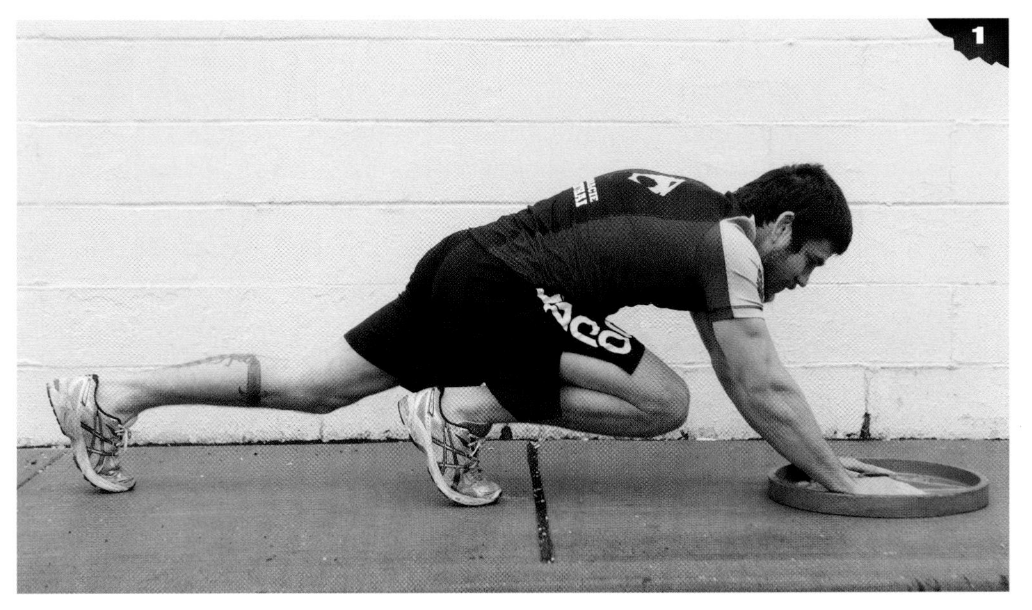

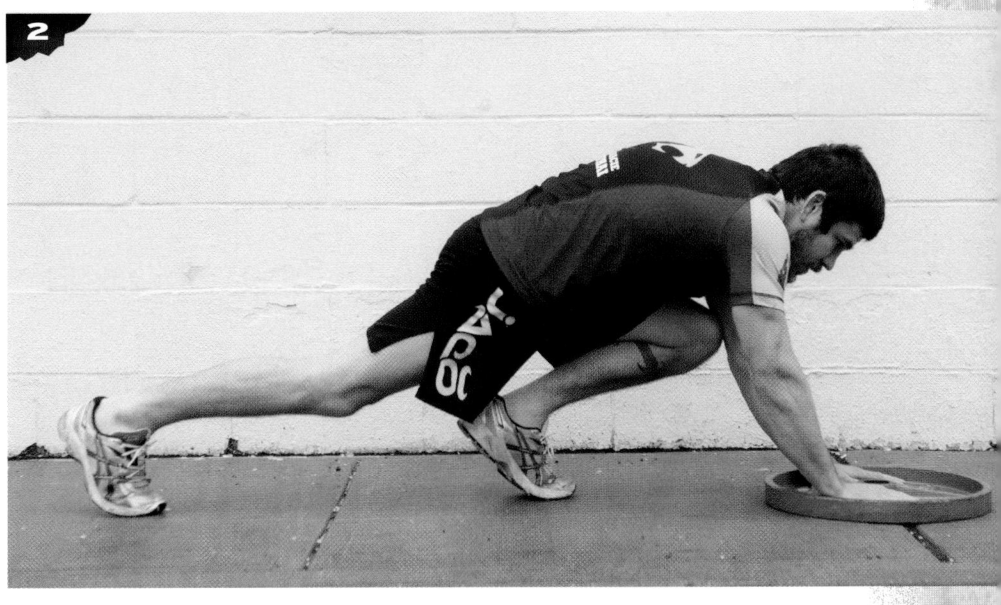

SLED ROUTINE FOR RECOVERY

The aim of the wise is not to secure pleasure, but to avoid pain.

—Aristotle

Over the last decade of training, I have had a lot of people throw different training "myths" out at me. Whether it was "lifting stunts your growth" or "eating too much protein shuts down your kidneys" or "too much strength will hurt your martial arts," I have heard them all. Two myths that are probably the most common are about soreness and training. First, people think that if you are not really sore after a workout, you have done nothing, or that the sorer you are, the better. Second is that lactic acid is the cause for the soreness in the muscles a few days after training. I am sure we have all experienced this post-training pain phenomenon, and some of you martial athletes out there probably even seek it out on a regular basis.

When my athletes are sore from a previous workout, I have put together "shuttle" workouts to help minimize additional damage and possibly assist in faster healing. These workouts shuttle blood to the sore areas of the body, and increase circulation and muscle temperature without damaging the muscle with high eccentric tensions. We use these workouts often, with great results. Even though after 3 to 7 days, soreness will naturally be gone if you just rest, this may not be practical in your training. The shuttle workout allows the fighters to feel that they are not taking the day off, and still getting in a workout. To accomplish this, I use the sled that I commonly use for heavy pulling movements to strengthen our legs, hearts, and minds. During the recovery routine, I use a lower-friction surface and less weight. The magic behind the sled work is that it uses concentric contraction only. This means that you are working the muscle by shortening it, but not ripping it apart with lengthening tension.

Below is a list of my favorite exercises and how to perform them. As you will see, the sled is a very versatile tool and there are many exercises that you can create to help work around the pain. Each exercise can be performed for sets of 20 reps, or you can just cover a certain distance like I do—25 yards per set.

D. SLED RECOVERY WORKOUT

1. CLEAN PULL

Begin facing the sled, pull the straps toward the body, and raise the arms up overhead as you stand and lean back.

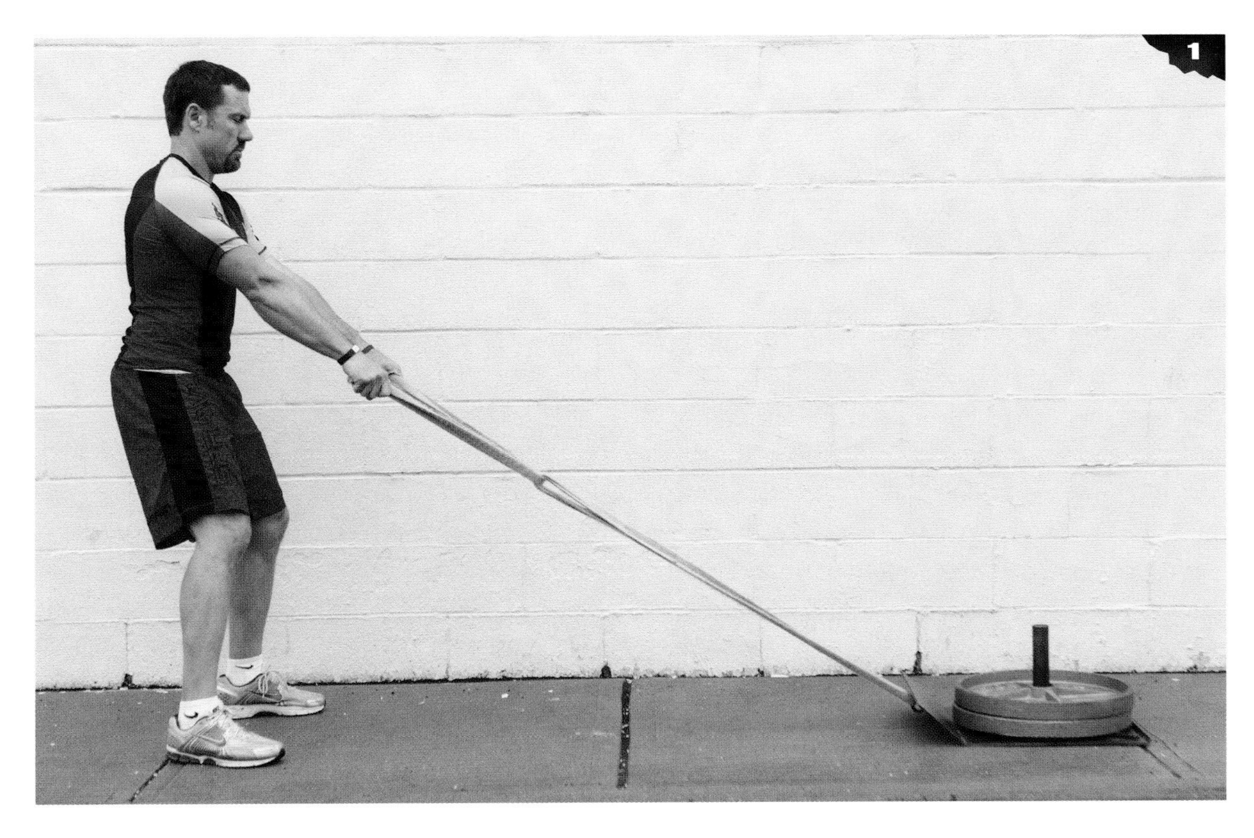

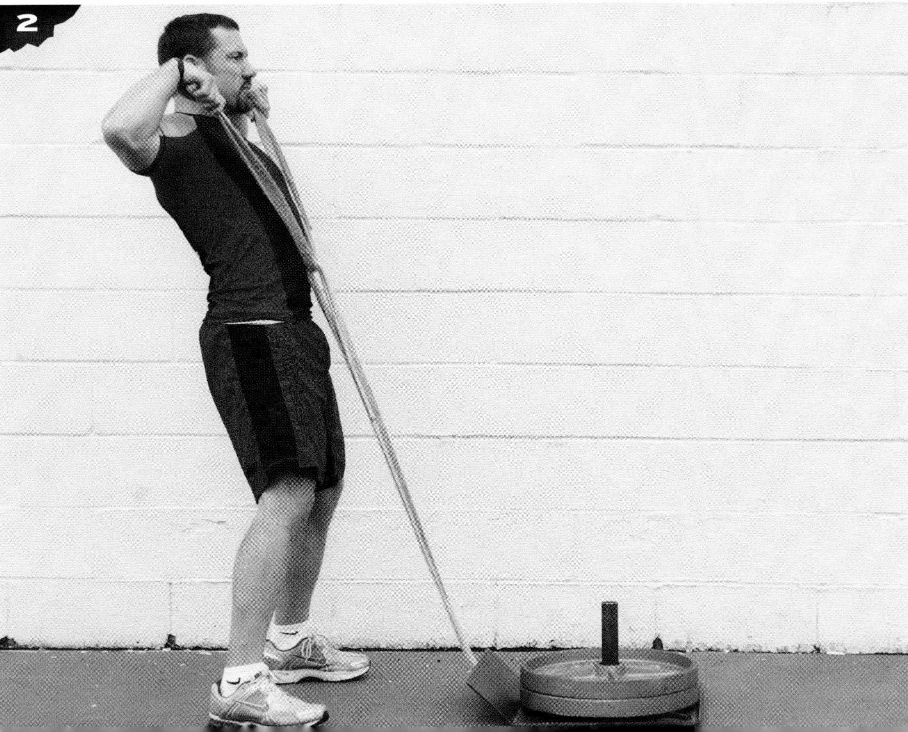

2. BICEP/CHEST PRESS

Begin facing away from the sled and first curl the weight forward, then raise the arms up and press them out in front of the body.

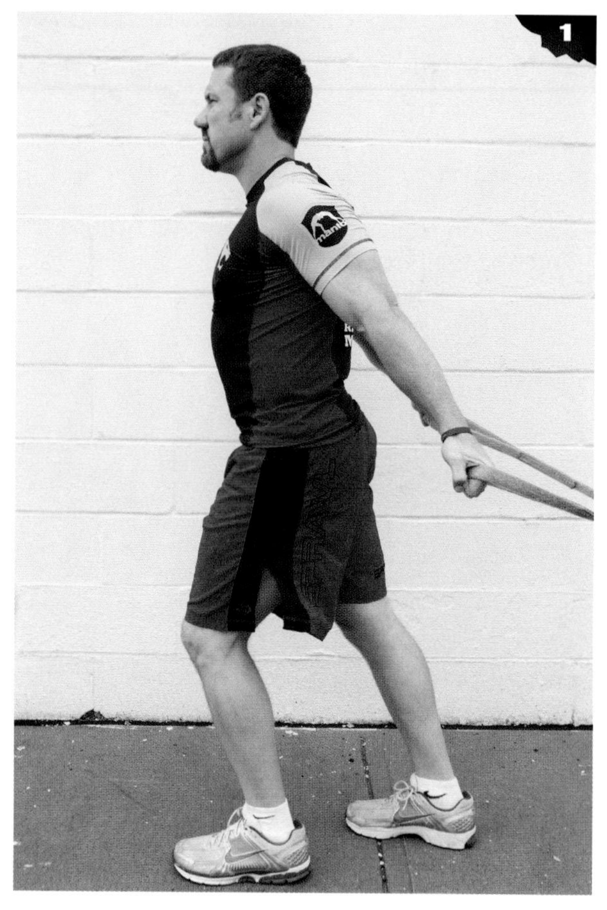

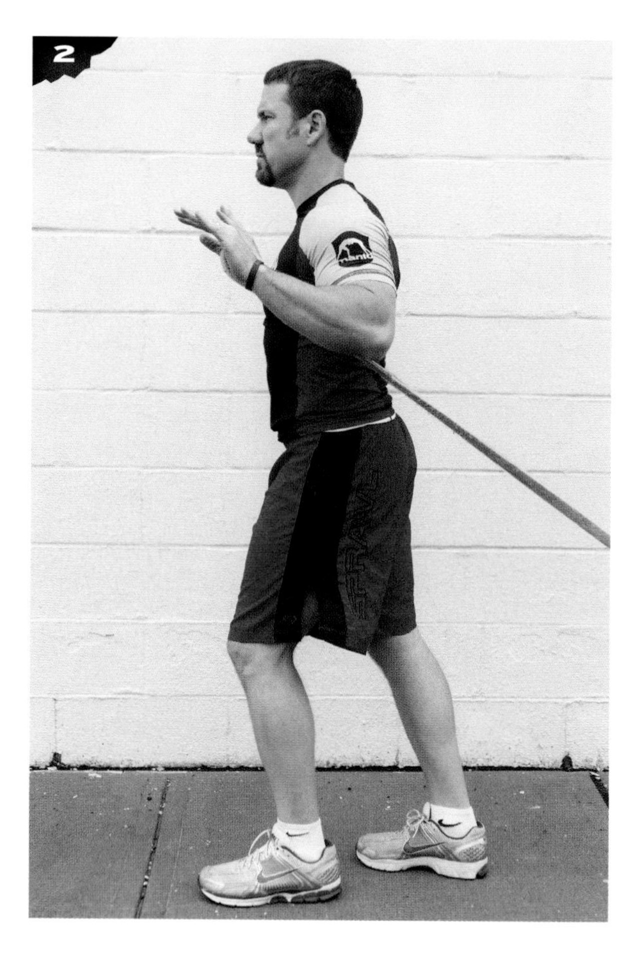

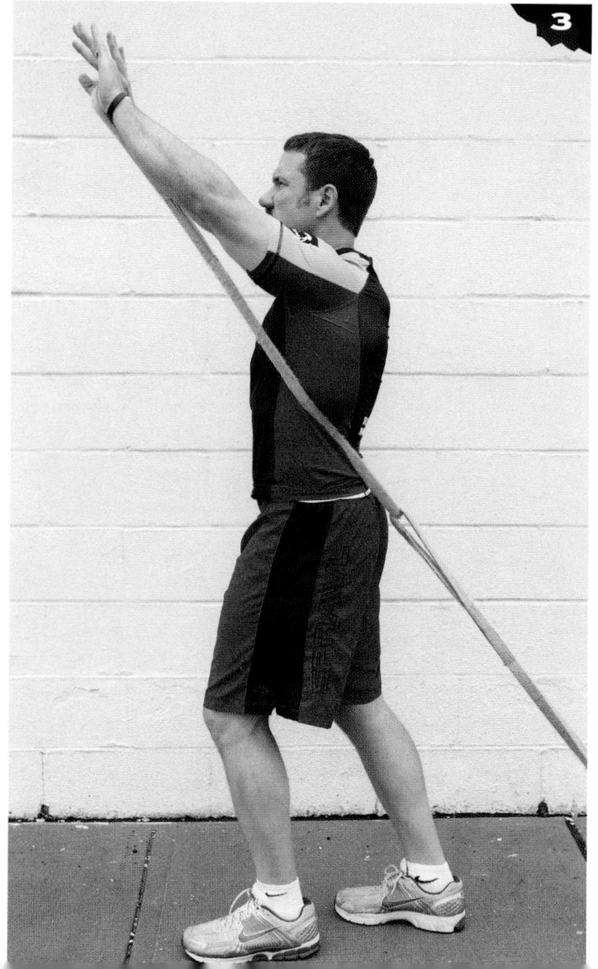

3. SWIM STROKE

Begin facing the sled and start with the body bent at the waist and hands held out front. Then "swim" the arms past the body and then up and back.

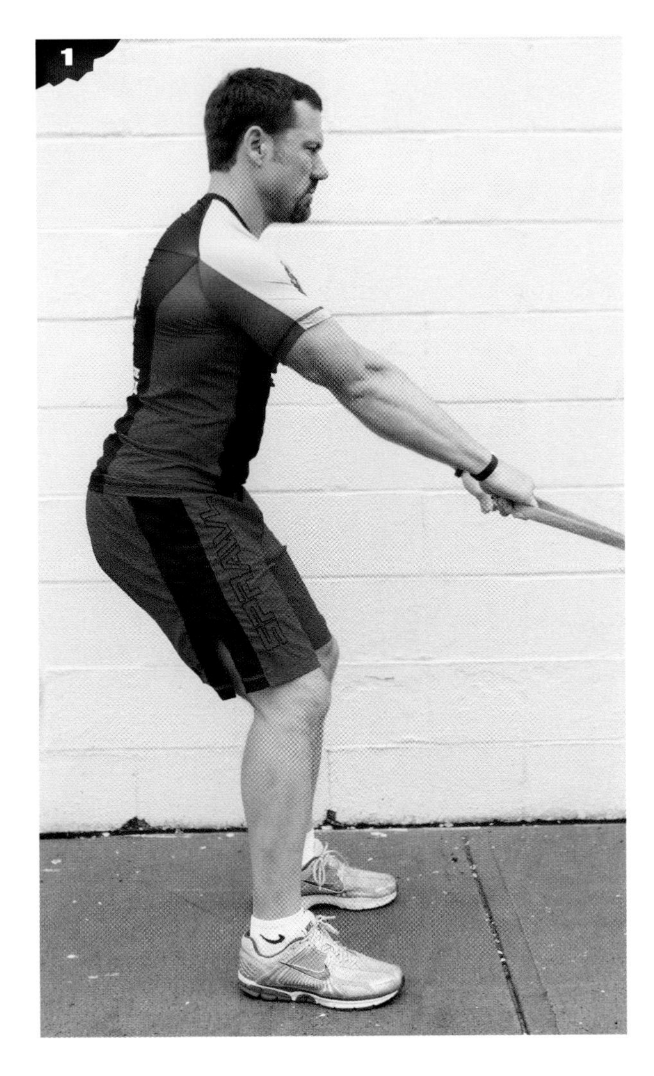

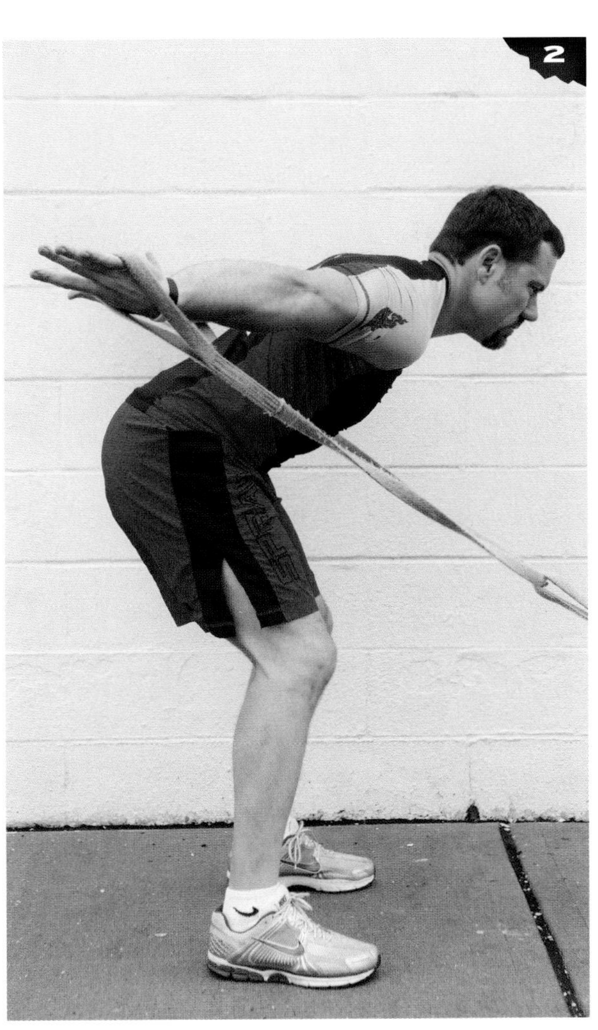

4. UPPER-BACK FLY

Begin facing the sled and start with arms out front, which is then turned into external rotation at the shoulder as the hands are brought up and palms turned to the sky.

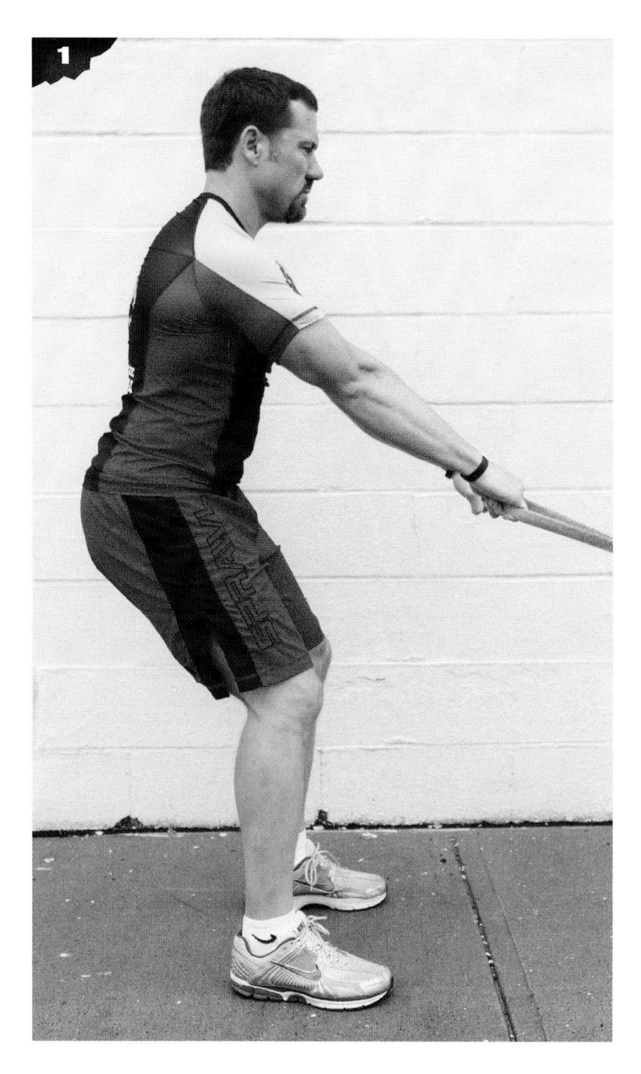

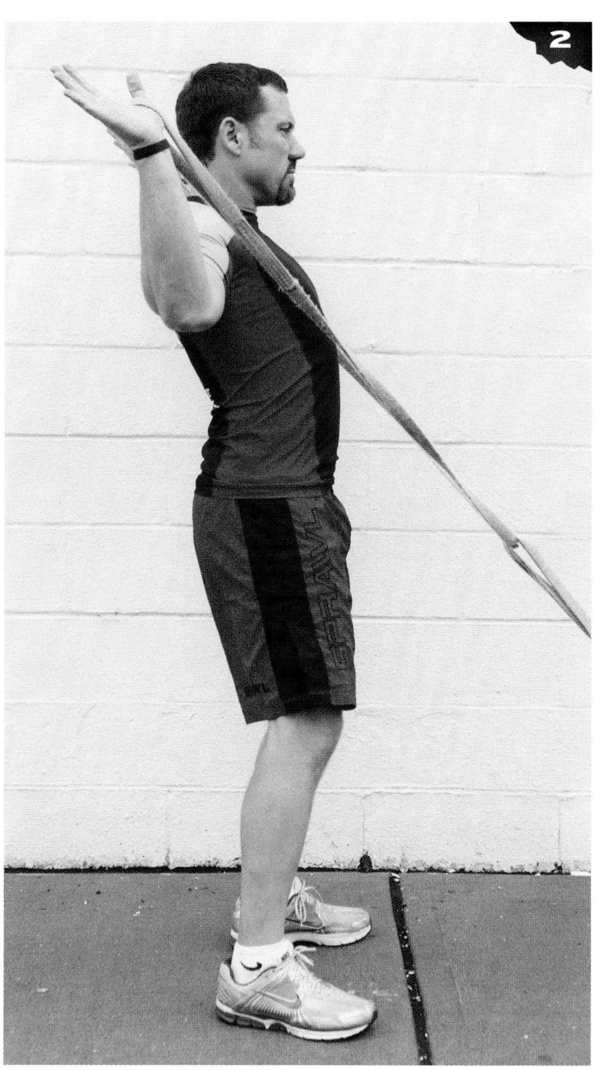

5. CORE ROTATION

Begin facing sideways to the sled and start with the feet pointed slightly forward, but with the arms reaching back to the sled. Then, keeping the foot position, twist the arms and torso to move the sled.

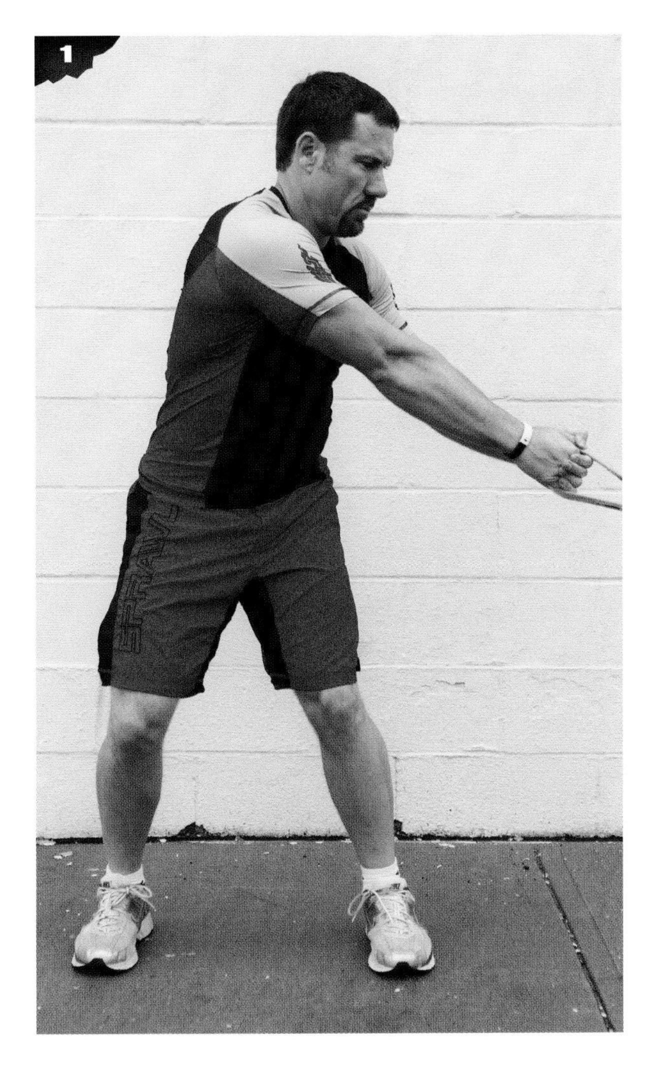

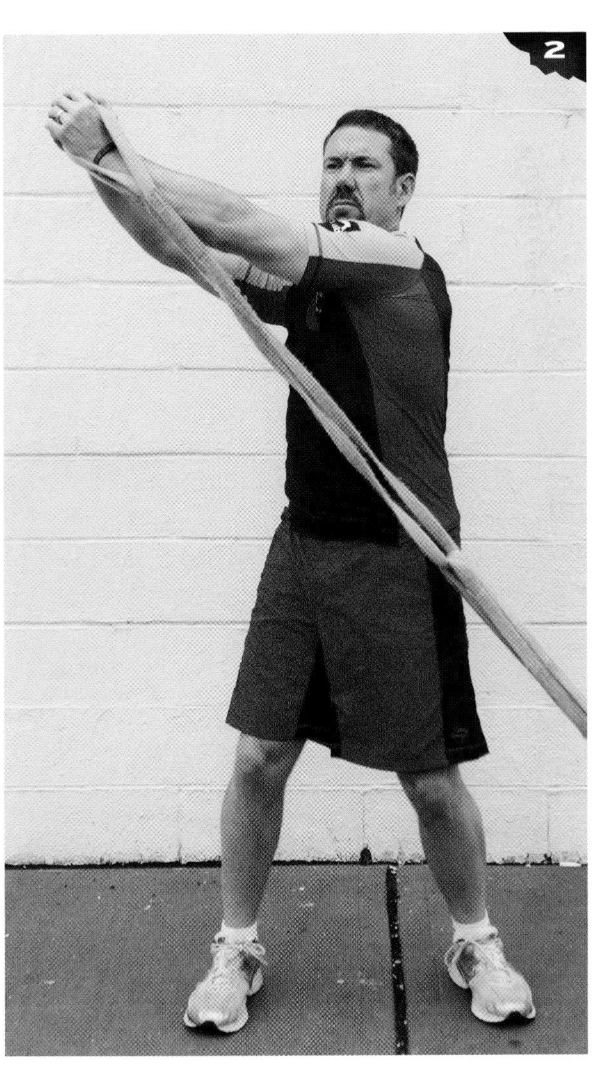

6. TRICEP

Begin facing away from the sled with the triceps stretched. Press the hands forward, pull the sled, and then repeat.

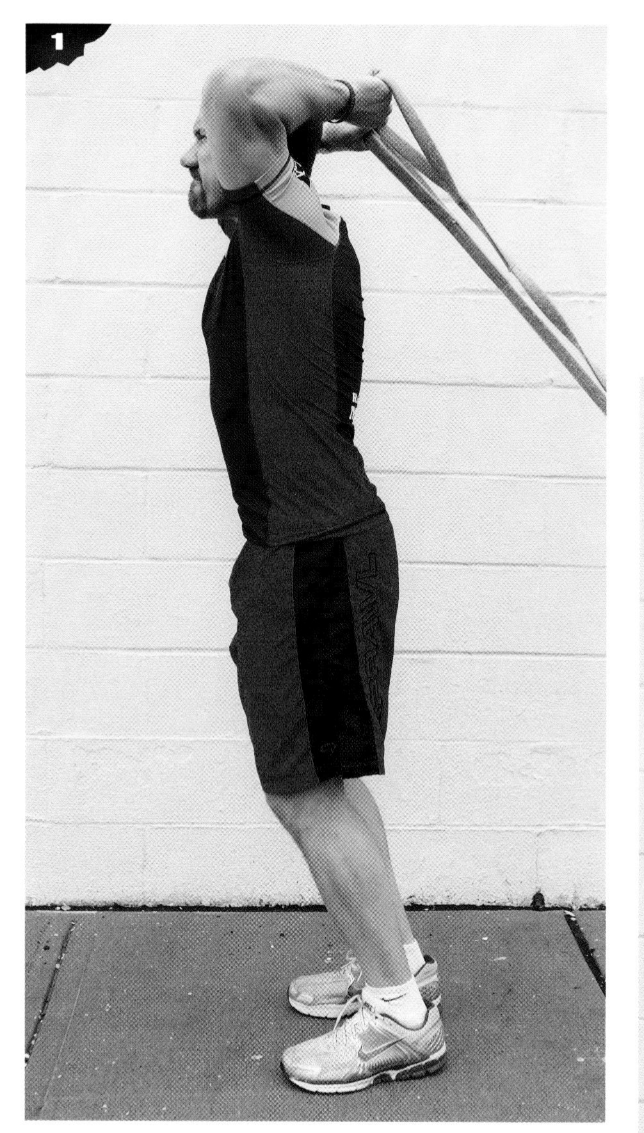

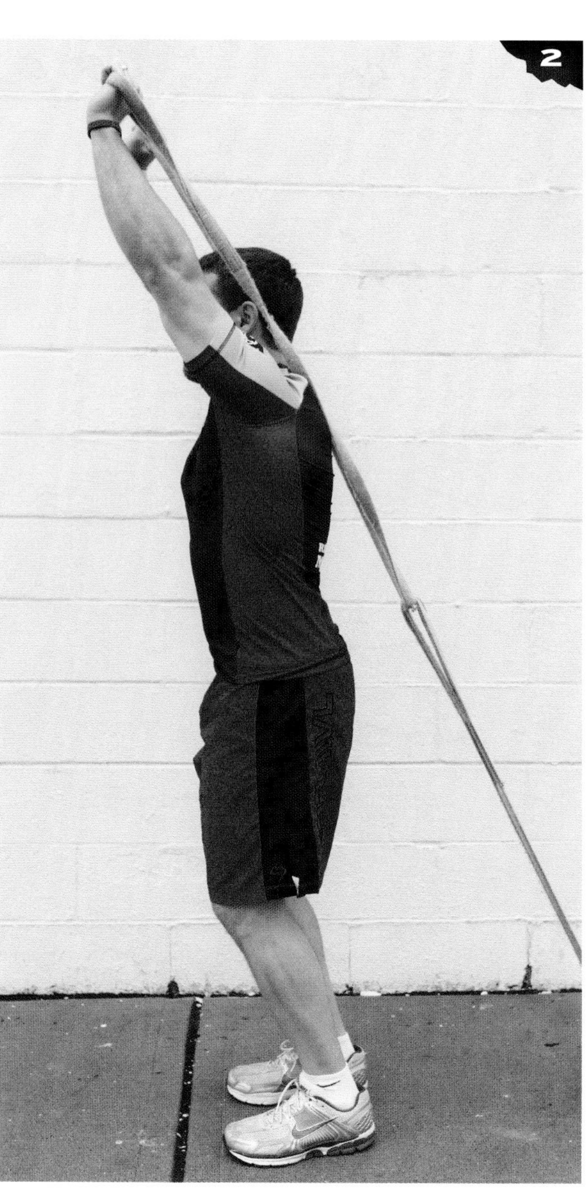

7. ABDOMINAL CURL

Begin facing away from the sled with the straps riding over the shoulders. Flex at the waist to pull the sled forward. Stand up, re-create tension, and repeat.

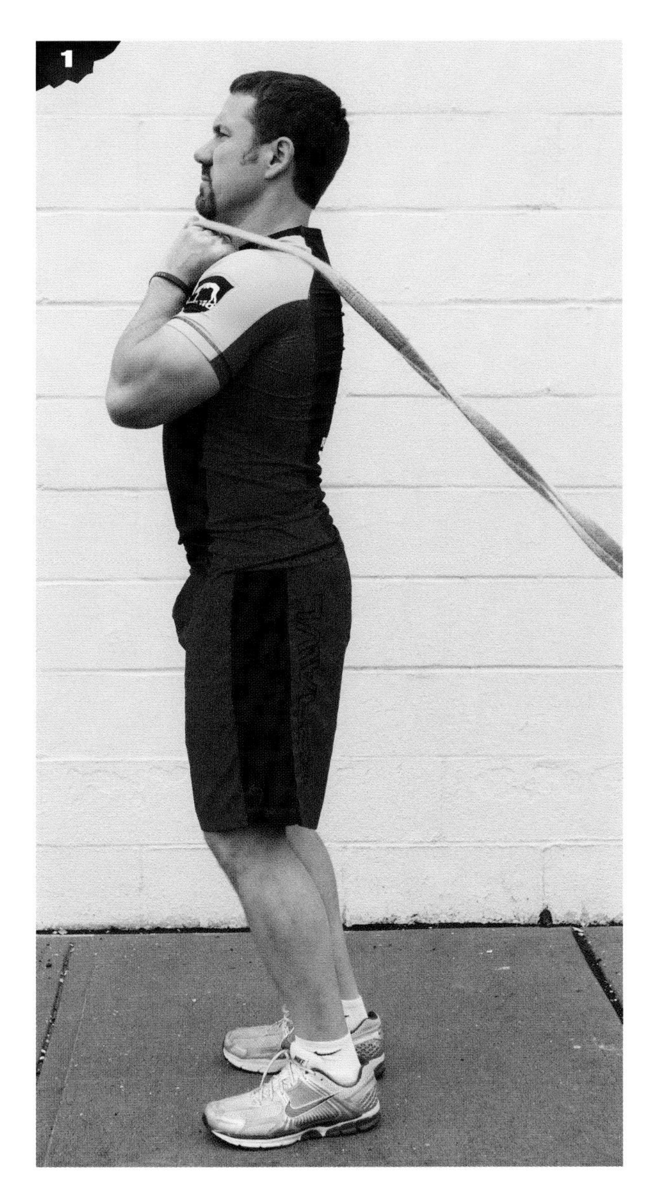

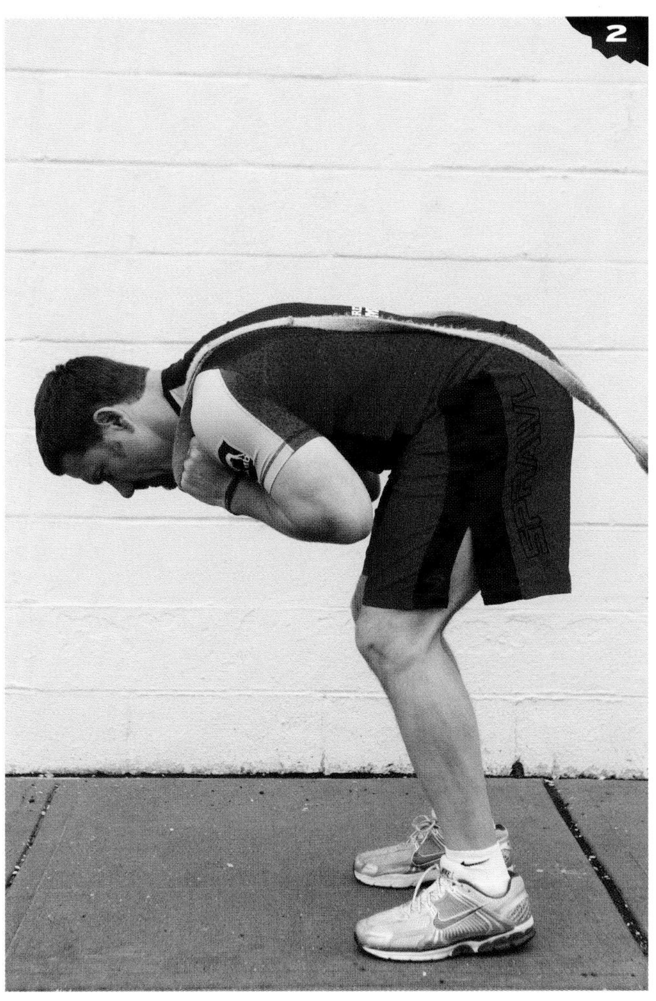

8. T-ROW

Begin facing the sled with the arms extended out front. With the elbows extended and the arms parallel to the ground, bring the hands straight backward.

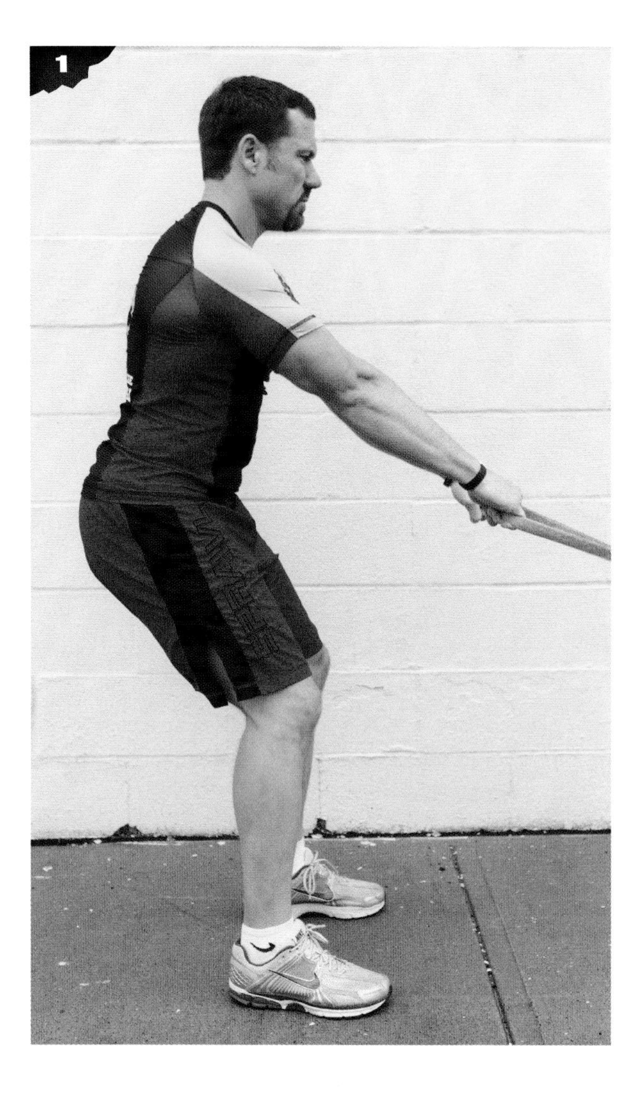

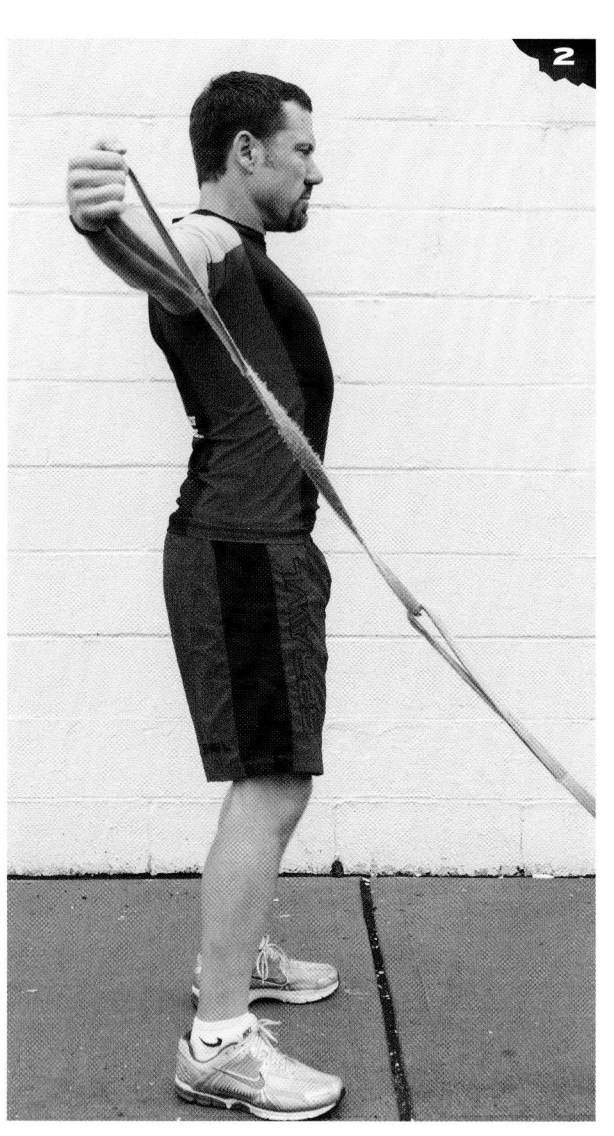

SLED RECOVERY WORKOUT CHEATSHEET

1. CLEAN PULL

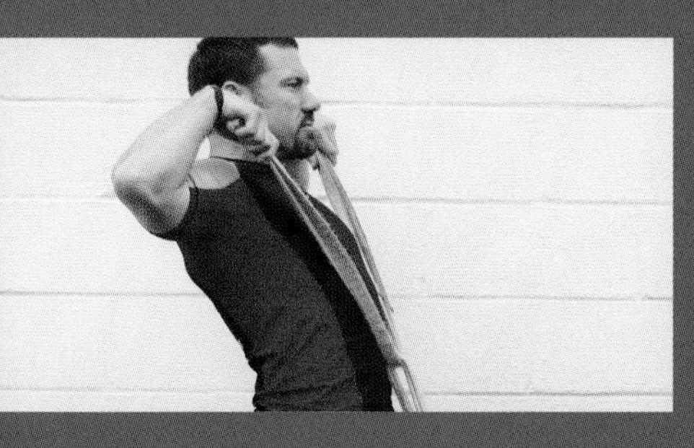

2. BICEP/CHEST PRESS

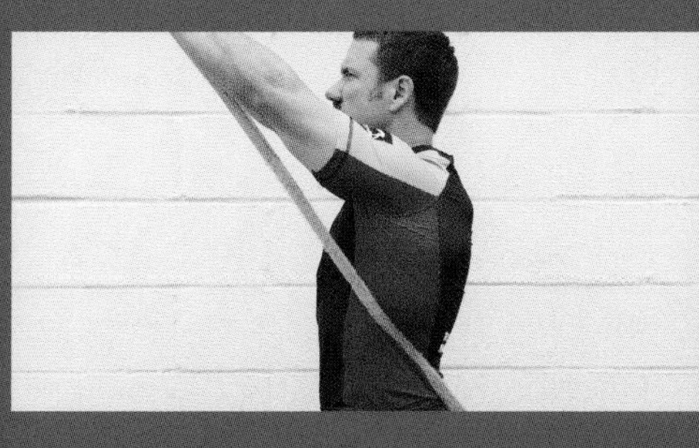

3. SWIM STROKE

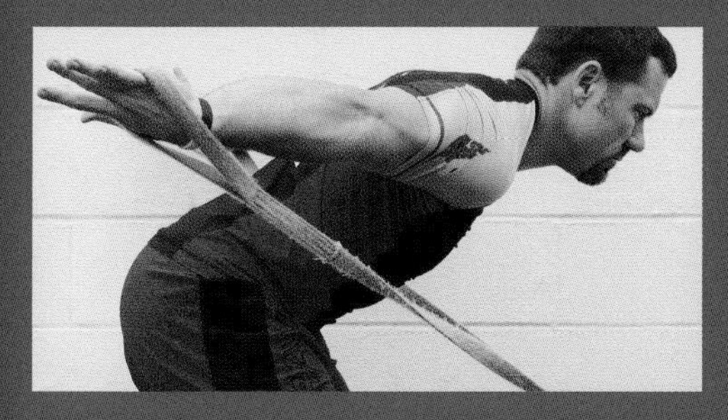

4. UPPER-BACK FLY

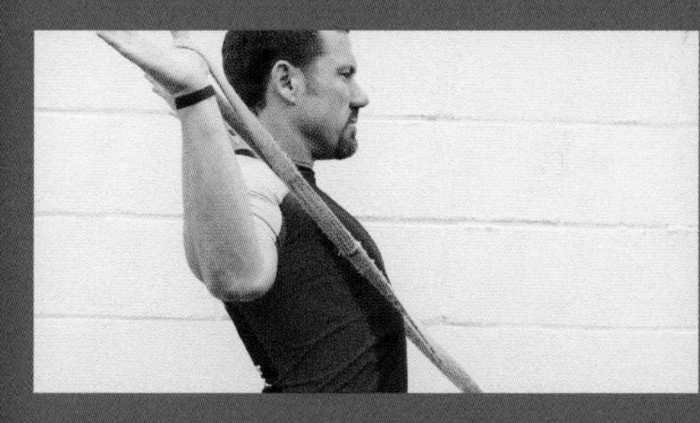

5. CORE ROTATION

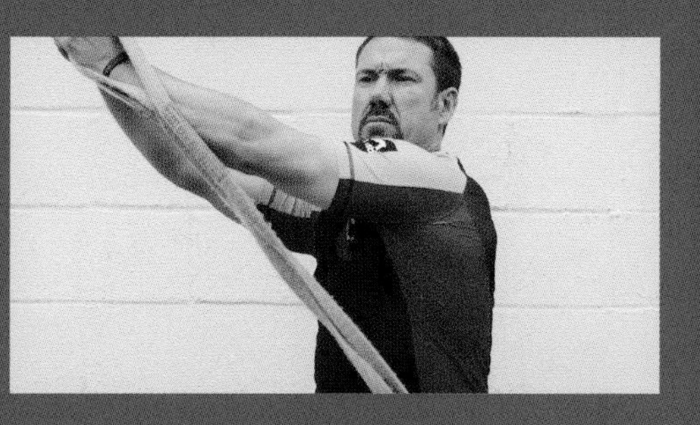

6. TRICEP

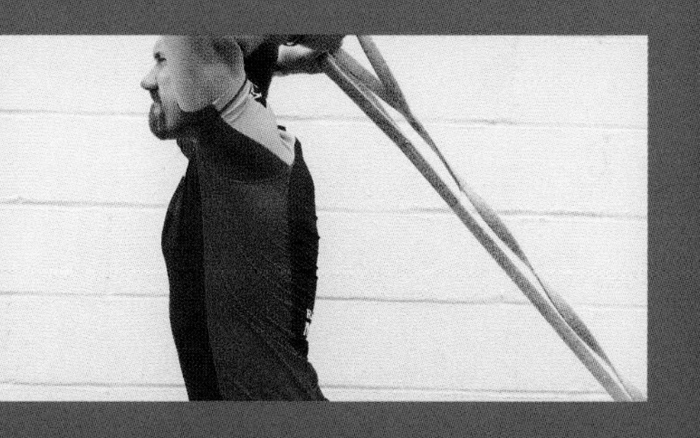

7. ABDOMINAL CURL

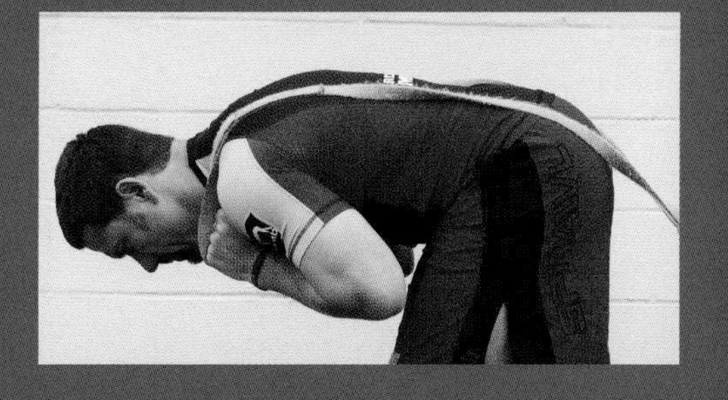

8. T-ROW

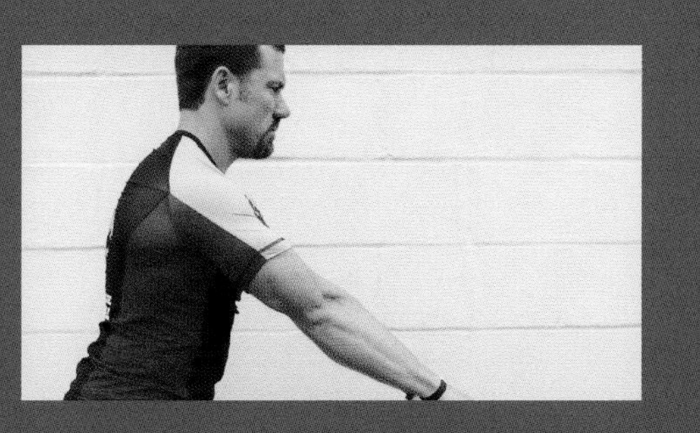

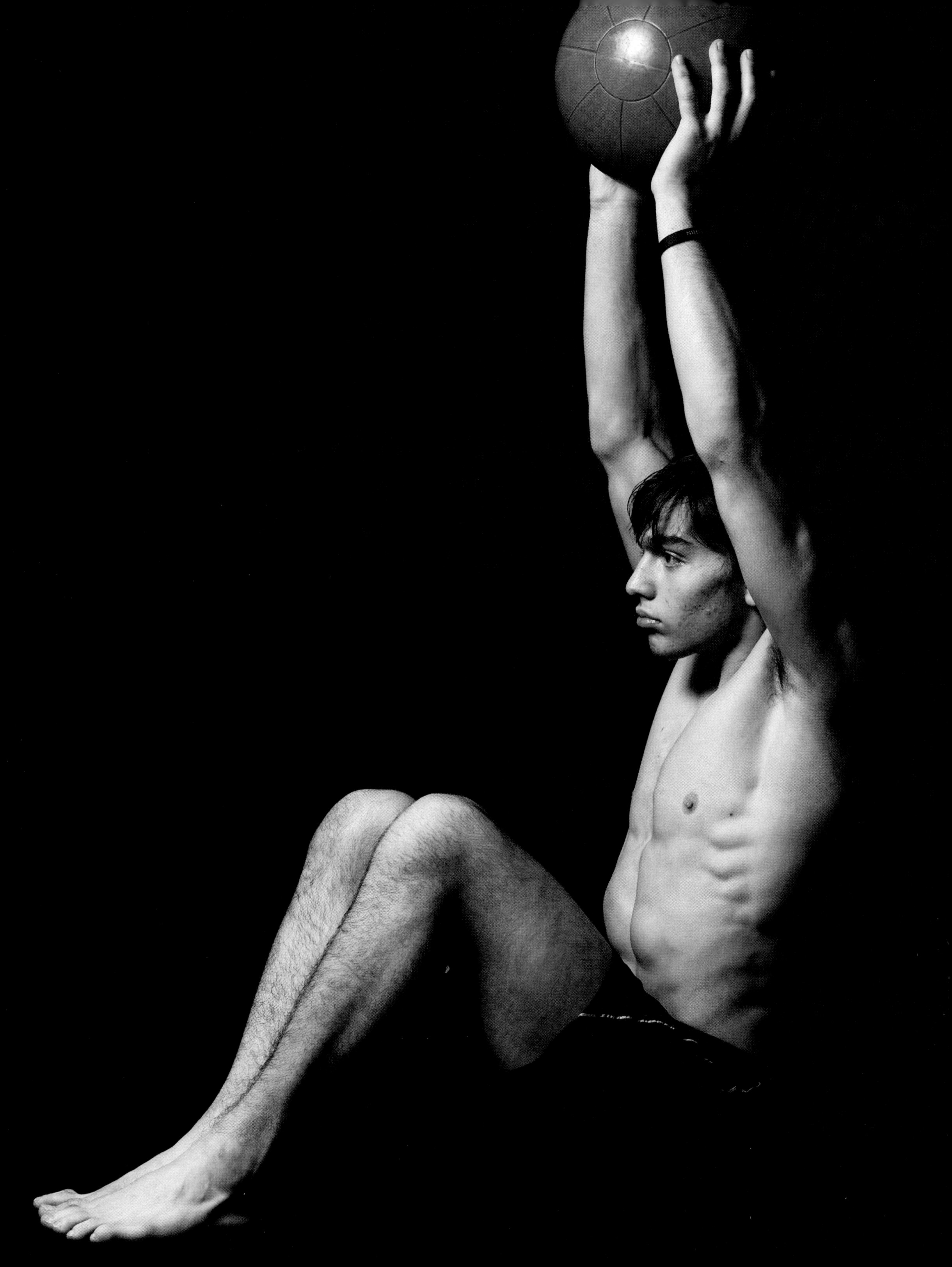

15

CORE TRAINING WORKOUTS

In the last decade, the "core" has become perhaps the hottest topic in fitness. This style of training has evolved from sit-ups to crunches to planks, with a thousand variations of each exercise in between. There are new pieces of training equipment produced almost daily that claim to somehow give you the rock-hard and lean midsection of which you've always dreamed.

To be precise, the core is defined as the region of the body in between the hips and the shoulders. So, even though we pay particular attention to the abdominal muscles in the front of our bodies, the core also includes the muscles on the sides and the back.

The muscles of the core must be strong to stabilize the body as well as be strong enough to transfer the forces from our lower body to our upper body during normal and athletic movement. Without a strong and stable core, decreased performance and injury may occur.

During many of the workouts contained in this book, the core region of the body is being challenged. Movements like pushups, chin-ups, sledgehammer swings, and deadlifts all recruit and develop the core. As a result of this, I have decided to place the core training circuits at the end of the book. These are to be performed at the end of Warrior Cardio sessions to bring both the heart rate back down and the session to a close.

The goal of these routines is not to challenge the heart, but to develop some strength and stability in the core. Although these exercises are often skipped, the execution of these routines will enhance your fitness and better prepare you for future workouts.

A. REGULAR PLANK CIRCUIT

To perform the circuit, perform the exercises in a row for 40 seconds each. If the exercise is unilateral, perform it on each side for 20 seconds. Perform the circuit for 2 total sets.

1. PLANK

Begin lying on your stomach with the elbows at the sides. Press into the ground with the elbows and toes, and lift the stomach from the ground while keeping the core tight and the back straight.

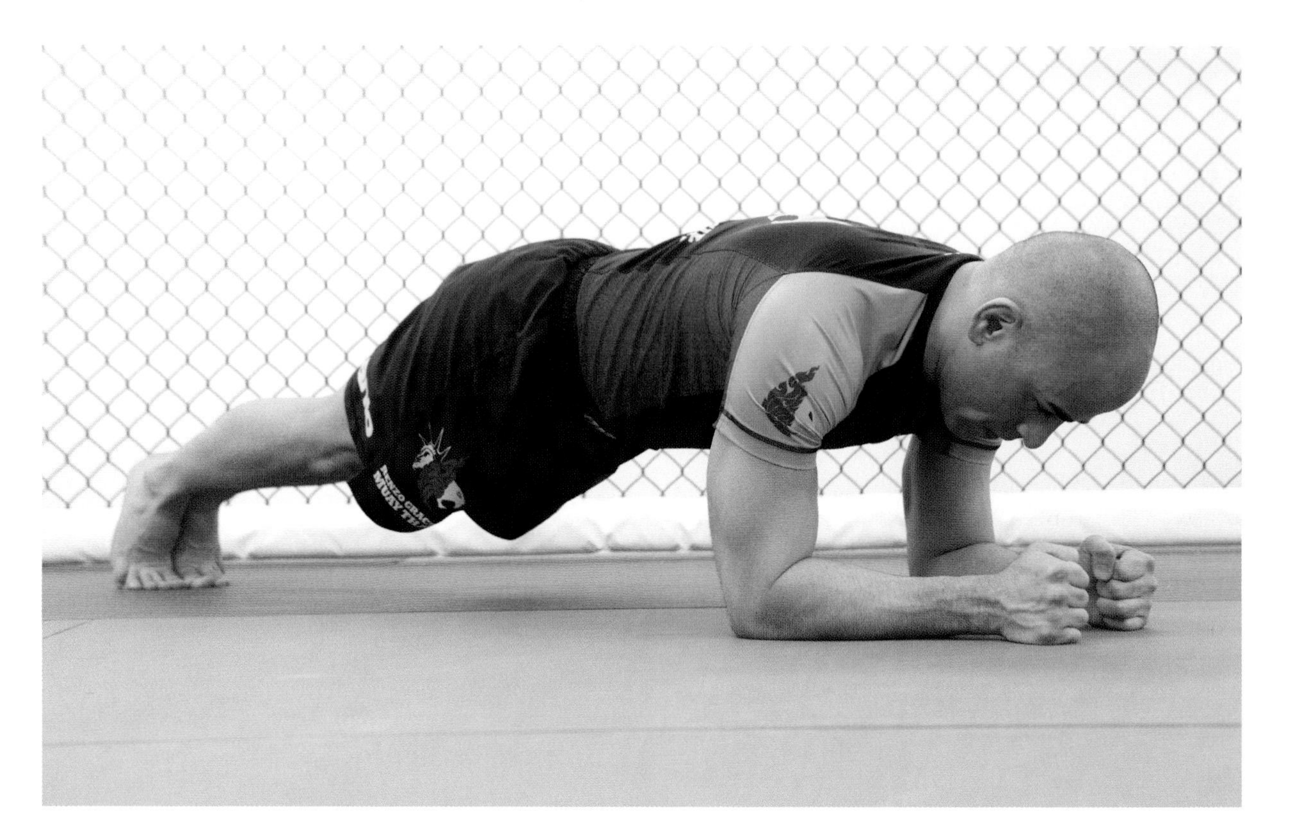

2. SINGLE-ARM PLANK

Begin lying on your stomach with the elbows at the sides. Press into the ground with the elbows and toes and lift the stomach from the ground while keeping the core tight and the back straight. Extend one arm out in front of the body.

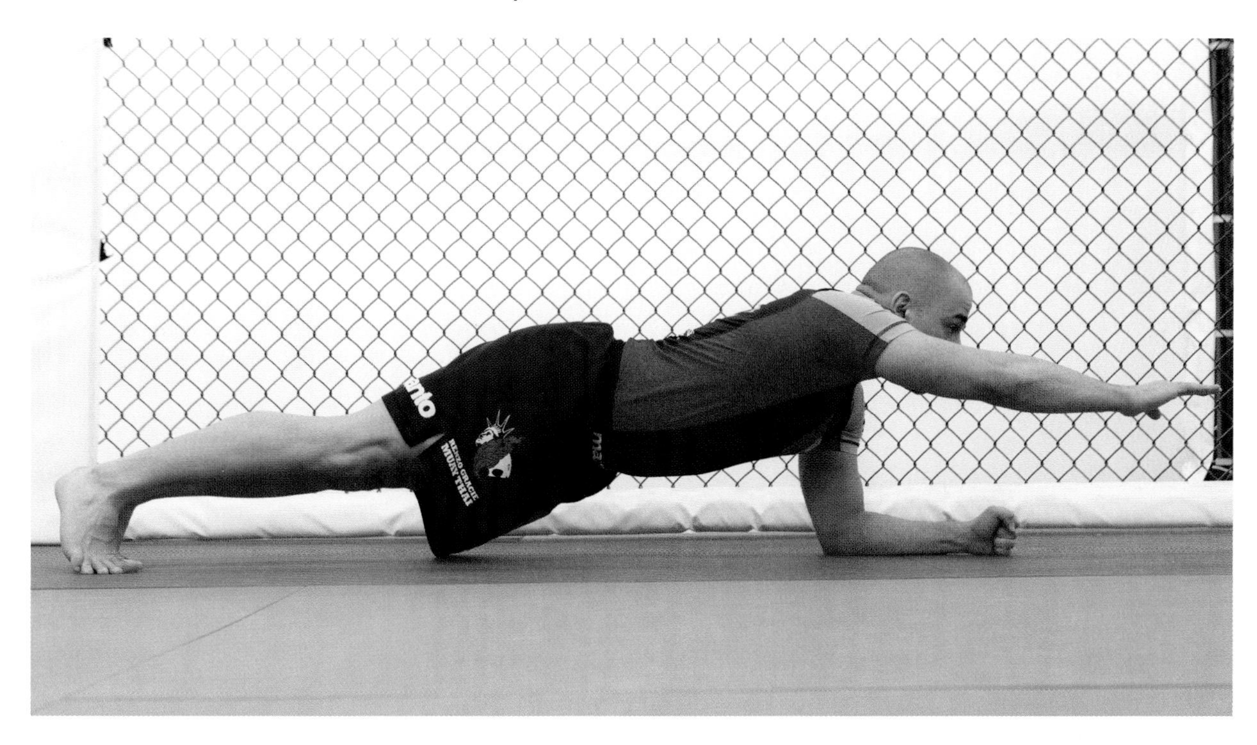

3. SINGLE-LEG PLANK

Begin lying on your stomach with the elbows at the sides. Press into the ground with the elbows and toes, and lift the stomach from the ground while keeping the core tight and the back straight. Lift one leg while keeping the knee straight.

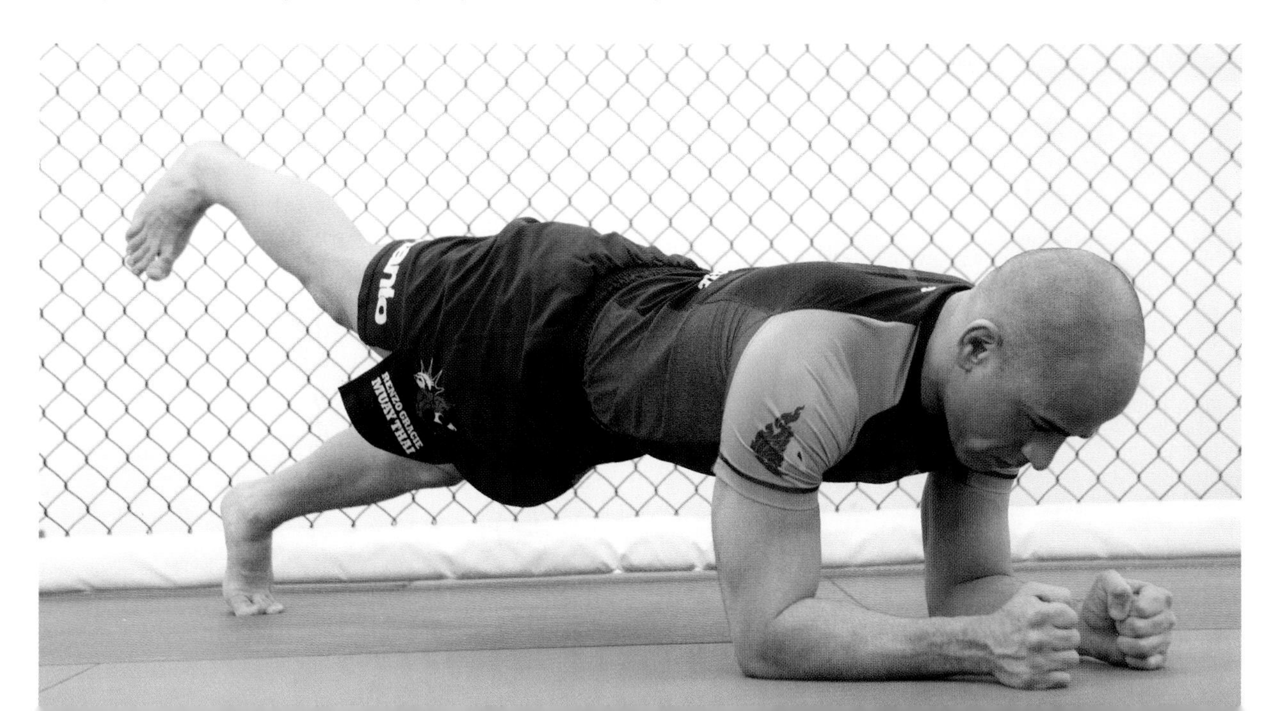

4. SINGLE-ARM AND SINGLE-LEG PLANK

Begin lying on your stomach with the elbows at the sides. Press into the ground with the elbows and toes, and lift the stomach from the ground while keeping the core tight and the back straight. Extend one arm out in front of the body and lift the opposite leg while keeping the knee straight.

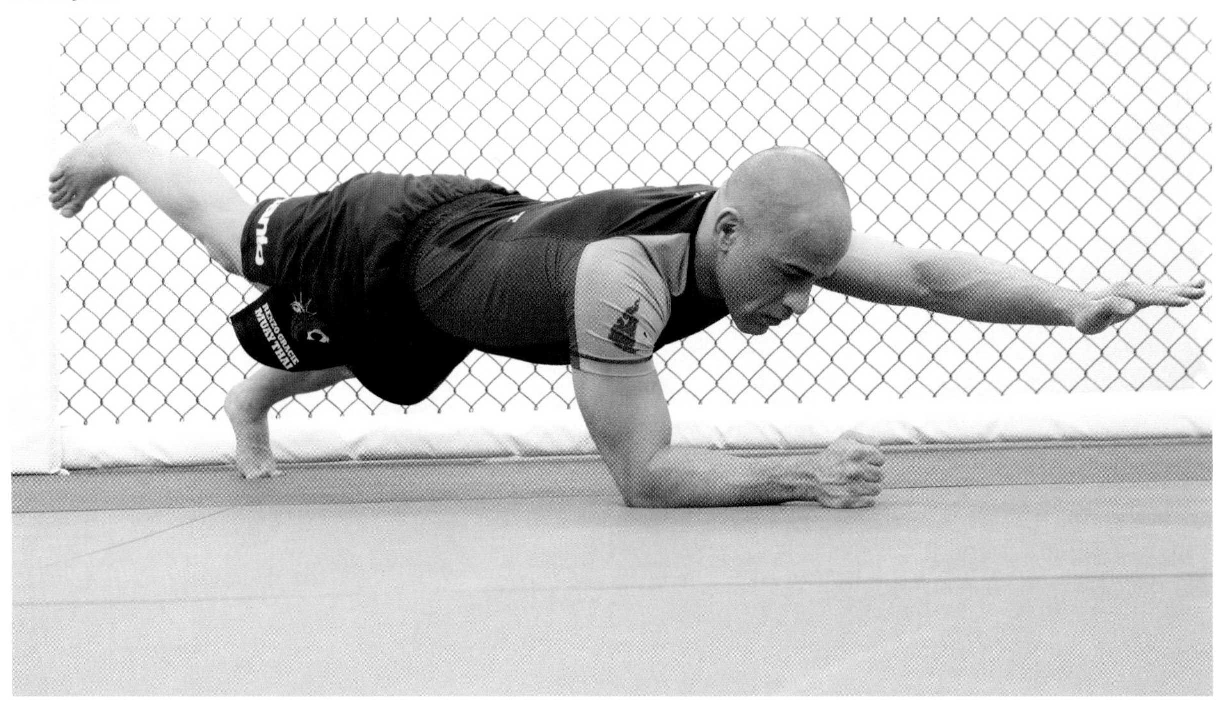

5. ROWING PLANK

Begin lying on your stomach with the elbows at the sides. Press into the ground with the elbows and toes, and lift the stomach from the ground while keeping the core tight and the back straight. Grab onto the band and row with one arm for the desired number of repetitions.

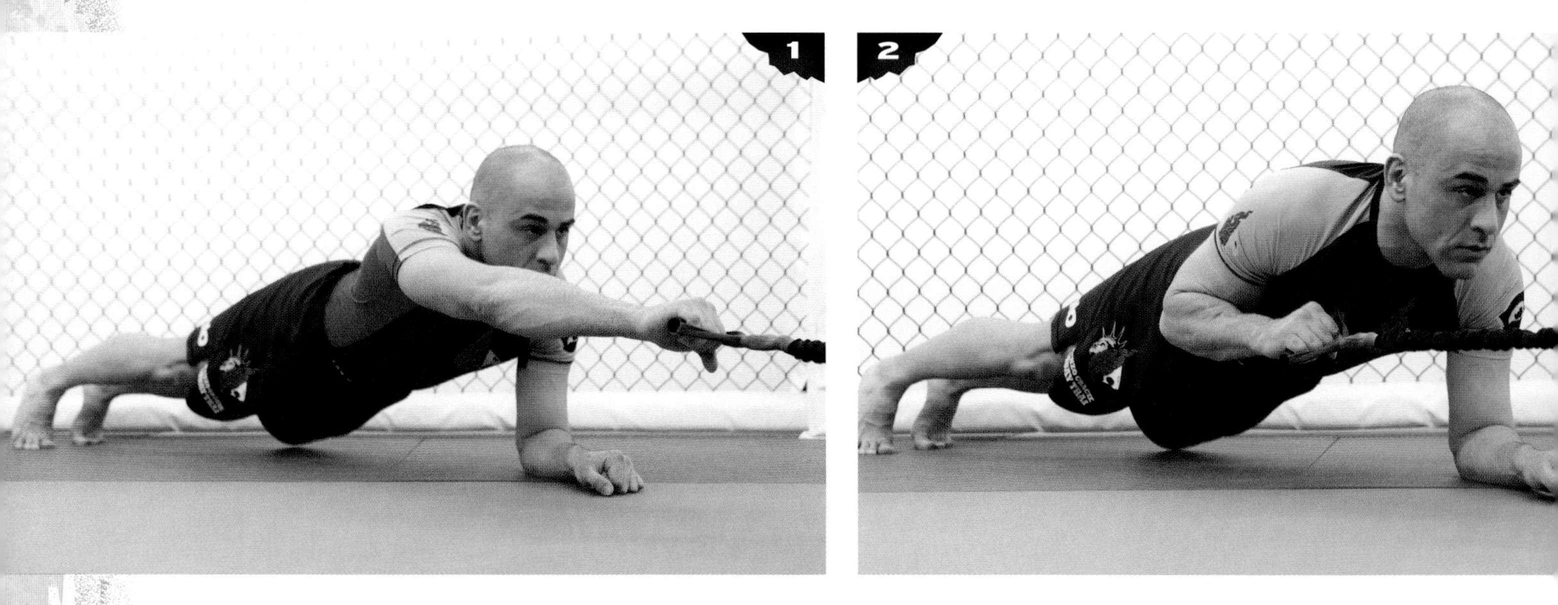

B. PUSHUP PLANK CIRCUIT

To perform the circuit, perform the exercises in a row for 40 seconds each. If the exercise is unilateral, perform it on each side for 20 seconds. Perform the circuit for 2 total sets.

1. PUSHUP HOLD

Begin lying on your stomach with the hands at the sides. Press into the ground with the hands and toes, and lift the torso from the ground while keeping the core tight and the back straight. Lock out at the elbows and hold the position.

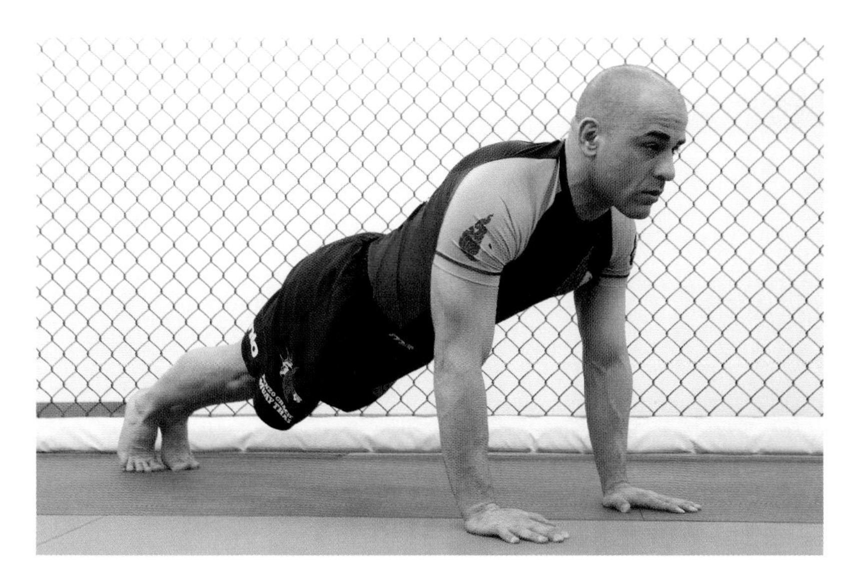

2. SINGLE-ARM PUSHUP HOLD

Begin at the top position of the Pushup Hold. Raise one hand out in front of the body and extend at the elbow.

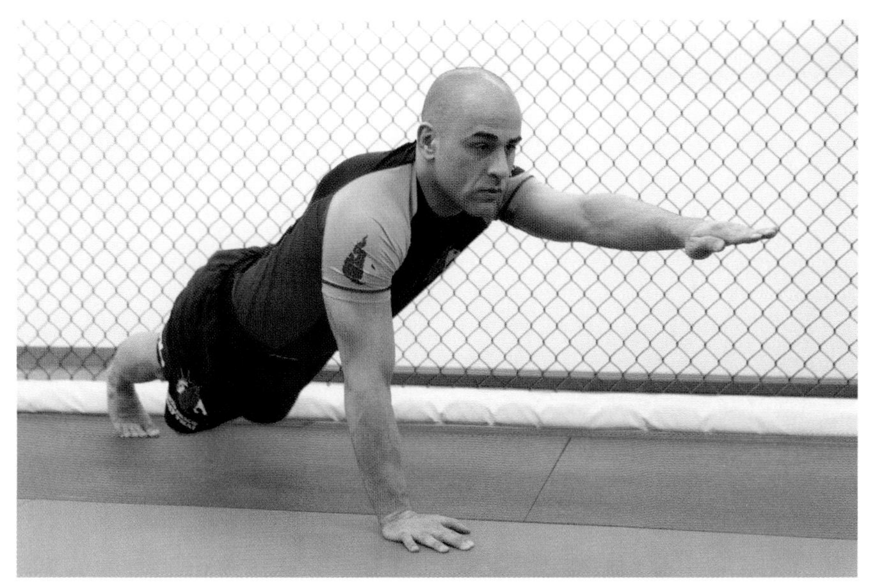

3. SINGLE-ARM SINGLE-LEG PUSHUP HOLD

Begin at the top position of the Single-Arm Pushup Hold. Raise the opposite foot in the air while keeping the knee straight.

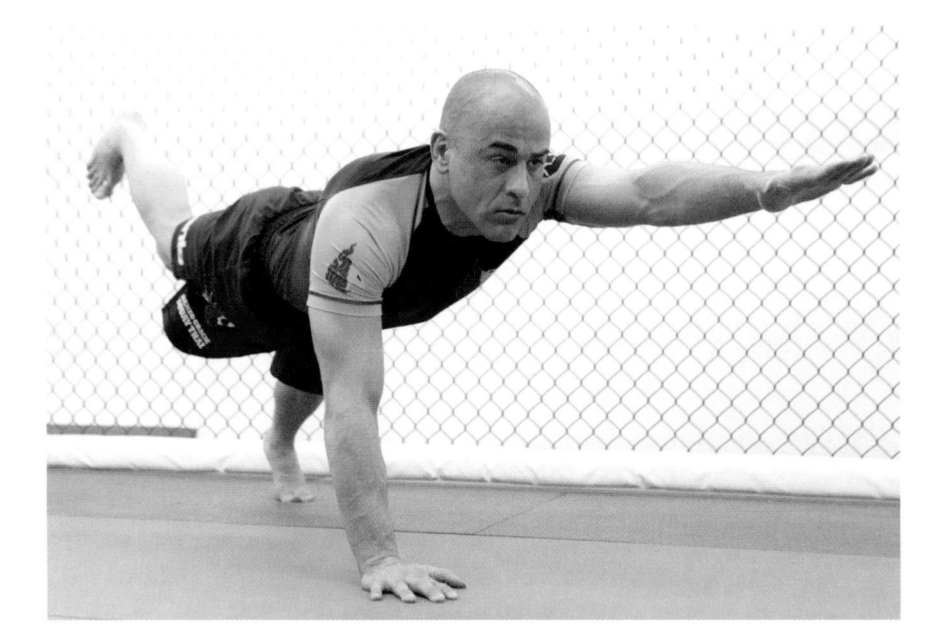

4. KNEE-TO-SIDE PUSHUP HOLD

Begin at the top position of the Pushup Hold. While keeping the back straight and the core tight, bring one knee up to the elbow on the same side.

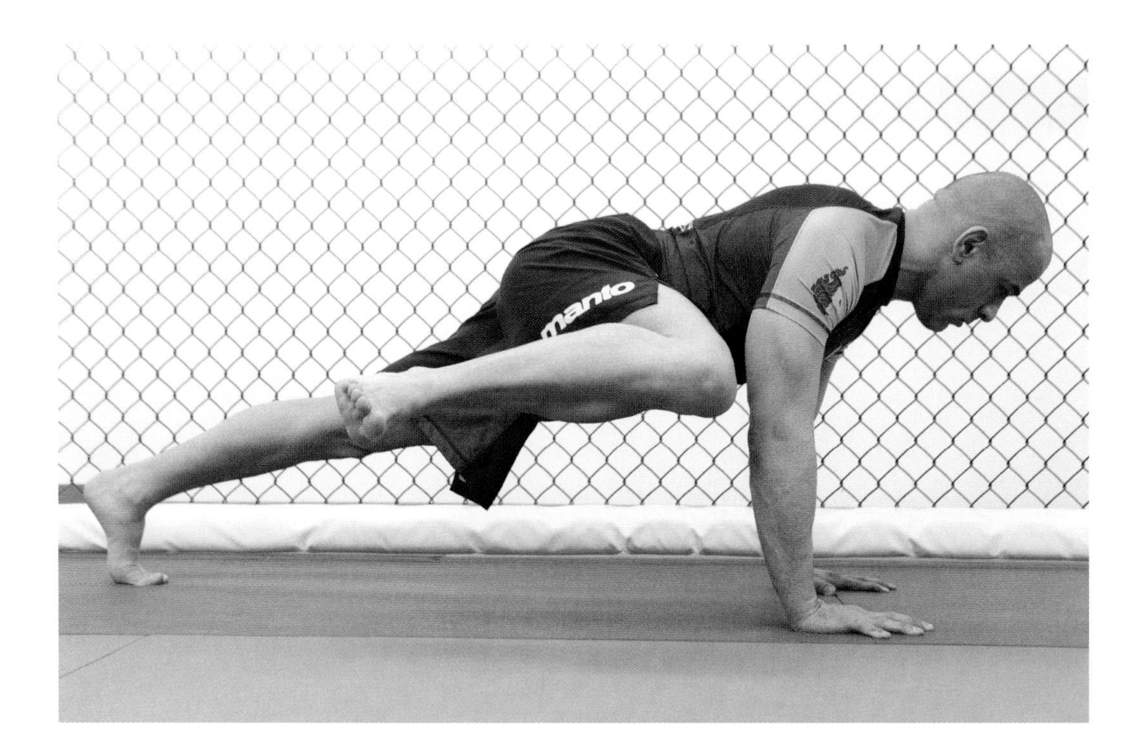

5. FOOT-TO-SIDE PUSHUP HOLD

Begin at the top position of the Pushup Hold. While keeping the back and knee straight, bring one leg out to the side.

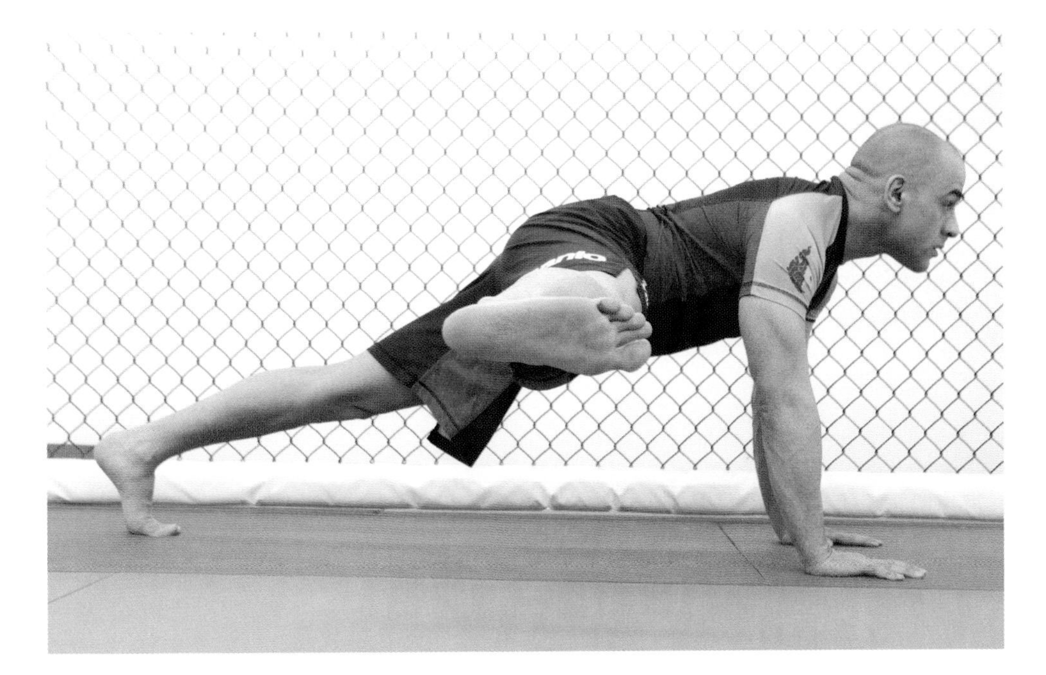

6. KNEE-TO-OPPOSITE-ELBOW PUSHUP HOLD

Begin at the top position of the Pushup Hold. While keeping the back and knee straight, bring the knee to the opposite forearm.

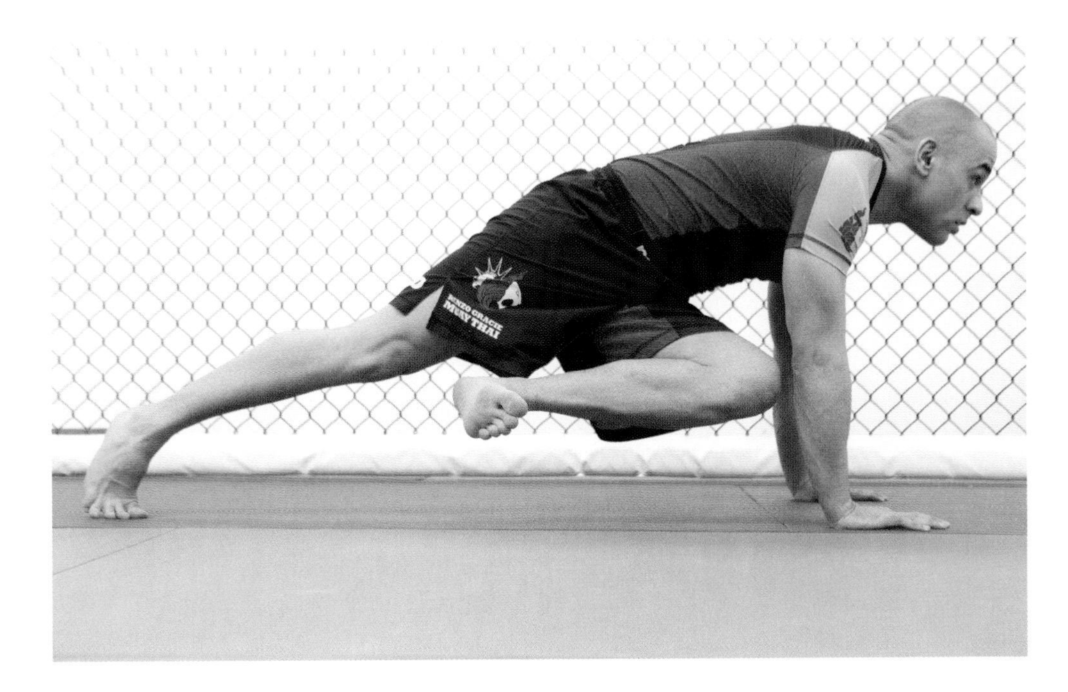

C. MED BALL PLANK CIRCUIT

To perform the circuit, perform the exercises in a row for 40 seconds each. If the exercise is unilateral, perform it on each side for 20 seconds. Perform the circuit for 2 total sets.

1. MED BALL PLANK

Begin lying on your stomach with the hands on a med ball. Press into the ground with the hands and toes, and lift the torso from the ground while keeping the core tight and the back straight. Lock out at the elbows and hold the position.

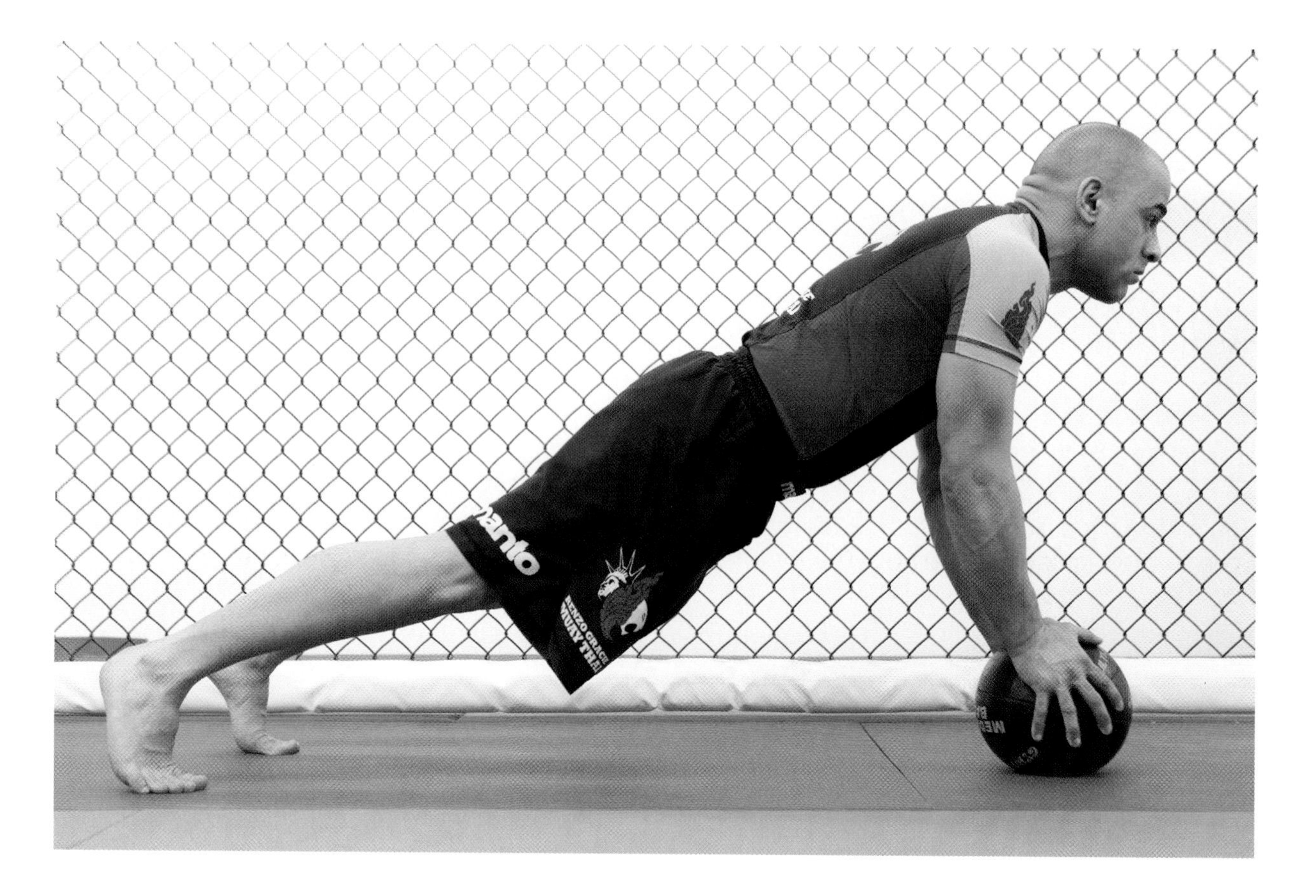

2. SINGLE-LEG MED BALL PLANK

Begin at the top position of the Med Ball Plank. Raise one foot in the air while keeping the knee straight.

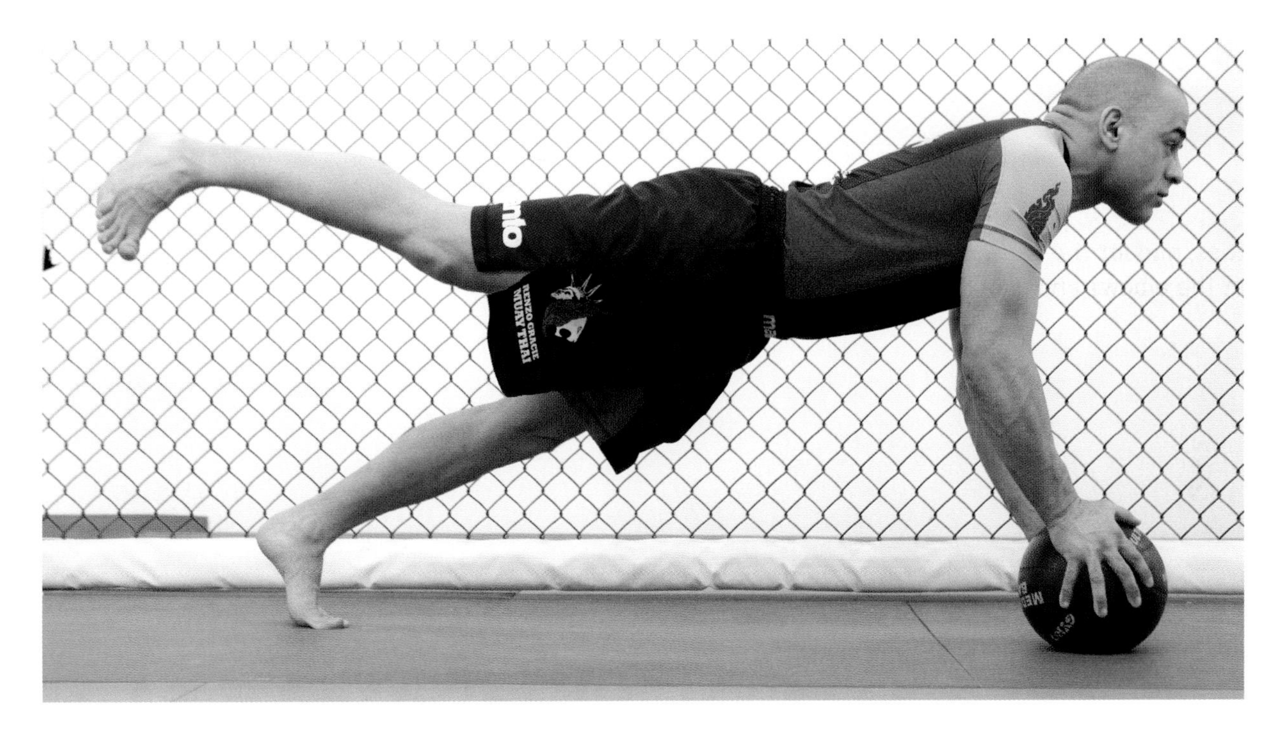

3. KNEE-FORWARD MED BALL PLANK

Begin at the top position of the Med Ball Plank. Bring one knee as far forward in between the elbows as possible without letting that foot touch the ground.

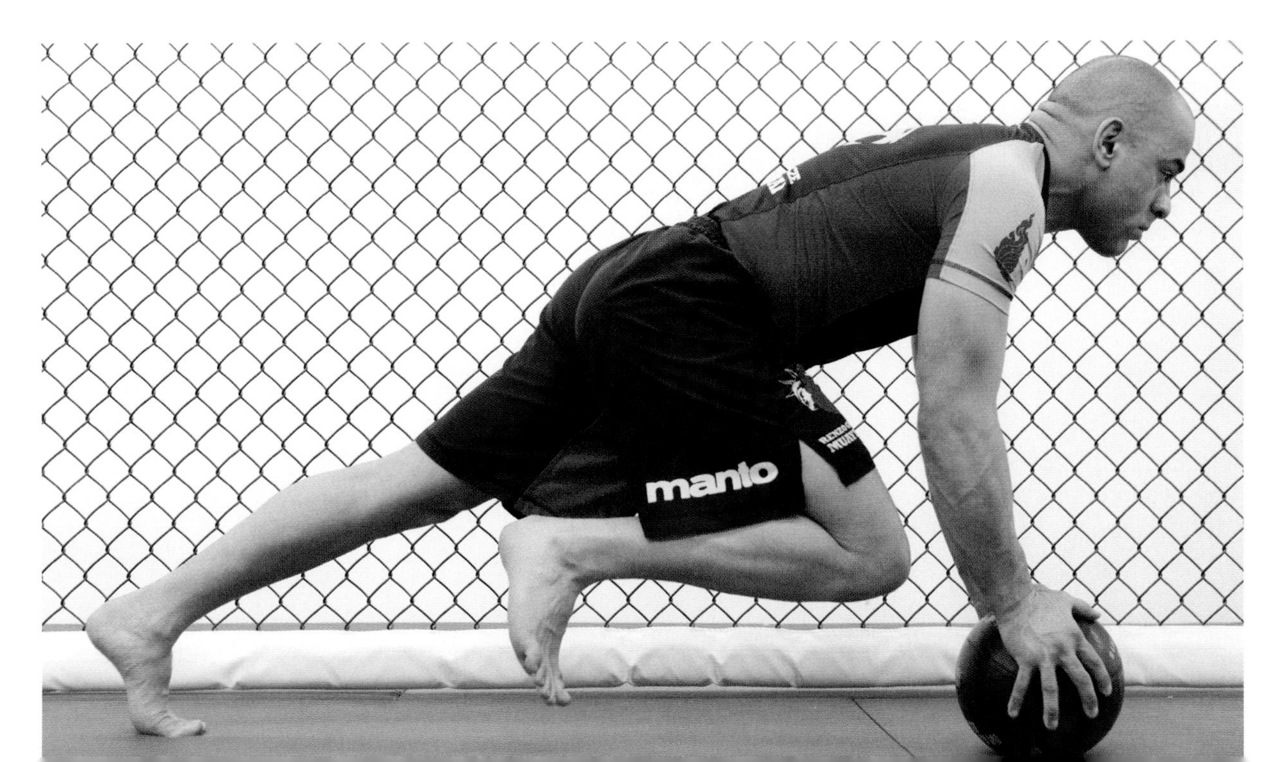

4. KNEE-TO-SIDE MED BALL PLANK

Begin at the top position of the Med Ball Plank. Bring one knee as far forward out to the side as possible.

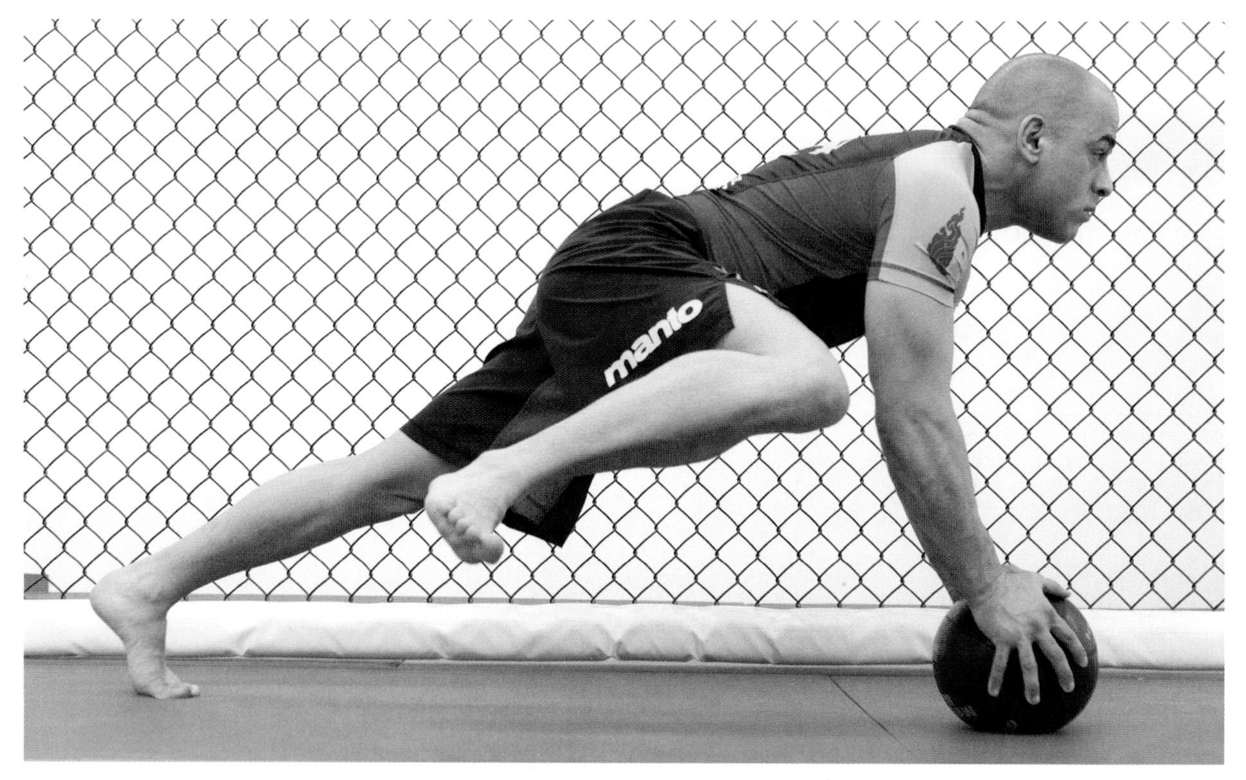

5. FOOT-TO-SIDE MED BALL PLANK

Begin at the top position of the Med Ball Plank. Bring one leg as far forward out to the side as possible without letting that foot touch the ground.

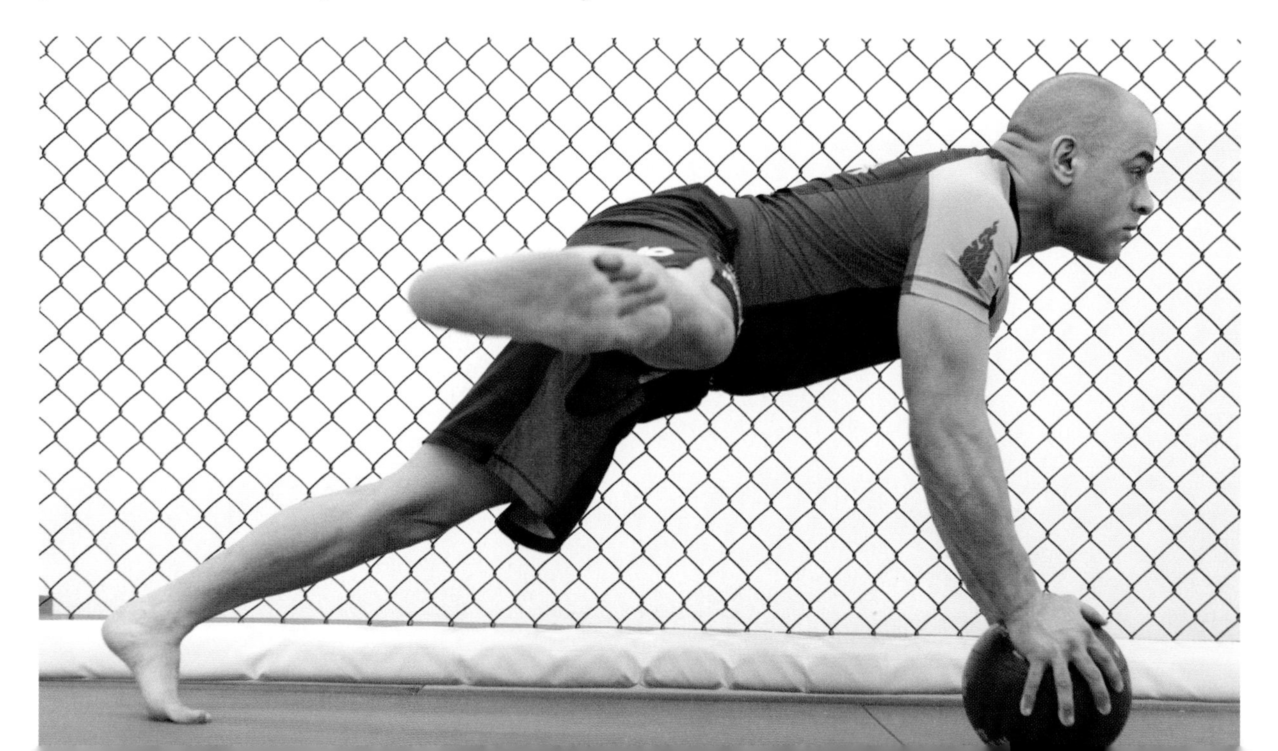

D. ELEVATED PLANK CIRCUIT

To perform the circuit, perform the exercises in a row for 40 seconds each. If the exercise is unilateral, perform it on each side for 20 seconds. Perform the circuit for 2 total sets.

1. ELEVATED PLANK

Begin lying on your stomach with the elbows at the sides and the feet up on a bench. Press into the ground with the elbows and toes, and lift the stomach from the ground while keeping the core tight and the back straight.

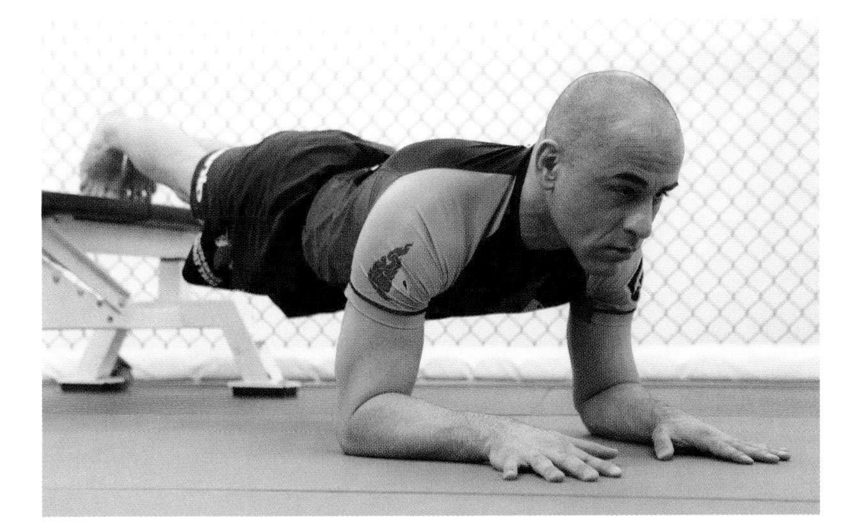

2. SINGLE-LEG ELEVATED PLANK

Begin in the top position of the Elevated Plank. Lift one leg while keeping the knee straight.

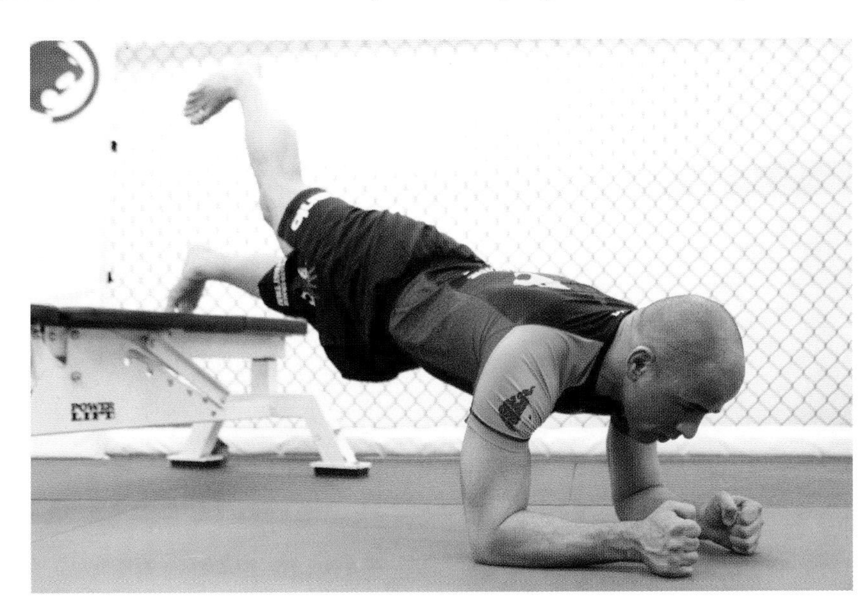

3. SINGLE-ARM ELEVATED PLANK

Begin in the top position of the Elevated Plank. Lift one arm out to the front while keeping the elbow extended.

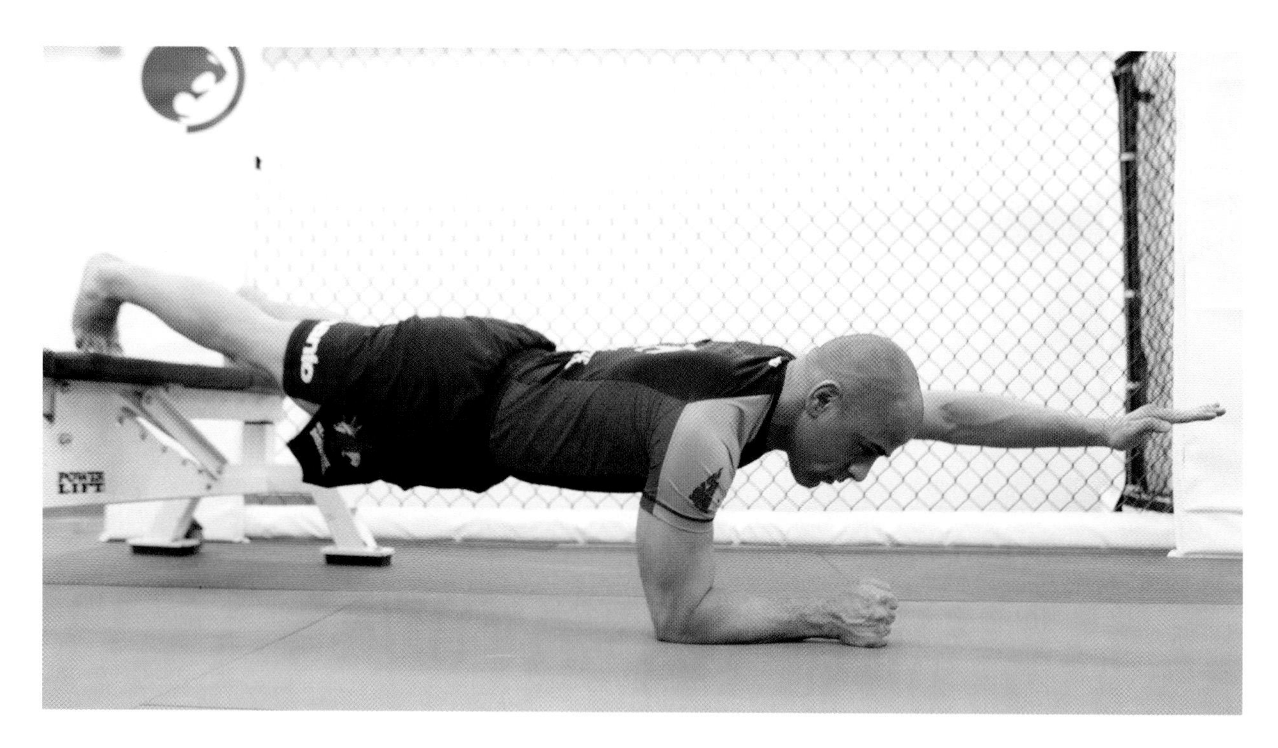

4. SINGLE-ARM SINGLE-LEG ELEVATED PLANK

Begin at the top position of the Single-Arm Elevated Plank. Raise the opposite foot in the air while keeping the knee straight.

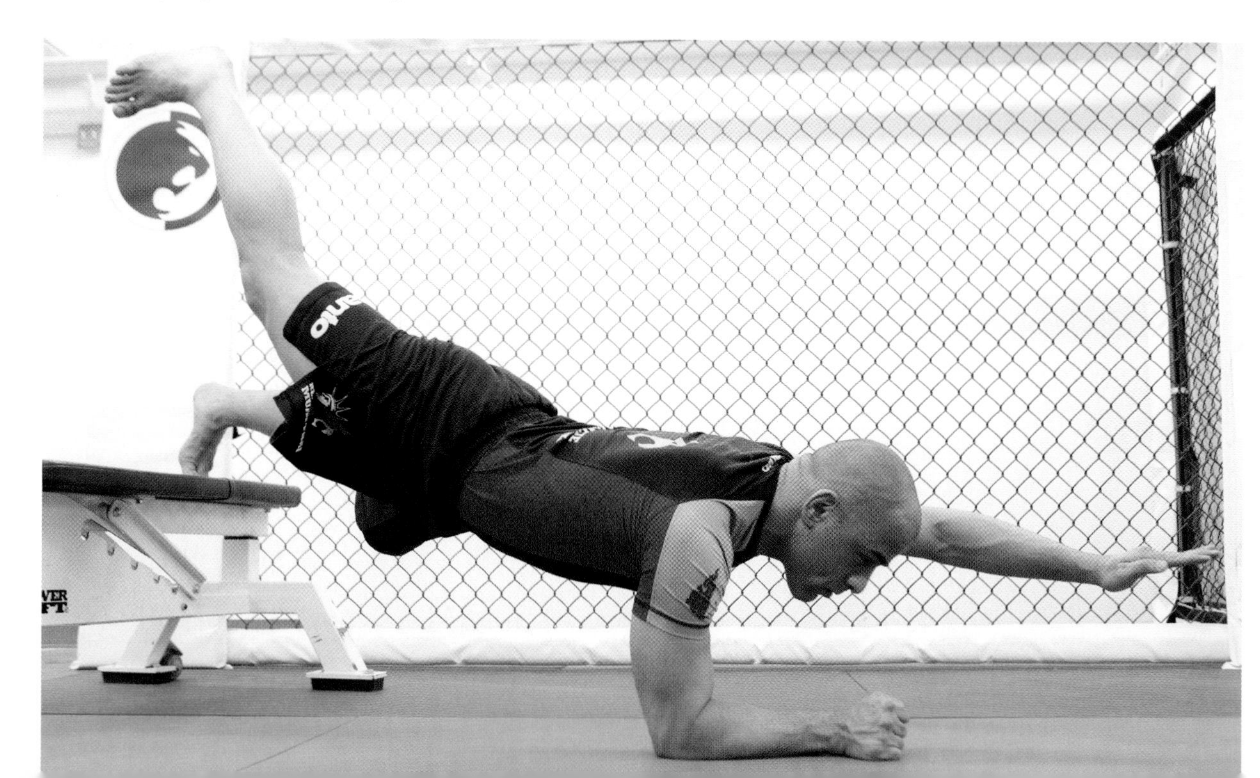

E. SWISS BALL PLANK CIRCUIT

To perform the circuit, perform each exercise in a row for 40 seconds. If the exercise is unilateral, perform it on each side for 20 seconds. Perform the circuit for 2 total sets.

1. SWISS BALL PLANK

Begin lying on your stomach with the elbows on the Swiss Ball. Press into the ball with the elbows and toes, and lift the stomach from the ground while keeping the core tight and the back straight.

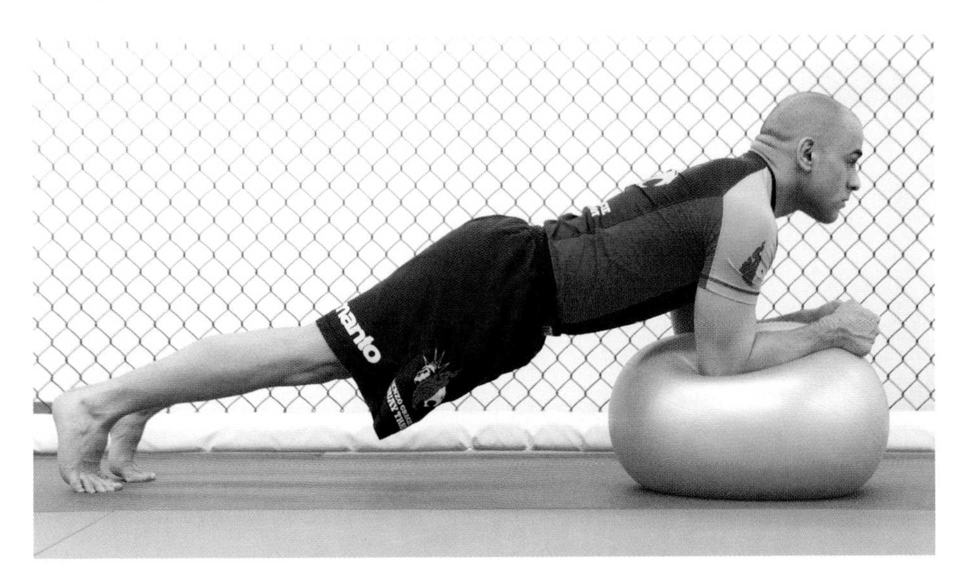

2. SINGLE-LEG SWISS BALL PLANK

Begin in the top position of the Swiss Ball Plank. Lift one leg while keeping the knee extended.

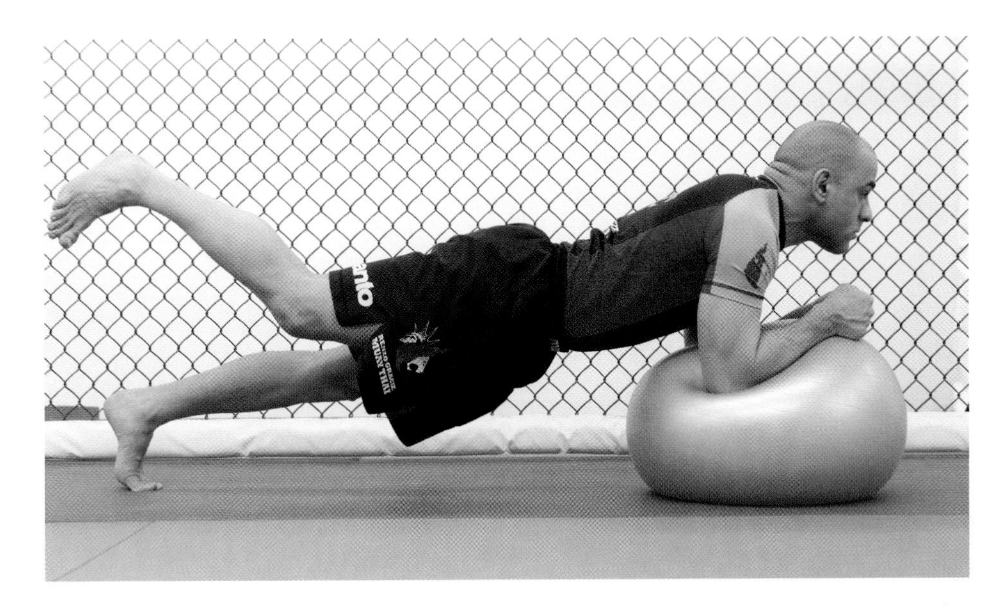

3. SWISS BALL PUSHUP HOLD

Begin lying on your stomach with the hands on the ball. Press into the ball with the hands and toes, and lift the torso from the ground while keeping the core tight and the back straight. Lock out at the elbows and hold the position.

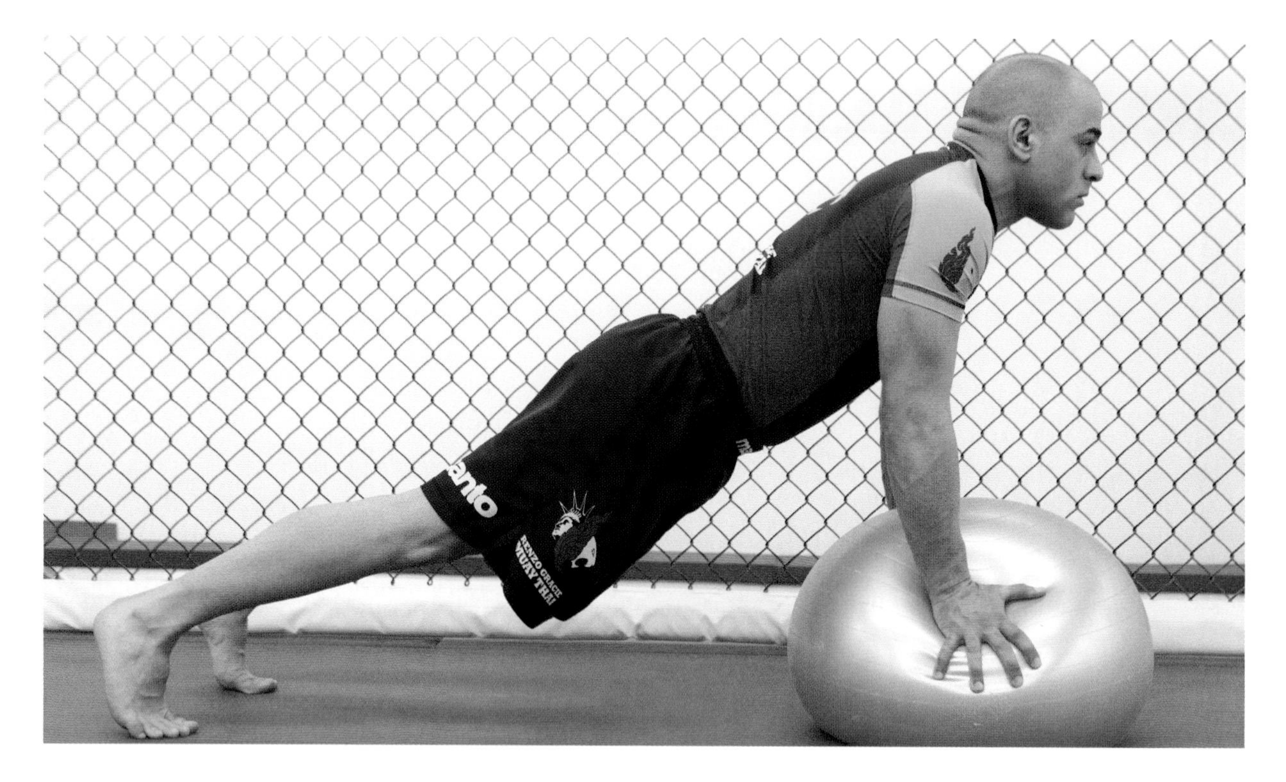

4. SWISS BALL KNEE-FORWARD PUSHUP HOLD

Begin at the top position of the Swiss Ball Pushup Hold. Bring one knee as far forward in between the elbows as possible without letting that foot touch the ground.

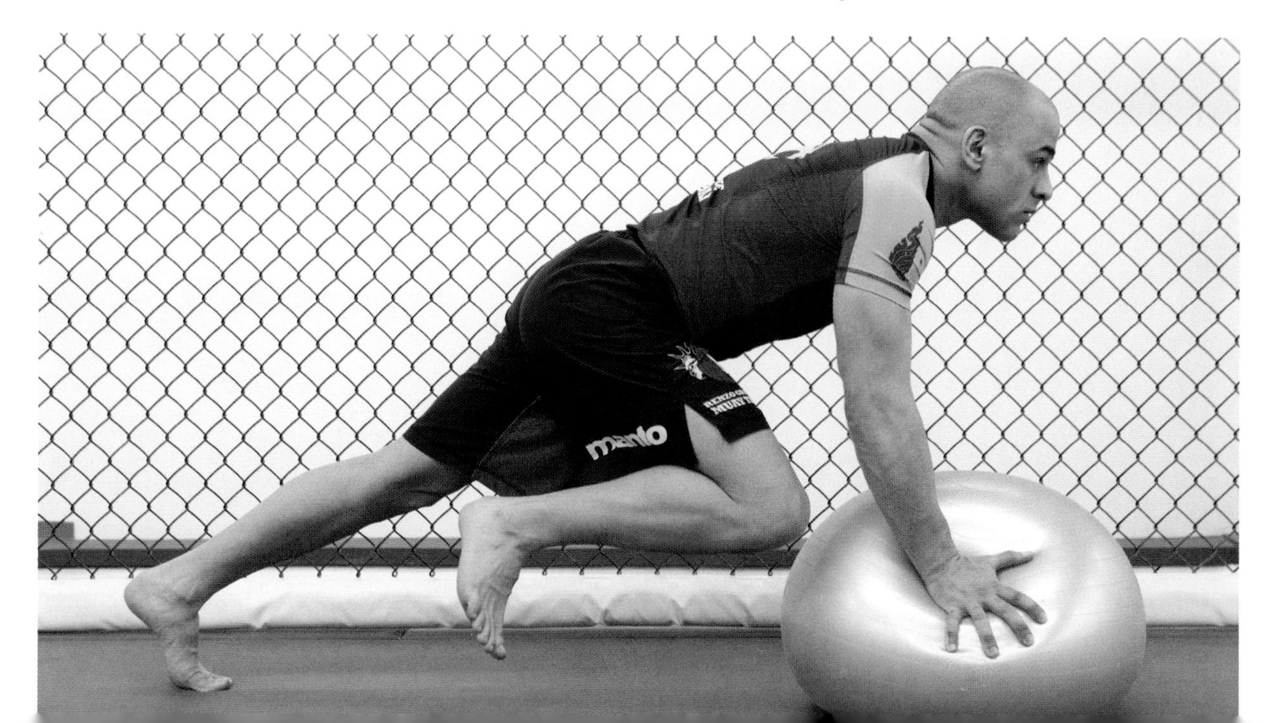

5. SWISS BALL KNEE-TO-SIDE PUSHUP HOLD

Begin at the top position of the Swiss Ball Pushup Hold. Bring one knee as far forward out to the side as possible.

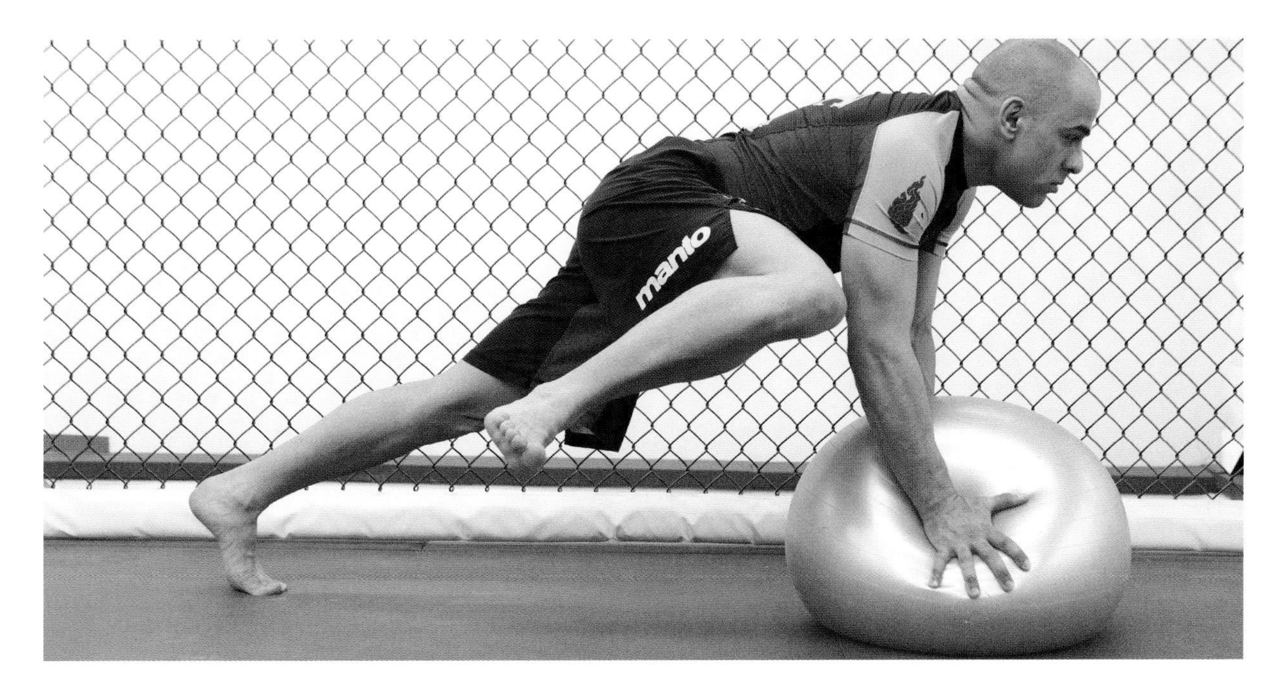

F. SIDE PLANK CIRCUIT

To complete a circuit, each exercise is to be performed in a row for 2 reps of 20 seconds on each side. Perform each circuit for 2 sets.

1. SIDE PLANK

Begin on one side, lying on the elbow with the top hand lying on the hip. Lift the hips into the air by pressing into the floor with the elbow and the bottom foot. Keep the core tight and the back and neck straight.

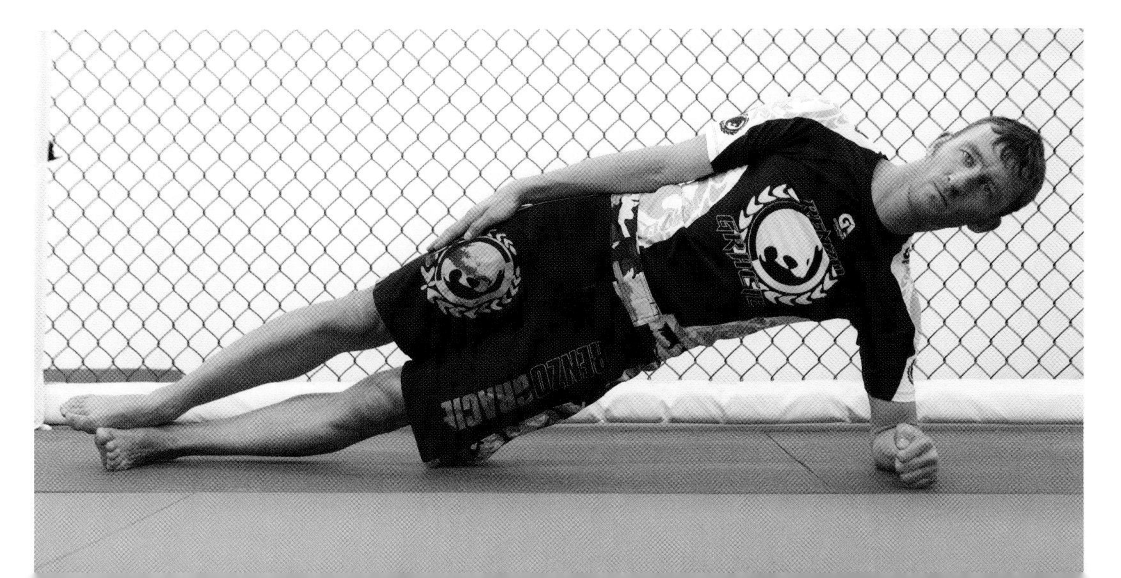

2. SIDE PLANK WITH ARM UP

Begin in the top position of the Side Plank. Raise the top arm up to the ceiling while keeping the elbow straight.

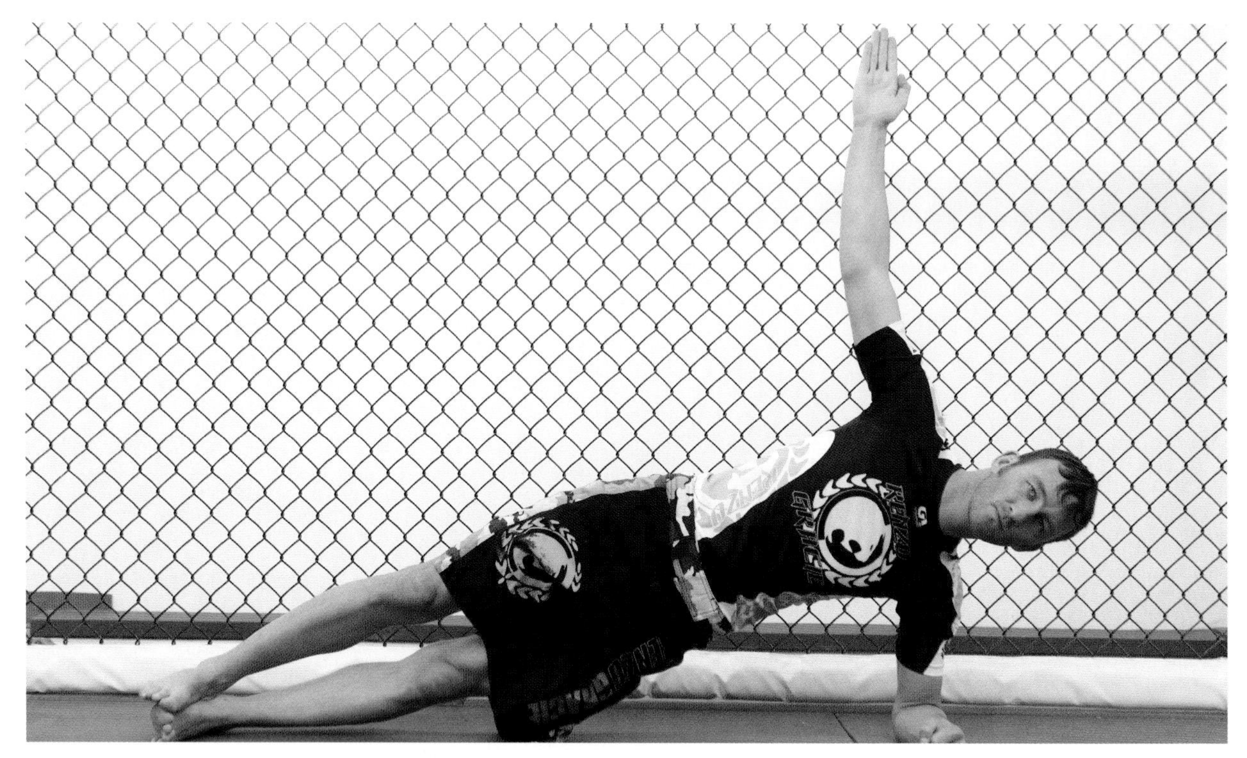

3. SIDE PLANK WITH ARM AND LEG UP

Begin in the top position of the Side Plank. Raise both the top arm and the top leg while keeping the elbow and knee extended.

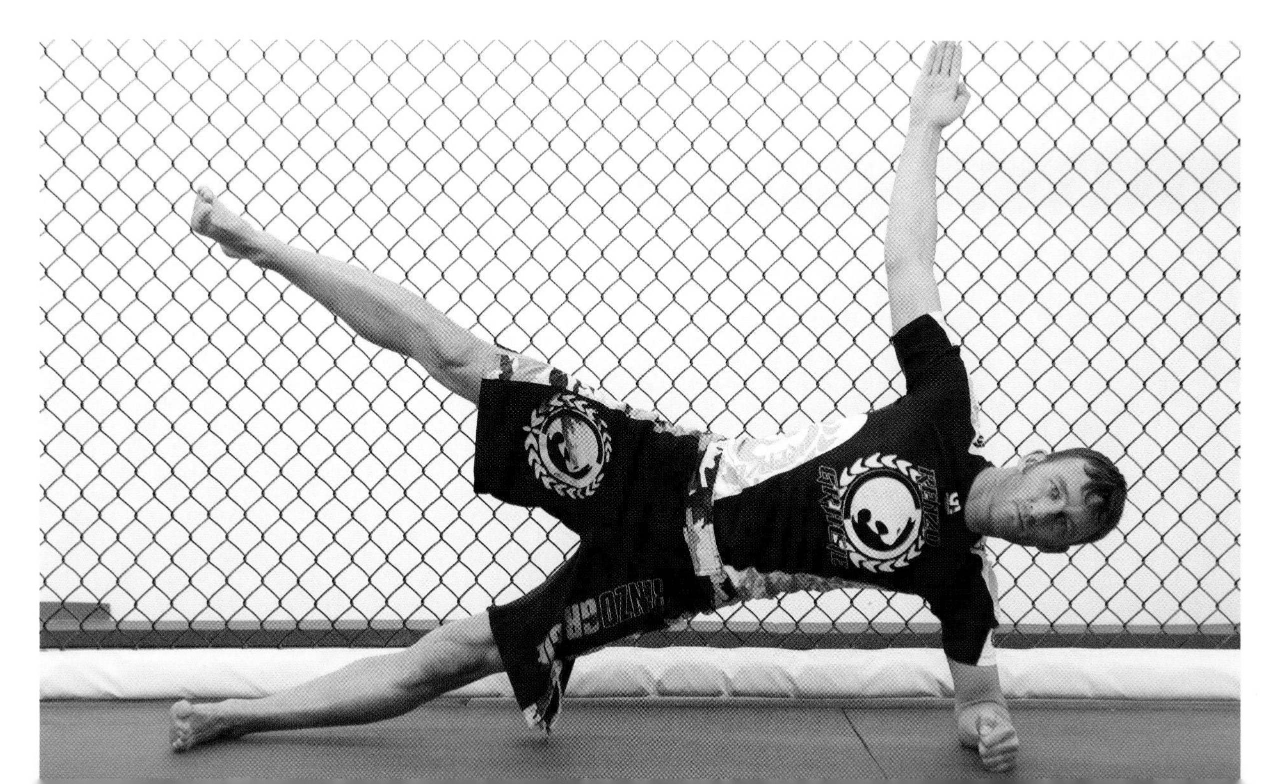

4. SIDE PLANK WITH KNEE UP

Begin in the top position of the Side Plank. Bring the bottom knee forward while keeping the core tight and the back and neck straight.

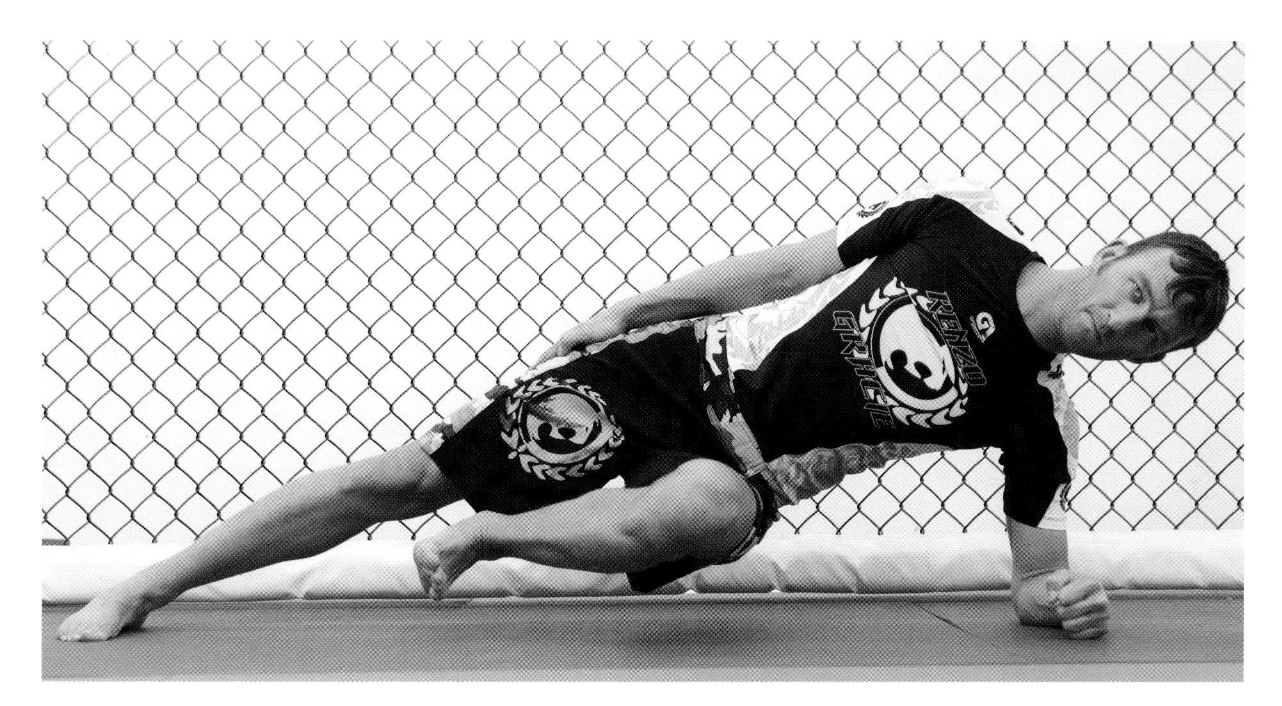

5. SIDE PLANK WITH KNEE AND ARM UP

Begin in the top position of the Side Plank. Bring the bottom knee forward and raise the top arm to the ceiling while keeping the core tight and the back and neck straight.

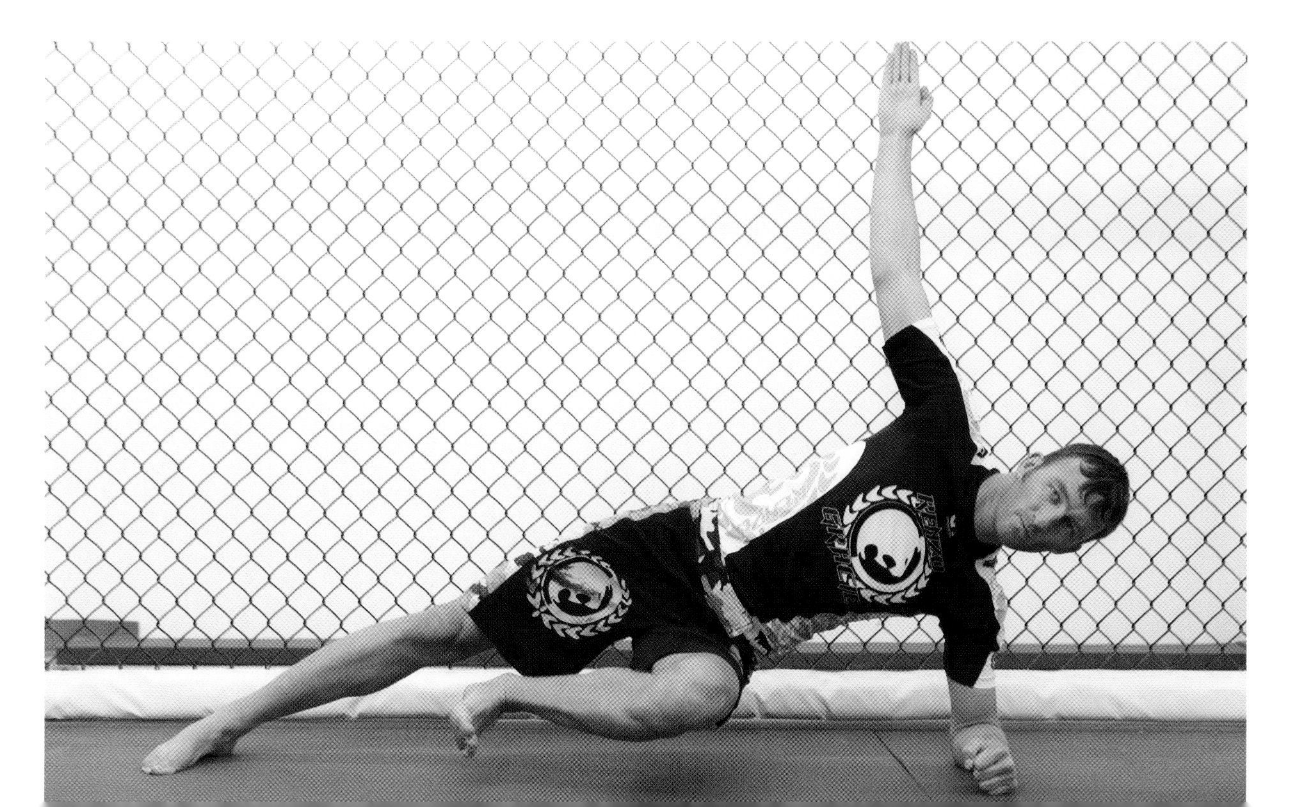

G. ELEVATED SIDE PLANK CIRCUIT

To complete a circuit, each exercise is to be performed in a row for 2 reps of 20 seconds on each side. Perform each circuit for 2 sets.

1. ELEVATED SIDE PLANK

Begin on one side, lying on the elbow with the top hand resting on the hip and the feet on a bench. Lift the hips into the air by pressing into the floor with the elbow and into the bench with the bottom foot. Keep the core tight and the back and neck straight.

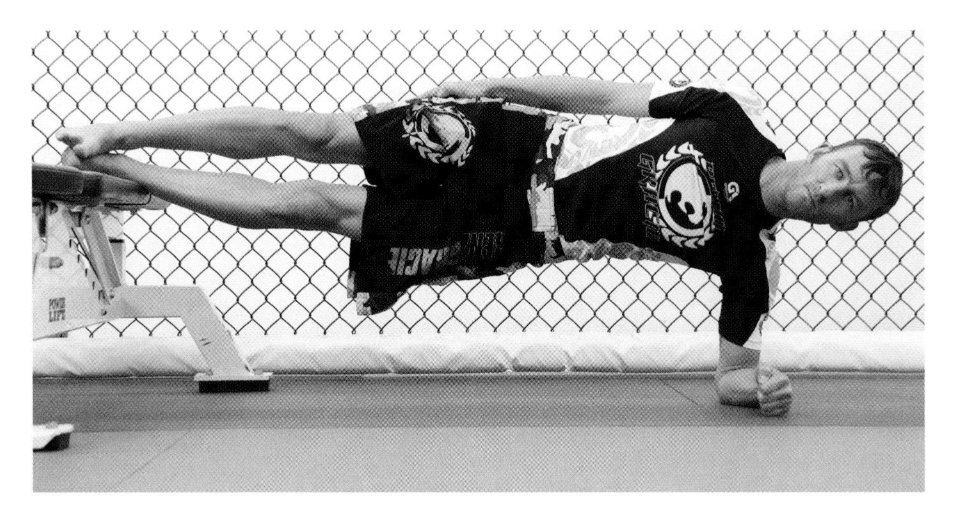

2. ARM-UP ELEVATED SIDE PLANK

Begin in the top position of the Elevated Side Plank. Lift the arm toward the ceiling and keep the elbow extended and the core tight.

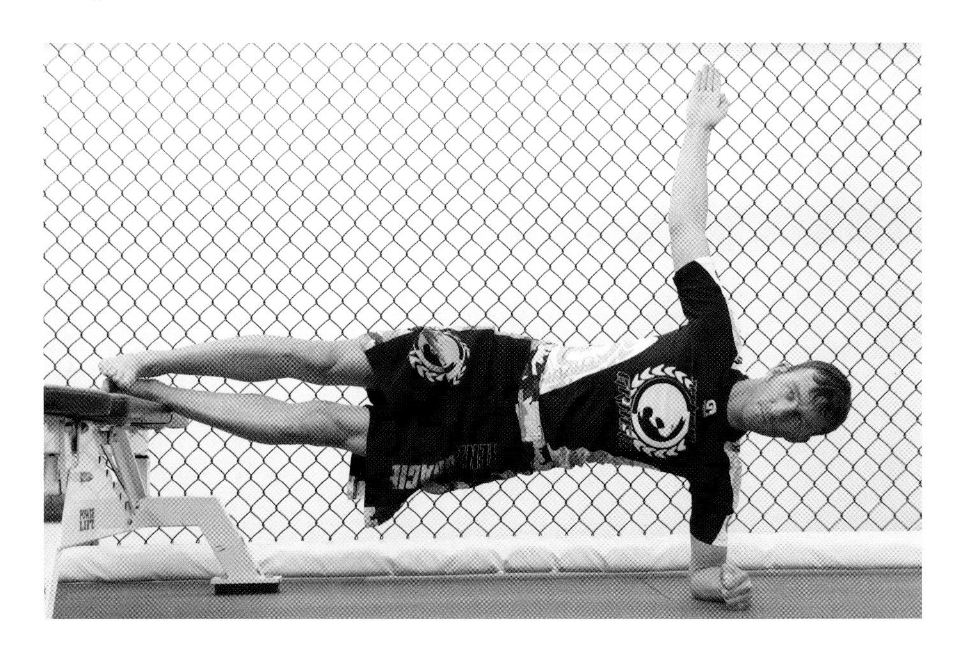

3. ARM- AND LEG-UP ELEVATED SIDE PLANK

Begin in the top position of the Elevated Side Plank. Raise both the top arm and the top leg while keeping the core tight and the elbow and knee extended.

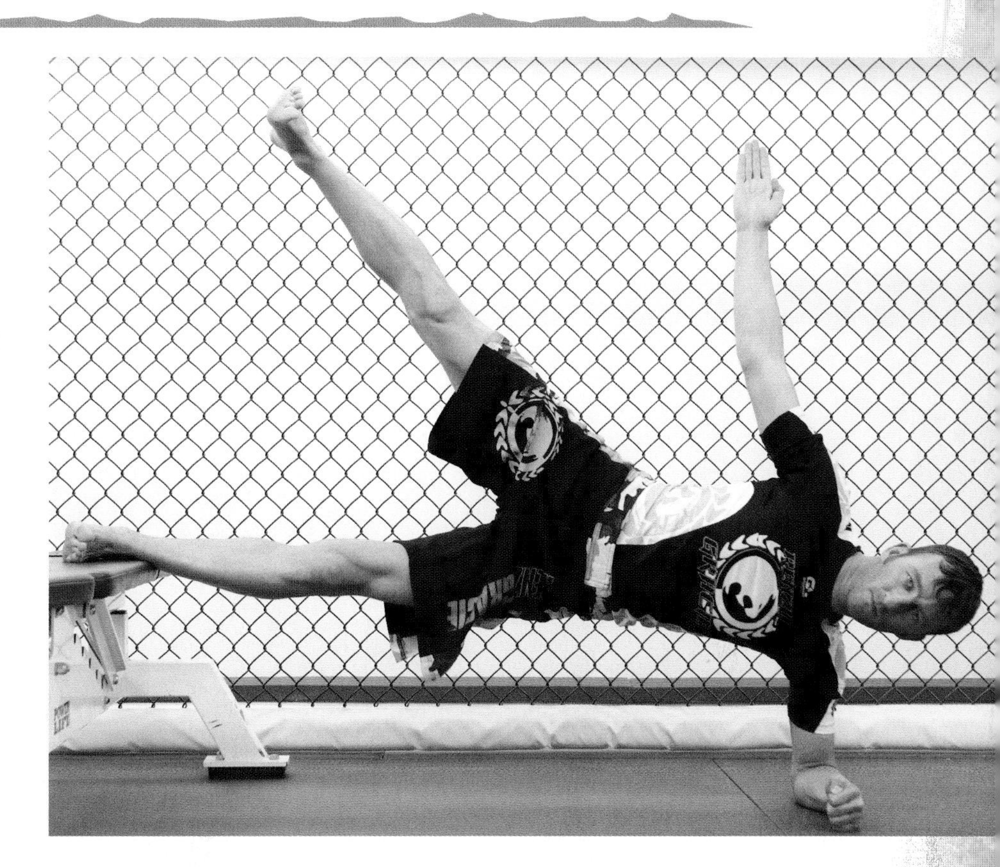

4. SWISS BALL ARM-UP SIDE PLANK

Begin on one side, lying on the elbow with the top hand lying on the hip and a Swiss Ball between the feet. Lift the hips into the air by pressing into the floor with the elbow and squeezing the ball with the feet. Raise the arm while keeping the core tight and the back and neck straight.

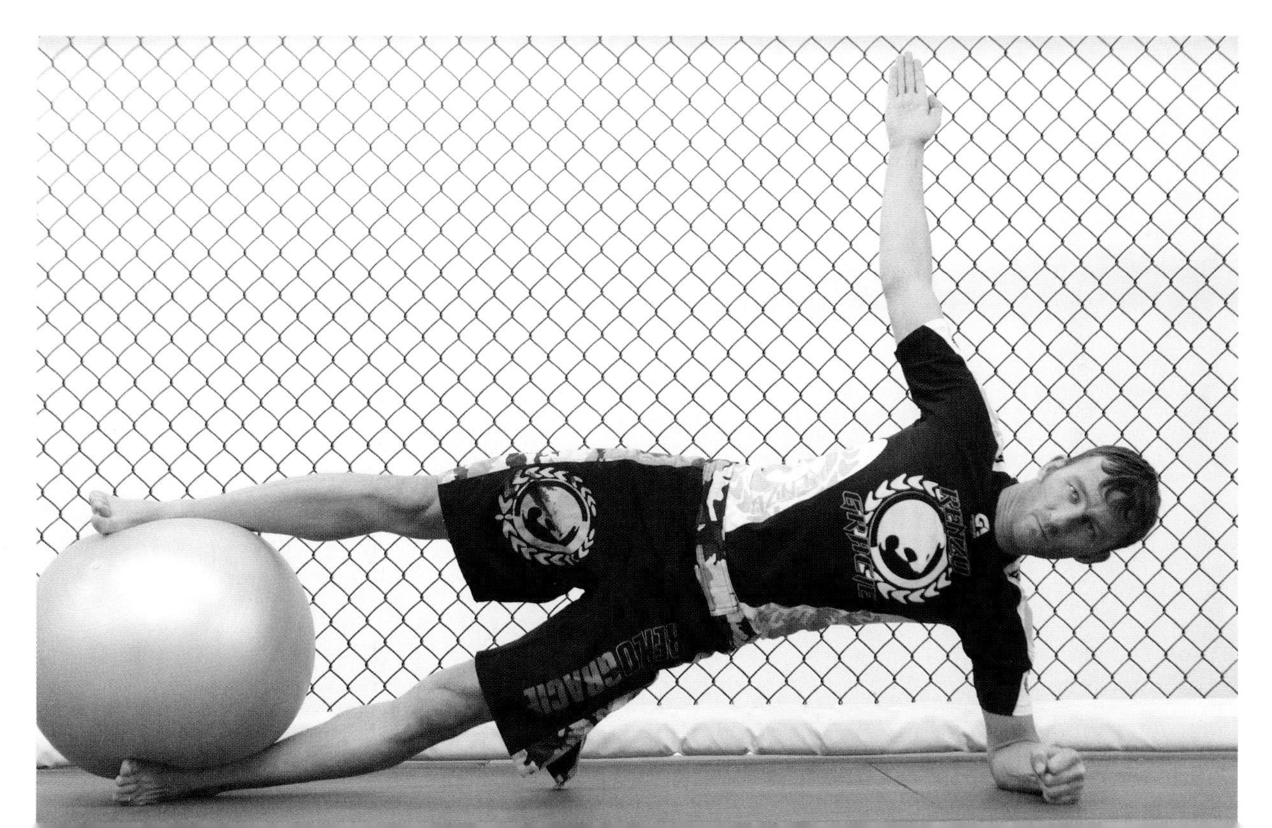

5. SIDE PLANK ROW

Begin in the top position of the Side Plank while holding a band with the top hand. Row the hand to the chest and hold the position.

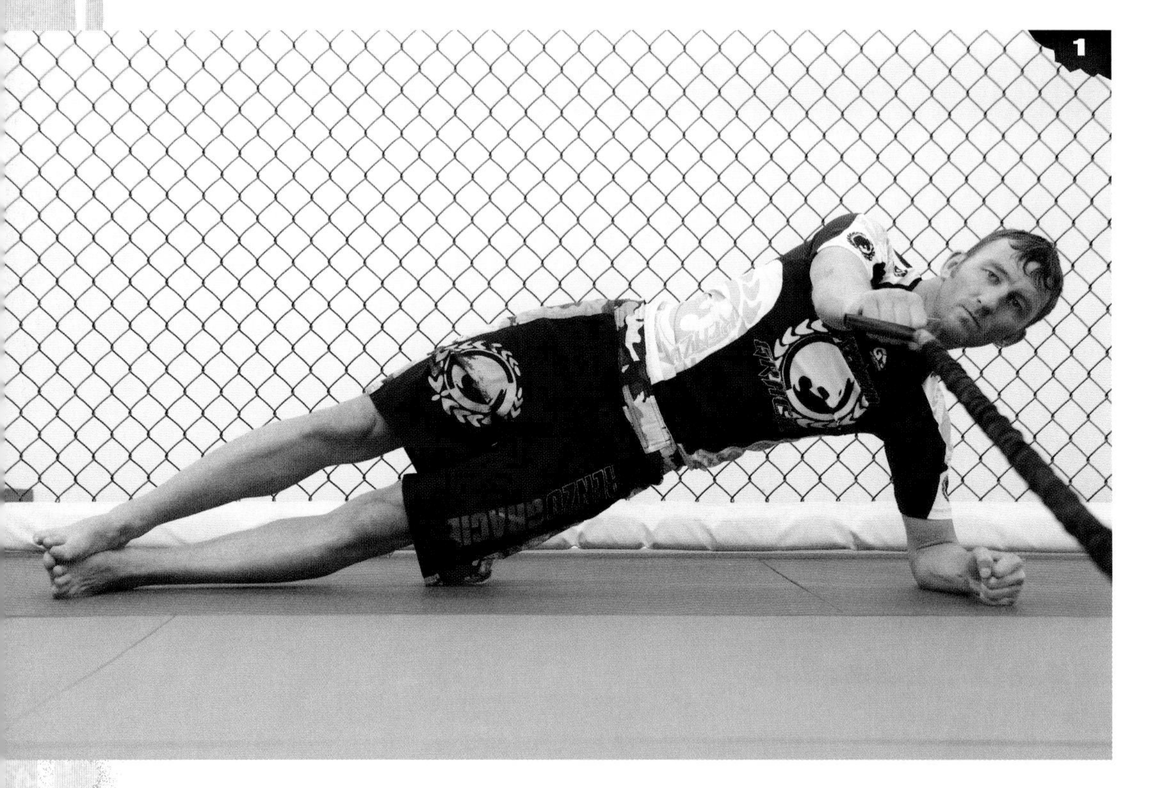

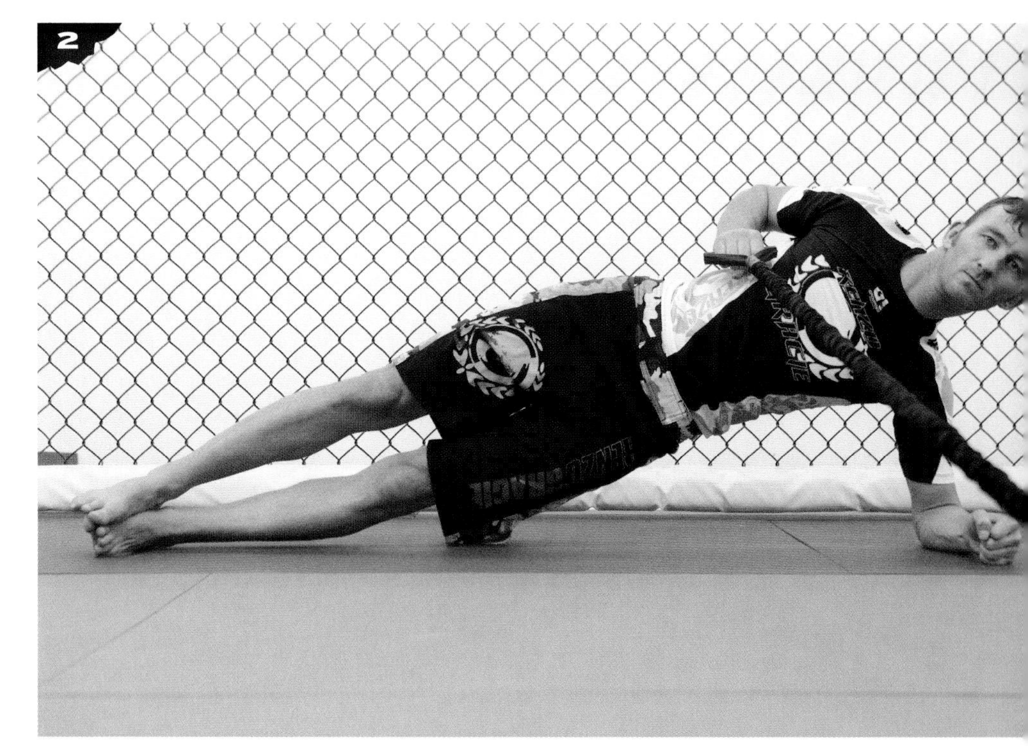

6. KNEE-TO-ELBOW SIDE PLANK

Begin in the top position of the Side Plank with the arm extended overhead and the weight on the top foot. Bring the bottom knee and the top elbow together while keeping the core tight. Return to the top position.

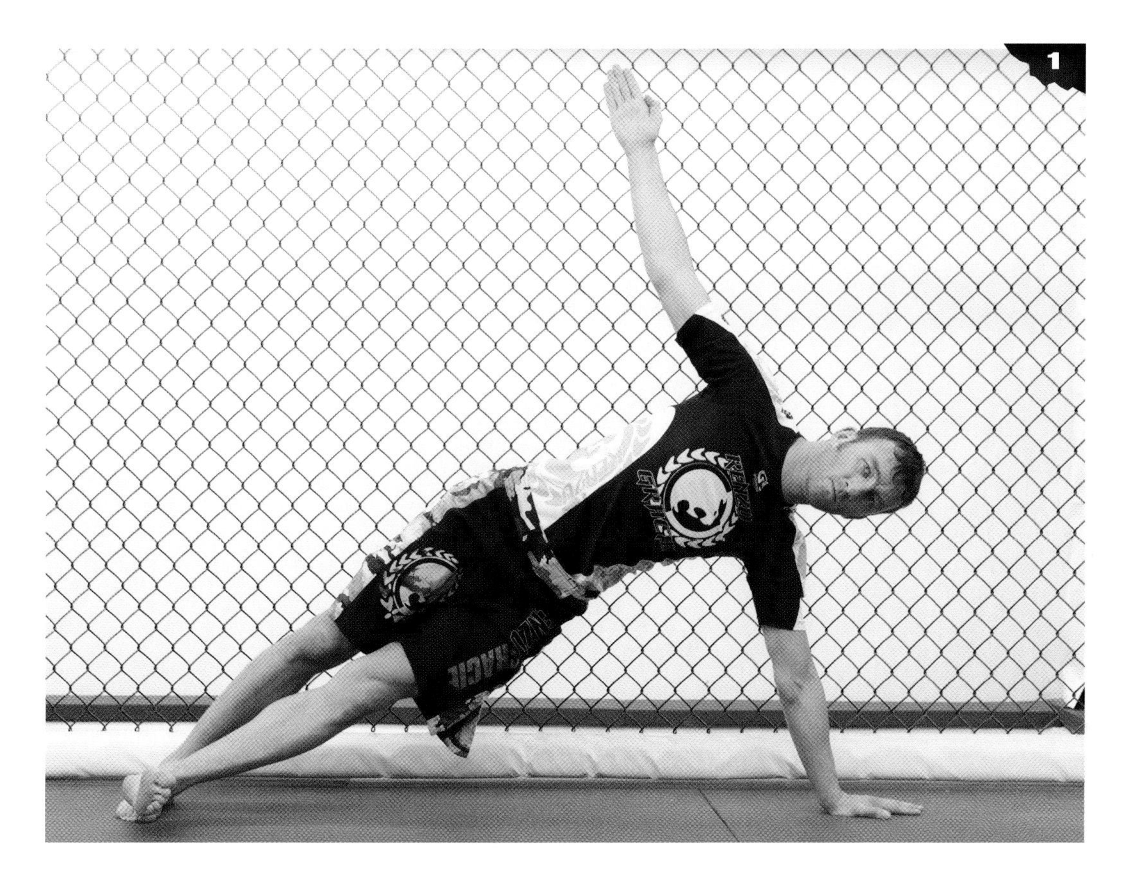

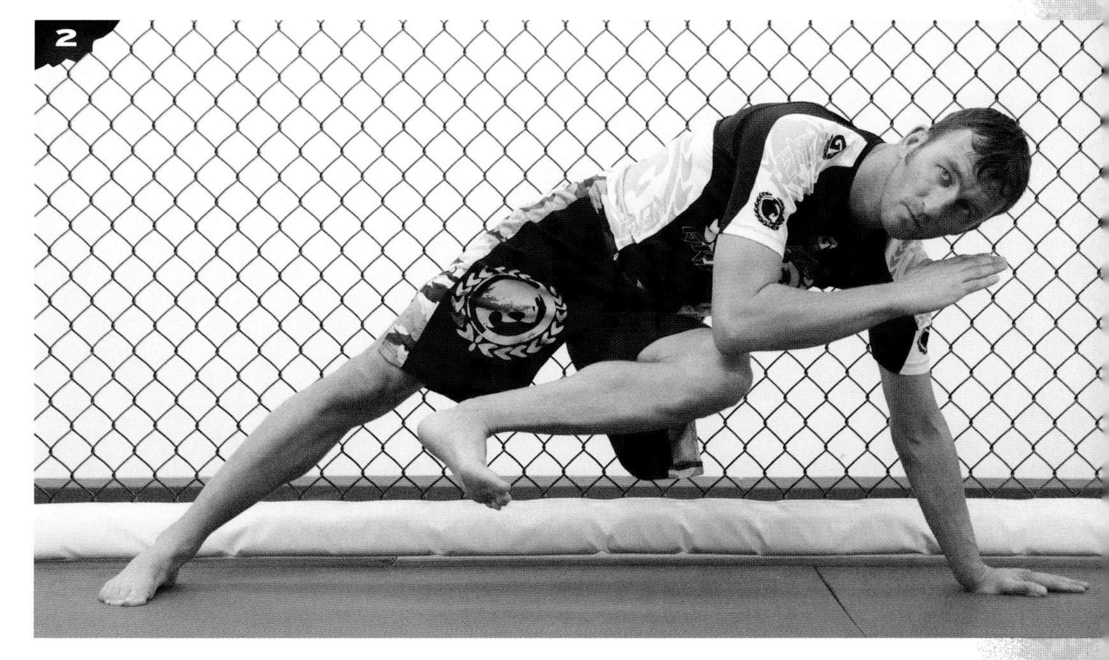

H. ADVANCED STABILIZATION CIRCUIT

To complete a circuit, exercises 1 through 3 are to be performed for 30 seconds and then exercises 4 through 6 are performed as described. Complete 2 circuits.

1. KETTLEBELL PUSHUP PLANK

Begin lying on your stomach with the hands gripping the kettlebells. Press into the ground with the hands and toes, and lift the torso from the ground while keeping the core tight and the back straight. Lock out at the elbows and hold the position.

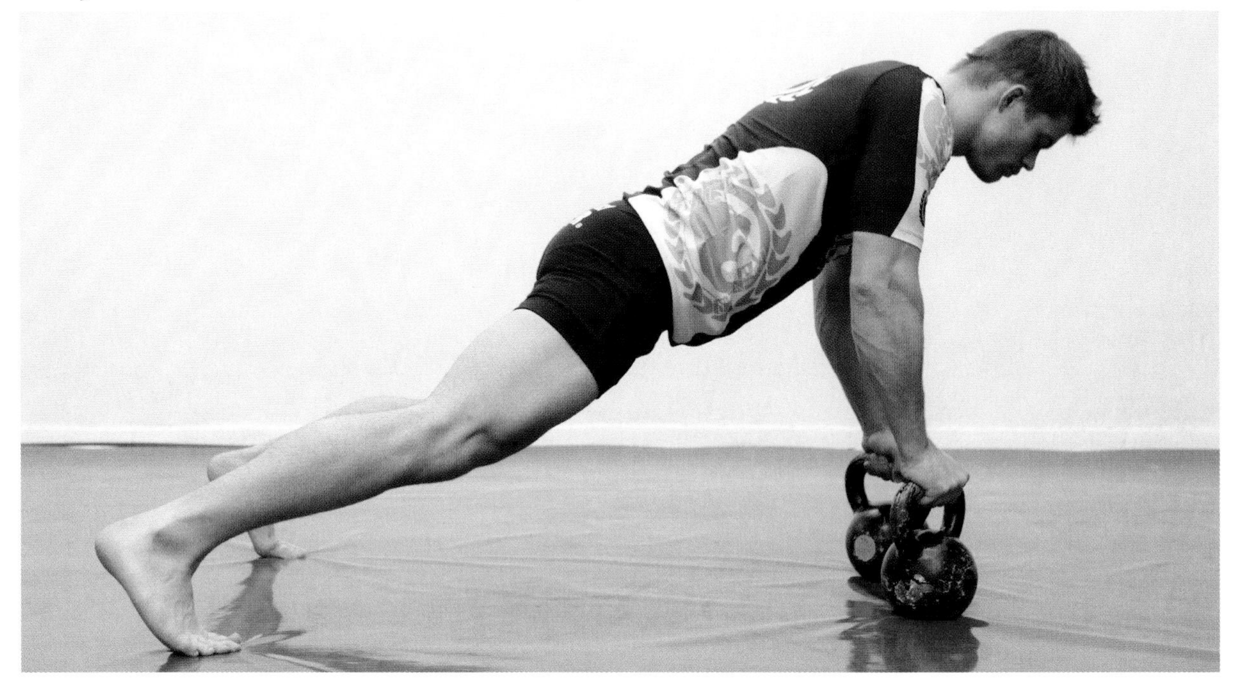

2. KNEE-FORWARD KETTLEBELL PUSHUP PLANK

Begin at the top position of the Kettlebell Plank. Bring one knee as far forward in between the elbows as possible without letting that foot touch the ground.

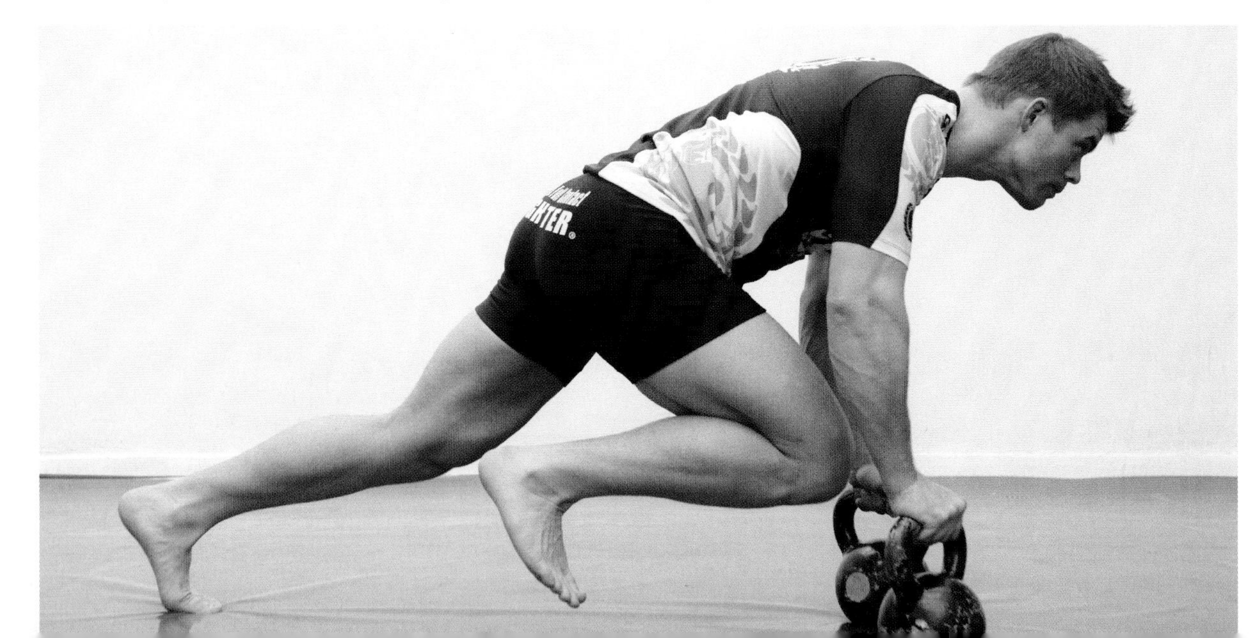

3. KNEE-TO-SIDE LOW KETTLEBELL PUSHUP PLANK

Begin in the top position of the Kettlebell Plank. Lower the chest to the kettlebells and bring one knee out to the side toward the hand.

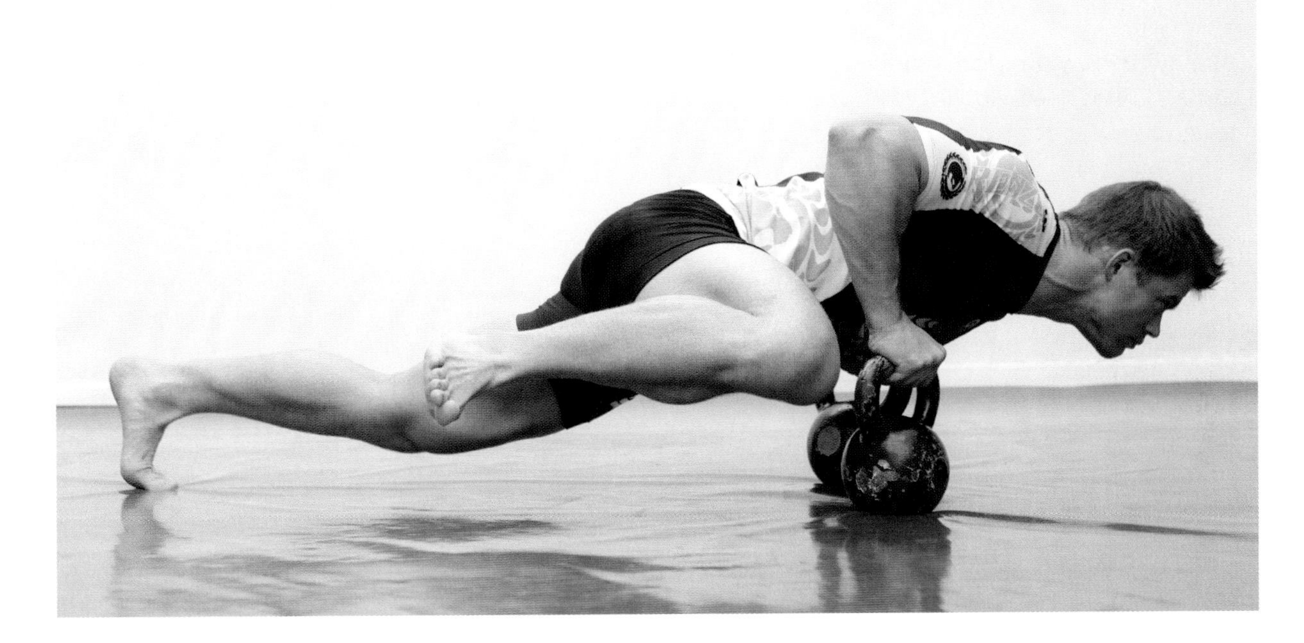

4. KETTLEBELL PUSHUP PLANK ROW

Begin in the top position of the Kettlebell Plank. Row one kettlebell up to the chest while keeping the core tight and the back flat. Perform 8 reps on each side.

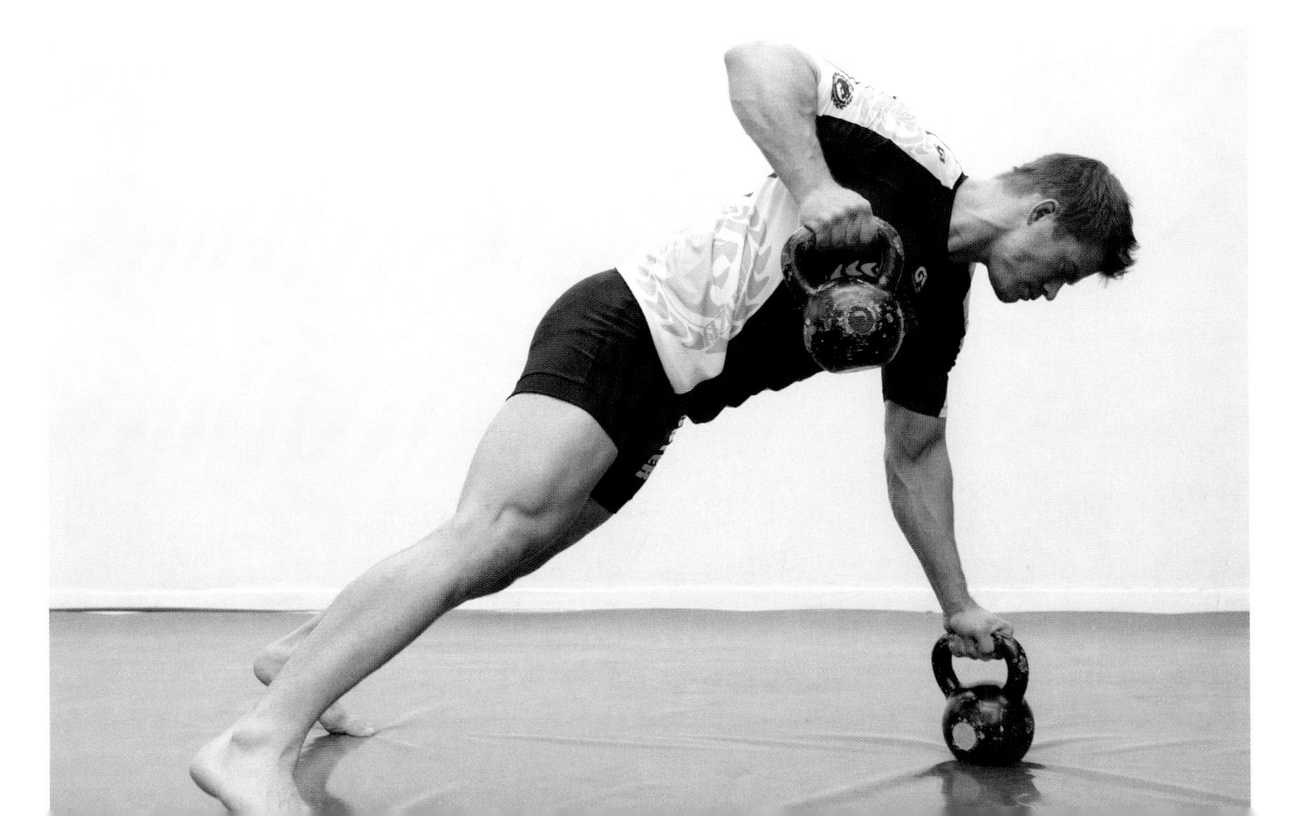

5. BARBELL ROLLOUT

Begin on the knees with the hands resting on a barbell shoulder width apart. Roll the bar forward on the ground while keeping the arms and lower back straight. Roll the bar until the body is horizontal, and then return to kneeling by reversing the motion. Perform 10 reps.

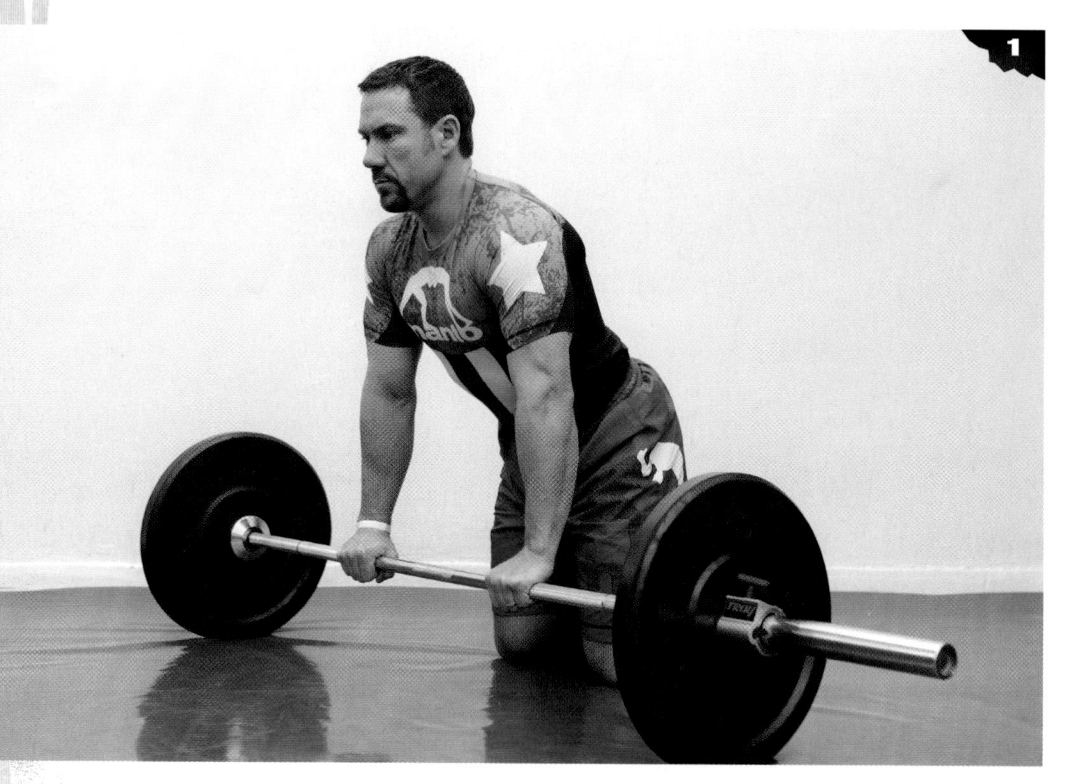

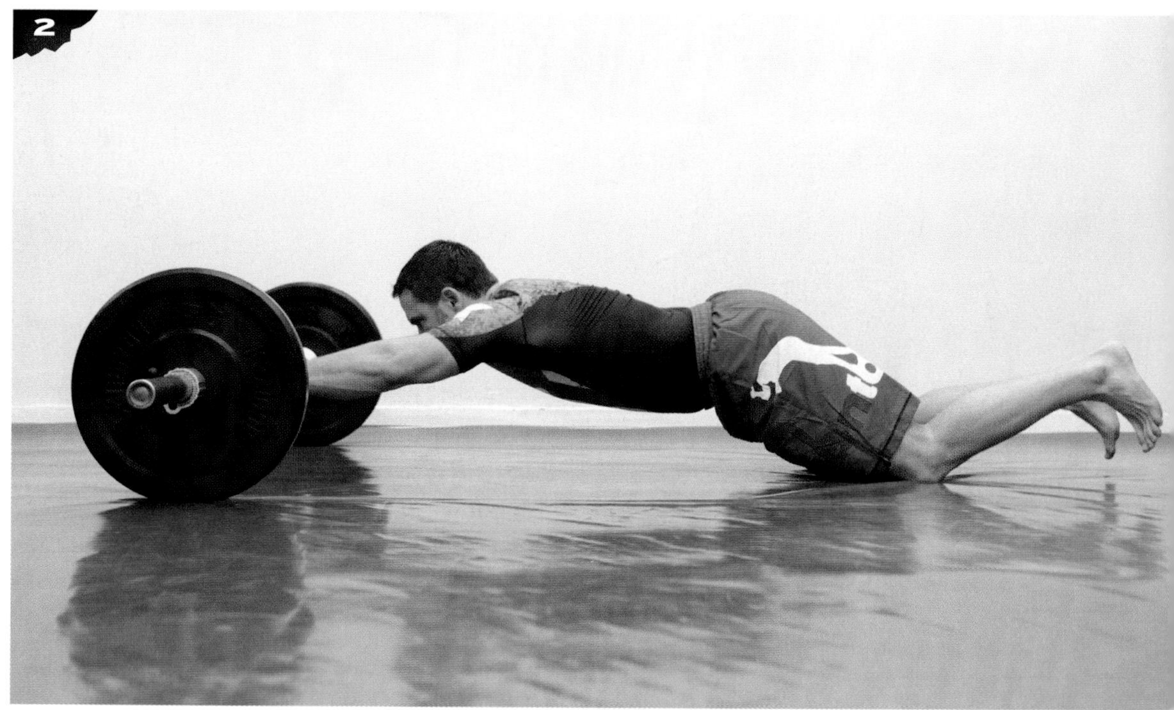

6. BARBELL OBLIQUE HOLDS

Begin lying on the back with a barbell pressed over the chest and the legs in the air. From this position, slowly lower the bar slightly to one side and the legs to the other side and hold. Perform 3 holds for 10 seconds on each side.

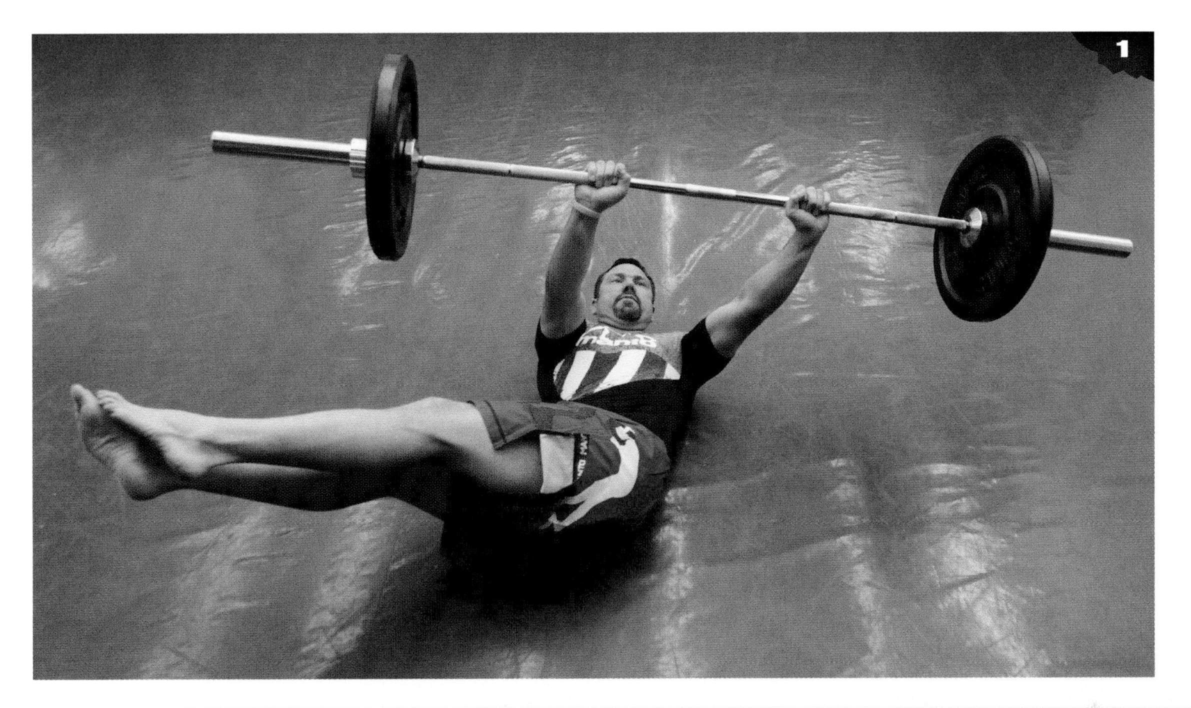

1

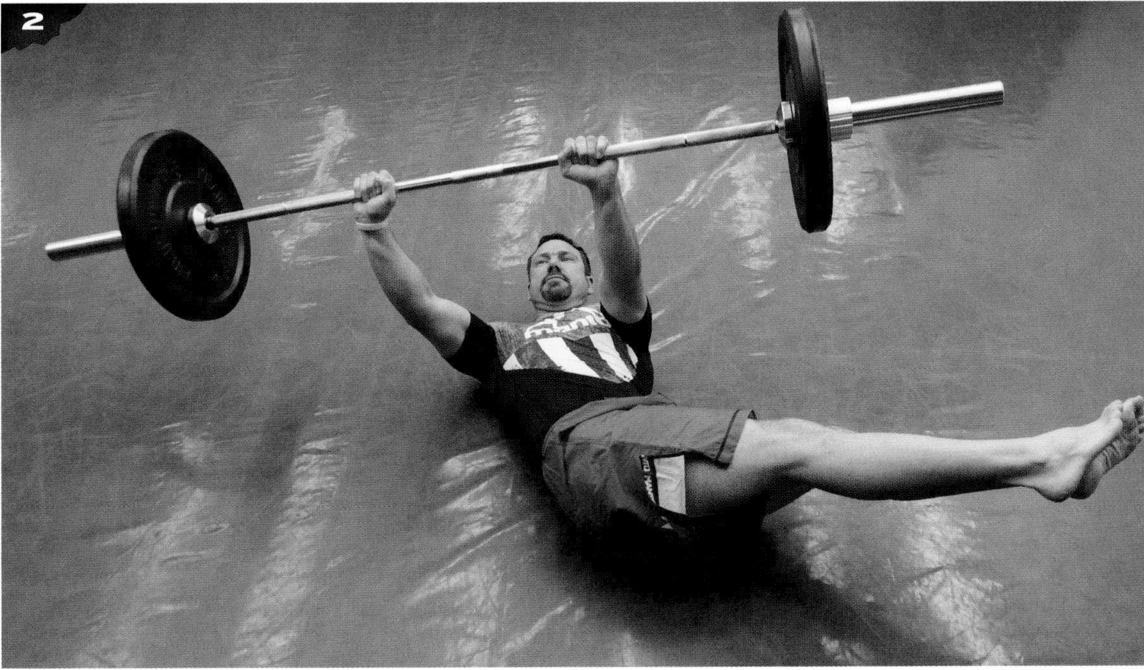

2

I. OBLIQUES CIRCUIT

Exercise 1 through 4 are to be performed for 2 sets of 10 reps on each side. Exercise 5 is to be performed for 3 sets of 10 reps.

1. SIDE CRUNCH

Begin lying on one side with the legs straight and bottom arm across the chest. By pushing into the ground with the bottom elbow, lift up the chest and bring the knees up. Lower back under control and repeat.

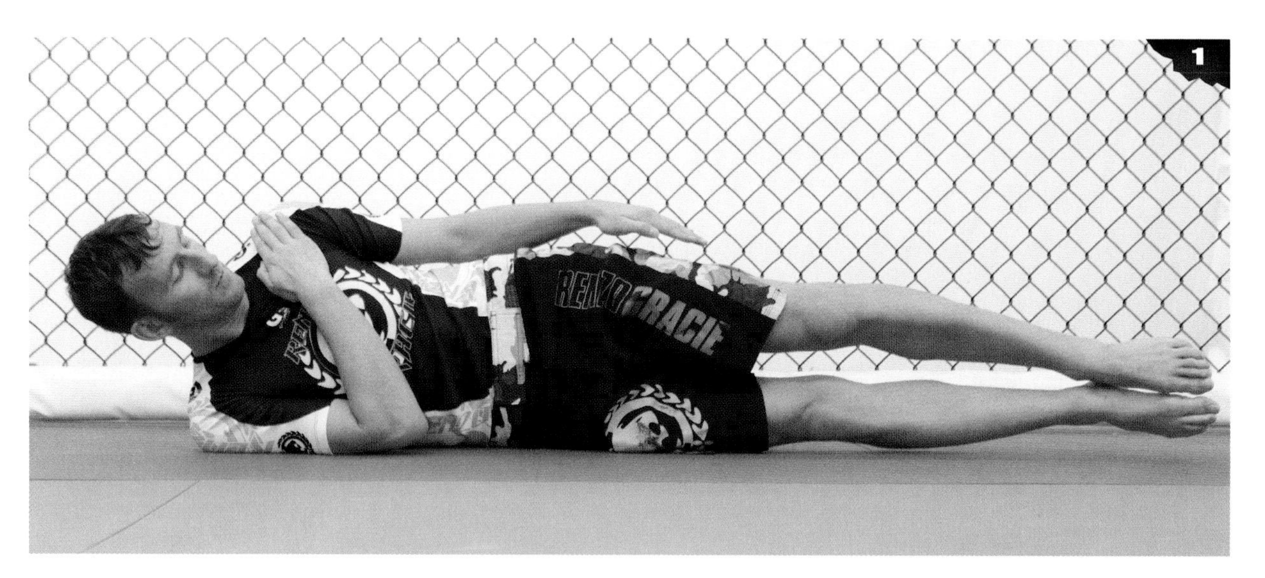

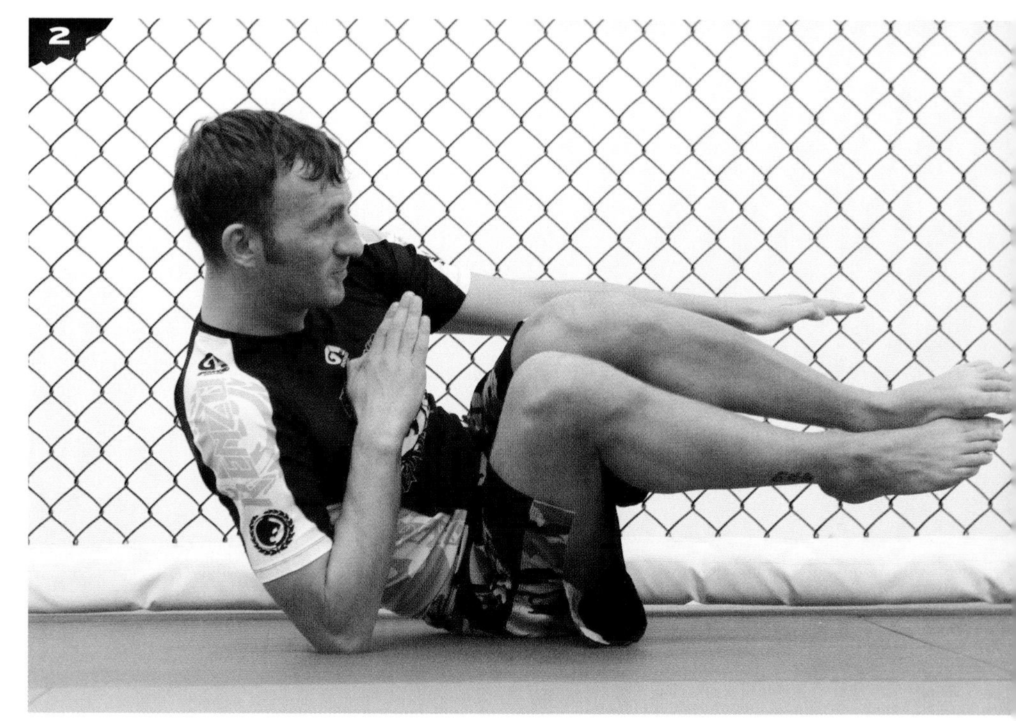

2. SIDE PRESS-UP

Begin lying on one side with the legs straight and the top hand on the ground by the waist. Lift the chest from the floor by contracting the core and pressing the hand into the ground. Lower under control and repeat.

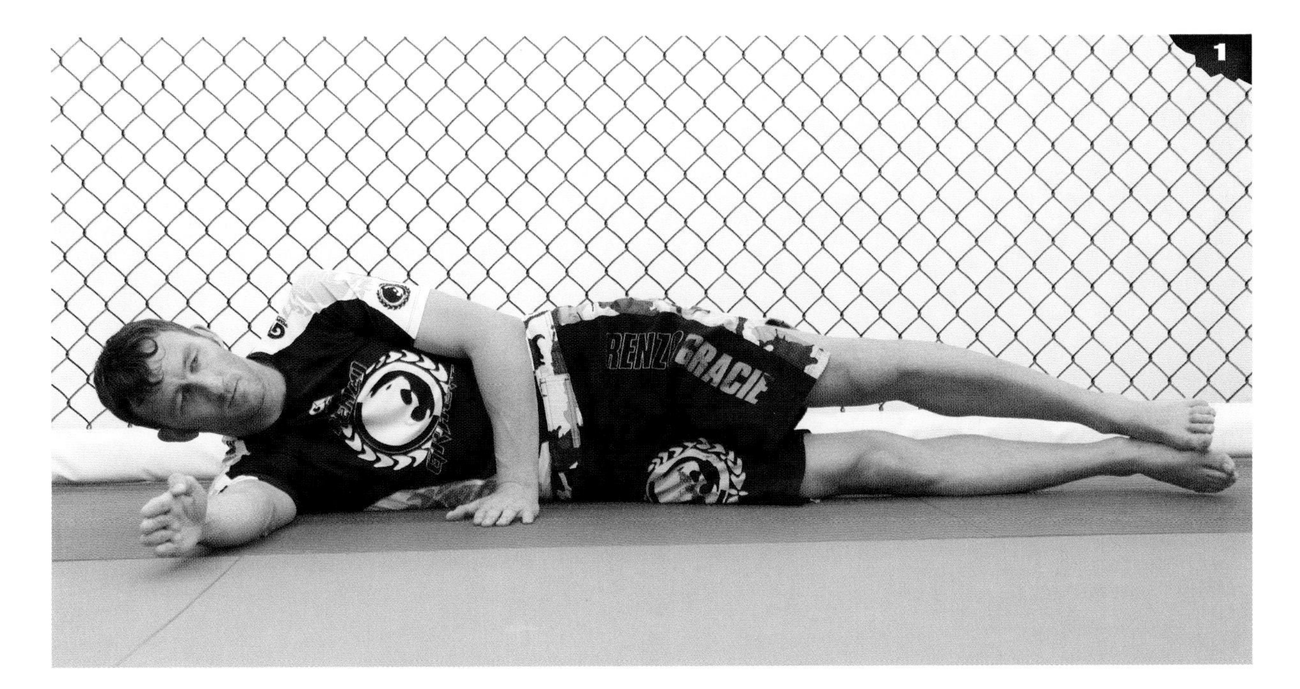

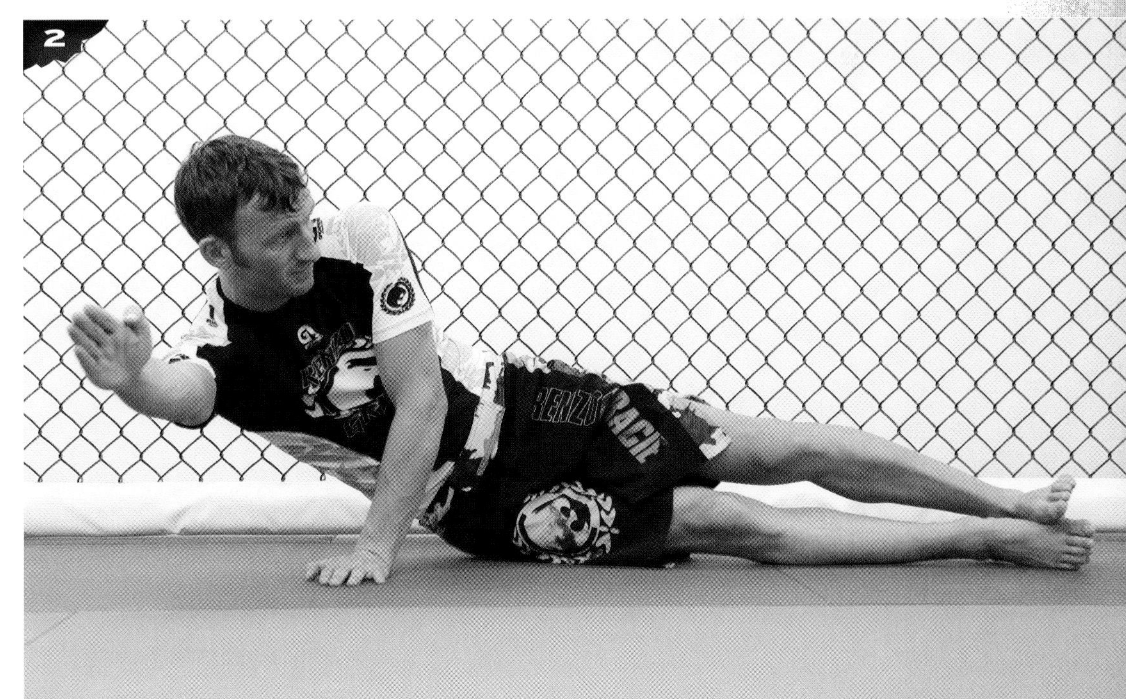

3. SIDE PRESS-UP WITH KNEE UP

Perform a Side Press-up and in the top position, bring up the top knee toward the chest. Lower under control and repeat.

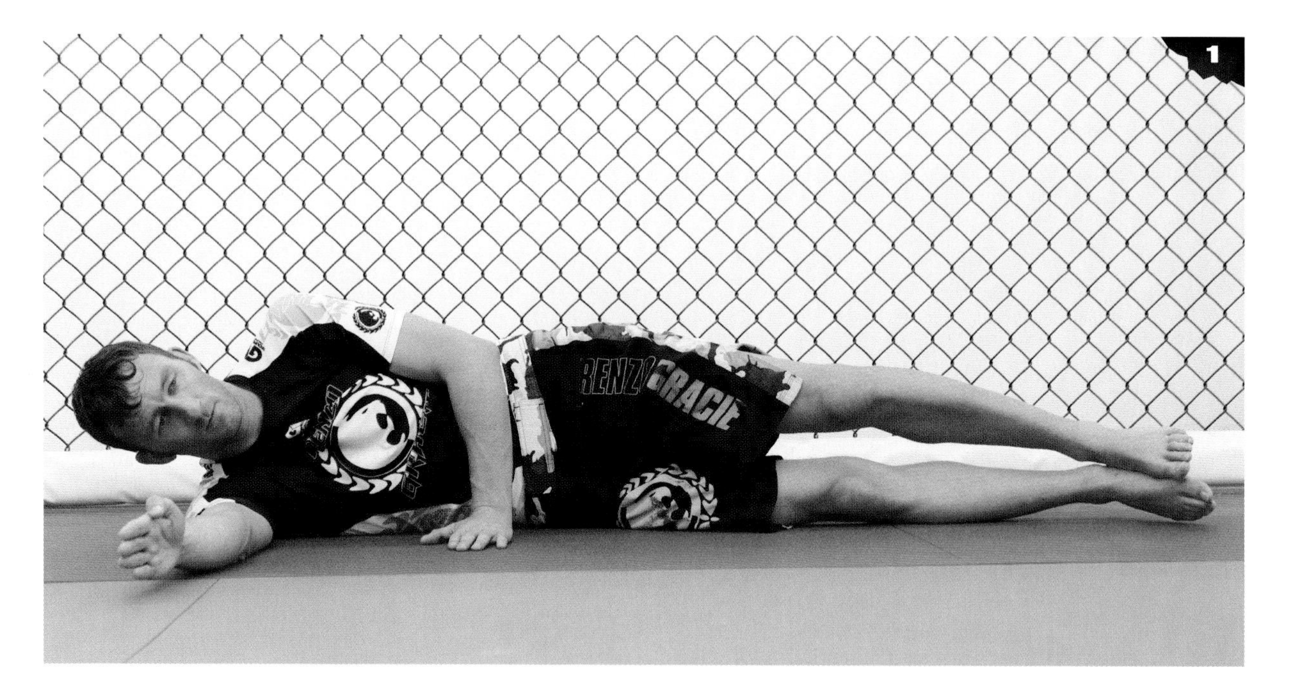

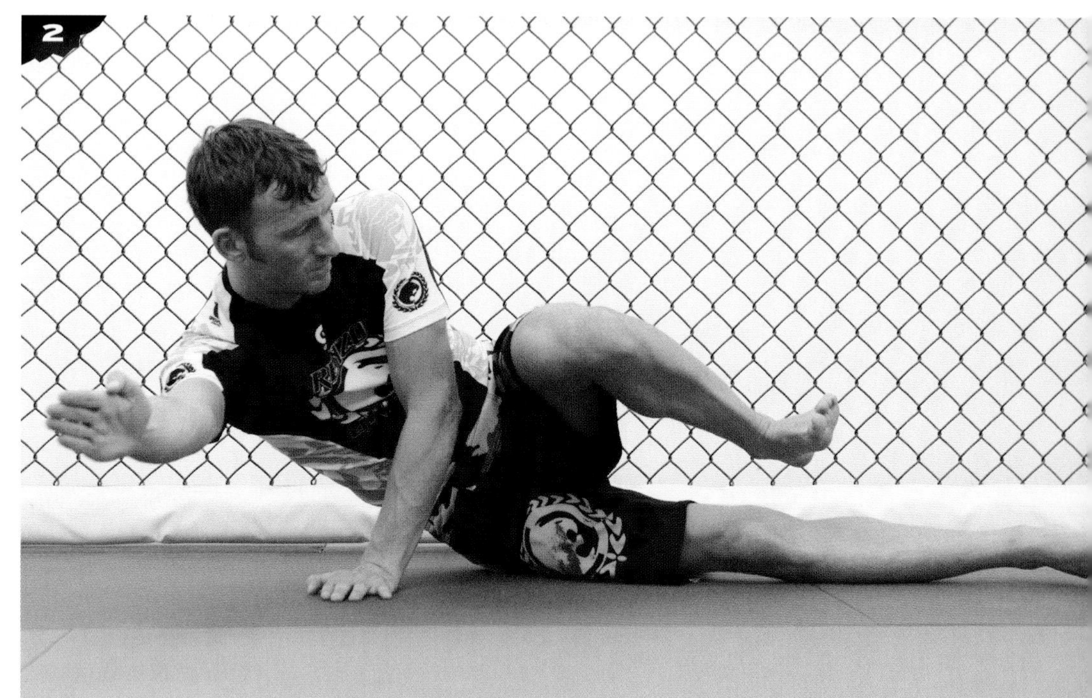

4. SEATED SIDE CRUNCH

Begin seated on one hip with the hands behind the body for support and the feet in the air with the knees extended. While keeping the core tight, bring the knees up toward the chest. Return to the start position and repeat.

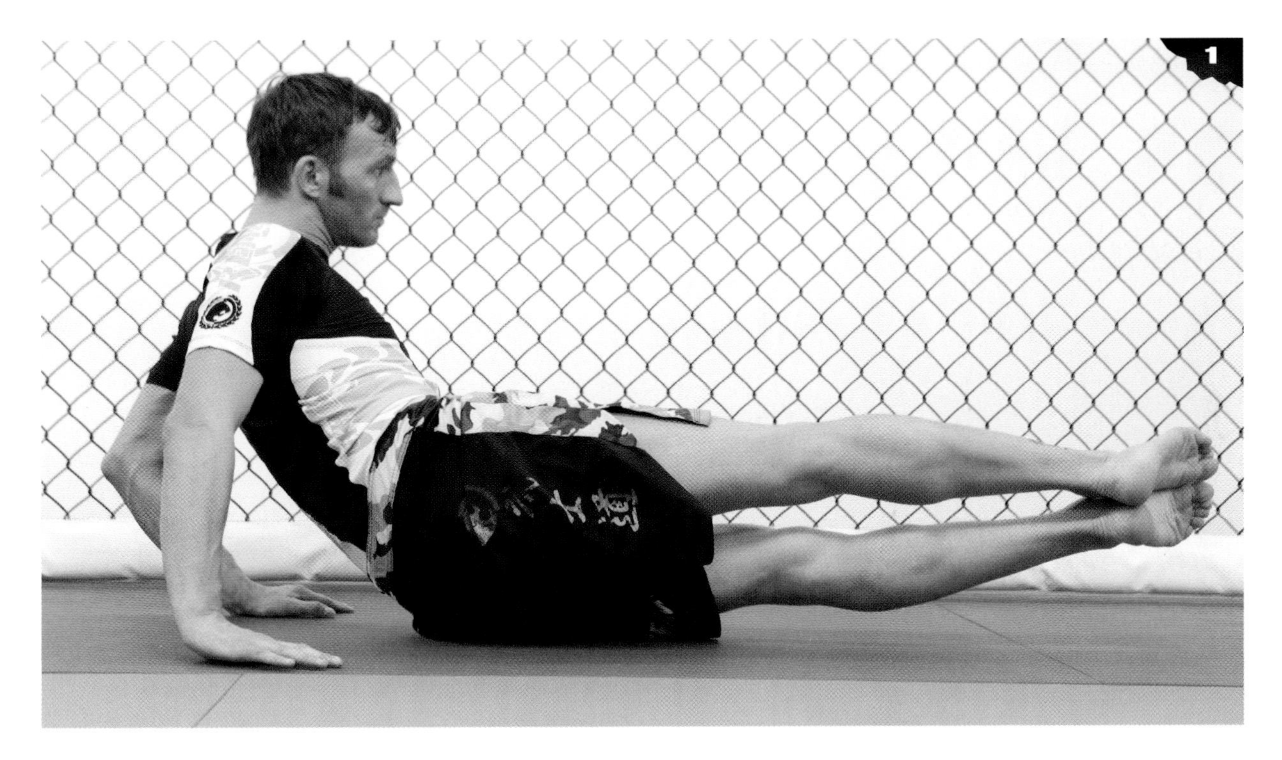

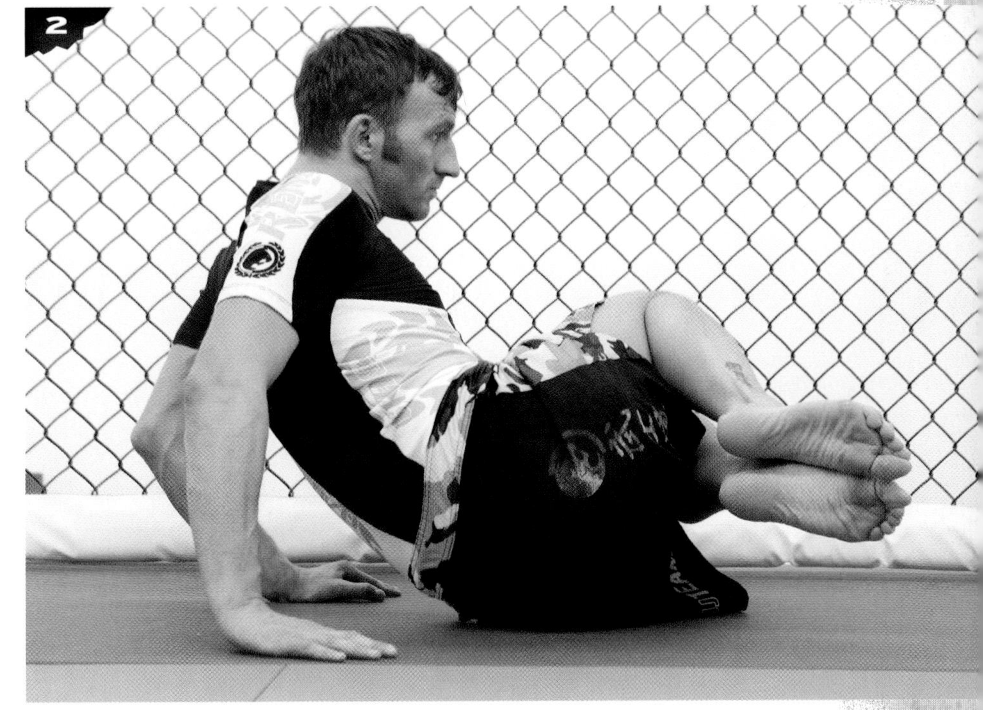

5. SEATED CRUNCH

Begin seated with the hands behind the head and the feet in the air with the knees extended. While keeping the core tight, bring the knees up and touch them with the elbows. Return to the original position and repeat.

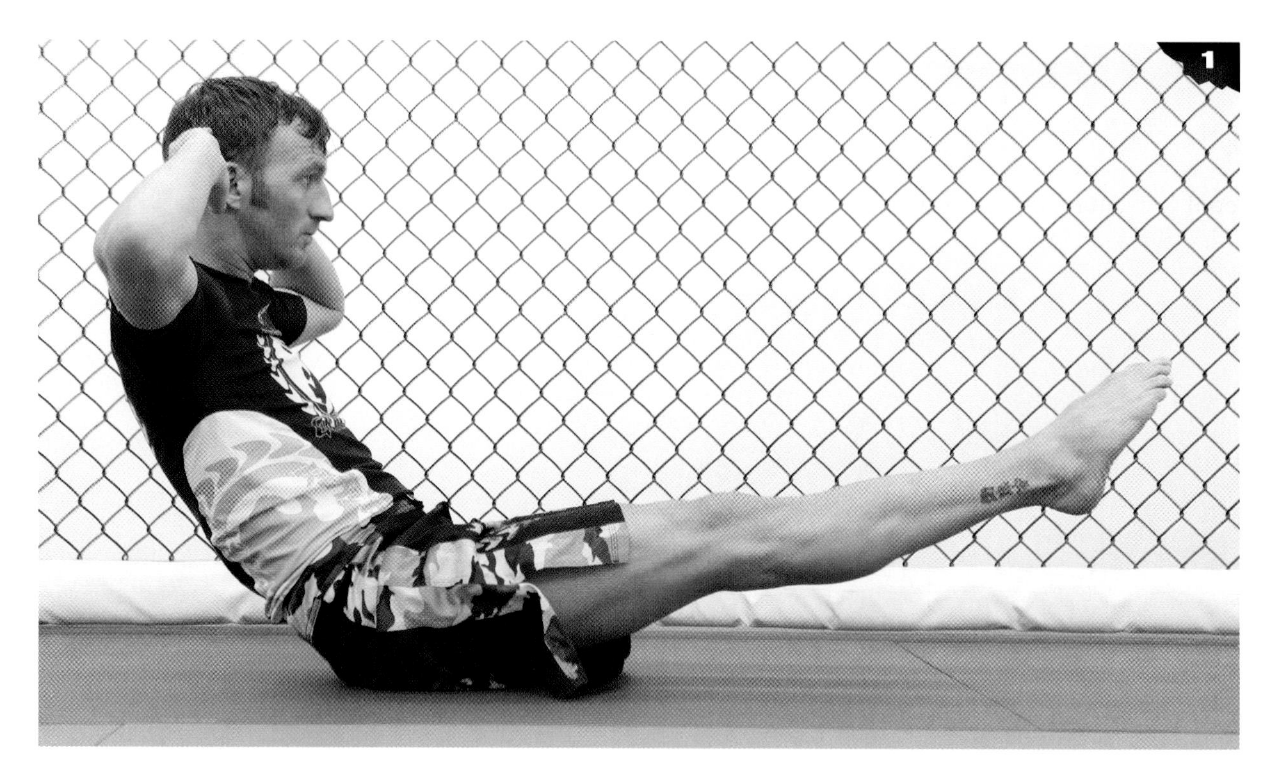

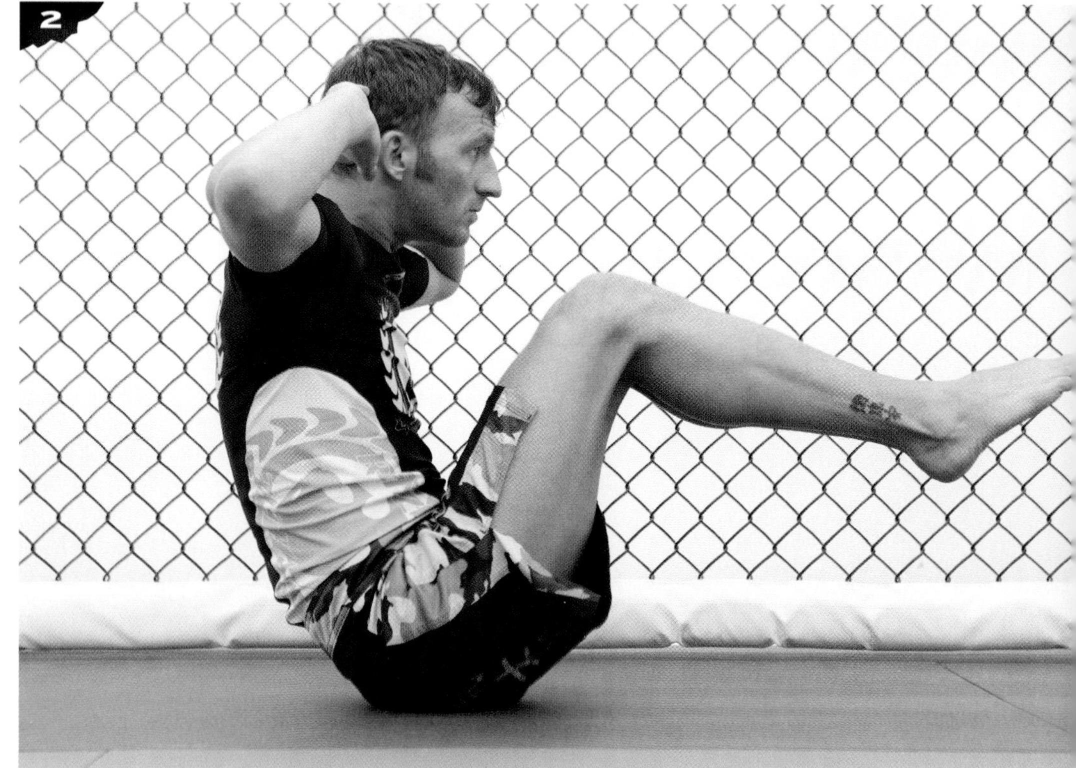

J. HIP FLEXOR CIRCUIT

To complete a circuit, exercises 1 through 3 are to be performed for 15 reps on each side. Exercise 4 is to be performed for 15 complete revolutions. Perform the circuit for 3 total sets.

1. ROPE CLIMB

Begin sitting with the feet in the air and one knee pulled up and the other leg extended. The arm on the side of the extended leg should reach up to the ceiling and row down on the side of the bent leg. Alternate back and forth while keeping the core tight.

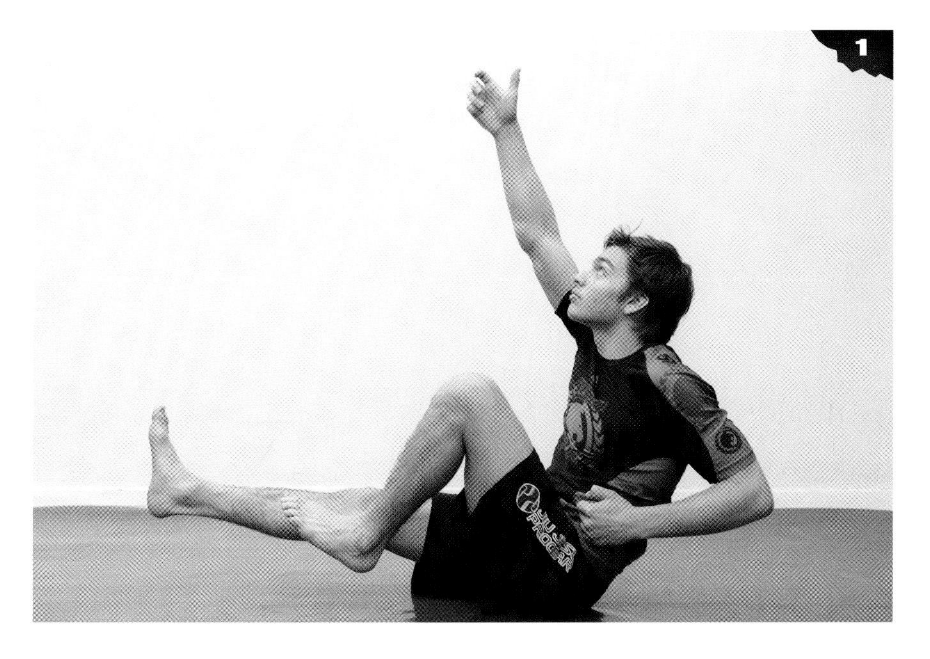

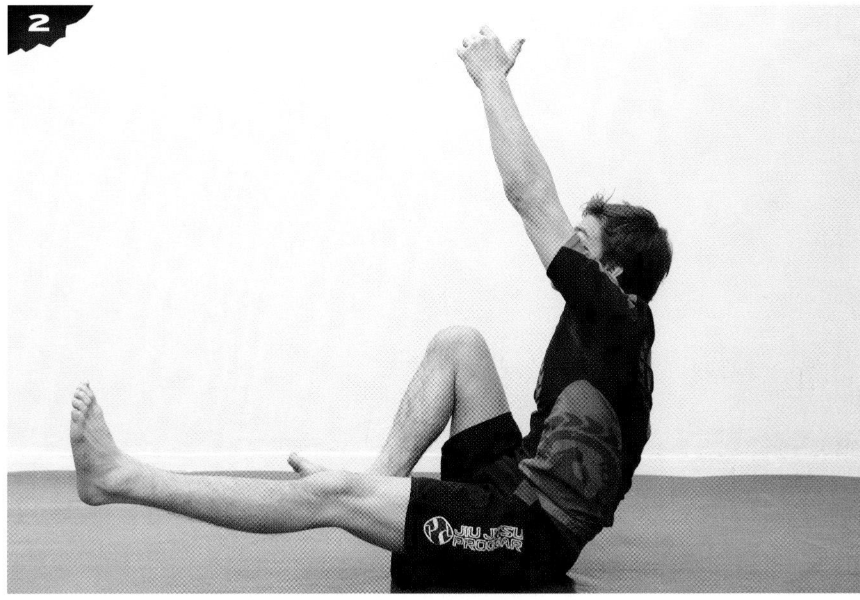

2. ROPE PULL

Begin sitting with the feet in the air and one knee pulled up and the other leg extended. The arm on the side of the extended leg should reach forward and row back on the side of the bent leg. Alternate back and forth while keeping the core tight.

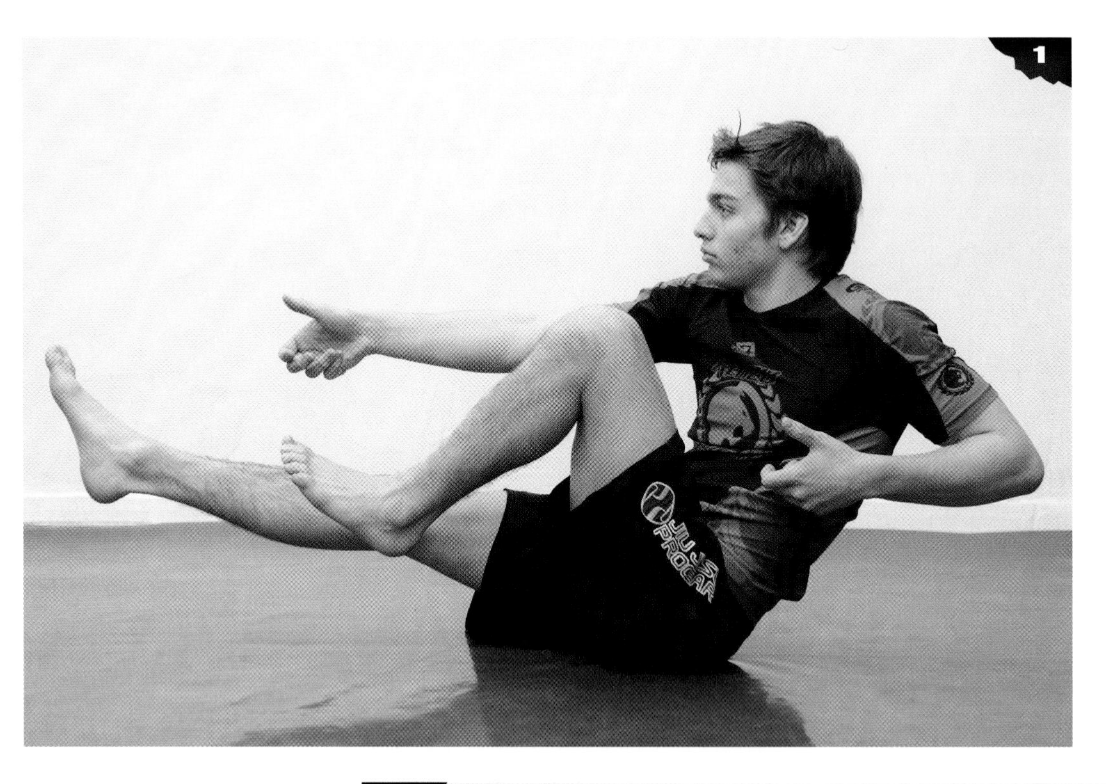

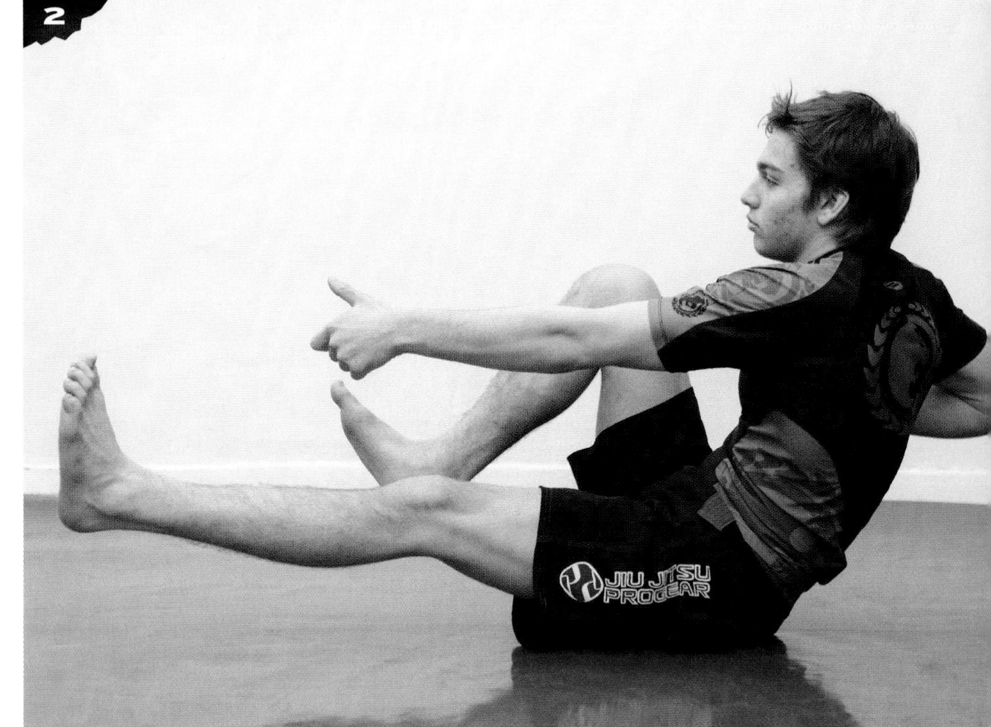

3. FOOT GRABS

Begin sitting with the feet in the air and the hands held out to the sides. Quickly pull one foot up and grab it with the opposite hand. Return to the original position and then repeat on the other leg.

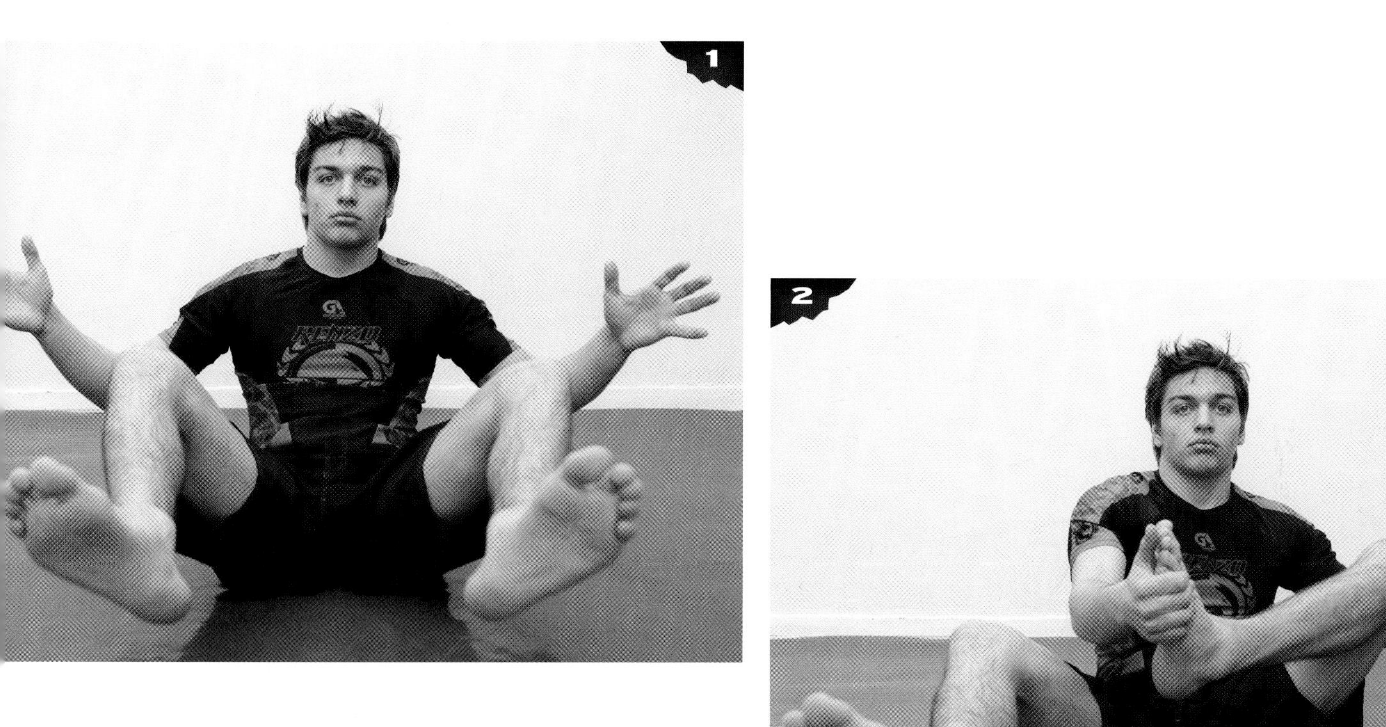

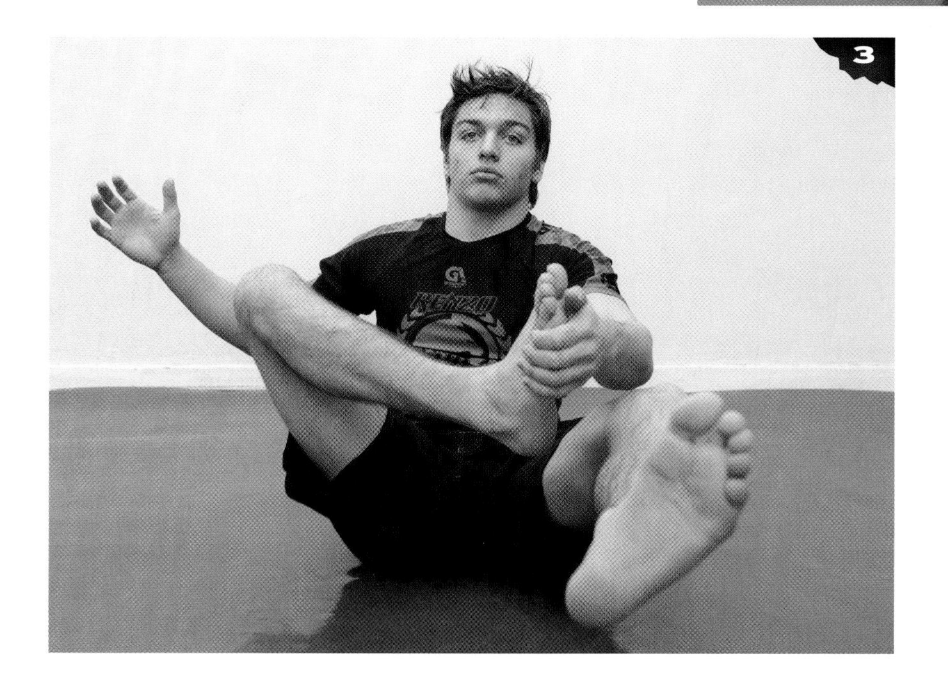

4. MED BALL SCISSORS

Begin in a seated position, holding the feet in the air and the med ball with one hand. Bring one knee up while extending the other leg. Pass the ball under the bent knee and over the lower leg. Switch the positions of the legs and then pass the ball under the bent knee.

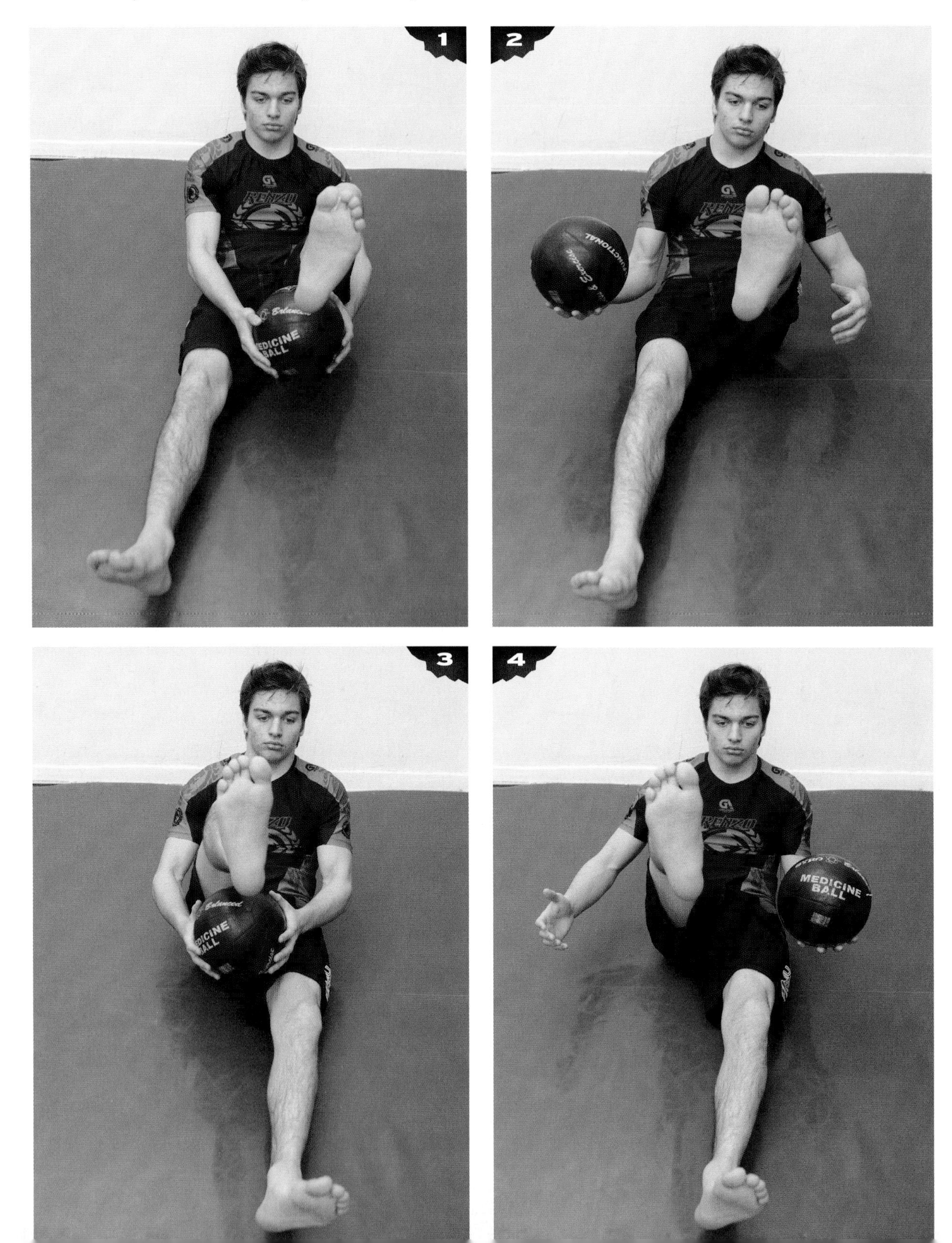

K. PARTNER CORE DRILLS CIRCUIT

To complete a circuit, perform the exercises in a row as described. Perform the circuit for 3 total sets.

1. PARTNER CRUNCH ROLLS

One partner lies on the ground in the crunch position with the elbows held touching the knees. The standing partner grabs the lying partner's ankles and pulls them forward and down so the partner's chest begins to rise. Once the feet touch the floor, the standing partner lowers the lying partner back to the starting position. The goal of the lying partner is to not allow the elbows to move from the knees. Perform for 8 reps.

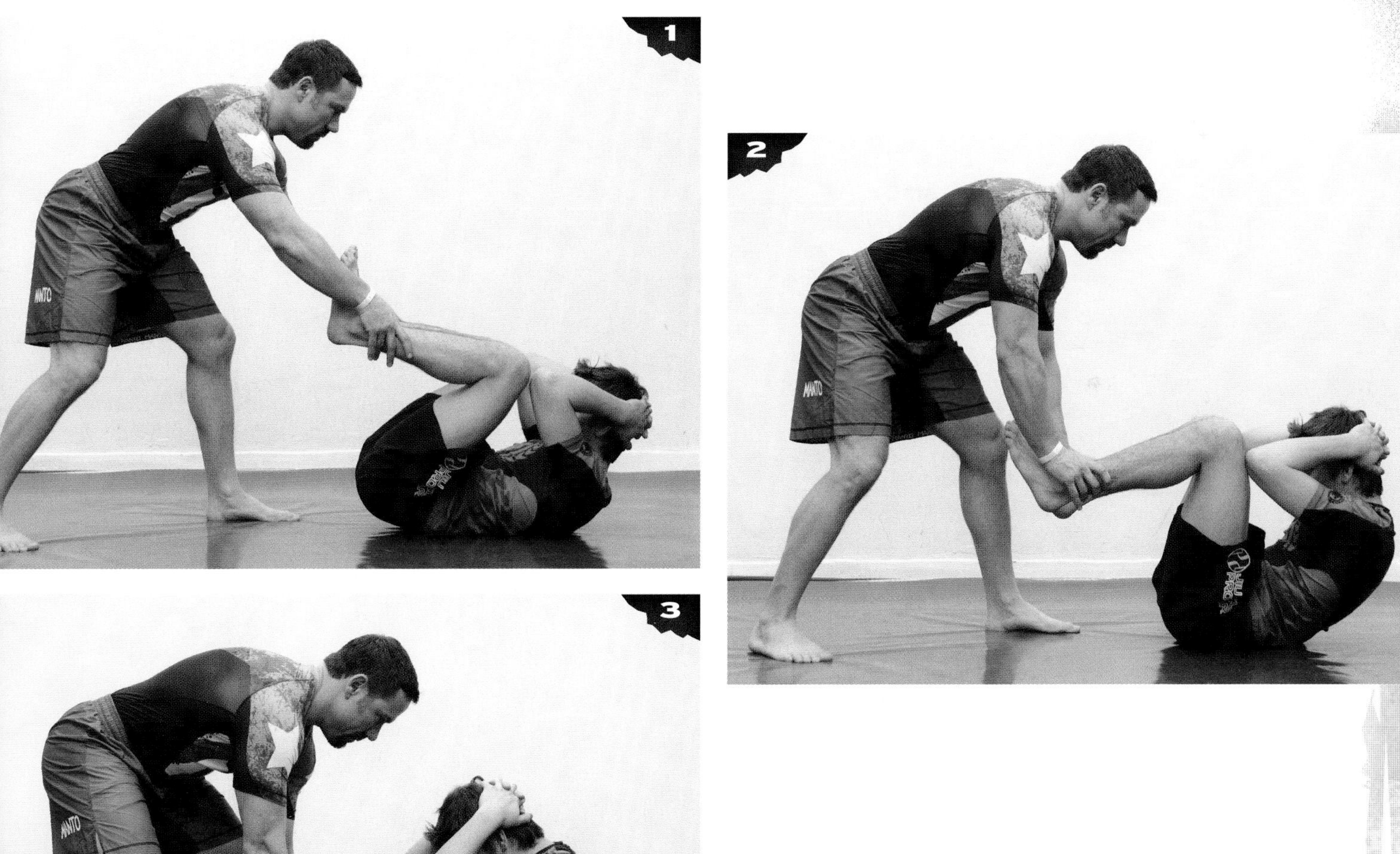

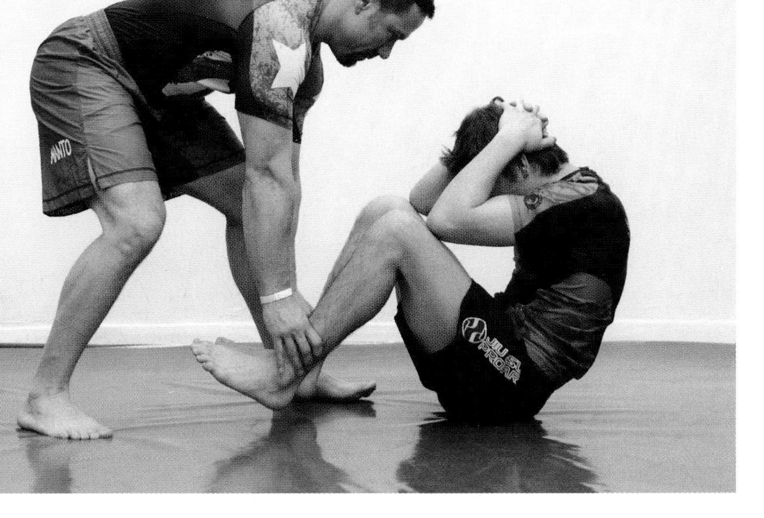

2. PARTNER STRAIGHT-LEG THROWS

The lying partner grabs the ankles of the standing partner and kicks his legs up toward the standing partner's hands. The standing partner receives the feet and quickly throws them straight forward and back to the ground. The goal of the lying partner is to slow the legs and repeat. Perform for 20 throws.

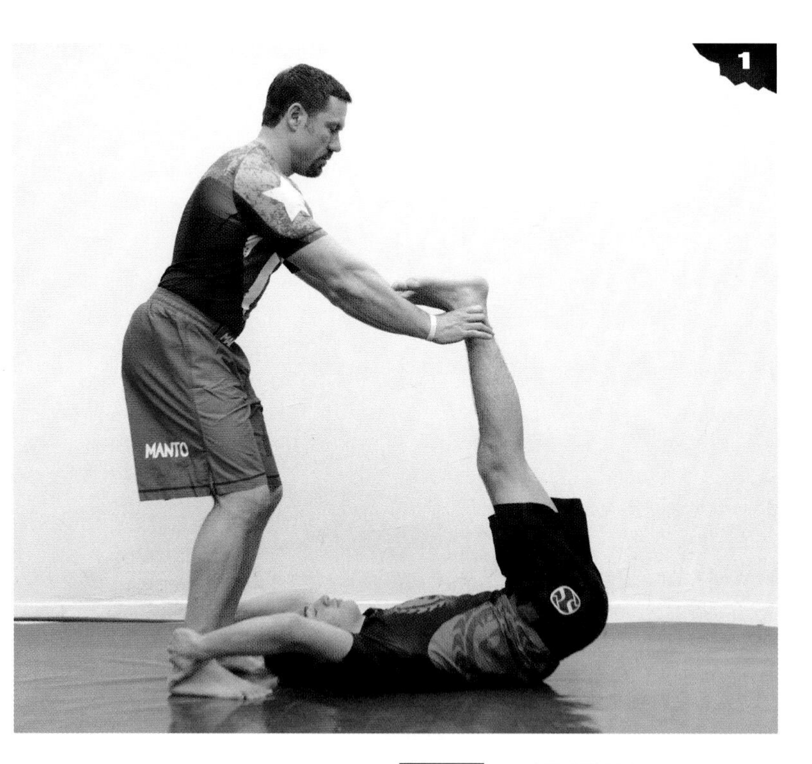

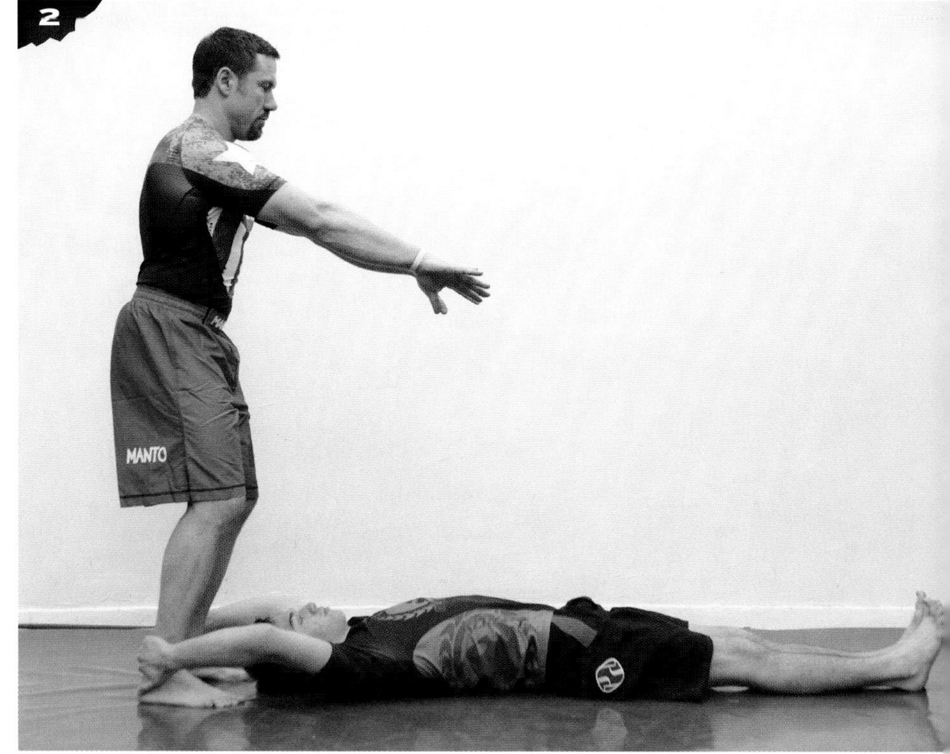

3. PARTNER SIDE LEG THROWS

The lying partner grabs the ankles of the standing partner and kicks his legs up toward the standing partner's hands. The standing partner receives the feet and quickly throws them out to the side and back to the ground. The goal of the lying partner is to slow the legs and repeat. Perform for 15 throws to each side.

1

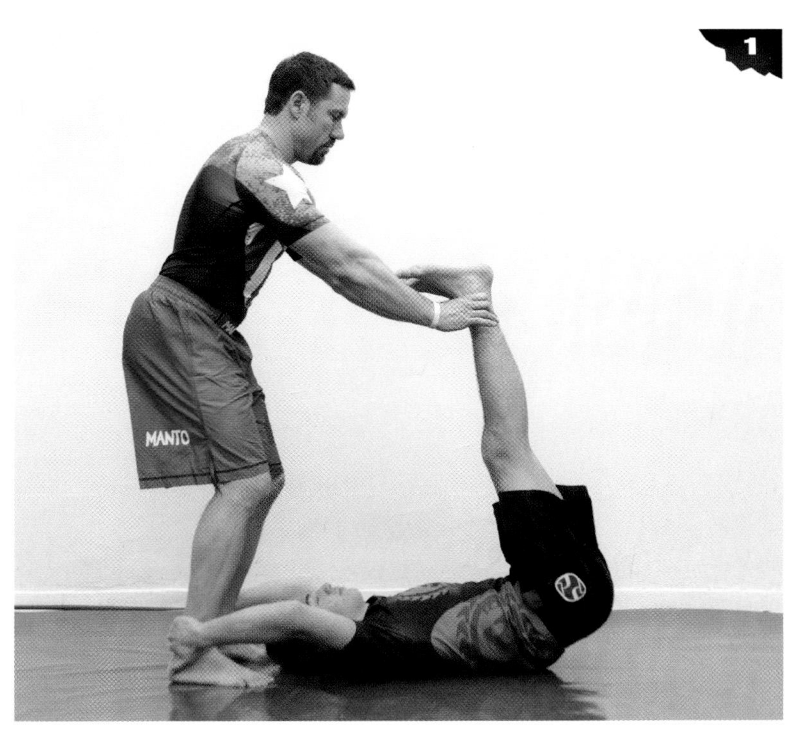

2

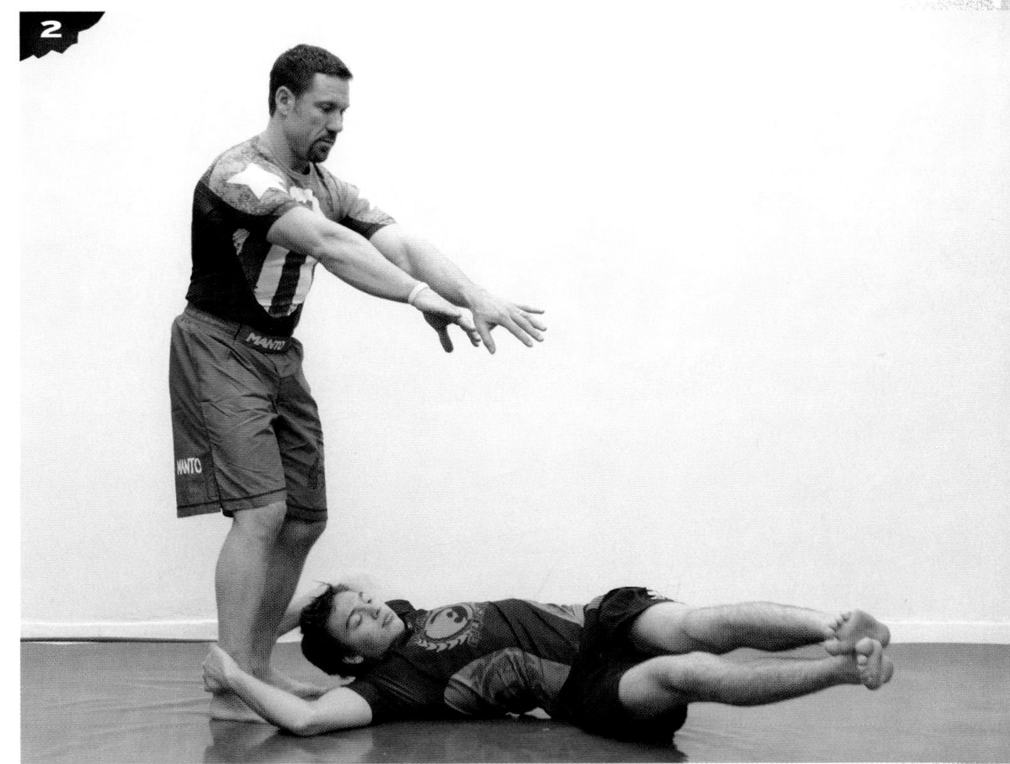

4. PARTNER SIT AND PUNCH

One partner lies on the back facing the standing partner with hands at the chin and knees bent. The lying partner sits up quickly and throws a punch at the standing partner's hands. He then quickly returns to the start position and repeats. Perform for 10 punches to each side.

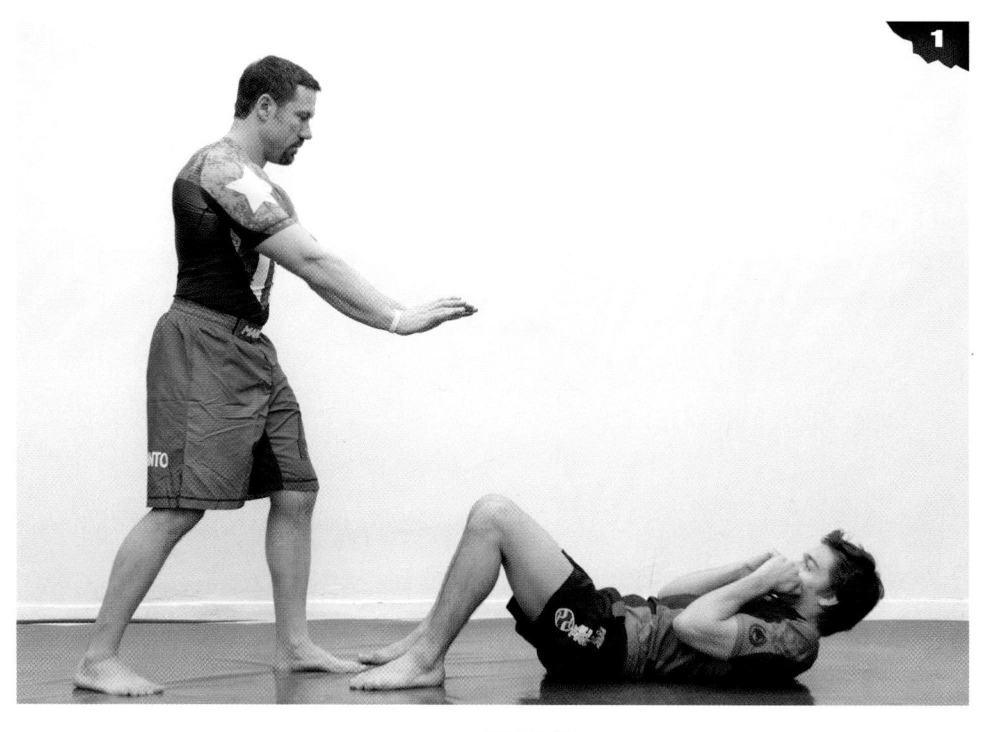

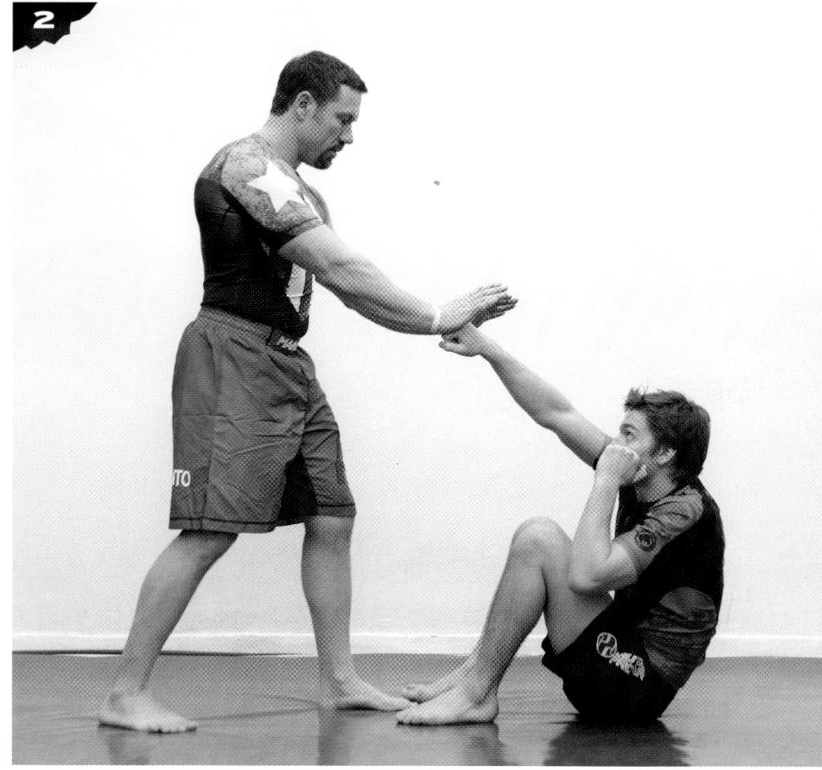

L. PARTNER MEDICINE BALL CIRCUIT

TAKE A DOSE OF THE MEDICINE BALL

During a recent workout, an MMA athlete asked why a medicine ball is called a medicine ball. Having used medicine balls for 20 years, I was surprised to realize I did not know. After some research, I was reminded that although the medicine ball is a popular core training tool, it is also the stuff of legend. The term "medicine ball" is said to have originated on U.S. transatlantic ships during World War I. Since the confined crew was bored from lack of exercise and seasick from long times at sea, the medical staff needed a way to work both their bodies and minds. These medics decided to stuff some basketballs with rags in order to weight them and created ball exercises to work the crew. The balls were referred to as "medicine" balls because exercise remedied the crews' symptoms as well as traditional pills.

Today we know there are two major advantages to medicine ball training. First, the medicine ball can be used in many different planes of motion. Since the ball is free to move anywhere, it can help to develop strength in many directions and angles. Second, a medicine ball can be thrown and released quickly, which allows an athlete to develop explosiveness.

To complete a circuit, exercises 1 through 3 are to be performed for 20 throws and 4 through 6 are to be performed for 15 throws on each side. Perform the circuit for 2 total sets.

1. PARTNER SEATED CHEST THROWS

Sit on the floor with the feet in the air. Pass the ball via chest passes with the standing partner.

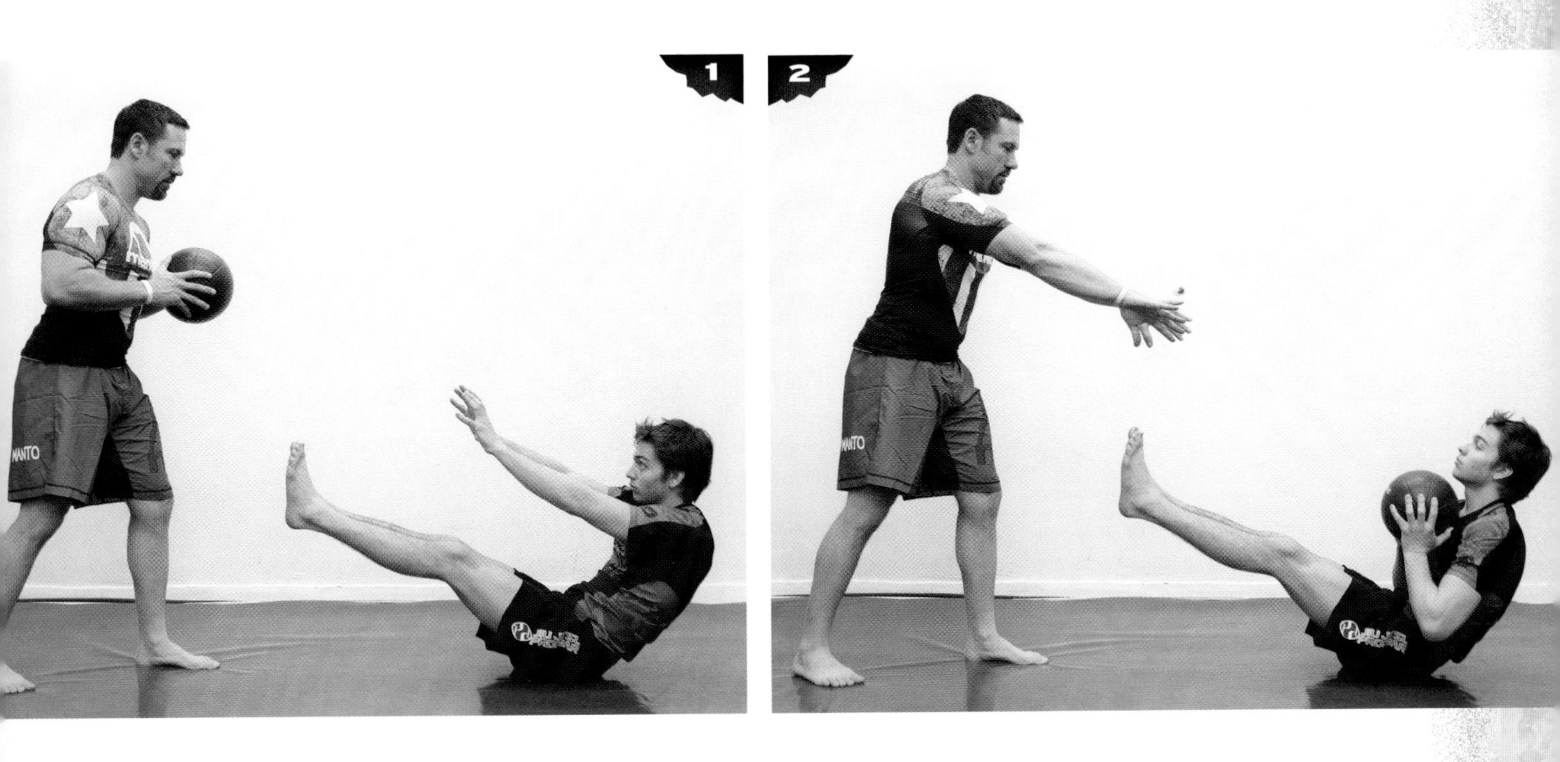

2. PARTNER KNEELING OVERHEAD THROWS

Begin kneeling, facing the standing partner with the ball held overhead. Throw the ball to the partner and wait to receive it back.

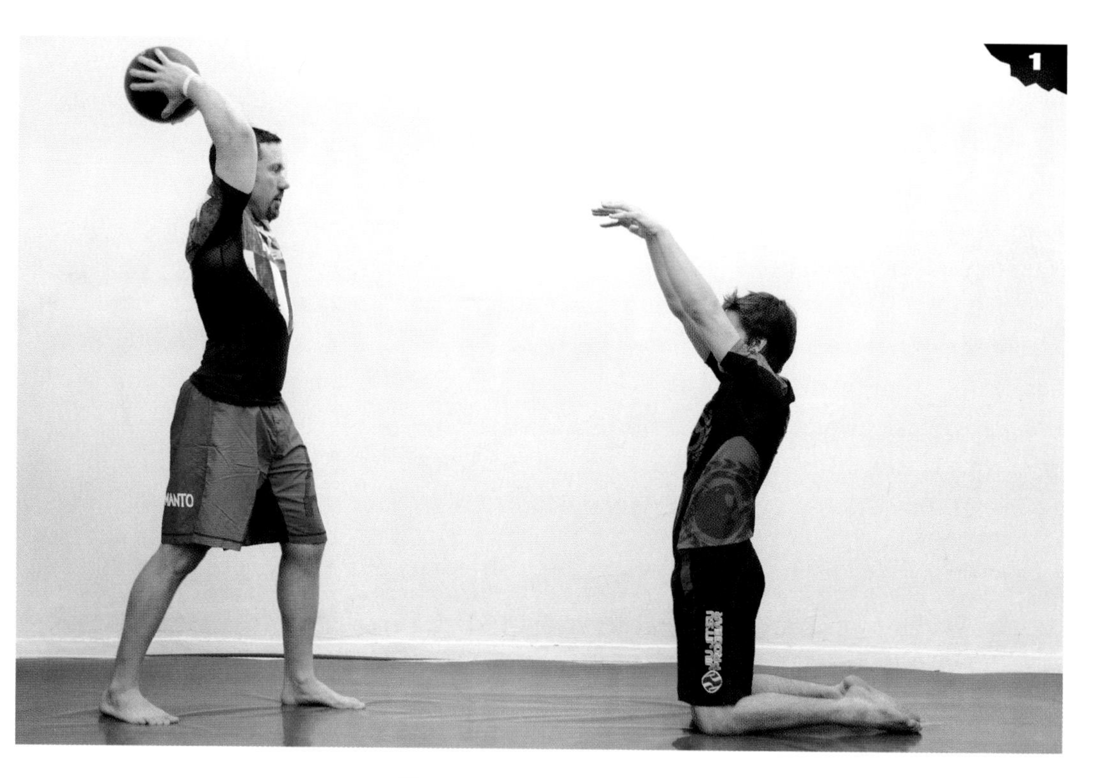

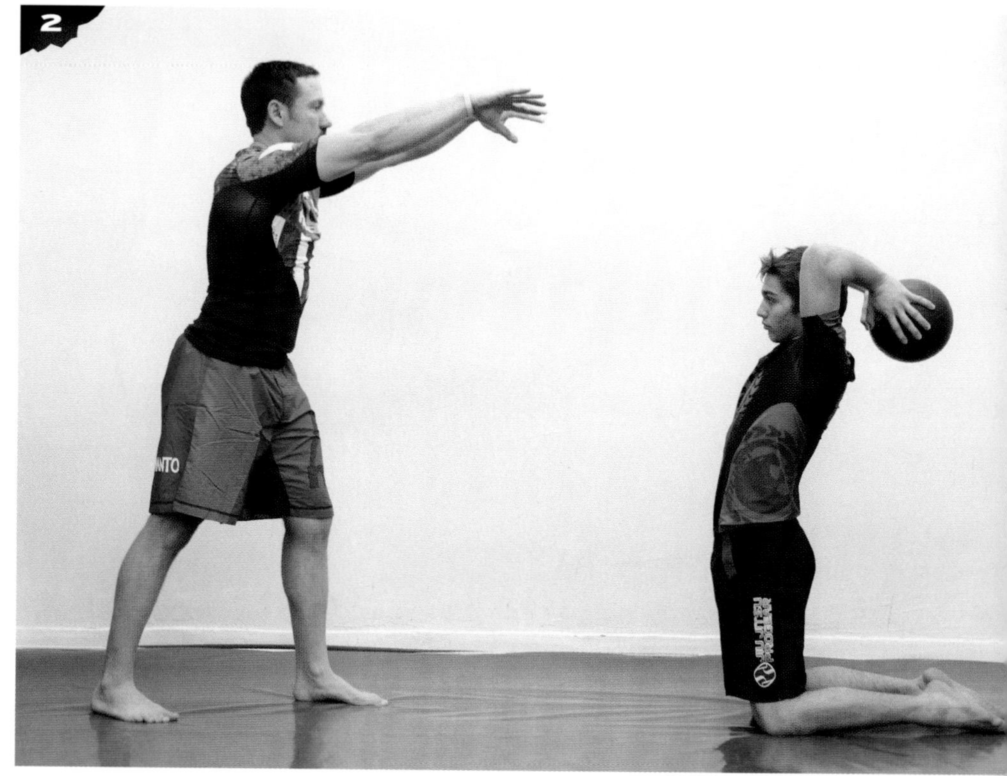

3. PARTNER LYING OVERHEAD THROWS

Begin seated facing the standing partner with the hands overhead. Receive the ball, lie back down, and then reverse the motion and throw the ball back to the partner.

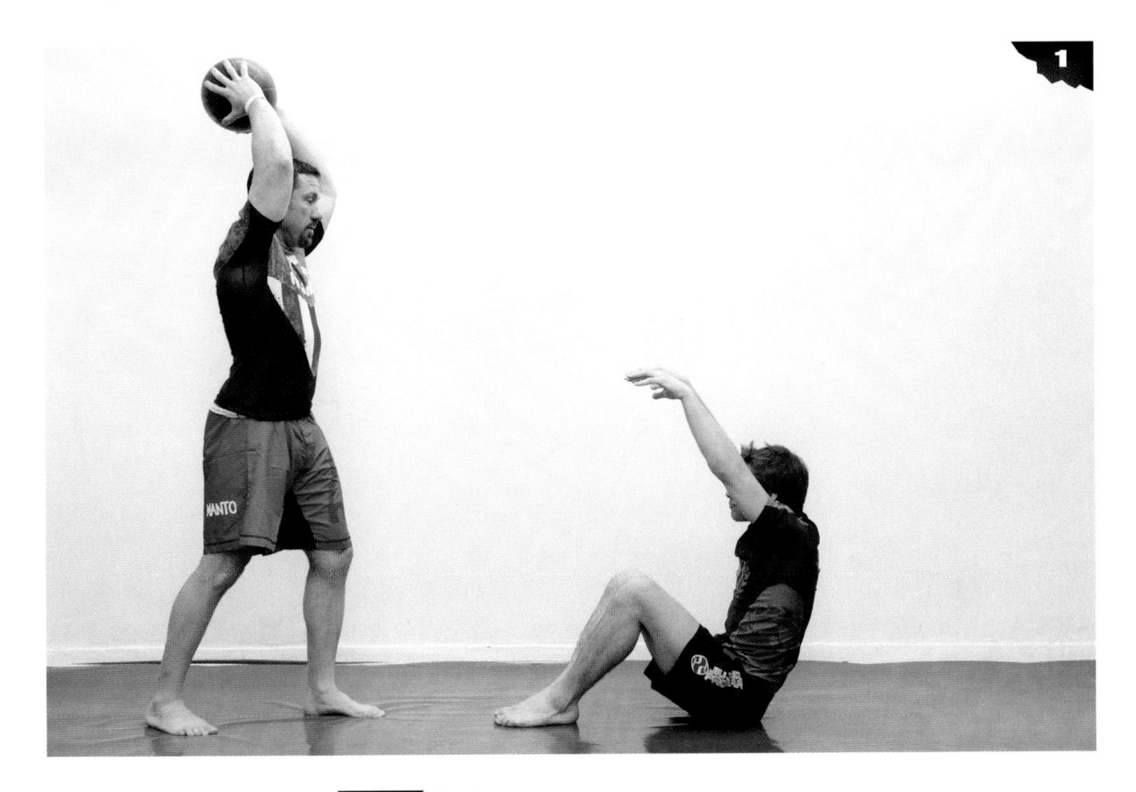

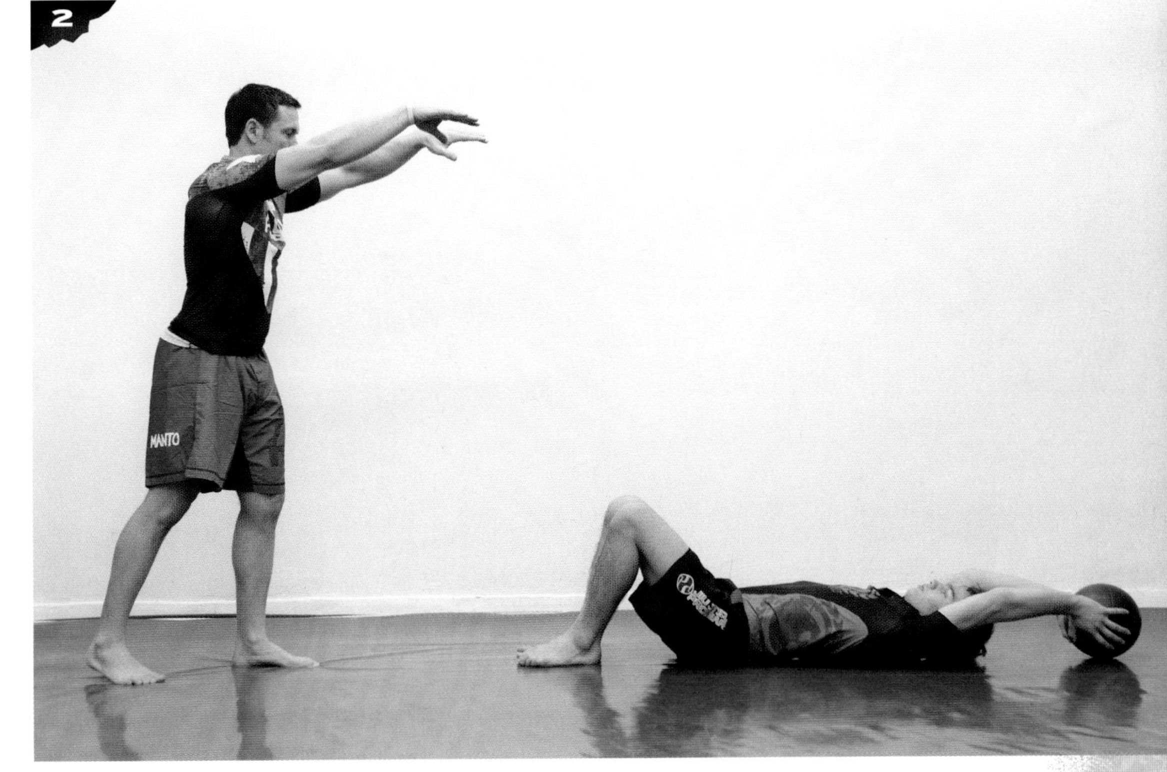

4. PARTNER SEATED SIDE THROWS

Begin seated on the floor perpendicular to the standing partner. Catch the ball and twist away from the partner. Then twist back and throw the ball back as if throwing a bucket of water.

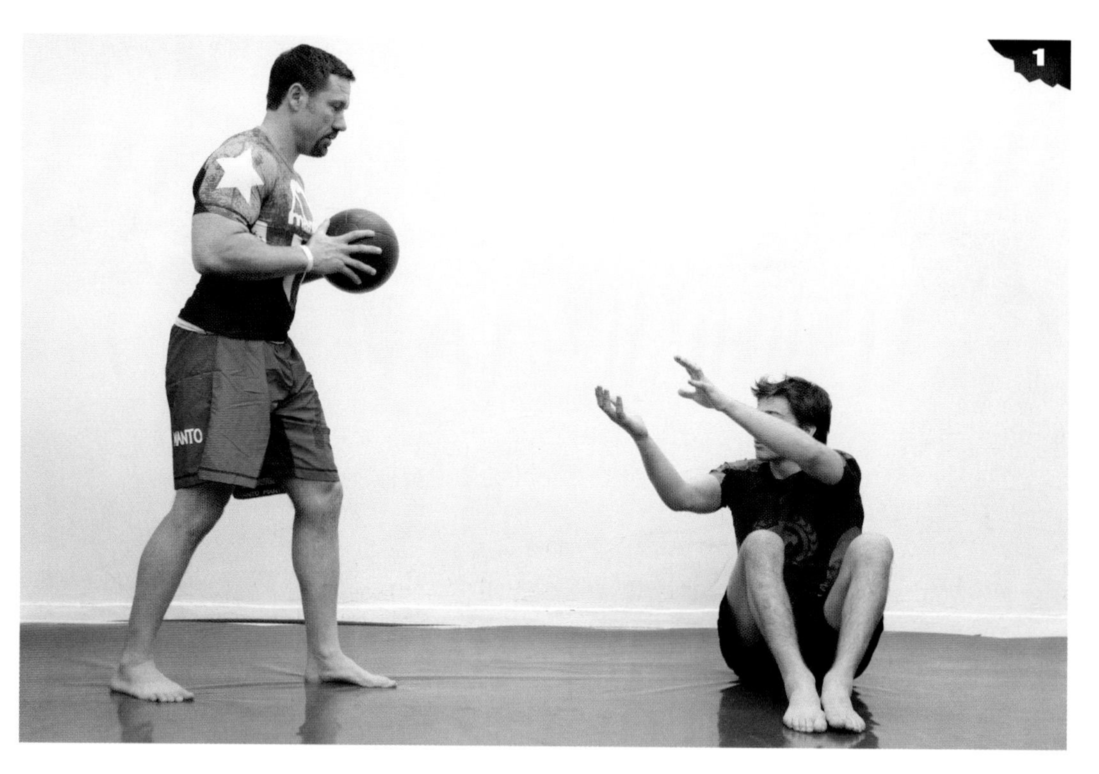

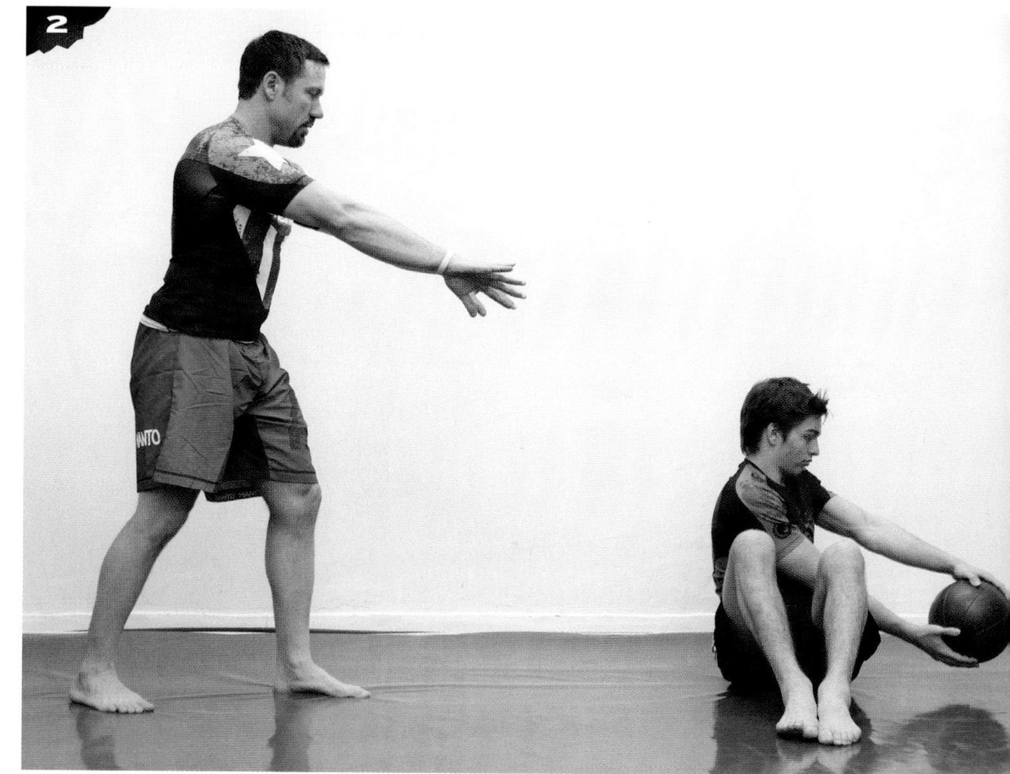

5. PARTNER SINGLE-ARM THROWS

Begin seated facing the standing partner with feet off the floor and the ball in one hand. Press the ball to the partner and then wait to receive it back.

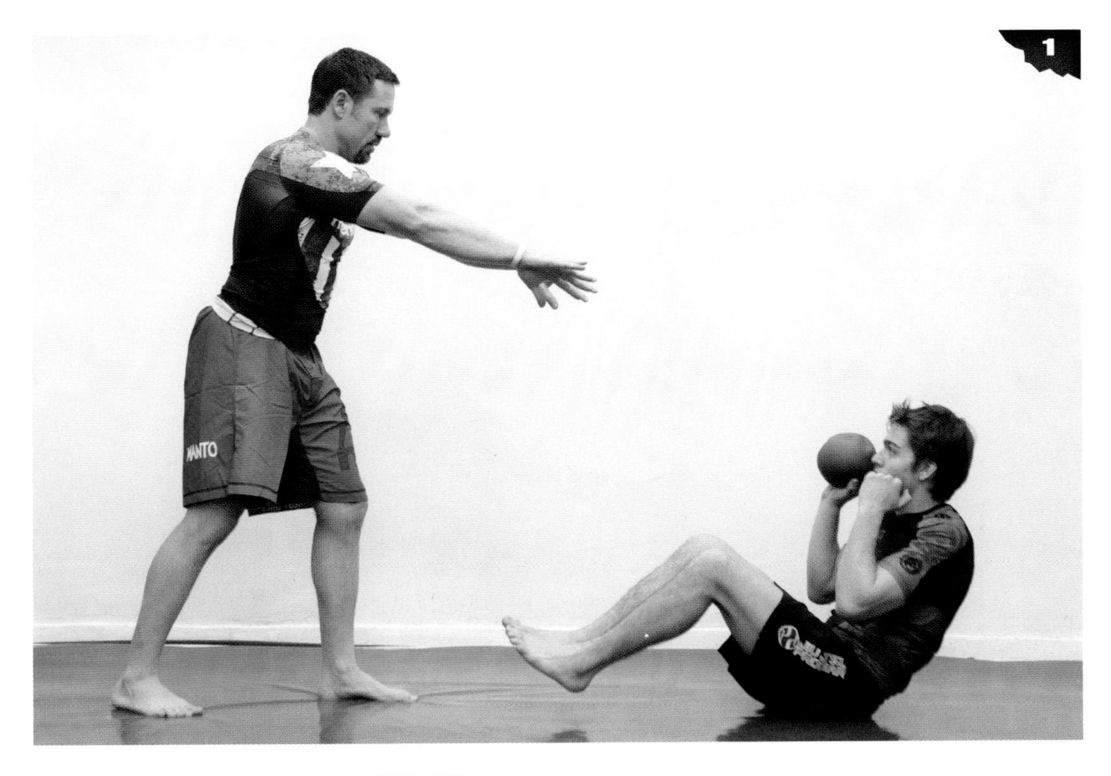

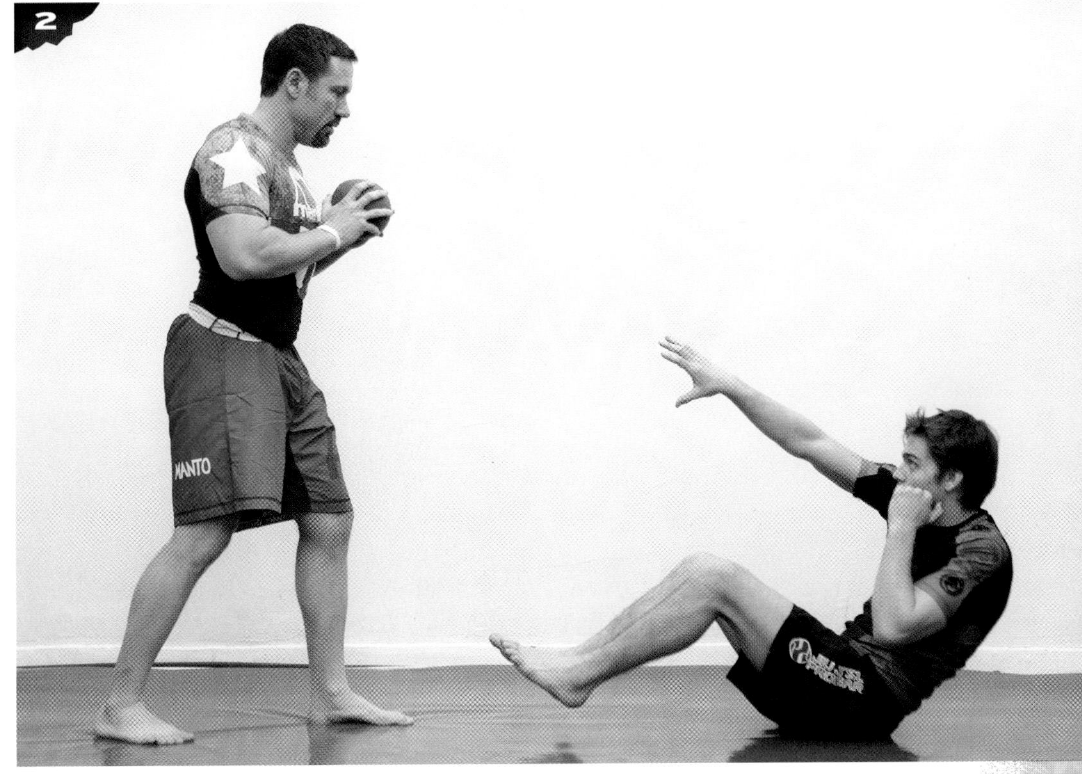

6. PARTNER KNEELING BACKWARD THROWS

Begin kneeling, facing away from the standing partner with the ball held out front. Twist and throw the ball to the partner and wait to receive it back.

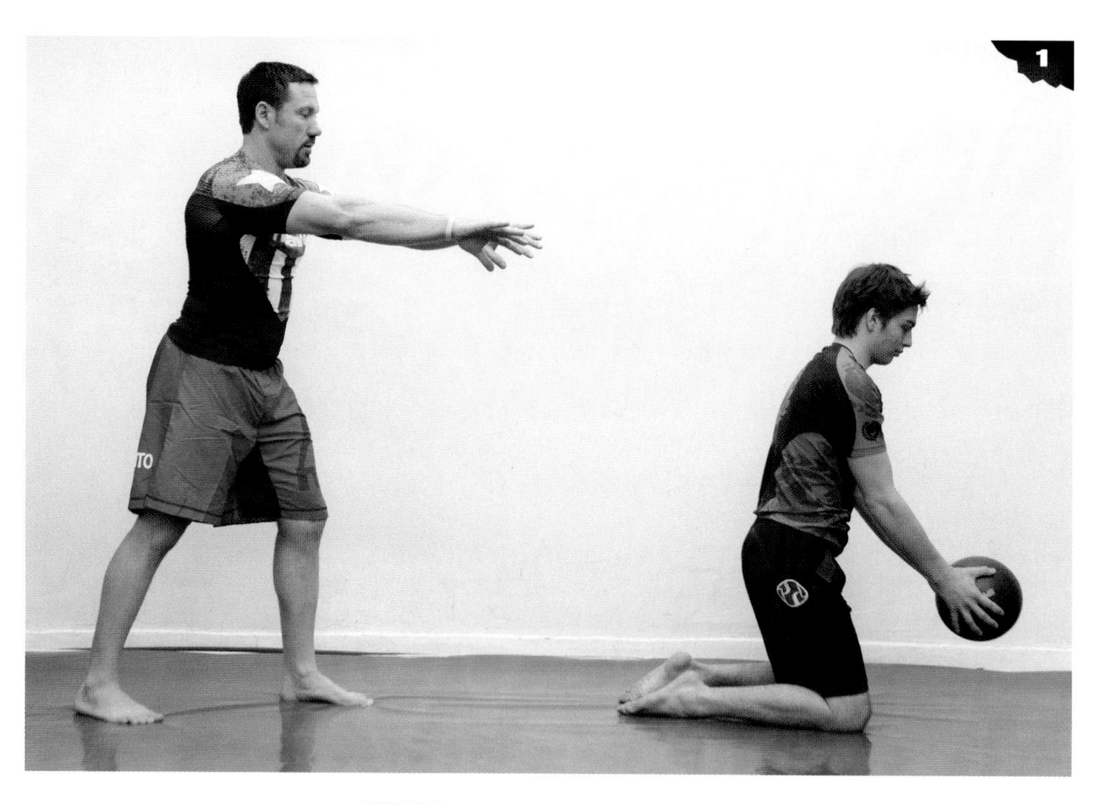

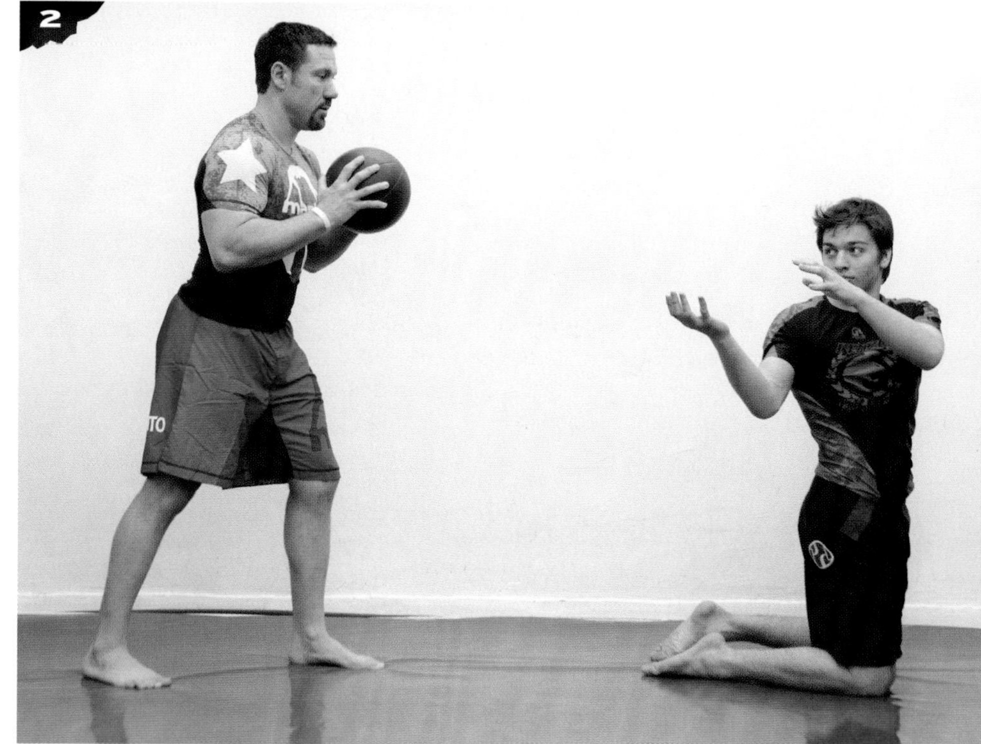

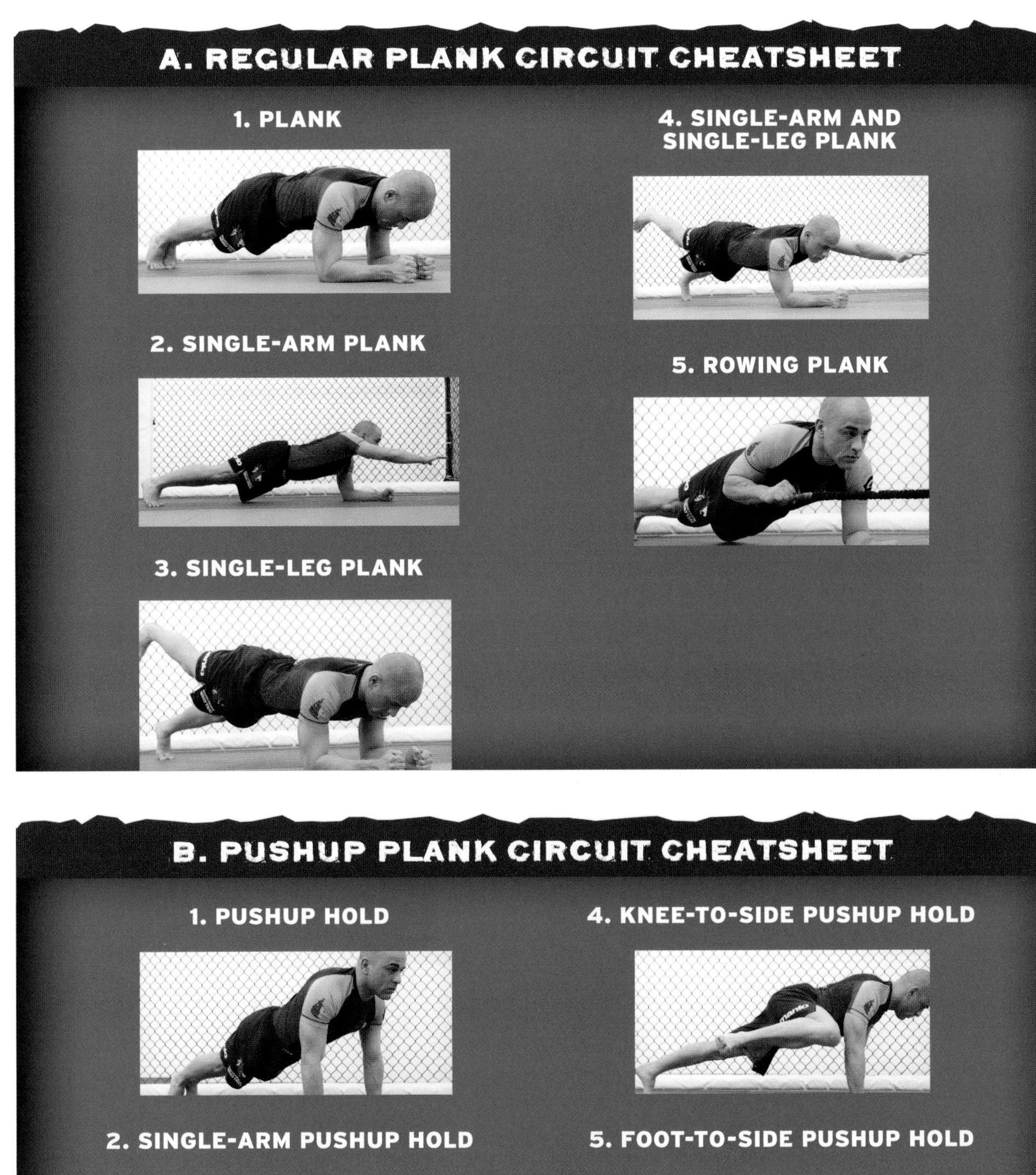

A. REGULAR PLANK CIRCUIT CHEATSHEET

1. PLANK

2. SINGLE-ARM PLANK

3. SINGLE-LEG PLANK

4. SINGLE-ARM AND SINGLE-LEG PLANK

5. ROWING PLANK

B. PUSHUP PLANK CIRCUIT CHEATSHEET

1. PUSHUP HOLD

2. SINGLE-ARM PUSHUP HOLD

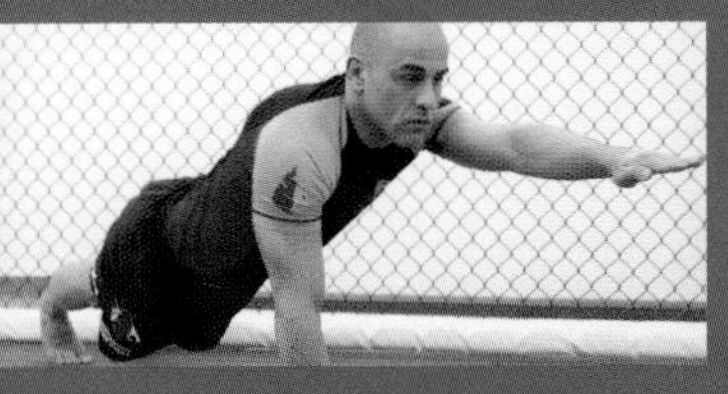

3. SINGLE-ARM SINGLE-LEG PUSHUP HOLD

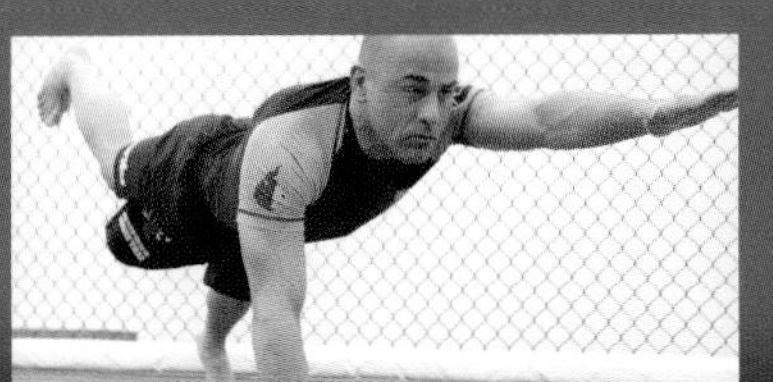

4. KNEE-TO-SIDE PUSHUP HOLD

5. FOOT-TO-SIDE PUSHUP HOLD

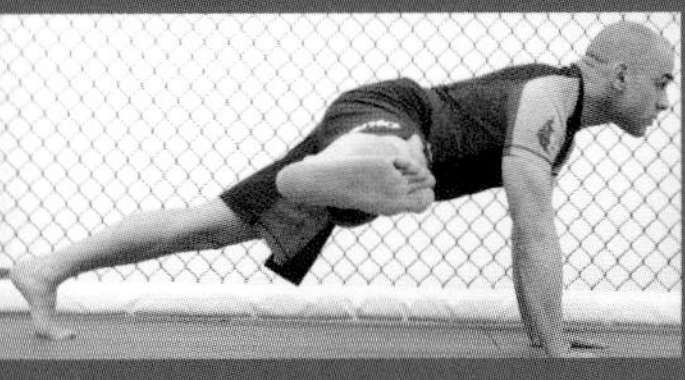

6. KNEE-TO-OPPOSITE-ELBOW PUSHUP HOLD

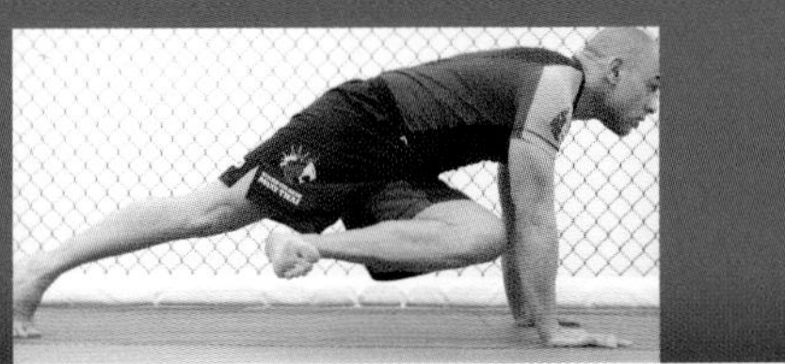

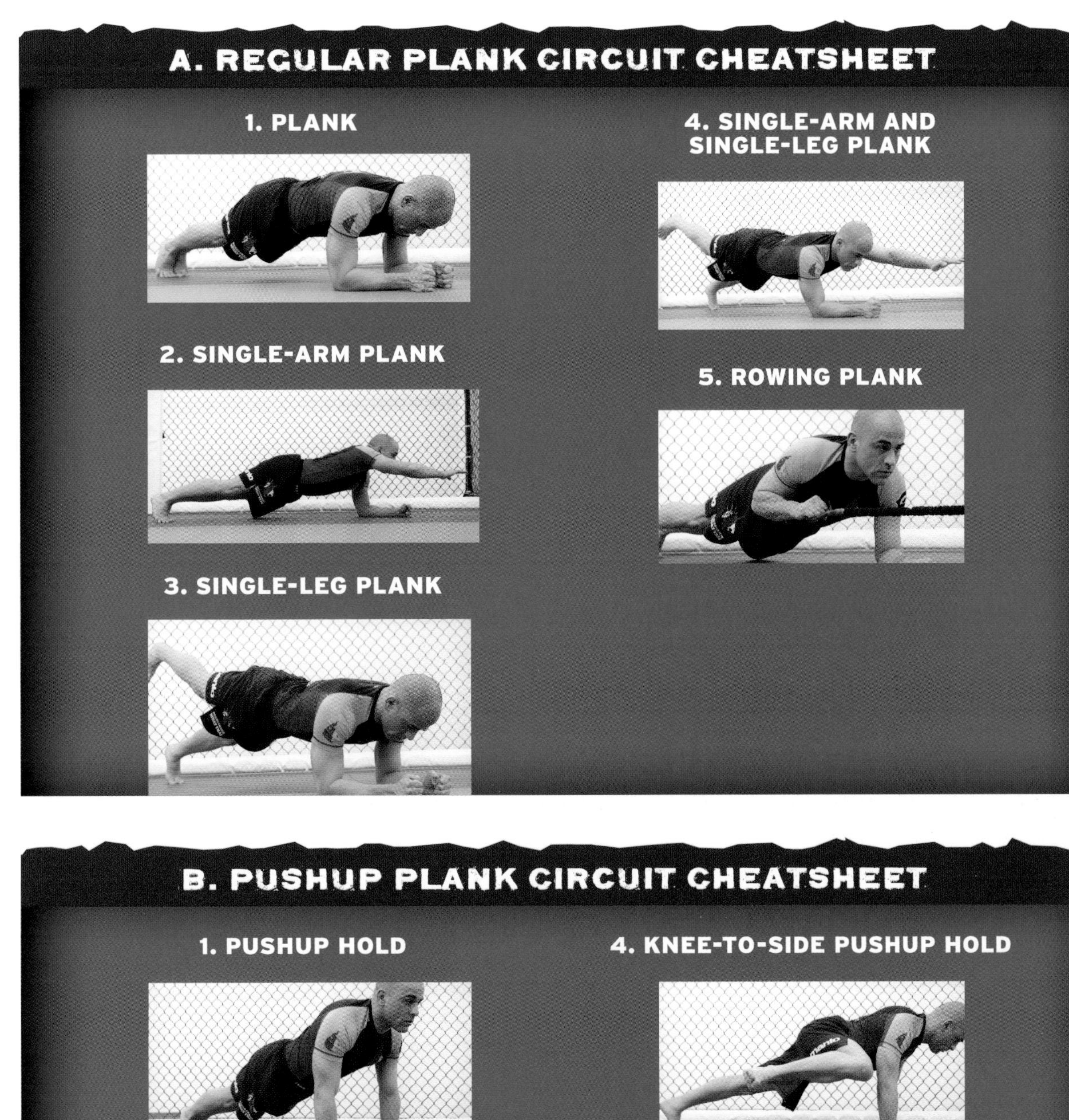

A. REGULAR PLANK CIRCUIT CHEATSHEET

1. PLANK

2. SINGLE-ARM PLANK

3. SINGLE-LEG PLANK

4. SINGLE-ARM AND SINGLE-LEG PLANK

5. ROWING PLANK

B. PUSHUP PLANK CIRCUIT CHEATSHEET

1. PUSHUP HOLD

4. KNEE-TO-SIDE PUSHUP HOLD

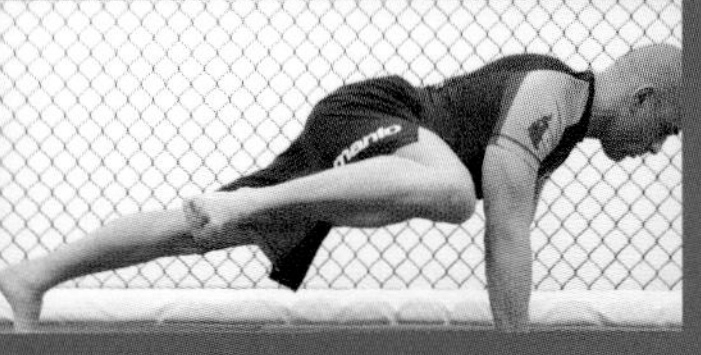

2. SINGLE-ARM PUSHUP HOLD

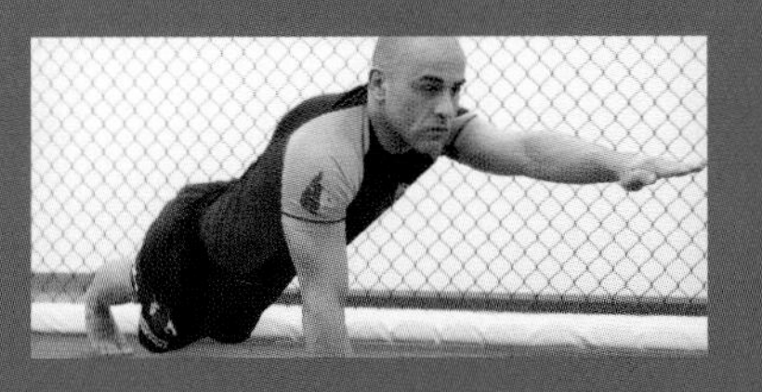

5. FOOT-TO-SIDE PUSHUP HOLD

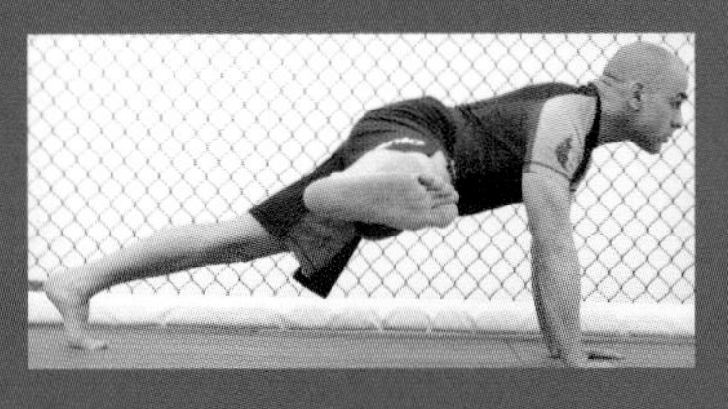

3. SINGLE-ARM SINGLE-LEG PUSHUP HOLD

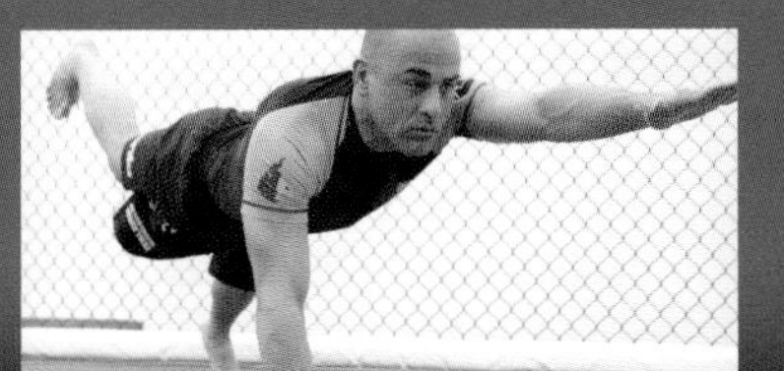

6. KNEE-TO-OPPOSITE-ELBOW PUSHUP HOLD

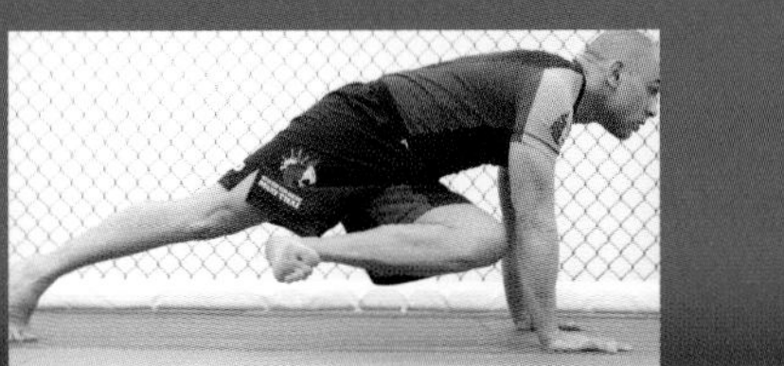

C. MED BALL PLANK CIRCUIT CHEATSHEET

1. MED BALL PLANK

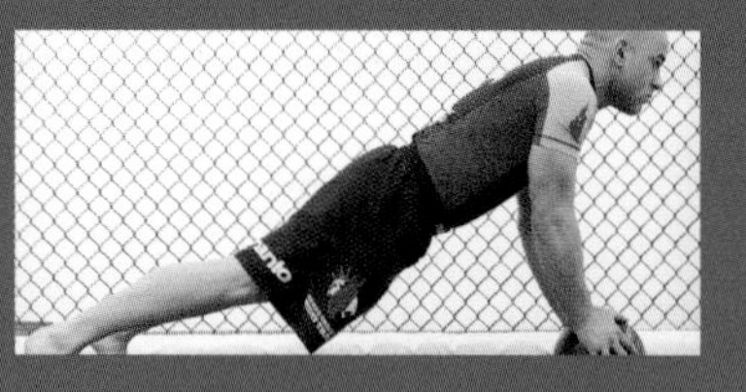

2. SINGLE-LEG MED BALL PLANK

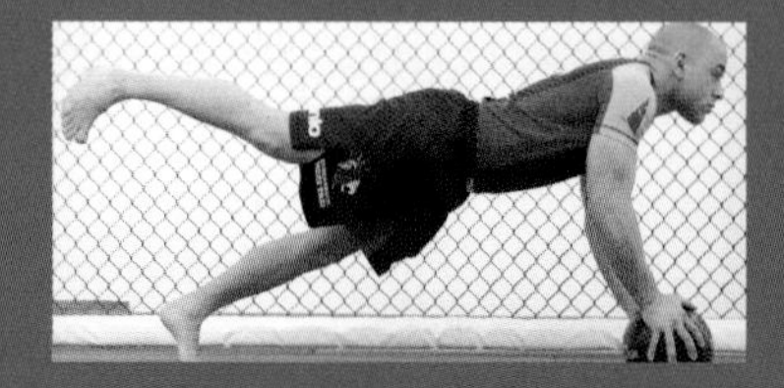

3. KNEE-FORWARD MED BALL PLANK

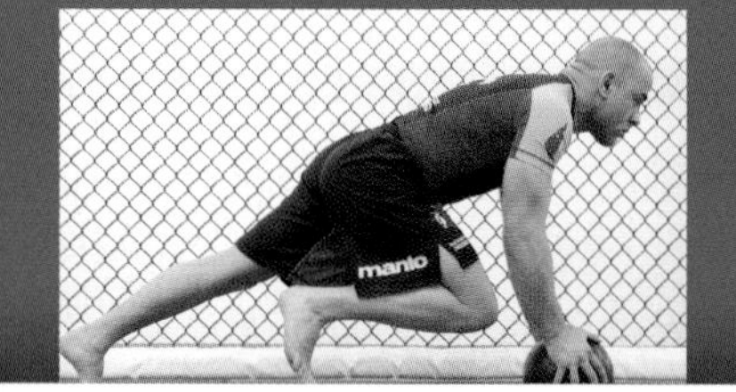

4. KNEE-TO-SIDE MED BALL PLANK

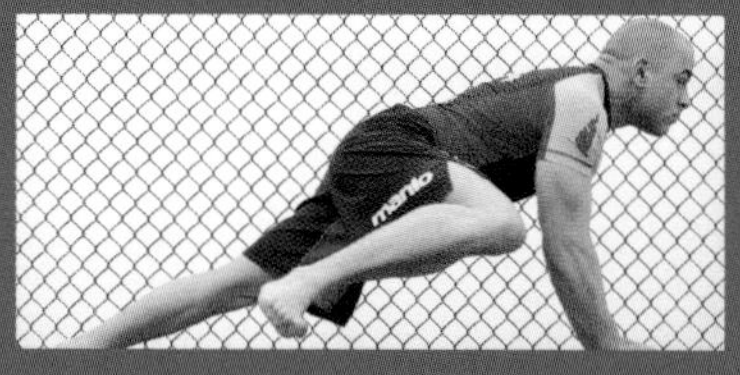

5. FOOT-TO-SIDE MED BALL PLANK

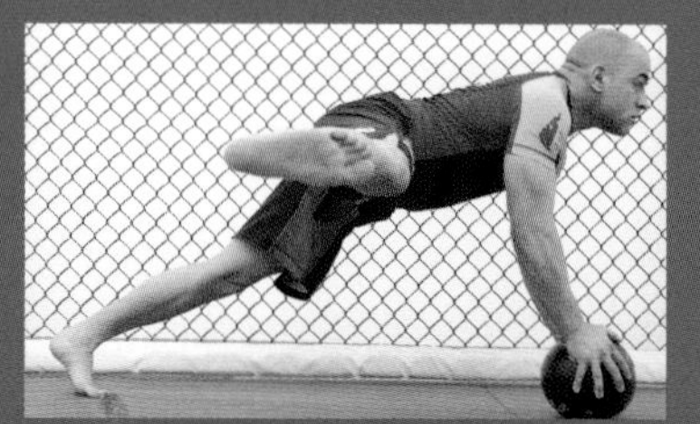

D. ELEVATED PLANK CIRCUIT CHEATSHEET

1. ELEVATED PLANK

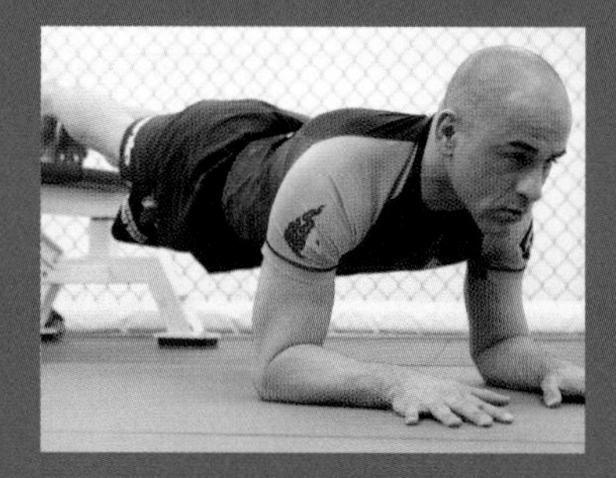

2. SINGLE-LEG ELEVATED PLANK

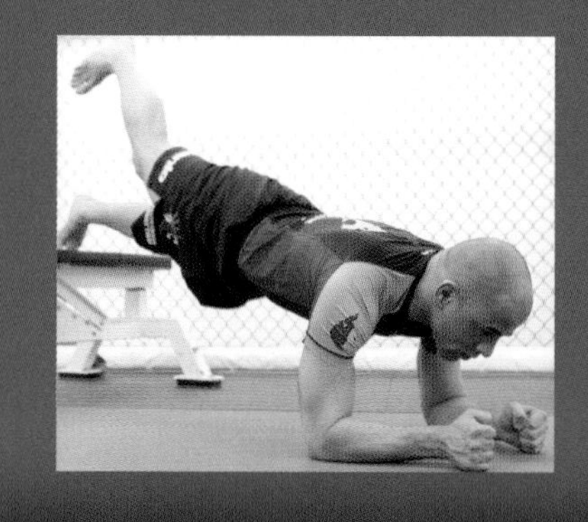

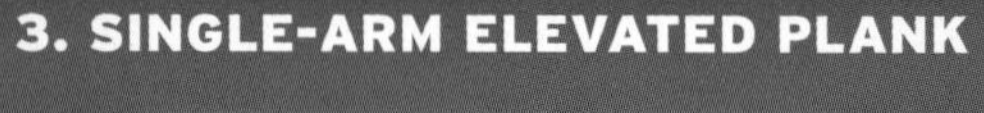

3. SINGLE-ARM ELEVATED PLANK

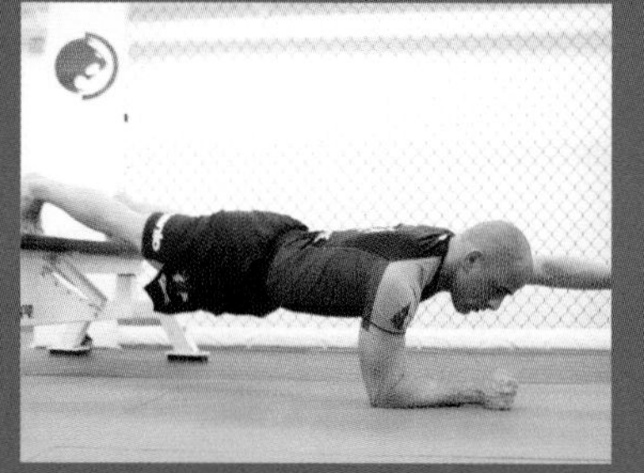

4. SINGLE-ARM SINGLE-LEG ELEVATED PLANK

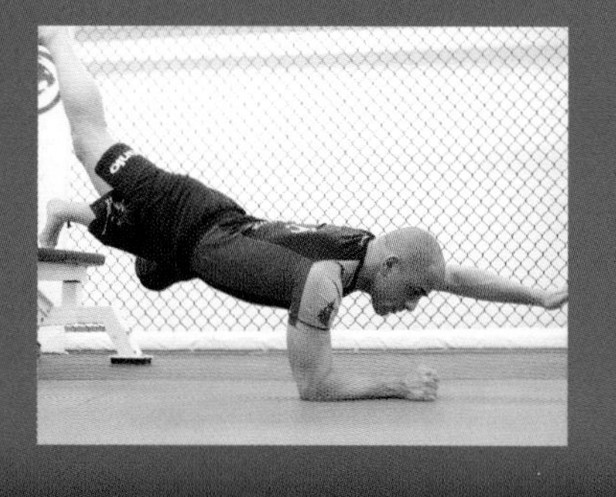

E. SWISS BALL PLANK CIRCUIT CHEATSHEET

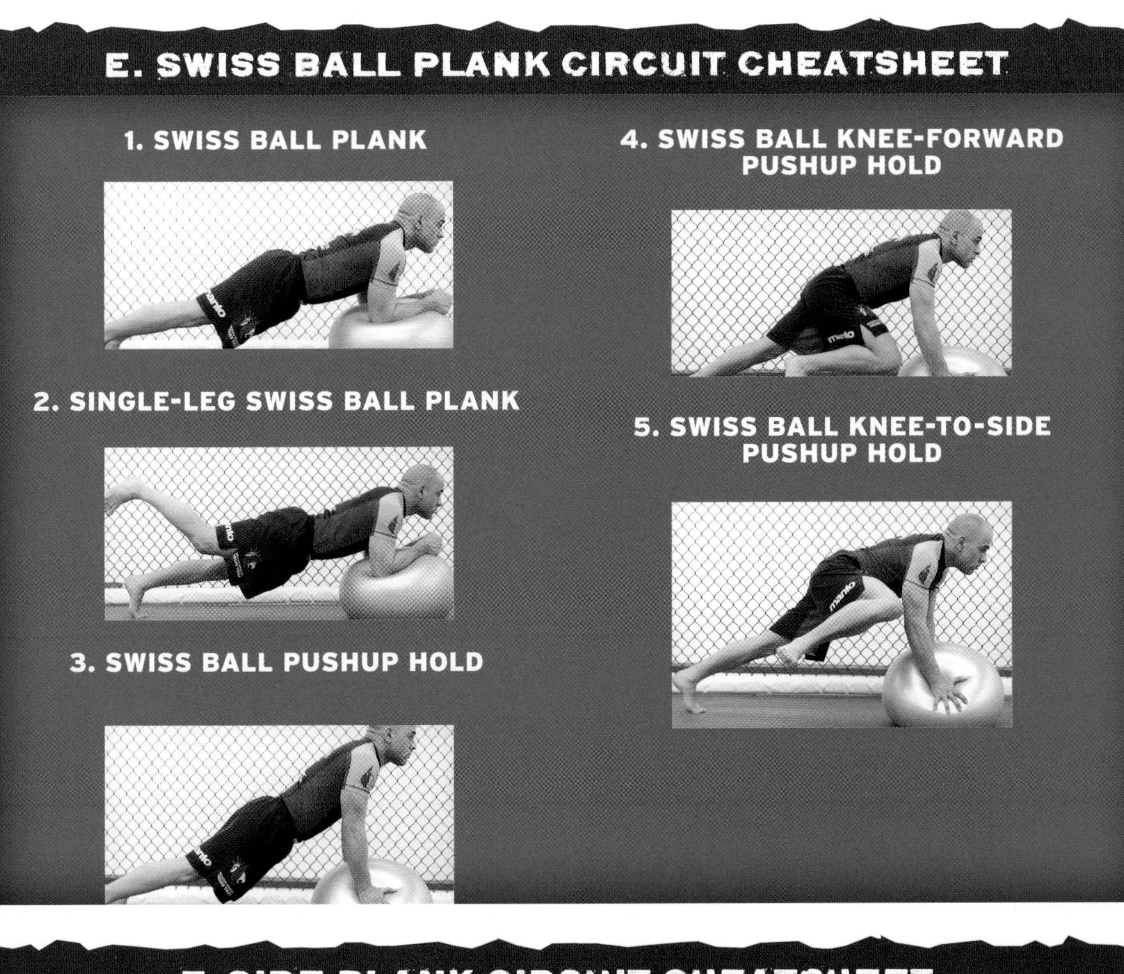

1. SWISS BALL PLANK

2. SINGLE-LEG SWISS BALL PLANK

3. SWISS BALL PUSHUP HOLD

4. SWISS BALL KNEE-FORWARD PUSHUP HOLD

5. SWISS BALL KNEE-TO-SIDE PUSHUP HOLD

F. SIDE PLANK CIRCUIT CHEATSHEET

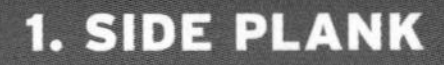

1. SIDE PLANK

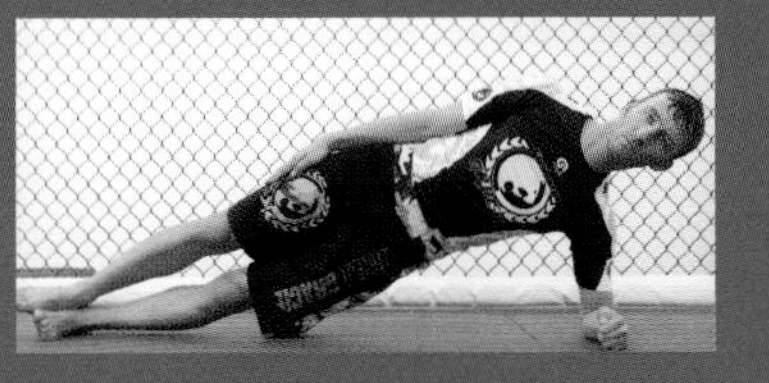

2. SIDE PLANK WITH ARM UP

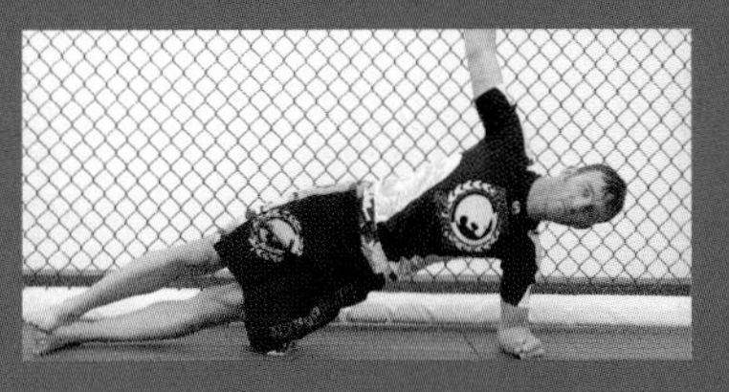

3. SIDE PLANK WITH ARM AND LEG UP

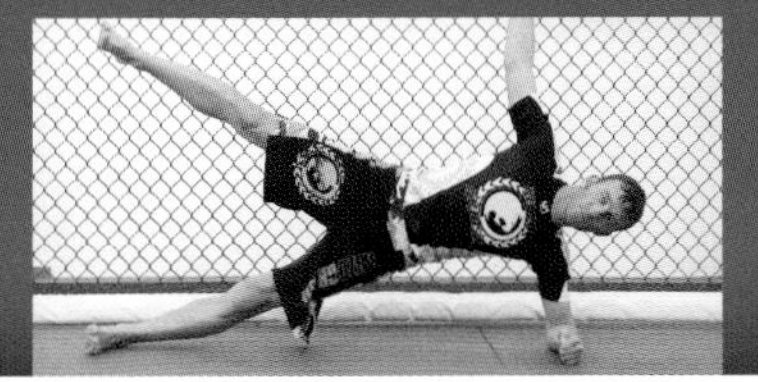

4. SIDE PLANK WITH KNEE UP

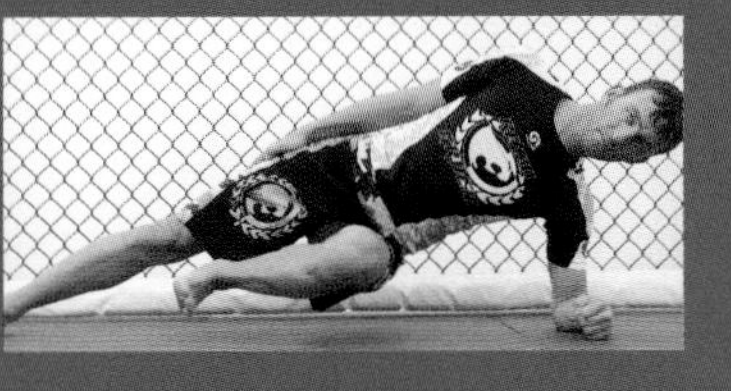

5. SIDE PLANK WITH KNEE AND ARM UP

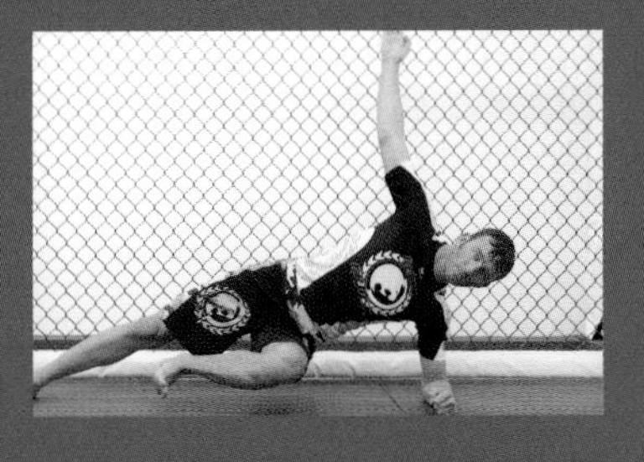

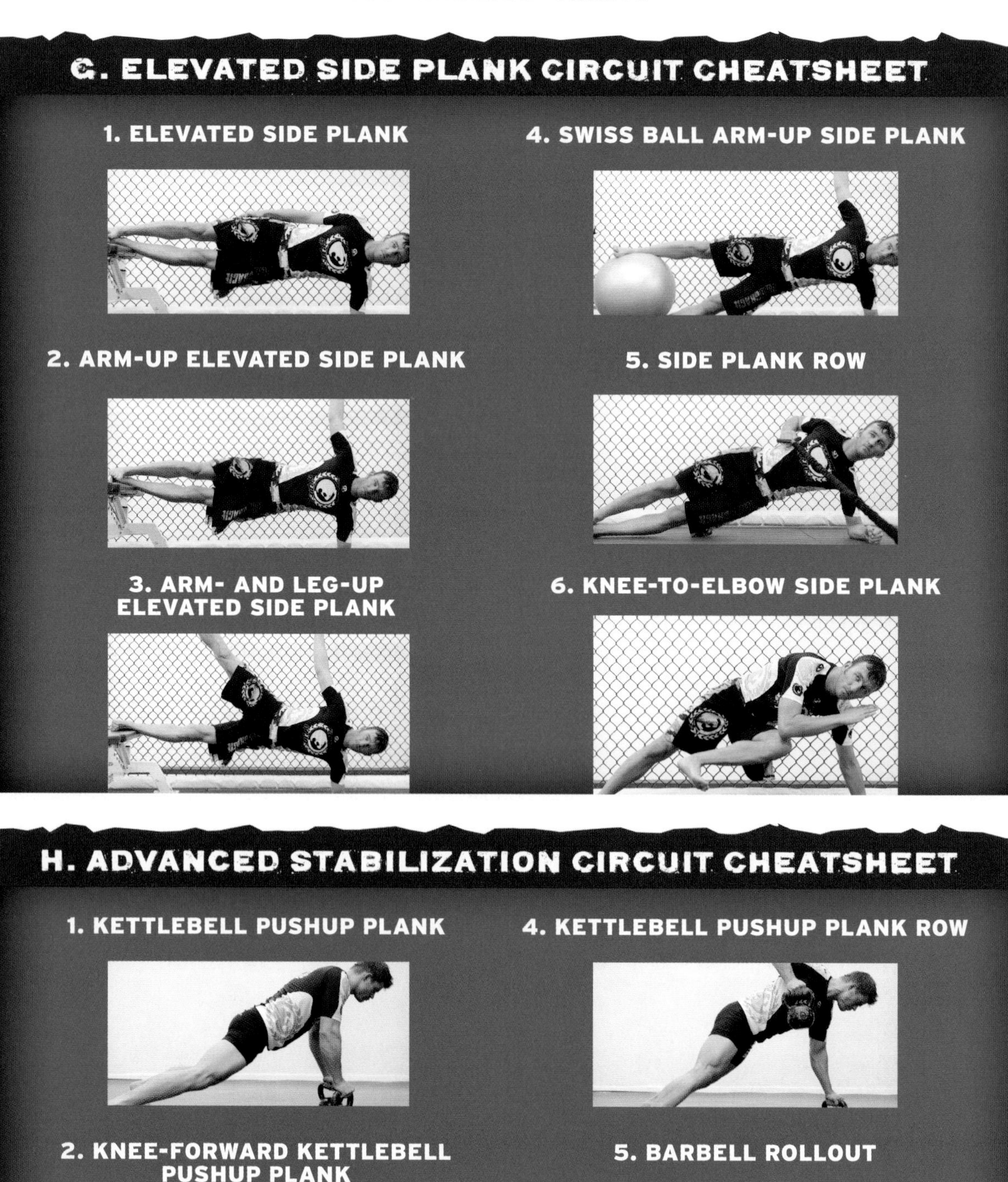

G. ELEVATED SIDE PLANK CIRCUIT CHEATSHEET

1. ELEVATED SIDE PLANK
2. ARM-UP ELEVATED SIDE PLANK
3. ARM- AND LEG-UP ELEVATED SIDE PLANK
4. SWISS BALL ARM-UP SIDE PLANK
5. SIDE PLANK ROW
6. KNEE-TO-ELBOW SIDE PLANK

H. ADVANCED STABILIZATION CIRCUIT CHEATSHEET

1. KETTLEBELL PUSHUP PLANK

2. KNEE-FORWARD KETTLEBELL PUSHUP PLANK

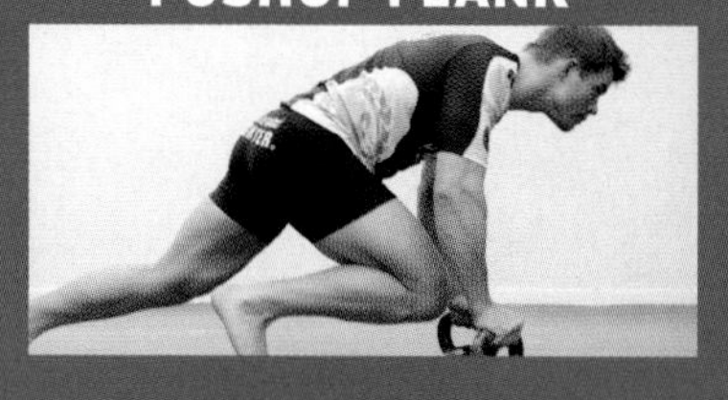

3. KNEE-TO-SIDE LOW KETTLEBELL PUSHUP PLANK

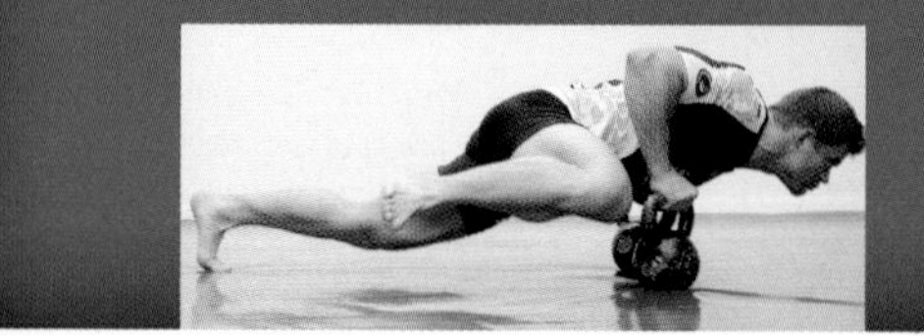

4. KETTLEBELL PUSHUP PLANK ROW

5. BARBELL ROLLOUT

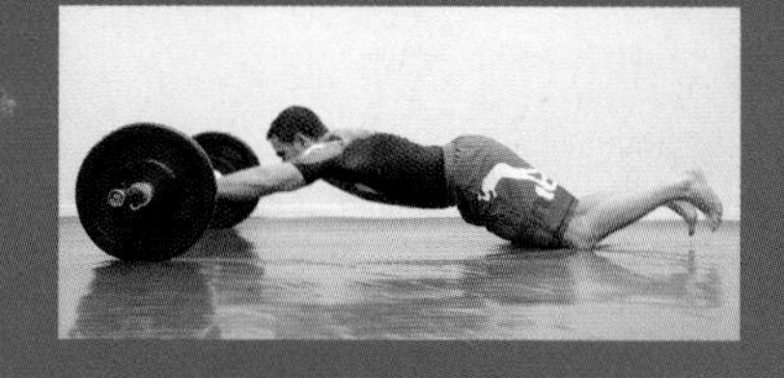

6. BARBELL OBLIQUE HOLDS

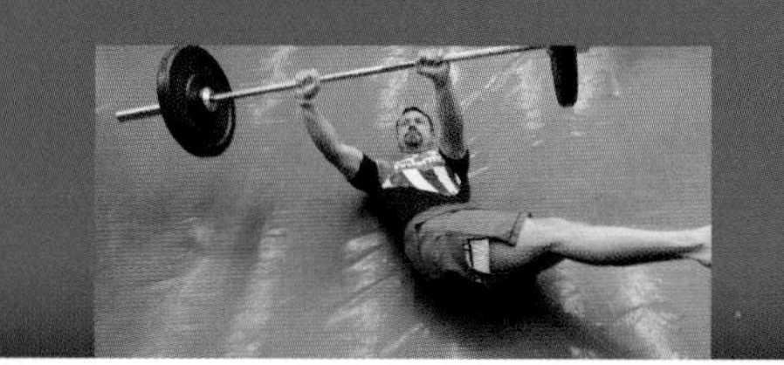

I. OBLIQUES CIRCUIT CHEATSHEET

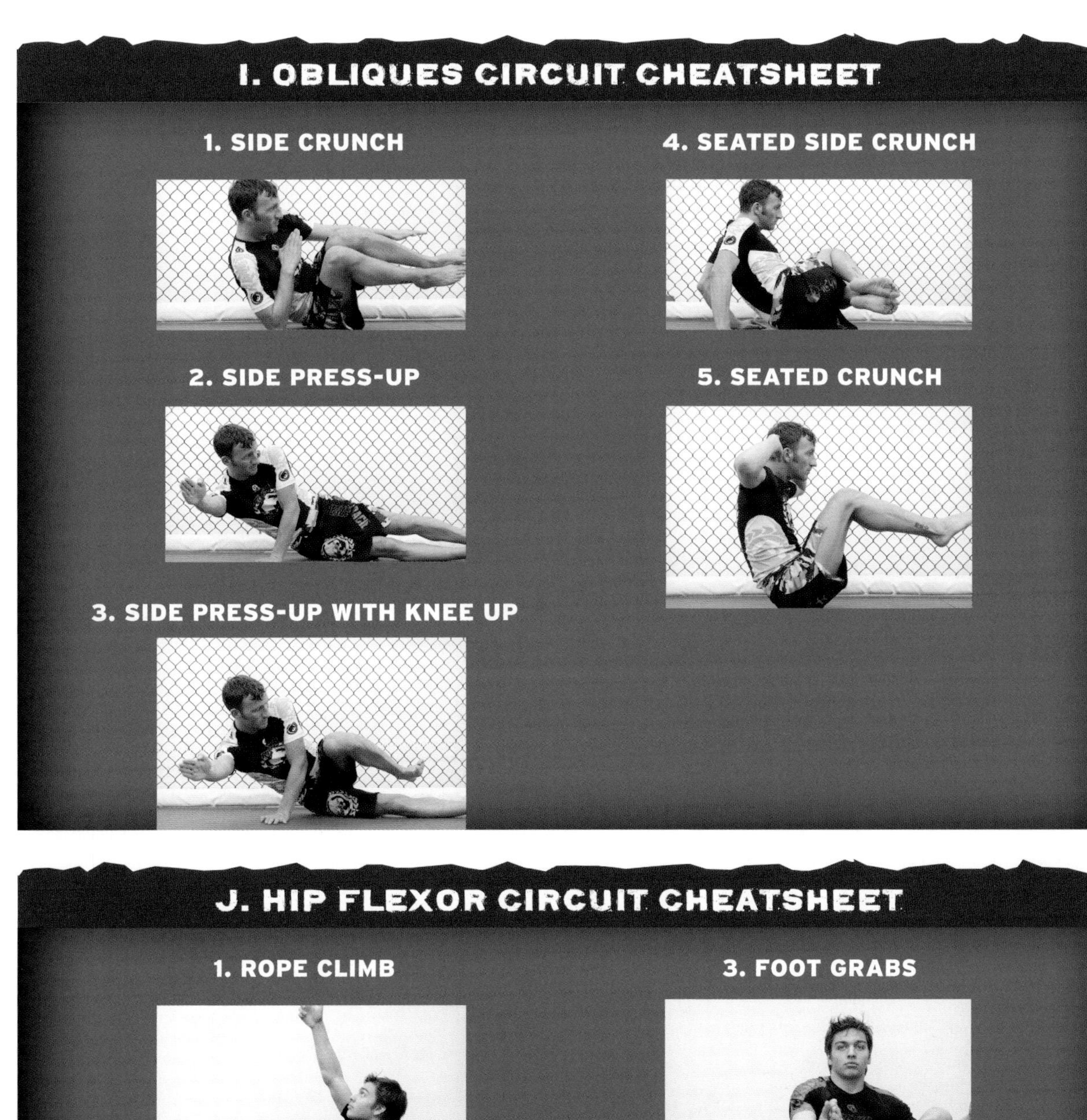

1. SIDE CRUNCH

2. SIDE PRESS-UP

3. SIDE PRESS-UP WITH KNEE UP

4. SEATED SIDE CRUNCH

5. SEATED CRUNCH

J. HIP FLEXOR CIRCUIT CHEATSHEET

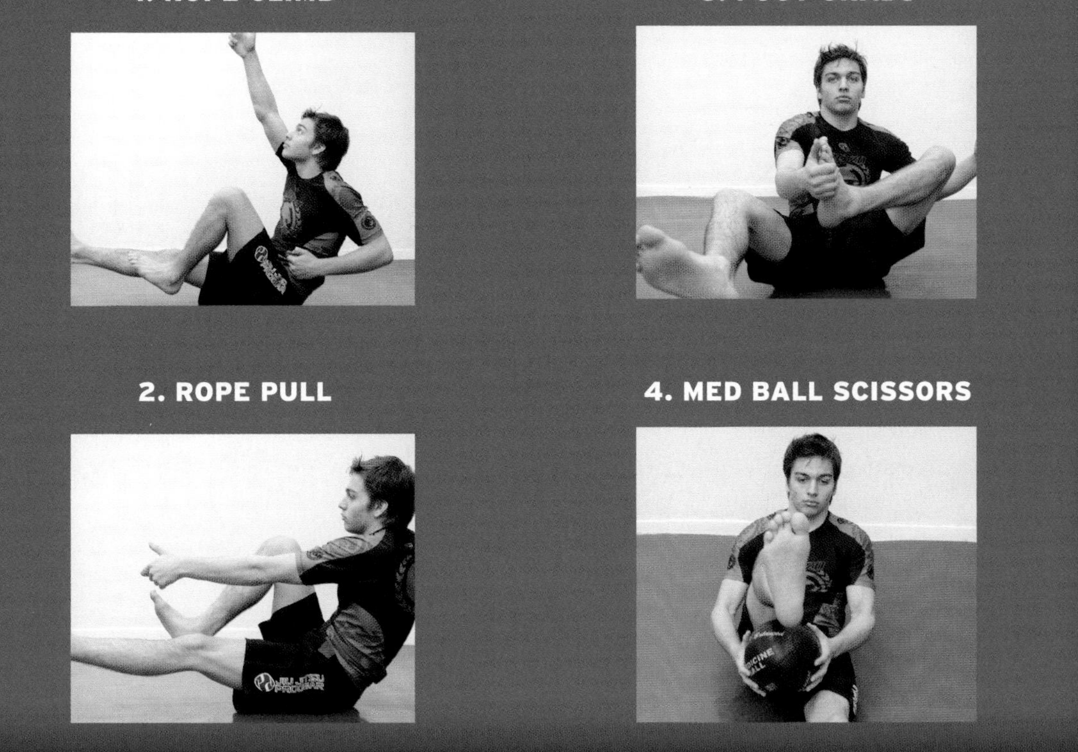

1. ROPE CLIMB

2. ROPE PULL

3. FOOT GRABS

4. MED BALL SCISSORS

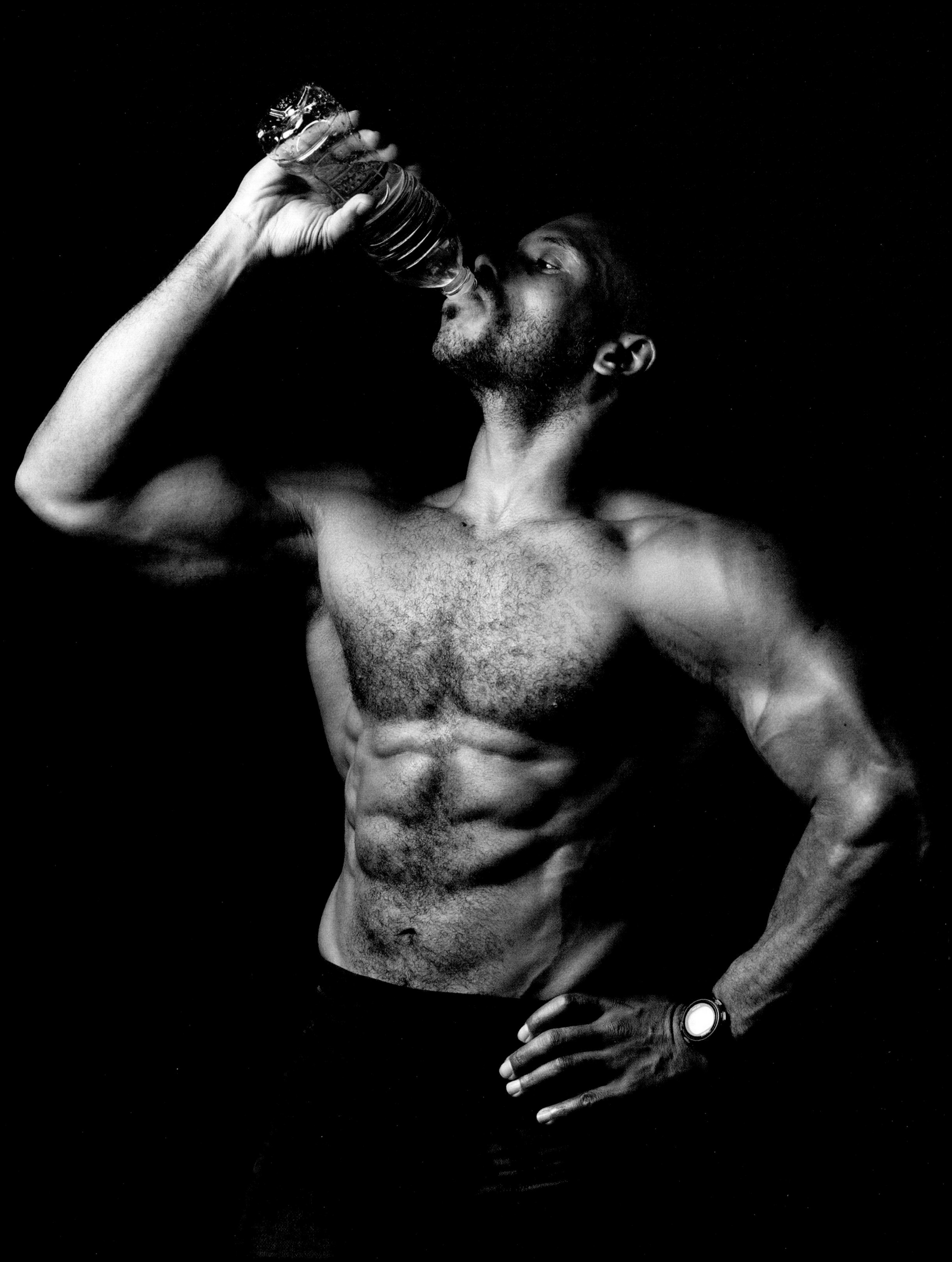

16

NUTRITION FOR WARRIORS

BY JOHN BERARDI, PhD

WITH NATE GREEN AND KRISTA SCOTT-DIXON

In 2009, during an interview with *MMA Weekly*, Georges St. Pierre—arguably the best pound-for-pound fighter in the world—leaned back in his chair, sipped a bottle of water, and talked about how he was working on his nutrition to improve his fighting.

His nutrition.

You have to realize how ridiculous that sounded at the time. Here was a guy who was already the undisputed Ultimate Fighting Championship welterweight champion, with a staggering nineteen wins and only two losses. And he was going to eat more broccoli to become a better fighter. Yeah, right.

"What do you think eating better will do for you?" asked the interviewer.

Georges smiled. "I have good genetics and I've never had to diet," he said. "But I think eating well from now on will help me become a better fighter. I think it'll help me gain quality muscle. It will help me recover and heal faster. It will give me more energy and explosion. That's why I started working with John Berardi and Precision Nutrition." (That's us.)

Eight weeks after the interview—after following the same eating habits you'll learn in this chapter—Georges had gained 10 pounds of lean muscle mass. Most important, he continued to win. To the rest of the world, Georges was simply the same dominating fighter he had always been, albeit with more muscle. But Georges knew that along with his superior skill and intense training, eating the right foods at the right times gave him an extra edge over the rest of the competition. He could feel it.

Around the same time, Martin Rooney started working with Dan and Jim Miller. According to Martin, the Miller brothers were the epitome of bad eating habits. Tough-as-nails, sure. Hard workers, yes. But the guys loved themselves some McDonald's.

At the time, Jim was a small, 160-pound scrappy fighter who fought in the 155-pound division. At only 5 pounds above fighting weight, Jim was small for his division, an extreme disadvantage within a group of fighters who routinely cut down from 175 to make weight. His brother Dan was a heavy 215 pounds who fought at 185. When it was time to cut for a fight, Dan would lose precious muscle along with the fat, decreasing his strength and power.

Both were talented UFC hopefuls. But to get to the next level, Martin knew they needed more than raw skill. So he started manipulating their nutrition by making small, simple changes, just like the ones you'll learn in this chapter. These small changes made a big difference in their physiques and performance. Now, Jim walks around at 175 pounds and still competes in the 155-pound class. His extra muscle mass helps him dominate his opponents in the cage. Dan stays at a healthy, lean 200 pounds. When he cuts to make it down to 185, he maintains his muscle, power, and speed.

By adding healthy eating habits and smart training to their natural talent and skill, the Miller brothers not only rose to UFC superstardom, they also became the winningest brothers in UFC history.

Why do elite fighters like Georges and the Miller brothers focus on what they put in their bodies?

Because they know their success depends on what their bodies can do—and what they can't do. They understand that when all else is equal, the fighter with more energy, more power, and better recovery will be the last one standing.

The good news: whether you're a fighter, an athlete, or anyone looking to get in better shape, you can boost your energy, improve your recovery, and learn to easily (and safely) gain lean mass or drop weight, all with a few simple eating strategies, just like GSP and the Millers.

Over the next few pages you'll learn the "Warrior 20," our top twenty best foods for warriors of any kind. You'll also discover the "Warrior 10," our top ten no-BS supplements to help you get stronger, more explosive, and healthier.

As our elite athletes know, the most radical changes in body composition and performance happen by following small daily steps. So that's where we'll start. This isn't nutritional theory. These are nutritional strategies and tools that will help make you a better fighter—and you can start applying them immediately. Today.

THE WARRIOR 20

When we sat down to write this chapter, we first looked in our kitchens to see what kinds of food filled our fridges and cabinets—and what kinds of food *didn't* make an appearance.

Then we looked at our top-performing athletes to see what was in *their* kitchens.

Know what we found?

High-performing athletes, professional trainers, and nutritionists pretty much eat the same 20 foods. In no particular order:

PROTEIN

1. **Whole eggs**
2. **Lean meats, poultry, and game**
3. **Fatty fish**
4. **Fermented soy**

LEGUMES

5. **Beans**
6. **Lentils**

FRUITS AND VEGETABLES

7. **Tomatoes**
8. **Spinach**
9. **Cruciferous vegetables (e.g., broccoli, cabbage, cauliflower, Brussels sprouts)**
10. **Avocados**
11. **Citrus (orange, grapefruit)**
12. **Berries**

STARCHES AND WHOLE GRAINS

13. **Sweet potatoes/yams**
14. **Quinoa**
15. **Amaranth**

GOOD FATS

16. **Nuts (and nut butters)**
17. **Seeds (flax, hemp, chia)**
18. **Olive oil**

DRINKS

19. **Water**
20. **Green tea**

These twenty foods are at the head of the pack in terms of health and nutrition. The Warrior 20 are *power* foods, loaded with nutrients, vitamins, and minerals that help promote muscle growth and recovery as well as muscle/cardiovascular endurance. They help reduce painful and annoying inflammation so our bodies can heal, allowing us to get back on the mat more quickly. These are the twenty foods that you need to build more muscle, more power, and better endurance, and to cut the fat that is holding you back.

PROTEIN

If you've ever trained with weights, you've probably heard how important it is to "eat a lot of protein." Although "a lot" is relative to your body size and goals, more protein usually equals better muscle retention, better recovery, and increased energy—all good things for athletes.

Most people, however, consume only about 75% of their ideal protein needs per day. Since protein builds and repairs muscle, you're likely short-changing yourself in the muscle growth and recovery department.

Here are our top picks for protein:

1. WHOLE EGGS (NOT WHITES)

Eggs are one of the best sources of protein on the planet and also some of the cheapest. They're also very easy to prepare. You can hard boil, scramble, pan fry, or poach them—whichever method is easiest for you.

One thing to keep in mind: despite what you may have heard, the egg yolks—the yellow part inside of the egg—are actually *good* for you. They contain a nutrient called choline, which is essential for cardiovascular and brain function.

So ditch the egg-white omelet and go with the whole egg.

What to look for

Look for the words "free range," "cage-free," or "omega-3" on your egg cartons. These eggs come from healthier chickens and have more nutrients and lower risk of salmonella (though you should still cook the eggs).

2. LEAN MEATS

Lean meats like chicken, turkey, lean cuts of pork (e.g., tenderloin) and beef, along with wild game (buffalo, venison, elk, ostrich, rabbit, etc.), provide high-quality protein as well as other vitamins, nutrients, and healthy fats, especially if the meats are pasture-raised.

You can buy the meat ground or, if you have more time to cook, you can get steaks.

What to look for

If you have the option and the means, try looking for these phrases:
"Grass fed" (beef, bison)
"Free range" (chicken, turkey)
"Pasture raised" (all of the above)
"Organic" (all of the above)

If you don't have access to organic meats, don't worry; it won't make or break your progress.

3. FATTY FISH

Fatty fish like salmon, mackerel, sardines, and anchovies are high in protein and omega-3 fats. Omega-3s, which most of us don't get enough of, help increase mood and circulation while controlling and managing inflammation. (If you've ever suffered an acute injury, you know how annoying the healing process can be. Omega-3s speed your recovery.)

What to look for

"Wild caught" is often best. In the wild, fish like salmon (a natural carnivore) eat other fish, krill, and plankton. This leads to them producing higher levels of omega-3s.

Conversely, when a fish is "farm raised" it often eats *grain*—which, obviously, is not its natural diet.

If you can find "wild caught" or "sustainably raised" and can afford the extra cost, go for it. If you can't, don't worry. The farm-raised stuff still packs a good protein punch.

4. FERMENTED SOY

Tempeh is a traditional East Asian food made from the fermentation of cooked soybeans. It's high in protein, and the fermentation process produces natural antibiotic agents that are believed to increase the body's resistance to infections.

Note for vegetarians and vegans: Even if you don't eat meat, you still need protein. Most vegetarians and vegans drop meat without even thinking about how to add more protein, which can dramatically decrease recovery.

Note for meat-eaters: Adding vegetarian options like tempeh is a good way to get some variety in your diet. And the fermented kind doesn't affect your hormones.

FAQ about protein

How many grams of protein should I eat?

At least 1 gram per pound of bodyweight. To figure out your protein needs, simply match your bodyweight to grams of protein. Weigh 165 pounds? You need at least 165 grams of protein every day. Weigh 200 pounds? You need at least 200 grams of protein every day.

Do I really have to count protein grams?

Absolutely not. The fighters and other athletes we work with do one simple thing to figure out their protein need: they look at the palm of their hand.

Each palm is equal to about 30 grams of protein.

If you weigh 165 pounds and need 165 grams of protein, eat six palms of protein per day.

If you weigh 200 pounds and need 200 grams of protein, eat seven palms of protein per day.

How often should I eat protein?

Our athletes eat 30 to 60 grams (one to two palms) of protein with every meal. If you're smaller or female, opt for the lower end of the protein range. If you're a larger male, opt for the higher end.

The easiest way to get all your protein is to divide it up throughout the day.

If you weigh 165 pounds and need to get your six to eight palms of protein in, simply eat four meals per day with two palms of protein at each.

If you weigh 200 pounds and need to get your seven to ten palms of protein in, eat five meals with two palms of protein each.

Are tuna and other fish okay to eat?

Sure, but they don't make our Warrior 20 because they lack the significant amounts of omega-3 fats that the fatty fish have. Plus tuna and several other larger fish (such as swordfish) can be quite high in heavy metals and/or environmental contaminants. Eat big fish sparingly.

LEGUMES

Legumes are excellent sources of fiber, a key nutrient that helps you feel full, controls blood sugar, and prevents cravings for less nutritious foods in "dieting" phases.

While the recommended daily fiber intake is 35 grams, most athletes get only about 11 grams. If you don't eat enough fiber, you'll have poor digestion and constipation, which are two serious complications for athletes.

5. BEANS

Half a cup of beans contains roughly 10 grams of fiber and plenty of antioxidants, which can help prevent cellular damage and speed recovery.

Beans are also loaded with magnesium, iron, zinc, and potassium. Many fighters are deficient in these crucial vitamins and minerals, which decreases their strength and power.

A list of our favorites:

- Small red beans (adzuki)
- Kidney beans
- Garbanzo beans (chick peas)
- Black beans
- Pinto beans

You can even use refried beans if you prefer them.

6. LENTILS

Lentils are small, disk-shaped legumes and are a good source of fiber. They also lack sulfur, which is one of the main contributors to the bloated, gassy feeling some people get from beans.

Finally, lentils contain manganese, an important mineral that's essential for growth, wound healing, and peak brain function.

FAQ about legumes

How much should I eat? How often should I eat it?

Aim for ¼ cup of legumes (that's about the size of a golf ball) three to four times per day. You can add them to a salad, or just eat them alongside your protein.

Are canned beans and lentils okay?

Sure. Especially if you know you won't have the time (or patience) to soak, cook, and dry them. Just make sure to drain the murky water from the can and rinse the beans in water before heating and eating.

I hate beans. Is there any way to make them taste better?

Feel free to experiment with spices and condiments like garlic powder, salt, pepper, balsamic vinegar, hot sauce, or salsa.

How can I avoid gas?

Some people won't have any problems at all, but if you do feel bloated after eating beans, there are a couple of things you can do.

First, try eating lentils. Since they lack sulfur, they rarely cause gas problems. Second, make sure you rinse your beans with water and get rid of the murky stuff in which they've been sitting. Also, try a different kind of bean; different types have different effects.

Finally, you can always supplement with Beano.

VEGETABLES

Low in calories and loaded with vitamins, minerals, and fiber, vegetables are nutritional powerhouses.

7. TOMATOES

Tomatoes, though technically a fruit, make the Warrior 20 because of their high vitamin C, lutein, and lycopene content.

Vitamin C helps form collagen, which is the primary component of connective tissue, the stuff that holds your bones and muscles together. The more stress you put your body through, the stronger and healthier your connective tissue needs to be.

Lutein is a compound that may help keep your eyes safe from oxidative stress and improve vision. And lycopene, which is a pigment that gives tomatoes a red color, is a strong antioxidant.

Varieties to look for:

- Vine-ripened tomatoes
- Roma tomatoes
- Cherry or grape tomatoes
- Heirloom varieties (in season)

8. SPINACH

Green leafy vegetables like spinach provide a huge nutritional boost for a low amount of calories. One cup of raw spinach contains only 49 calories and is loaded with nutrients, one of which is vitamin K, which contributes to building strong bones.

9. CRUCIFEROUS VEGETABLES

Cruciferous vegetables like broccoli, cabbage, cauliflower, bok choy, and Brussels sprouts contain vitamins, minerals, and fiber that will help you feel fuller longer and may help protect against cancer development. They contain sulfur compounds that help boost the immune system and promote bone health. Also, these vegetables help clear estrogen from the body, which is good for both male and female athletes.

MUSHROOMS (HONORABLE MENTION)

Mushrooms are technically a fungus, of course, not a vegetable. Nevertheless they're highly nutritious. They have fiber plus trace minerals such as copper and manganese, and vitamins such as B vitamins.

Mushrooms—especially Asian varieties such as shiitake or maitake—also boost the immune system, which is important when training in close contact with other people, in gyms that can be marinating in bacteria, viruses, and nonfriendly fungi.

So, although mushrooms didn't make our Warrior 20 list, you should still consider adding them as part of your daily intake.

FAQ about vegetables

How much should I eat? How often should I eat it?

Make a fist and look at it. That's your portion size. For both men and women, have at least two fists of vegetables, four to five times per day. Just include vegetables as part of each meal.

Can I eat frozen or canned vegetables?

We recommend you try to find fresh vegetables and eat them as much as possible, but frozen and canned vegetables are fine if you don't want to eat them raw, or if you know you'll never actually cook them.

I hate the taste of vegetables! How can I make them taste better?

If you don't like the taste of raw veggies, try different methods of preparation such as steaming or grilling. Also, experiment with different spices, oils, and condiments.

One of our favorites is steamed broccoli with olive oil, salt, pepper, and red pepper flakes.

Another option is to mask the taste by throwing a cup of spinach in a blender with other ingredients to make a Super Shake (recipe on page 352).

Can I eat them raw?

Sure, but don't dip them in ranch or blue cheese dressing. Instead, try a blend of olive oil and balsamic vinegar.

FRUITS

Fruits, also known as "nature's candy," are usually sweet (although there are exceptions, such as avocado or cucumber) and are rich in vitamins, mineral, and fiber while being relatively low in calories.

10. AVOCADOS

Avocados contain monounsaturated fat, which lowers cholesterol and may help burn fat, and are an excellent source of potassium, which ensures proper muscle growth and regulates fluid levels in the body.

To pick the perfect avocado at the grocery store, find an avocado that yields to soft pressure (meaning you can squeeze it just a little and it's not rock solid).

11. CITRUS

Citrus fruits like oranges and grapefruit are full of vitamin C (which can help strengthen your connective tissue) and are loaded with more than 170 cancer-fighting phytochemicals (chemical compounds that occur naturally in plants).

One such phytochemical group is the limonoid family, which is believed to have therapeutic effects such as stopping the spread of bacteria and viruses.

FRUITS VS. VEGGIES

Although both fruits and veggies contain healthy nutrients and make an appearance in our Warrior 20, there are a few special considerations to think about before you dive into your meal plan. That's because fruits, while healthy and nutritious, contain more sugar (in the form of fructose) than vegetables. Fructose can make it more difficult to lose body fat while in a dieting phase, and is best used sparingly when weight loss is a goal.

WHAT'S YOUR GOAL?

Maintain Weight or Build Muscle
We recommend having vegetables and fruits with almost every meal.

Weight Loss
We recommend having vegetables with every meal and limiting your fruit consumption to your post-workout meal.

12. BERRIES

You can't go wrong with fiber-rich berries. A list of our favorites:

- Raspberries
- Blueberries
- Blackberries
- Strawberries
- Cranberries

Blueberries help the neurons in your brain communicate with one another more effectively, which staves off mental deterioration and protects memory. And both raspberries and strawberries contain ellagic acid, which helps fight cancer cells.

FAQ about fruits

How much should I eat? How often should I eat it?
Make a fist and look at it. For both men and women, we recommend having one fist of fruits once or twice per day. Because of their higher sugar content, fruits are best eaten after a workout. (For more info, check out the Anytime vs. Post-Workout Meals section on page 372.)

Can I eat frozen fruits?
We recommend you eat fresh fruits when possible, but frozen fruits are perfect to throw into a Super Shake (recipe on page 364).

What's the best way to eat avocados?
We like scooping them straight into our mouths, but you can try adding some sea salt and pepper. They're also great sliced over salads, or as part of a guacamole spread.

Is fruit juice okay?
Unless it's fresh-squeezed in front of you, fruit juice is usually a poor option because of the added sugar and lack of fiber. Fruit juice is processed food. Stick with whole fruit instead.

STARCHES AND WHOLE GRAINS

Grains—especially the white breads and rices we all grew up with—don't contain much nutrition and are generally high in calories, making them a sub-par choice for athletes.

But some grains and starchier carbohydrates can be helpful, especially when eaten after a workout. (See the Anytime vs. Post-Workout Meals section on page 372 for more information.)

13. SWEET POTATOES AND YAMS

Tuberous roots such as sweet potatoes are a plant's storage tank, so they're loaded with carbohydrate energy. Orange-fleshed sweet potatoes are loaded with vitamin A, which is important in the synthesis of protein, the main process of muscle growth. Vitamin A is also involved in the production of glycogen, the body's storage form of energy for high-intensity performance.

White sweet potatoes or other types of yam also have carbohydrate energy, but not as much of the other nutrients.

14. QUINOA

Quinoa (pronounced "KEEN-wah") was known by the Incas as the "mother of grains," and was one of their chief sources of nutrition. Though technically a seed, quinoa is higher in protein than most grains and can be a tasty replacement for rice. It's also gluten-free, making it a solid choice for those with a gluten intolerance.

15. AMARANTH

The seed of the amaranth plant was a staple food of the Aztecs. It's high in protein and iron, and contains three times more fiber than wheat. Amaranth, like quinoa, is gluten-free.

FAQ about starches and whole grains

How much should I eat? How often should I eat it?
Most men should have two golf-ball-size portions of grains/starches after a workout. And women should stick with one golf-ball-size portion.

Where can I find quinoa and amaranth?

Although these grains are becoming more popular, you may have a tough time finding them in your local grocery store. If that's the case, simply head to any health food store and ask.

How do I cook quinoa and amaranth?

1. *Rinse and strain the dry grains.*
2. *Put in a pot and add enough water to cover the grains by about 3 inches.*
3. *Cover and bring to a boil.*
4. *Reduce heat to low and simmer until cooked.*
5. *Test for doneness.*
6. *Drain if necessary.*
7. *Store cooked grains for several days in the fridge, or months in the freezer.*

HEALTHY FATS

Athletes need fat. Our bodies use fatty acids to do everything from building cell membranes, to keeping our sex hormones (including testosterone) revving, to performing key functions in our brains, eyes, and lungs.

Fats also help slow down the digestion process so our bodies have more time to absorb nutrients, and help provide a sustainable level of energy.

16. NUTS (AND NUT BUTTERS)

Many nuts (and nut butters) are rich in monounsaturated and omega-3 fatty acids, which can help reduce inflammation and even lead to better mood and mental processes.

Nuts are also a source of l-arginine, which is an amino acid that converts to nitric oxide (NO), a powerful neurotransmitter that helps improve circulation. Coconut is high

SUPER SHAKE

The Super Shake is a concept we developed that combines high-quality protein, fiber, good fats, antioxidants, and more in a tasty formula.

It can replace a meal when you're in a hurry, or give you some extra protein and calories when trying to build muscle mass.

SEVEN STEPS TO A TASTY SUPER SHAKE

For optimal mixing, flavor, and consistency, follow the steps in order. Mix and match as you like.

Step 1: Start with ice

- Use 1 to 4 cups for a thin, chilled shake.
- Use 5 to 10 cubes for a thicker shake with a pudding-like consistency.

Step 2: Pick a fruit from the Warrior 20

Don't be afraid to experiment with berries, since you've got lots of options here. If you like a thick shake, go with frozen over fresh.

Step 3: Toss in some spinach

Yeah, we know it sounds gross to put veggies in a shake, but if you use spinach, you'll barely taste it. If you use frozen veggies, buy them fresh, then freeze them. (For some reason, pre-frozen veggies don't taste as good as the ones you freeze yourself.)

Step 4: Scoop some protein

Add 1 to 2 scoops of a protein powder of your choice.

Step 5: Select a nut or seed

Make sure you're not allergic. Aim for 1/3 cup of nuts per shake.

- Walnuts, cashews, almonds, Brazil nuts, nut butter
- Flax, hemp, chia

Step 6: Pour in some liquid

How much depends on how thick or thin you want it. If you have a weak blender, more liquid makes it easier to blend.

- Water
- Chilled green tea
- Unsweetened milk alternative (almond, rice, hemp, coconut)

Step 7: Choose your topper

This step is optional, but it nicely finishes off any shake.

- Dark chocolate
- Ground coffee beans
- Coconut, oats, granola
- Cinnamon, vanilla extract

TWO SAMPLE SHAKE RECIPES

Berry Blast Shake

- *1 cup frozen, mixed berries*
- *1/2 cup fresh spinach*
- *2 scoops vanilla-flavored milk protein powder*
- *1 Tbsp raw mixed nuts*
- *1 Tbsp ground flax seeds*
- *1 cup almond milk (unsweetened)*

Chocolate Peanut Butter Shake

- *2 scoops chocolate-flavored milk protein powder*
- *2 Tbsp natural peanut butter*
- *1 Tbsp raw, mixed nuts*
- *1 Tbsp ground flax seeds*
- *1 cup of almond milk (unsweetened)*

in medium-chain triglycerides and a healthy form of saturated fat.

Some of our favorite nuts:

- Walnuts
- Almonds (almond butter)
- Cashews (cashew butter)
- Pecans
- Macadamias
- Pistachios
- Coconut

What to look for

Avoid the processed roasted nuts (which may lose a lot of their nutritional value) and instead look for *raw* nuts. If you're eating nut butter, look for the least processed version (and read the label for hidden sugar or other junk).

17. SEEDS

Like nuts, seeds contains good fats. Seeds are also rich in fiber, which can help you feel fuller longer.

Some of our favorites:

- Flax (ground)
- Hemp
- Chia
- Pumpkin

18. EXTRA-VIRGIN OLIVE OIL

Extra-virgin olive oil is high in antioxidants and contains monounsaturated fat, which has been shown to control LDL ("bad") cholesterol levels while raising HDL ("good") levels. The ancient Spartan warriors swore by olive oil (along with garlic), and they knew a thing or two about ass-kicking.

What to look for

Always go with "extra virgin," as it's the least processed type, generally tastes better, and has more nutritional benefits.

FAQ about fat

How much should I eat? How often should I eat it?

Add a little healthy fat to every meal—about 1 to 2 tablespoons (a tablespoon is about the size of your thumb) per meal. You can add avocado, mixed nuts, olive oil, coconut, or seeds.

What's the best way to eat olive oil?

Olive oil is okay to cook with as long as you use it only with low to medium temperatures (such as slow roasting). Anything hotter will destroy the nutritional benefits of the oil. That's why we usually cook with coconut oil instead (which also qualifies as a healthy fat).

We recommend you spend a little extra money, get a high-quality olive oil, and enjoy it fresh over salads or veggies. We've even had some brave athletes take straight spoonfuls of the stuff.

When the quality is good, you'll notice a big difference in the taste. (Millions of Southern European cooks—and the ancient Spartan warriors—back us up on this one.)

DRINKS

Since you need something to wash all that high-quality food down, here are our top two choices for Warrior-approved beverages.

19. WATER

Most of us walk around semi-dehydrated and don't consciously notice it. Since water makes up approximately 70% of our body and is crucial for every metabolic process, you'll perform your best when well hydrated.

20. GREEN TEA

Aside from water, tea is the most widely consumed beverage on the planet. Green tea in

ALCOHOL

Alcohol isn't a recovery drink. But you already knew that.

So how does it fit into your overall plan? Well, it depends on your goals and how often you drink.

HEALTH BENEFITS?

Some studies have shown that moderate drinkers (one to two drinks per day) have fewer heart attacks and strokes than abstainers or heavy drinkers. Moderate drinkers are also less likely to suffer diabetes, arthritis, and dementia.

All good things, of course. (Though the jury is still out as to whether those benefits are related to alcohol or other lifestyle factors not accounted for.)

So let's say alcohol—in moderation—*is* good for your "health."

What about your physique and performance?

WHAT HAPPENS WHEN YOU DRINK

Your Physique

When you consume alcohol, your body treats it much like a high-carbohydrate diet. In other words, your insulin levels spike, and your body has to first burn the alcohol for energy instead of any dormant fat stores.

If you need to lose some fat—or if you're trying to make weight for a fight—drinking alcohol can make it more difficult to do so.

It's also been shown that alcohol decreases the use of glucose and amino acids in your skeletal muscles, which can adversely affect muscle growth.

Your Sex Life

Alcohol is a depressant, which means it will curb your anxiety and tension. However, it can also kill your libido by lowering your testosterone levels.

Your Performance

Alcohol is a central nervous system depressant. Since your strength and power relies on having a high-functioning nervous system, alcohol can decrease your performance.

IT'S NOT ALL BAD

With all that information, it may seem as though we're totally against consuming alcohol. We're not. In fact, we enjoy a nice beer or glass of wine as much as the next person. What we frown upon is the *over*-consumption of alcohol *or* drinking too much when your physique or performance goals can be put at stake.

HOW TO MAKE IT WORK FOR YOU—A GENERAL RULE

If you don't already consume alcohol, you have no reason to start now.

But if you do enjoy an occasional drink, try to keep it to roughly five drinks per week. (It's better if you don't have all five in one night, either. Space them out and enjoy some wine with dinner or a beer with friends on the weekend.)

What constitutes a "drink"?

- 12-ounce serving of beer
- 5-ounce serving of wine
- 1½-ounce serving of liquor

A NOTE FOR COMPETITORS

Abstain from alcohol a week before your fight. You don't want to risk the chance of decreased performance or recovery. This is especially true if you're trying to make weight.

Before that one-week period and after, however, the general rule above applies.

particular is a great choice for athletes, thanks to a chemical called EGCG that can help lower cortisol (stress hormone) levels after a particularly stressful event like training. EGCG also helps boost your immune system.

FAQ about beverages

How much water should I drink?

We recommend our athletes drink 2 liters (about 8 cups) of water spread throughout the day. To ensure you're getting enough, buy a 2-liter container, fill it every night, put it in the fridge, and empty it by the end of the next day.

Spread your water intake throughout the day by having a glass or two with each meal—don't drink it all at once. And sip, don't gulp.

Are tea bags okay?

They're fine, especially if you're in a rush. Still, tea bags usually contain lower-quality "dust" tea, a sort of waste product left over from sorting the higher-quality loose leaf tea.

If you have tea that comes in bags, don't worry. It can still offer similar benefits. However, we encourage you to try loose tea (or some combination of loose and bagged) to see how you like it. The easiest way to prepare loose leaf tea is by purchasing a French press (which is usually reserved for coffee).

What about other kinds of tea?

Black, oolong, and rooibos teas all offer similar antioxidant benefits to green tea. However, "herbal teas," which are an infusion of leaves, flowers, fruits, and herbs, contain no actual "tea" and therefore none of the benefits of the teas listed above.

Is green tea okay to drink at night?

If you're relatively caffeine sensitive, we recommend you stop drinking green tea around 1 or 2 p.m. to give the caffeine enough time to wear off.

THE WARRIOR 10: SUPPLEMENTS

The supplement industry can be a shady place, especially for athletes. It seems every other product in this largely unregulated industry is riddled with some fancy new "muscle-blasting" technology that promises much but delivers little. Consumers are stuck being their own experts for what they should and shouldn't buy. As always, stick with the basics that offer the most benefit.

While there are a host of nice supplements besides the Warrior 10 that might be beneficial, getting too worried about supplements or bogged down in the details is a huge distraction. It's time that could be better spent on training, recovering, eating properly, and mastering your sport.

These are the 10 Warrior supplements that we believe make the biggest impact, and many of our elite athletes take them daily. Most supplement or health food stores should carry reputable brands of all of these supplements, or you can order online.

1. **Multivitamin**
2. **Vitamin D**
3. **Liquid Fish Oil**
4. **Healthy Oil Blend**
5. **Protein Blend**
6. **Post-Workout Drink**
7. **BCAA Drink**
8. **Creatine Monohydrate**
9. **Arginine, HMB, and Glutamine (for Injury Recovery)**
10. **Curcumin (for Inflammation)**

1. MULTIVITAMIN

Since most of us are deficient in one or more vitamins or minerals—approximately 68% of the general population is deficient in calcium, 90% in chromium, 75% in magnesium, and 80% in vitamin B6—a high-quality multivitamin is a great way to fill in the gaps and get the extra vitamins we may not get from food alone.

Vitamins, minerals, and nutrients play a role in normalizing bodily functions and cannot be made by the body alone (except for vitamin D, which we can get from the sun).

Our favorite brands:
- Multi+ by Genuine Health
- Super Easy Multi Plus (Men) by Platinum Naturals
- Training-Peak by Inner Armour

FAQ about multivitamin

How much should I take?
Follow the instructions on the back of whichever multivitamin you choose. Some you'll take once per day; others you'll take multiple times per day.

When should I take it?

If it's a once-per-day capsule, take it in the morning with breakfast. If it's supposed to be taken multiple times per day, pair it with breakfast and a late afternoon snack.

(While these are the recommended times, they're not etched in stone. In other words, just take your multivitamin whenever you remember to take your multivitamin.)

2. VITAMIN D

Vitamin D isn't a "true" vitamin, as we don't need food to attain it. Natural sunlight allows our body to create vitamin D.

However, it's estimated that anywhere from 30% to 80% of the U.S. population is vitamin D deficient, which can lead to the following problems:
- Increased loss of muscle strength and mass as we age
- Increased risk of cancers
- Lower levels of immunity

And other countries—even those that get "adequate" sunlight—still may be deficient.

If you live in an area where you can't get 15 minutes of direct sunlight daily, you'll greatly benefit from supplementing with vitamin D.

Our favorite brands:
- Vitamin D3 by NOW
- Vitamin D by Nature Made
- Vitamin D by GNC

FAQ about vitamin D

How much should I take?
We recommend 4,000 IUs (international units) per day. (It will say how many IUs per capsule on the bottle.)

When should I take it?

With your multivitamin.

3. LIQUID FISH OIL

It's estimated that 95% of people in the United States are deficient in omega-3 fatty acids. Omega-3s have a host of benefits such as improving insulin sensitivity (which can help with muscle growth and fat loss), increasing mood and circulation, and controlling and managing inflammation.

Since your body can't naturally create omega-3s, you must get them from food and supplement sources.

Taking liquid fish oil, which contains the powerful omega-3s docosahexaenoic acid

(DHA) and eicosapentaenoic acid (EPA), is an easy way to get your high-quality fats without needing to eat a few pounds of salmon.

Our favorite brands:
- o3mega by Genuine Health
- Carlson's Very Finest Fish Oil

FAQ about fish oil

How much should I take?

We recommend starting with 1 gram of fish oil per body-fat percentage every day for the first four weeks. So, if you're 12% body fat, you'll take 12 grams of fish oil. If you're 8% body fat, you'll take 8 grams of fish oil. And if you're 16% body fat, you'll take 16 grams of fish oil. (You get the idea.)

After those four weeks, cut that dose in half.

So if you're 12% body fat and taking 12 grams of fish oil the first four weeks, drop down to 6 grams of fish oil per day.

What does a gram of fish oil look like?

Well, a teaspoon is roughly 5 grams.

That's another reason why we recommend taking liquid fish oil instead of capsules, since 1 gram of fish oil is equal to about one capsule. (And who wouldn't rather take a teaspoon or two than pop a handful of pills?)

When should I take it?

We recommend splitting your fish oil evenly throughout the day and taking it with meals.

4. HEALTHY OIL BLEND

Since we know omega-3 and other unsaturated fatty acids are important for everything from muscle growth to fat loss, injury recovery, and mood enhancement, we really like to load up.

That's why we recommend our athletes take a good oil blend that contains a host of different healthy fat sources.

Our favorite brands:
- Udo's 3-6-9 Blend
- Barlean's Organic Master Blend

FAQ about oil blend

How much should I take?

We recommend taking 1 to 2 teaspoons per day. The easiest way to take your oil is to pour it directly into a teaspoon and swallow, or combine it with white or balsamic vinegar to make a salad dressing.

When should I take it?

We recommend taking your oil blend during meals.

5. PROTEIN BLEND

Proteins are the building blocks of muscle and aid in muscle repair, increased energy, and better recovery. Unfortunately, only 75% of us get enough protein every day.

A good protein powder blend can help you reach your protein needs when eating whole food is inconvenient.

Our favorite brands:
- Metabolic Drive by Biotest (milk protein blend)
- Vegan Proteins+ by Genuine Health (for vegetarians and vegans)
- Nitro-Peak by Inner Armour

If you're lactose intolerant or vegan/vegetarian, you can also supplement with rice, hemp, pumpkin seed, or pea protein. We don't recommend soy. FAQ about protein blend

How much should I take?

We recommend taking one to two scoops per day as part of a Super Shake.

When should I take it?

Whenever eating whole food is inconvenient, or when you need an extra meal.

6. POST-WORKOUT DRINK

When you're in the gym or on the mat, you're not actually building muscle—you're tearing it down.

Exercise breaks down our muscle carbohydrate stores and our muscle protein structures. Then our immune system comes in to clean up the mess. Finally, signals are generated to tell our body to rebuild.

A good post-workout drink—a mixture of high-quality protein and fast-acting carbohydrates—is your "rebuilding material."

A carb and protein drink is perfect for when you're trying to gain muscle or doing periods of intense exercise in the off-season or in between fights.

Our favorite brands:
- Surge Recovery by Biotest
- 2:1:1 Recovery by Optimum Nutrition
- Mass-Peak by Inner Armour

Be sure to read the label to ensure you're not getting a ton of sugar or other chemical additives you don't need.

FAQ about post-workout drink

How much should I take?

How much you should take depends on your body size.

If you're skinny and usually have a hard time putting on muscle, take:

45 g protein, 90 g carbs (520 cals) in 1,000 ml of water

If you put on fat very easily, take:

15 g protein, 30 g carbs (180 cals) in 500 ml of water

And if you're somewhere in between, take:

30 g protein, 60 g carbs (360 cals) in 750 ml of water

When should I take it?

The perfect time to take your post-workout shake is actually *during* the workout (yeah, we know it says "post-workout"). Our athletes mix their workout drink before they head to the gym and drink it during their session. By the end of the session, if they have any left over, they slam it back.

7. BCAA DRINK

A BCAA drink is a good replacement for a post-workout drink when you're dieting or trying to lose weight. This is because BCAAs don't contain any carbohydrates. BCAA stands for branched chain amino acid. Amino acids are the building blocks of protein, and make up 75% of your body. Think of them as Legos for your life. A high-quality BCAA supplement can help reduce the chance of muscle tissue breakdown, thus leading to better recovery and preservation of your lean muscle.

Our favorite brands:
- Instantized BCAA 5000 powder by Optimum Nutrition
- BCAA-Peak by Inner Armour

FAQ about BCAA drink

How much should I take?

BCAA powder usually comes with its own serving scoop. We recommend you mix 10 grams of BCAA powder (two level scoops) into 2 to 3 cups of cold water.

When should I take it?

The perfect time to take your BCAA drink is during your workout.

8. CREATINE MONOHYDRATE

Creatine, the most researched supplement in all of sports science, is a white, tasteless powder that can translate to more strength, muscle, and endurance.

While we all have creatine in our muscles already (about half of which is derived from eating creatine-rich meat), supplementing with creatine can have huge positive effects on your body, the most notable being increasing maximal force production of your muscles. (That means you can lift more weight more explosively.)

One thing to remember: you only want creatine *monohydrate*. There are other kinds of creatine out there that are simply not as effective.

Our favorite brands:

- Micronized German Creatine by Biotest
- Power-Peak by Inner Armour

FAQ about creatine monohydrate

How much should I take?

We recommend taking 10 grams (two scoops) of creatine per day.

When should I take it?

You can either mix it with green tea (it dissolves better in warm beverages) or include it in your post-workout drink or BCAA recovery drink.

9. ARGININE, HMB, AND GLUTAMINE (FOR INJURY RECOVERY)

When you're injured, you need to recover as quickly and effectively as possible. While most of your recovery will come from rest, proper food intake, and perhaps physical therapy, you can increase your rate of recovery by supplementing with arginine, HMB, and glutamine.

Arginine is an amino acid that may stimulate insulin and IGF (insulin-like growth factor) action. These powerful anabolic hormones may stimulate protein synthesis and collagen deposition. Arginine also stimulates nitric oxide production, which may increase blood flow to the injured area as well as help with "tissue clean-up."

HMB, a metabolite of the amino acid leucine, inhibits muscle protein breakdown

SUPPLEMENT SUMMARY

SUPPLEMENTS TO TAKE WHEN GAINING OR MAINTAINING WEIGHT

- Multivitamin
- Vitamin D
- Liquid fish oil
- Omega-3 blend
- Protein blend
- Post-workout drink
- Creatine monohydrate

SUPPLEMENTS TO TAKE WHEN LOSING WEIGHT

- Multivitamin
- Vitamin D
- Liquid fish oil
- Omega-3 blend
- Protein blend
- BCAA drink

SUPPLEMENTS TO TAKE WHILE INJURED

- Multivitamin
- Vitamin D
- Liquid fish oil
- Omega-3 blend
- Protein blend
- BCAA drink
- Curcumin
- Arginine, HMB, and glutamine

and increases net protein balance. This may mean more muscle mass.

Glutamine is an amino acid that is essential for the metabolism of rapidly renewing cells. Glutamine may also speed up wound healing, though it hasn't been shown to do it alone.

However, in one study, the combined administration of 14 grams arginine, 3 grams HMB, and 14 grams glutamine in two divided doses (two doses of 7 grams arginine, 1.5 grams HMB, 7 gram glutamine per day) for 14 days significantly increased collagen synthesis in adults.

In other words, these three supplements converge into a super-recovery elixir when combined.

FAQ about arginine, HMB, and glutamine

How much should I take?

If you take them individually, we recommend the following dosages:

ANYTIME VS. POST-WORKOUT MEALS

We break our meal choices into two categories: Anytime (AT) meals and Post-Workout (PW) meals. They're exactly what they sound like. AT meals can be eaten at any time of the day. PW meals should be eaten only after a workout.

THE DIFFERENCE BETWEEN AT AND PW MEALS

The difference is all in the carbs. As discussed in the science section at the beginning of this part, when you eat carbohydrates, your body breaks them down into simple sugars and uses them as an immediate source of energy. Once absorbed, these sugars go to the liver to fill energy stores. From there, they enter the bloodstream and venture out to the other cells of the body.

This is when a hormone called insulin is released to handle this "sugar load" on the body. Like a transport truck with that big load of sugar, insulin transports nutrients into cells for energy and storage.

The most important thing you need to know for your diet is this: If you can control insulin, you can control your body composition and your energy.

Insulin is a tricky hormone. Sometimes, such as after a workout, a large insulin response can be a good thing since it helps us shuttle nutrients to all the right places. Carbs eaten post-workout will ensure better recovery, fat loss, and energy because our body will use those carbohydrates for repairing our muscle tissue. But at other times a large insulin response can be a bad thing, since it can lead to excess fat gain. (You might also notice it makes you feel tired or sluggish.) When your body hasn't undergone any stress (as from a workout), it doesn't need extra carbs for energy. But if you give it starchy carbs anyway, your body decides to store that energy as fat so you can use it later.

The bottom line: If you control your insulin response by eating the "right" carbs at the "right" times, you'll be able to fuel your performance, gain lean muscle, and lose fat.

Anytime meals are lower in carbs, have a minimal effect on insulin, and can be eaten at any time of the day. This way, you provide your body with energy without that energy leading to fat gain.

Post-workout meals contain more carbs, will have a bigger effect on insulin, and should be eaten within two to three hours after your workout. This way, the carbs will be put to work to help your body recover and repair.

Arginine—7 grams twice per day
HMB—1.5 grams twice per day
Glutamine—7 grams twice per day

When should I take it?

If you're taking Pro Science Armor by EAS, we recommend taking one packet twice per day.

10. CURCUMIN (FOR INFLAMMATION)

Another supplement that can help with injury recovery by controlling inflammation is curcumin, the active ingredient of the Indian spice turmeric.

Turmeric has long been used as an anti-inflammatory agent in wound healing, and current research is showing how helpful curcumin can be for mild, temporary pain.

Our favorite brands:

- Curcumin by Biotest
- Bio-Enhanced BCM-95 Curcumin by Genceutric Naturals

FAQ about curcumin

How much should I take?
About 500 mg per day of curcumin is the right amount for managing inflammation.
When should I take it?
With meals.

SAMPLE MEAL PLANS

Let's take what we've learned about the Warrior 20 foods and Warrior 10 supplements and combine them to make a day's worth of meals.

The following "Training Day" and "Off Day" sample meal plans were designed for a hypothetical male fighter who weighs between 175 and 215 pounds and wants to improve his body composition (slightly less fat, slightly more muscle) while fueling his training sessions.

If you fit our hypothetical male example, great! If not, don't worry. With a few simple tweaks, you can easily make this plan work for you by either:

- slightly reducing the amount of food you eat to further fat loss (replace your grains with greens, consume a lower-calorie post-workout shake), or
- slightly adding more food to further muscle growth (add in one more Super Shake, add 1 to 2 cups of fruit in the morning, consume a higher-calorie post-workout shake).

A FEW REMINDERS ABOUT THE MEAL PLAN

The following information can be found throughout this chapter (and we encourage you to read through it all), but here's an abbreviated version:

- "Anytime" meals consist of mostly protein, vegetables, and high-quality fat and are good to eat anytime.
- "Post-workout" meals consist of mostly protein, vegetables, and carbs and are good to eat directly post-workout.
- Forget counting protein grams and instead look at the palm of your hand. Fighters who weigh under 170 pounds should consume one palm-sized protein portion per meal, and fighters above 170 should consume two palm-sized protein portions per meal.

- You should have at least two fists of vegetables with every meal.
- You should have at least 1 to 2 teaspoons of high-quality fat with every meal (in the form of avocado, fish oil, olive oil, raw nuts, and/or nut butters).
- Don't like broccoli? Not a fan of beef? Try finding a few new ways to prepare them and/or experiment with other similar options you *do* enjoy. Stick with the Warrior 20 as much as possible, however.
- Does dairy make you feel bloated? Make sure to read our small section about milk alternatives. (That's why we prefer to use unsweetened almond milk as the base of our Super Shakes.)
- Beans not agreeing with you? Try eating lentils (they lack the sulfur that can cause gas problems) and make sure to rinse your canned beans with fresh water to get rid of the murky stuff in which they've been sitting.
- Don't skimp on the water. Try and drink at least 1 to 2 cups with every meal.
- Don't waste your money on supplements that (a) don't work, (b) are too expensive, or (c) are dangerous. Rest assured: if it's not on the Warrior 20, our elite fighters likely don't use it.

SAMPLE TRAINING DAY EATING PLAN

MEAL 1—ANYTIME

- Breakfast scramble with 4 whole eggs, 1 cup spinach, ½ red or yellow bell pepper, ½ tomato
- ¼ cup lentils or beans (kidney, garbanzo, pinto, black, or red)
- ½ avocado on the side
- 2 cups water or green tea
- 1 multivitamin (once a day)
- 4,000 IU Vitamin D3

MEAL 2—ANYTIME

- Super Shake made with 1 to 2 scoops of vanilla protein blend, ½ cup mixed frozen berries (raspberries, blueberries, blackberries, strawberries), 1 cup spinach, 1 Tbsp nut butter, and 2 cups almond milk
- 1 tsp liquid fish oil

MEAL 3—ANYTIME: BIG BOWL SALAD WITH PROTEIN

- 2 cups broccoli, coleslaw, and/or carrot blend (found in bags in the salad section of your grocery aisle)
- 2 palm-size portions of seasoned grilled chicken, lean beef, fish, or fermented soy
- ¼ cup beans (kidney, garbanzo, pinto, black, or red)
- ¼ cup raw mixed nuts (almonds, cashews, pecans, walnuts, or pistachios)
- 2 Tbsp oil blend mixed with 2 Tbsp white wine vinegar to make salad dressing
- 2 cups water or green tea

MEAL 4—ANYTIME: PRE-WORKOUT SHAKE

- Small Super Shake made with ½ cup canned pumpkin, 1 scoop vanilla protein blend, 2 Tbsp heavy cream, sprinkle of cinnamon, sprinkle of stevia or Splenda to taste, and 1½ cups water

WORKOUT SHAKE

- Post-workout shake made with 30 g protein and 60 g carbs in 750 ml water
- 2 scoops (10 g) of creatine monohydrate

MEAL 5—POST-WORKOUT

- 2 palm-size portions of seasoned fish, chicken, beef, or fermented soy
- 2 cups steamed vegetables (broccoli, cauliflower, Brussels sprouts)
- 1 Tbsp olive oil to drizzle over vegetables
- 2 golf-ball-size portions of cooked quinoa or 1 small sweet potato
- ¼ cup lentils or beans (kidney, garbanzo, pinto, black, or red)
- 1 orange for dessert
- 2 cups water
- 1 tsp liquid fish oil

SAMPLE OFF-DAY EATING PLAN

MEAL 1—ANYTIME

- Breakfast omelet made with 3 whole eggs, ½ cup lean ground beef, 1 cup spinach, and ½ tomato, topped with 2 Tbsp salsa
- ¼ cup lentils or beans (kidney, garbanzo, pinto, black, or red)
- ½ avocado on the side
- 2 cups green tea with 2 scoops (10 g) of creatine monohydrate mixed in
- 1 multivitamin (once a day)
- 4,000 IU Vitamin D3

MEAL 2—ANYTIME

- Super Shake made with 1 to 2 scoops of vanilla protein blend, ½ cup mixed frozen berries (raspberries, blueberries, blackberries, strawberries), 1 cup spinach, 1 Tbsp nut butter, and 2 cups almond milk
- 1 tsp liquid fish oil

MEAL 3—ANYTIME: BIG BOWL SALAD WITH PROTEIN

- 2 cups broccoli, coleslaw, and/or carrot blend (found in bags in the salad section of your grocery aisle)
- 2 palm-size portions of seasoned grilled chicken, lean beef, fish, or fermented soy
- ¼ cup beans (kidney, garbanzo, pinto, black, or red)
- ¼ cup raw mixed nuts (almonds, cashews, pecans, walnuts, or pistachios)
- 2 Tbsp oil blend mixed with 2 Tbsp white wine vinegar to make salad dressing
- 2 cups water or green tea

MEAL 4—ANYTIME

- Super Shake made with 1 to 2 scoops of chocolate protein blend, ⅓ cup cottage cheese, 2 tsp ground flax seeds, 1 cup spinach, 1 tsp cocoa, 3 drops mint extract, ¼ cup pecans, 1 cup water, and a handful of ice cubes
- 1 tsp liquid fish oil

MEAL 5—ANYTIME

- 2 palm-size portions of seasoned fish, chicken, beef, or fermented soy
- 2 cups steamed vegetables (broccoli, cauliflower, Brussels sprouts)
- 1 Tbsp olive oil to drizzle over vegetables
- ¼ cup lentils or beans (kidney, garbanzo, pinto, black, or red)
- 2 cups water
- 1 tsp liquid fish oil

GAINING AND LOSING WEIGHT

Depending on your fitness needs, your goals may be focused more on losing weight or on gaining muscle. Neither of these is as hard as you'd think. You don't have to track your calories, spend your life in the gym, or take expensive supplements.

Instead, just follow a few simple habits.

HOW TO LOSE WEIGHT

Replace your grains with greens.

Remember how we divide our meals into "Anytime" (AT) and "Post-Workout" (PW) options? The main difference is the amount of carbohydrates. PW meals are higher in carbs (to replenish your glycogen stores after intense exercise), while AT meals are lower in carbs to minimize fat gain.

But sometimes we have clients who "forget" that PW meals should be, well, *post*-workout. They mindlessly eat carbs at random times of the day, often without noticing it.

One easy solution is to look at your plate whenever you sit down for a meal and replace your grains (rice, bread, corn, and other starchy carbs such as potatoes) with greens (leafy greens like spinach, or cruciferous vegetables such as broccoli).

The simple mantra "replace grains with greens" will help keep your AT meals effective for weight loss.

Eat slowly.

When is the last time you timed how long it took you to eat a meal? (What? You've never done that?)

We'll save you the trouble: you probably ate it *way* too fast. Because the breakdown of enzymes and nutrients in your food is a slow process, it takes your brain a full 20 minutes to register that you're full. If you scarf down your meal in less than 20 minutes, you're probably consuming more calories than your body really needs.

The next time you sit down to eat, take your time. Chew your food slowly. Set your fork and knife down between bites. Drink some water. You may just find you're full before you know it. You can get away with eating less without being hungry. And you'll enjoy the meal more, too.

Eat till 80% full.

If you've ever leaned back in your chair and said, "Man, I'm full," you know what it feels like to *overeat*. Trouble is, most of us do it multiple times per week. (And sometimes every day.) Most of us eat—or continue eating—regardless of whether we need to. In our minds, we have no such thing as a "food quota." But our bodies say otherwise. They do have a quota.

In other words, hunger is linked more to our minds and less to an actual biological need to feed ourselves. We *want* food even if we don't really *need* food. That's why starting today, at every meal, we want you stop eating a little sooner than you normally would. We want you to stop eating at "80% full."

You can do this two ways:

- Leave a couple of extra bites of your meal on your plate and save the rest in the fridge for later.
- Plan what you're going to eat, then slightly reduce the total amount. In other words, if you were going to eat one chicken breast with rice and vegetables today, eat half a chicken breast with less rice and vegetables. You'll finish the meal sooner (but you're eating more slowly, right?). And stop at about 80% full.

HOW TO GAIN WEIGHT

Consume an extra Super Shake.

The number one reason people have trouble putting on weight? They don't eat nearly enough. And that's because eating 3,000+ calories per day is difficult with whole food. Since you already know how to make a Super Shake, we want to help you take full advantage of its power. If you're currently drinking one calorie-rich Super Shake per day, start drinking *two*.

If you're already drinking two Super Shakes per day, have *three*. (There's no reason to go above three, however.)

Just one protein- and fiber-filled Super Shake can bump up your calories by 800 or more.

Add a bowl of morning oatmeal.

If you've already added an extra Super Shake (up to a maximum of three per day) and still need to gain more weight, you can break the "post-workout" meal rule for breakfast by adding a bowl of oatmeal with fruit.

These extra carbohydrates in the morning will supply your body with a few hundred calories, which will help kick-start your day.

Doctor John's Oatmeal

¼ cup rolled oats (slow-cooked on the stovetop for 5 minutes)
1 scoop of vanilla protein powder
⅓ cup mixed nuts
½ cup frozen berries

Add fat.

If adding extra carbohydrates makes you feel too bloated but you'd still like to add mass, then consider adding more fat to your diet for additional calories instead. Saturated fats in particular will help keep sex hormone production going strong and your moods upbeat, which can be especially important when your body and emotions are stressed from training.

Add two to three small portions per day of the following:

- Fattier fish such as salmon
- Fattier cuts of meat (*if* the meat is grass-fed or wild; otherwise keep the meat lean)
- Avocados
- Nuts, seeds, and nut butters
- Heavy whipping cream (for coffee, or small amounts in Super Shakes)
- Raw coconut, coconut milk, and extra-virgin coconut oil
- High-quality extra-virgin olive oil
- Cold-pressed fresh oils such as hemp, flax, or pumpkin seed
- Butter (grass-fed if possible)

Avoid processed/refined fats such as cooking or vegetable oil, margarine, cooking spray, commercial peanut butter, palm oil, or the coconut oil that appears in processed foods (it's been chemically altered, so it's not healthy like fresh coconut).

Remember that carbs and fat are like two sides of a scale. Don't bring carbs and fat up together; that's a recipe for body-fat gain. Instead, increase either one *or* the other, while keeping protein constant.

Eat two post-workout meals.

If you've added an extra Super Shake and morning oatmeal but *still* want to gain more weight—you've got the metabolism of a hummingbird, don't you?—try having one more post-workout meal after your training session.

Simply follow our post-workout meal guidelines (add two golf-ball-size portions of quinoa, amaranth, or sweet potato to your protein and veggies) and dig in.

WHAT TO EAT BEFORE TRAINING

Working out on a full stomach can be uncomfortable and slow you down. Doing it on an empty stomach isn't much better. The best option?

A light "Anytime" meal with slightly more carbs one to two hours before your training session. Make sure to get a balance of protein, slower-digesting carbs (e.g., lentils or higher-fiber veggies), and a little fat. This supplies your body with enough energy to fuel your workouts, but not enough meal volume to harm your performance (or send you running for the puke bucket).

Here are a few of our favorite pre-training meals:

Pumpkin Pie Shake

A small Super Shake—about half the size you'd normally consume—is a quick, easy meal. We like a "Pumpkin Pie Shake," which bumps up the higher-fiber carbs with sweet squash. Sip it, don't chug it.

½ cup canned pumpkin or butternut squash
1 scoop of vanilla protein powder
2 Tbsp coconut milk or heavy cream
A sprinkle each of cinnamon and nutmeg
Sweetener (such as stevia or Splenda) to taste
1½ to 2 cups water

Spinach, Lentil, and Walnut Salad

The fat in the dressing and nuts will help your body absorb the vitamins and minerals in the greens, while the vinegar, fat, and fiber slow the digestion, so you'll be ready for action like Popeye by the time you roll on to the mat.

2–3 handfuls of mixed greens or baby spinach
3–4 oz lean protein (such as chicken breast, fish, or lean meat)
2 Tbsp cooked lentils
1–2 Tbsp olive oil
Splash of balsamic vinegar
Sprinkle of chopped walnuts

Breakfast of Champions

Early morning workout? This one's easily eaten out of a Tupperware container on the way to the gym.

1 cup cottage cheese
1 cup berries
2 Tbsp ground flax seeds
1–2 oz mixed chopped nuts and seeds

SPECIAL TOPIC FOR FIGHTERS: CUTTING WEIGHT

If you're a fighter, when it comes to cutting weight before a fight, you can do it either of two ways: the smart way or the stupid way.

The stupid way is to starve yourself, take a lot of diuretics, not drink any water, and wear trash bags. This leads to fast weight loss. It also leads to fast muscle loss, decreased energy and power, and one bad temper.

The smart way involves simple carbohydrate, water, and sodium manipulation that can help you shed excess water weight, maintain most of your muscle, and ensure you can rehydrate back up to a heavy fighting weight.

Unfortunately, a lot of people pick the stupid way. You're gonna be different.

SOME THOUGHTS ON WEIGHT CUTTING

Weight cutting isn't magic. It won't save your butt if you're a lousy fighter. In fact, if you're

CHART OF GRAPPLER'S WEIGHT LOSS PROTOCOL

SUNDAY

Carbohydrates	Less than 50 g; no fruits, starches, or sugars
Protein and Fat	As much as you want
Water	1/2 gallon
Salt	Salt food normally
Diuretics	None
Laxative	None
Exercise	Light exercise taper
Immersion	None

MONDAY

Carbohydrates	Less than 50 g; no fruits, starches, or sugars
Protein and Fat	As much as you want
Water	1 gallon
Salt	Salt food normally
Diuretics	None
Laxative	None
Exercise	Light exercise taper
Immersion	None

TUESDAY

Carbohydrates	Less than 50 g; no fruits, starches, or sugars
Protein and Fat	As much as you want
Water	1 gallon
Salt	Salt food normally
Diuretics	None
Laxative	None
Exercise	Light exercise taper
Immersion	None

WEDNESDAY

Carbohydrates	Less than 50 g; no fruits, starches, or sugars
Protein and Fat	As much as you want
Water	1/2 gallon
Salt	No salt
Diuretics	None
Laxative	None
Exercise	Light exercise taper
Immersion	None

THURSDAY

Carbohydrates	Less than 50 g; no fruits, starches, or sugars
Protein and Fat	As much as you want until noon, then eat light until weigh-In
Water	1/4 gallon
Salt	No salt
Diuretics	Herbal; 1 dose with breakfast, lunch, and dinner
Laxative	1 bottle magnesium citrate at 7 p.m. if necessary
Exercise	Light exercise taper
Immersion	Hot water immersion if necessary

FRIDAY

Carbohydrates	Less than 50 g; no fruits, starches, or sugars
Protein and Fat	Eat lightly until weight-in
Water	None until after weigh-in
Salt	No salt until after weigh-in
Diuretics	Herbal; 1 dose with breakfast, lunch, and dinner
Laxative	None
Exercise	No exercise
Immersion	Hot water immersion if necessary

inexperienced, it's a lot smarter to lose weight slowly in the several weeks before your fight than to try to manage an opponent while freshly dehydrated and brain-dead from severe cutting.

Always improve your skill, fitness, and competition readiness *first* before relying on weight cutting for the extra edge.

Expect to be mentally sluggish and low-energy when weight cutting, and build that "buffer zone" into your preparations. Don't expect to be able to cram physically, emotionally, and mentally for a fight while you're sitting in a sauna dreaming of ice water. And don't show up for a competition with 2 or 3 pounds left to lose, unless you want to waste a lot of fighting energy running around the parking lot and spitting. Do your prep work—for *everything*, including cutting—well in advance.

Realize that you're setting yourself up for some disordered eating and metabolic disruption with frequent weight cutting, especially if it's drastic. If you find yourself stuck in a vicious cycle of constantly battling to cut weight and then binge eating afterward, consider two options:

- Drop the weight/fat permanently so that you're walking around lean, and within 5 pounds of your fighting weight.
- Take several months to focus on adding quality muscle mass and power; go up a weight class and make all that mass count for something.

HOT WATER IMMERSION

If required, fill a bathtub with water that doesn't burn the hand but causes moderate pain if the hand is underwater. Submerge your entire body and head so that only your face is exposed to the air. Stay in the tub for 10 minutes. Exit the tub at the 10-minute mark and place an ice pack over your head and neck to cool off. Don't shower afterward, as you'll start absorbing that water. Do this twice on Friday if necessary.

HOW TO CUT WEIGHT

WEIGH-IN 24 HOURS BEFORE THE FIGHT

Pro fighters typically weigh in at least a day before they fight, so they have time to rehydrate and re-feed.

The following is the exact same cutting and rehydration protocol we use with dozens of fighters before and after weigh-ins.

(In fact, if done precisely, it's easy for some athletes to drop 30 pounds in the week leading up to the fight, and to get all that weight back on during the 24 hours between the weigh-in and the fight.)

ONE WEEK BEFORE THE FIGHT (ASSUMING A SATURDAY EVENT)

Carbs

Keep carbs below 50 grams, which helps deplete your muscle glycogen levels and flush water.

One gram of carbohydrate pulls 2.7 grams of water into the muscle, which is why we minimize carbohydrates the week prior.

Protein and fat

Because you gotta eat *something*.

This is the perfect opportunity to load up on the protein and fat sources from the Warrior 20. Also, leafy vegetables (like spinach) and cruciferous vegetables (like broccoli and cauliflower) are fine to have at every meal.

Water

You don't lose weight by not drinking water, at least not at first. Instead, you put your body into flushing mode by drinking lots of water (which will down-regulate aldosterone, a hormone that acts to conserve sodium and secrete potassium) and then by cutting water intake suddenly at the end.

That's why you'll be consuming 1 to 2 gallons per day before tapering down.

Salt

Since your body likes to hold on to sodium (which will hold on to water), you'll continue to salt your foods normally for the first part of the week, but will try to eliminate salt completely once you start cutting your water.

Diuretics

This step isn't necessary, but when we use a diuretic we always use a natural one, such as H_2O Lean or dandelion root.

Laxative

Use this step only in cases where you're very close to not making your weight.

Exercise

The week before a fight, you won't be in a position to gain muscle or get any stronger or more powerful. The best thing you can do is light weight training and medium-paced striking/grappling and technique drilling sessions.

Immersion

We sweat a lot in hot environments. However, we sweat the most in hot, humid environments. Since hot water offers both heat and 100% humidity, you can lose more water in a hot immersion tub than in a sauna.

DAY OF WEIGH-IN

Before weigh-in

You'll keep your carbs low and eat small amounts of protein and fat so you won't be hungry. Drink absolutely no water before the weigh-in. You can help keep your saliva going by chewing on sugar-free gum or swishing out your mouth with water.

After weigh-in

Now is the time to rehydrate and get back up to your normal weight.

Eat as much as you want, as long as you're eating healthy meals. (Eating a bunch of crap and upsetting your stomach is the worst thing you could do after all that hard work.)

Consume 1 liter of water for every hour you're awake after your weigh-in. We recommend mixing ½ scoop of Biotest brand Surge Workout Fuel—a blend of rehydrating carbs and acid buffers—into each liter of water.

On average, the body can absorb only about 1 liter (2.2 pounds) of fluid an hour, so don't drink any more than that. Also, roughly 25% will be lost as urine.

No exercise today. (Work on your mental prep.)

FIGHT DAY

Now that the big day has arrived, you should be close to your initial weight before you started the cutting protocol.

Eat small meals that include carbs, protein, and fat. Don't try any new or stomach-upsetting foods today—stick with a routine that you know works for you, and don't forget to eat slowly. Unless your fight name is Nerves of Steel, your stomach will probably be doing backflips, so go easy.

Continue with your 1 liter of water per hour awake, up until three hours before the fight starts.

No exercise today, but stay loose.

Oh, and kick some ass.

RINGSIDE OR MORNING OF WEIGH-IN

In an attempt to eliminate radical weight-cutting practices or simply to cut down on time-consuming processes, many tournaments and competitions will have morning or ringside weigh-ins. This means you may have only a few hours—or worse, only a few *minutes*—before you fight.

In this case, we recommend you reduce your weight *gradually* in the weeks leading up to your fight. Trying to fight while drastically dehydrated is a recipe for disaster. See our tips on losing weight on pages 380–81.

If you weigh in on the morning of a tournament or competition, you can implement the suggestions mentioned in a less drastic fashion. Ideally, start your dehydration week within no more than 5 pounds of your weight class and dehydrate/cut more moderately.

Then, after you've weighed in and during the ensuing hours before you fight, sip (don't chug) a solution of sodium, glucose, and water (something like Gatorade or Pedialyte is a good start). Have a small meal of protein and carbohydrate (such as a half-size Super Shake), eating familiar foods that you know you can easily tolerate.

Throughout the day, nibble at small meals that have a little salt and are balanced in carbohydrates, fat, and protein. And keep drinking moderately, but not so much that you'll have to run out for a whiz just as the fight announcer is calling your name.

For a ringside weigh-in, it's okay to be *slightly* dehydrated, but start sipping at a sodium, glucose, and water solution as immediately as possible.

TRANSITIONING AFTER CUTTING

The weight-cutting process doesn't end with your fight or when you step on the scale. Your body will experience a "rebound" effect.

Expect that your appetite signals are going to be off for at least a week after cutting. The adrenaline of competition combined with the body's compensation mechanisms will mean that you'll probably be ravenous and inclined to eat weird things, like a sandwich using two pizzas for the bread and peanut butter ice cream for the filling.

As much as possible, resist the urge to stuff yourself silly after your fight day. You'll feel lousy, and pack on extra pounds that you don't need.

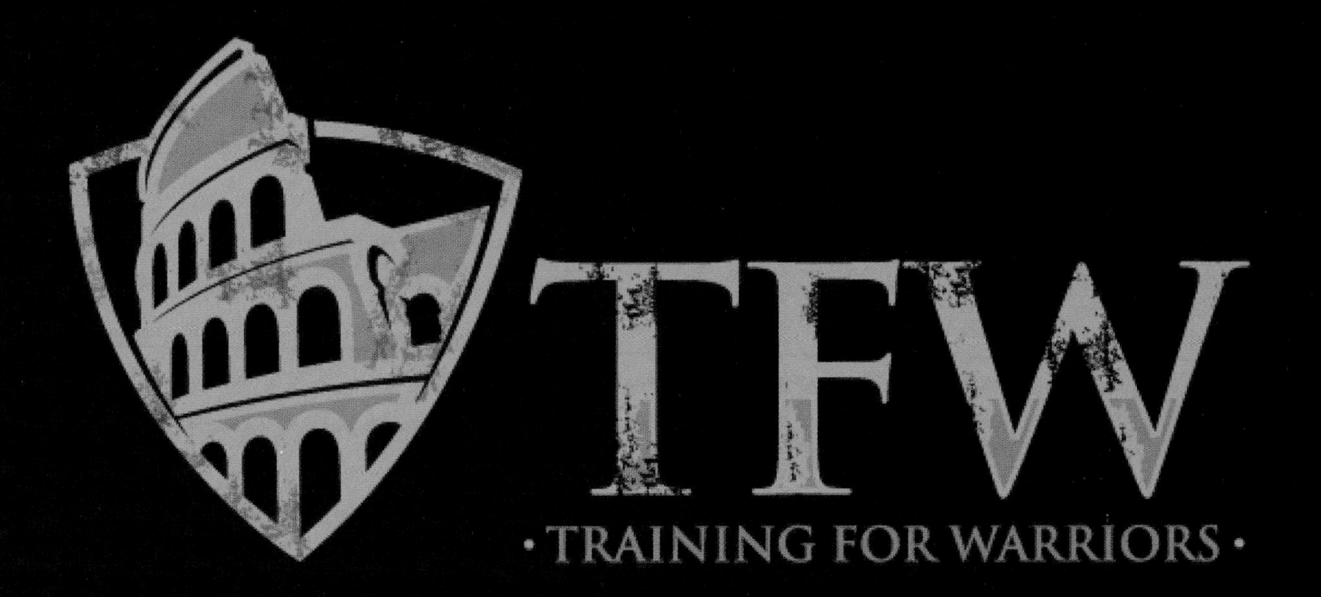
TFW
· TRAINING FOR WARRIORS ·

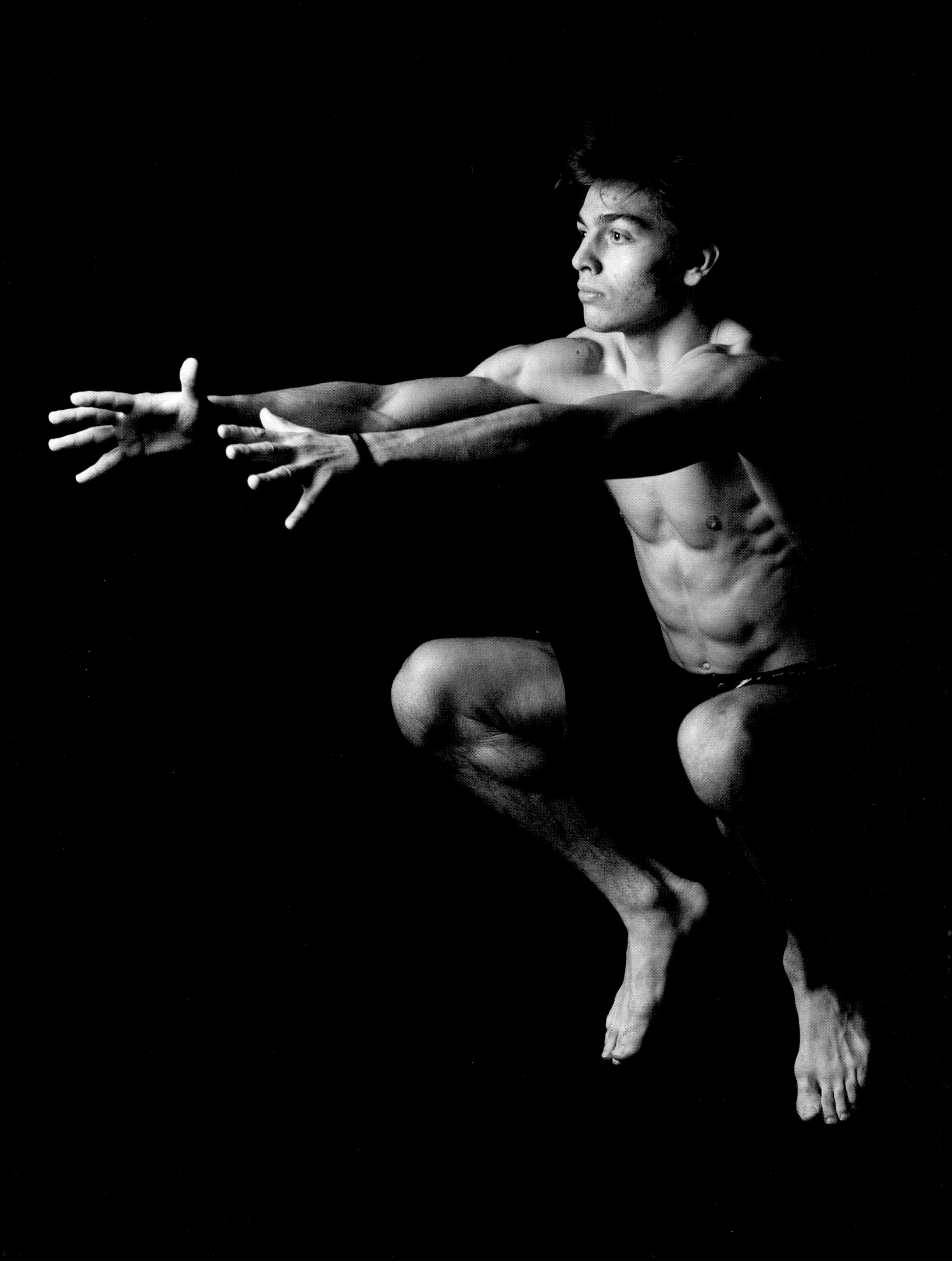

17

WARRIOR CARDIO 12-WEEK WORKOUT

This chapter contains a 12-week workout featuring the exercises contained in this book. These workouts were designed to improve your strength, speed, and flexibility in addition to your cardiovascular capacity.

Each workout begins with the TFW Prehab 15, which is followed by the Warrior Warmup. I strongly suggest that you do not skip this portion of the workout. These two sections, when applied over time, will pay huge dividends.

Following the Warrior Warmup, each workout will feature some form of Metabolic Training. During every circuit that is performed, I recommend that you monitor your heart rate before starting a circuit, at the end of each circuit, and again at the beginning of the next circuit following recovery. This monitoring will allow you to determine the cardiovascular demand in terms of intensity (maximum heart rate attained) as well as the heart's capacity to recover, or heart rate variability (the amount of beats the heart rate reduced in the rest period). All of this data should be recorded at every workout to determine if there is actual improvement in metabolic capacity taking place.

After the Metabolic Training, every session concludes with Core Training. This section was designed to improve both strength and stability. Although the Core Training is saved for last during the workouts, this does not mean that it is less important than the other sections. Make sure to stay the course during each workout and work your core.

When you have completed the 12 weeks, you will be stronger, leaner, and more physically and mentally prepared to face any challenge.

WEEK 1

The Warrior 7 Performance Evaluation Tests

MONDAY

1. **Prehab 15, 15 Minutes**
   All Prehab 15 Drills (pp. 35-48)
2. **Warrior Warmup, 20 Minutes**
   All Mini Plyo Hops and Movement Drills (pp. 53-73) All TFW Hip Circuit (pp. 74-83) All Upper-Body Band Routine (pp. 84-89)
3. **Metabolic Training, 25 Minutes**
   Category 1 Hurricane (p. 130)
4. **Core Training, 10 Minutes**
   Regular Plank Circuit (pp. 306-8)

WEDNESDAY

1. **Prehab 15, 15 Minutes**
   All Prehab 15 Drills (pp. 35-48)
2. **Warrior Warmup, 20 Minutes**
   All Stationary Warmup Drills (pp. 43-48 in *Training for Warriors*) 2 sets of 10 reps All Movement Warmup Drills (pp. 48-50 in *Training for Warriors*) 2 sets of 20 yards All Muscle Activation Exercises (pp. 51-58 in *Training for Warriors*) 1 set of 8 reps (on each side if necessary)
3. **Metabolic Training, 25 Minutes**
   Upper-Body Barbell Complex for 3 sets (pp. 148-50)
4. **Core Training, 10 Minutes**
   Pushup Plank Circuit (pp. 309-12)

FRIDAY

1. **Prehab 15, 15 Minutes**
   All Prehab 15 Drills (pp. 35-48)
2. **Warrior Warmup, 20 Minutes**
   All Mini Plyo Hops and Movement Drills (pp. 53-73) TFW Hip Circuit (pp. 73-83) Upper-Body Band Routine (pp. 84-89)
3. **Metabolic Training, 25 Minutes**
   Power Circuit for 3 total sets (pp. 107-11)
4. **Core Training, 10 Minutes**
   Med Ball Plank Circuit (pp. 312-14)

WEEK 2

MONDAY

1. **Prehab 15, 15 Minutes**
   All Prehab 15 Drills (pp. 35-48)
2. **Warrior Warmup 20 Minutes**
   All Stationary Warmup Drills (pp. 43-48 in *Training for Warriors*) 2 sets of 10 reps All Movement Warmup Drills (pp. 48-50 in *Training for Warriors*) 2 sets of 20 yards All Muscle Activation Exercises (pp. 51-58 in *Training for Warriors*) 1 set of 8 reps (on each side if necessary)
3. **Metabolic Training, 25 Minutes**
   Category 1 Hurricane (p. 130)
4. **Core Training, 10 Minutes**
   Elevated Plank Circuit (pp. 315-16)

WEDNESDAY

1. **Prehab 15, 15 Minutes**
   All Prehab 15 Drills (pp. 35-48)
2. **Warrior Warmup, 20 Minutes**
   All Mini Plyo Hops and Movement Drills (pp. 53-73) TFW Hip Circuit (pp. 74-83) Upper-Body Band Routine (pp. 84-89)
3. **Metabolic Training, 25 Minutes**
   Lower-Body Barbell Complex for 3 sets (pp. 145-47)
4. **Core Training, 10 Minutes**
   Obliques Circuit (pp. 330-34)

FRIDAY

1. **Prehab 15, 15 Minutes**
   All Prehab 15 Drills (pp. 35–48)
2. **Warrior Warmup, 20 Minutes**
   All Stationary Warmup Drills (pp. 43–48 in *Training for Warriors*) 2 sets of 10 reps All Movement Warmup Drills (pp. 48–50 in *Training for Warriors*) 2 sets of 20 yards All Muscle Activation Exercises (pp. 51–58 in *Training for Warriors*) 1 set of 8 reps (on each side if necessary)
3. **Metabolic Training, 25 Minutes**
   Tire Circuit for 3 sets (pp. 117–21)
4. **Core Training, 10 Minutes**
   Hip Flexor Circuit (pp. 335–38)

WEEK 3

MONDAY

1. **Prehab 15, 15 Minutes**
   All Prehab 15 Drills (pp. 35–48)
2. **Warrior Warmup, 20 Minutes**
   All Mini Plyo Hops and Movement Drills (pp. 53–73) All TFW Hip Circuit (pp. 74–83) Upper-Body Band Routine (pp. 84–89)
3. **Metabolic Training, 25 Minutes**
   Category 2 Hurricane Work-to-Rest Method (pp. 131–33)
4. **Core Training, 10 Minutes**
   Swiss Ball Plank Circuit (pp. 317–19)

WEDNESDAY

1. **Prehab 15, 15 Minutes**
   All Prehab 15 Drills (pp. 35–48)
2. **Warrior Warmup, 20 Minutes**
   All Stationary Warmup Drills (pp. 43–48 in *Training for Warriors*) 2 sets of 10 reps All Movement Warmup Drills (pp. 48–50 in *Training for Warriors*) 2 sets of 20 yards All Muscle Activation Exercises (pp. 51–58 in *Training for Warriors*) 1 set of 8 reps (on each side if necessary)
3. **Metabolic Training, 25 Minutes**
   Full-Body Barbell Complex for 3 sets (pp. 151–56)
4. **Core Training, 10 Minutes**
   Side Plank Circuit (pp. 319–21)

FRIDAY

1. **Prehab 15, 15 Minutes**
   All Prehab 15 Drills (pp. 35–48)
2. **Warrior Warmup, 20 Minutes**
   All Mini Plyo Hops and Movement Drills (pp. 53–73) All TFW Hip Circuit (pp. 74–83) Upper-Body Band Routine (pp. 84–89)
3. **Metabolic Training, 25 Minutes**
   Fighter Circuit for 3 sets (pp. 112–16)
4. **Core Training, 10 Minutes**
   Elevated Side Plank Circuit (pp. 322–25)

WEEK 4

The Warrior 7 Performance Evaluation Tests

MONDAY

1. **Prehab 15, 15 Minutes**
   All Prehab 15 Drills (pp. 35–48)
2. **Warrior Warmup, 20 minutes**
   All Stationary Warmup Drills (pp. 43–48 in *Training for Warriors*) 2 sets of 10 reps All Movement Warmup Drills (pp. 48–50 in *Training for Warriors*) 2 sets of 20 yards All Muscle Activation Exercises (pp. 51–58 in *Training for Warriors*) 1 set of 8 reps (on each side if necessary)
3. **Metabolic Training, 25 Minutes**
   Category 2 Hurricane Work-to-Rest Method (pp. 131–33)
4. **Core Training, 10 Minutes**
   Partner Medicine Ball Circuit (pp. 343–48)

WEDNESDAY

1. **Prehab 15, 15 Minutes**
   All Prehab 15 Drills (pp. 35-48)
2. **Warrior Warmup, 20 Minutes**
   All Mini Plyo Hops and Movement Drills (pp. 53-73) All TFW Hip Circuit (pp. 74-83) Upper-Body Band Routine (pp. 84-89)
3. **Metabolic Training, 25 Minutes**
   10-Exercise Barbell Complex for 3 sets (pp. 157-66)
4. **Core Training, 10 Minutes**
   Partner Core Drills Circuit (pp. 339-42)

FRIDAY

1. **Prehab 15, 15 Minutes**
   All Prehab 15 Drills (pp. 35-48)
2. **Warrior Warmup, 20 Minutes**
   All Stationary Warmup Drills (pp. 43-48 in *Training for Warriors*) 2 sets of 10 reps All Movement Warmup Drills (pp. 48-50 in *Training for Warriors*) 2 sets of 20 yards All Muscle Activation Exercises (pp. 51-58 in *Training for Warriors*) 1 set of 8 reps (on each side if necessary)
3. **Metabolic Training, 25 Minutes**
   Strongman Circuit for 3 sets (pp. 102-6)
4. **Core Training, 10 Minutes**
   Advanced Stabilization Circuit (pp. 326-29)

WEEK 5

MONDAY

1. **Prehab 15, 15 Minutes**
   All Prehab 15 Drills (pp. 35-48)
2. **Warrior Warmup, 20 Minutes**
   All Mini Plyo Hops and Movement Drills (pp. 53-73) All TFW Hip Circuit (pp. 74-83) Upper-Body Band Routine (pp. 84-89)
3. **Metabolic Training, 25 Minutes**
   Category 3 Hurricane Work-to-Rest Method (pp. 134-36)
4. **Core Training, 10 Minutes**
   Regular Plank Circuit (pp. 306-8)

WEDNESDAY

1. **Prehab 15, 15 Minutes**
   All Prehab 15 Drills (pp. 35-48)
2. **Warrior Warmup, 20 Minutes**
   All Stationary Warmup Drills (pp. 43-48 in *Training for Warriors*) 2 sets of 10 reps All Movement Warmup Drills (pp. 48-50 in *Training for Warriors*) 2 sets of 20 yards All Muscle Activation Exercises (pp. 51-58 in *Training for Warriors*) 1 set of 8 reps (on each side if necessary)
3. **Metabolic Training, 25 Minutes**
   The Gauntlet for 2 sets (pp. 258-63) Chin-up Series for 2 sets (pp. 252-54)
4. **Core Training, 10 Minutes**
   Pushup Plank Circuit (p. 309-12)

FRIDAY

1. **Prehab 15, 15 Minutes**
   All Prehab 15 Drills (pp. 35-48)
2. **Warrior Warmup, 20 Minutes**
   All Mini Plyo Hops and Movement Drills (pp. 53-73) All TFW Hip Circuit (pp. 74-83) Upper-Body Band Routine (pp. 84-89)
3. **Metabolic Training, 25 Minutes**
   The Climber Tabata for 1 set (pp. 211-14) Four-Way Lunge Circuit for 1 set (pp. 233-36) Prowler Finishers for 6 reps of 20 yards (pp. 291-92)
4. **Core Training, 10 Minutes**
   Med Ball Plank Circuit (pp. 312-14)

WEEK 6

MONDAY

1. **Prehab 15, 15 Minutes**
   All Prehab 15 Drills (pp. 35-48)
2. **Warrior Warmup, 20 Minutes**
   All Stationary Warmup Drills (pp. 43-48 in

Training for Warriors) 2 sets of 10 reps All Movement Warmup Drills (pp. 48–50 in *Training for Warriors*) 2 sets of 20 yards All Muscle Activation Exercises (pp. 51–58 in *Training for Warriors*) 1 set of 8 reps (on each side if necessary)

3. **Metabolic Training, 25 Minutes**
   Category 3 Hurricane Best-Time Method (pp. 134–36)
4. **Core Training, 10 Minutes**
   Elevated Plank Circuit (pp. 315–16)

WEDNESDAY

1. **Prehab 15, 15 Minutes**
   All Prehab 15 Drills (pp. 35–48)
2. **Warrior Warmup, 20 Minutes**
   All Mini Plyo Hops and Movement Drills (pp. 53–73) All TFW Hip Circuit (pp. 74–83) Upper-Body Band Routine (pp. 84–89)
3. **Metabolic Training, 25 Minutes**
   The Gauntlet for 2 sets (pp. 258–63) Chin-up Series for 2 sets (pp. 252–54)
4. **Core Training, 10 Minutes**
   Obliques Circuit (pp. 330–34)

FRIDAY

1. **Prehab 15, 15 Minutes**
   All Prehab 15 Drills (pp. 35–48)
2. **Warrior Warmup, 20 Minutes**
   All Stationary Warmup Drills (pp. 43–48 in *Training for Warriors*) 2 sets of 10 reps All Movement Warmup Drills (pp. 48–50 in *Training for Warriors*) 2 sets of 20 yards All Muscle Activation Exercises (pp. 51–58 in *Training for Warriors*) 1 set of 8 reps (on each side if necessary)
3. **Metabolic Training, 25 Minutes**
   The Lunger Tabata for 1 set (pp. 215–16) The Squatter Tabata for 1 set (p. 217) Prowler Finishers for 6 reps of 20 yards (pp. 291–92)
4. **Core Training, 10 Minutes**
   Hip Flexor Circuit (pp. 335–38)

WEEK 7

MONDAY

1. **Prehab 15, 15 Minutes**
   All Prehab 15 Drills (pp. 35–48)
2. **Warrior Warmup, 20 Minutes**
   All Mini Plyo Hops and Movement Drills (pp. 53–73) All TFW Hip Circuit (pp. 74–83) Upper-Body Band Routine (pp. 84–89)
3. **Metabolic Training, 25 Minutes**
   Category 2 Hurricane Best-Time Method (pp. 131–33)
4. **Core Training, 10 Minutes**
   Swiss Ball Plank Circuit (pp. 317–19)

WEDNESDAY

1. **Prehab 15, 15 Minutes**
   All Prehab 15 Drills (pp. 35–48)
2. **Warrior Warmup, 20 Minutes**
   All Stationary Warmup Drills (pp. 43–48 in *Training for Warriors*) 2 sets of 10 reps All Movement Warmup Drills (pp. 48–50 in *Training for Warriors*) 2 sets of 20 yards All Muscle Activation Exercises (pp. 51–58 in *Training for Warriors*) 1 set of 8 reps (on each side if necessary)
3. **Metabolic Training, 25 Minutes**
   The Doubler for 2 sets (pp. 255–57) Dumbbell Shoulder Circuit for 2 sets (pp. 264–67)
4. **Core Training, 10 Minutes**
   Side Plank Circuit (pp. 319–21)

FRIDAY

1. **Prehab 15, 15 Minutes**
   All Prehab 15 Drills (pp. 35–48)
2. **Warrior Warmup, 20 Minutes**
   All Mini Plyo Hops and Movement Drills (pp. 53–73) All TFW Hip Circuit (pp. 74–83) Upper-Body Band Routine (pp. 84–89)
3. **Metabolic Training, 25 Minutes**
   Lower-Body Dumbbell Complex for 2 sets (pp. 145–47) The Jumper Tabata for 1 set

(p. 218) Sled Dragging 2 sets of each drag for 20 yards (pp. 288–90)

4. **Core Training, 10 Minutes**
   Elevated Side Plank Circuit (pp. 322–25)

WEEK 8

The Warrior 7 Performance Evaluation Tests

MONDAY

1. **Prehab 15, 15 Minutes**
   All Prehab 15 Drills (pp. 35–48)
2. **Warrior Warmup, 20 Minutes**
   All Stationary Warmup Drills (pp. 43–48) in *Training for Warriors*) 2 sets of 10 reps All Movement Warmup Drills (pp. 48–50 in *Training for Warriors*) 2 sets of 20 yards All Muscle Activation Exercises (pp. 51–58 in *Training for Warriors*) 1 set of 8 reps (on each side if necessary)
3. **Metabolic Training, 25 Minutes**
   Category 2 Hurricane Best-Time Method (pp. 131–33)
4. **Core Training, 10 Minutes**
   Partner Medicine Ball Circuit (pp. 343–48)

WEDNESDAY

1. **Prehab 15, 15 Minutes**
   All Prehab 15 Drills (pp. 35–48)
2. **Warrior Warmup, 20 Minutes**
   All Mini Plyo Hops and Movement Drills (pp. 53–73) All TFW Hip Circuit (pp. 74–83) Upper-Body Band Routine (pp. 84–89)
3. **Metabolic Training, 25 Minutes**
   The Doubler for 2 sets (pp. 255–57) Dumbbell Shoulder Circuit for 2 sets (pp. 264–67)
4. **Core Training, 10 Minutes**
   Partner Core Drills Circuit (pp. 339–42)

FRIDAY

1. **Prehab 15, 15 Minutes**
   All Prehab 15 Drills (pp. 35–48)
2. **Warrior Warmup, 20 Minutes**
   All Stationary Warmup Drills (pp. 43–48) in *Training for Warriors*) 2 sets of 10 reps All Movement Warmup Drills (pp. 48–50 in *Training for Warriors*) 2 sets of 20 yards All Muscle Activation Exercises (pp. 51–58 in *Training for Warriors*) 1 set of 8 reps (on each side if necessary)
3. **Metabolic Training, 25 Minutes**
   Single Dumbbell Complex for 2 sets (pp. 176–81) The Burper Tabata for 1 set (p. 219) Sled Dragging 2 sets of each drag for 20 yards (pp. 288–90)
4. **Core Training, 10 Minutes**
   Advanced Stabilization Circuit (pp. 326–29)

WEEK 9

MONDAY

1. **Prehab 15, 15 Minutes**
   All Prehab 15 Drills (pp. 35–48)
2. **Warrior Warmup, 20 Minutes**
   All Mini Plyo Hops and Movement Drills (pp. 53–73) All TFW Hip Circuit (pp. 74–83) Upper-Body Band Routine (pp. 84–89)
3. **Metabolic Training, 25 Minutes**
   Category 3 Hurricane Work-to-Rest Method (pp. 134–36)
4. **Core Training, 10 Minutes**
   Regular Plank Circuit (pp. 306–8)

WEDNESDAY

1. **Prehab 15, 15 Minutes**
   All Prehab 15 Drills (pp. 35–48)
2. **Warrior Warmup, 20 Minutes**
   All Stationary Warmup Drills (pp. 43–48) in *Training for Warriors*) 2 sets of 10 reps All Movement Warmup Drills (pp. 48–50 in *Training for Warriors*) 2 sets of 20 yards All Muscle Activation Exercises (pp. 51–58 in *Training for Warriors*) 1 set of 8 reps (on each side if necessary)

3. **Metabolic Training, 25 Minutes**
   Sadiv Set Bench Press (p. 251) Advanced Pushup Circuit for 1 set (pp. 237–41) Chin-up Series for 2 sets (pp. 252–54)
4. **Core Training, 10 Minutes**
   Pushup Plank Circuit (pp. 309–12)

FRIDAY

1. **Prehab 15, 15 Minutes**
   All Prehab 15 Drills (pp. 35–48)
2. **Warrior Warmup, 20 Minutes**
   All Mini Plyo Hops and Movement Drills (pp. 53–73) All TFW Hip Circuit (pp. 74–83) Upper-Body Band Routine (pp. 84–89)
3. **Metabolic Training, 25 Minutes**
   Sadiv Set Deadlift (p. 250) 80 Rep Circuit for 2 sets (pp. 220–23)
4. **Core Training, 10 Minutes**
   Med Ball Plank Circuit (pp. 312–14)

WEEK 10

MONDAY

1. **Prehab 15, 15 Minutes**
   All Prehab 15 Drills (pp. 35–48)
2. **Warrior Warmup, 20 Minutes**
   All Stationary Warmup Drills (pp. 43–48) in *Training for Warriors*) 2 sets of 10 reps All Movement Warmup Drills (pp. 48–50 in *Training for Warriors*) 2 sets of 20 yards All Muscle Activation Exercises (pp. 51–58 in *Training for Warriors*) 1 set of 8 reps (on each side if necessary)
3. **Metabolic Training, 25 Minutes**
   Category 3 Hurricane Best-Time Method (pp. 134–36)
4. **Core Training, 10 Minutes**
   Elevated Plank Circuit (pp. 315–16)

WEDNESDAY

1. **Prehab 15, 15 Minutes**
   All Prehab 15 Drills (pp. 35–48)
2. **Warrior Warmup, 20 Minutes**
   All Mini Plyo Hops and Movement Drills (pp. 53–73) All TFW Hip Circuit (pp. 74–83) Upper-Body Band Routine (pp. 84–89)
3. **Metabolic Training, 25 Minutes**
   Sadiv Set Bench Press (p. 250) Advanced Pushup Circuit for 1 set (pp. 237–41) Chin-up Series for 2 sets (pp. 252–54)
4. **Core Training, 10 Minutes**
   Obliques Circuit (pp. 330–34)

FRIDAY

1. **Prehab 15, 15 Minutes**
   All Prehab 15 Drills (pp. 35–48)
2. **Warrior Warmup, 20 Minutes**
   All Stationary Warmup Drills (pp. 43–48) in *Training for Warriors*) 2 sets of 10 reps All Movement Warmup Drills (pp. 48–50 in *Training for Warriors*) 2 sets of 20 yards All Muscle Activation Exercises (pp. 51–58 in *Training for Warriors*) 1 set of 8 reps (on each side if necessary)
3. **Metabolic Training, 25 Minutes**
   Sadiv Set Deadlift (p. 250) 80 Rep Circuit for 2 sets (pp. 220–23)
4. **Core Training, 10 Minutes**
   Hip Flexor Circuit (pp. 335–38)

WEEK 11

MONDAY

1. **Prehab 15, 15 Minutes**
   All Prehab 15 Drills (pp. 35–48)
2. **Warrior Warmup, 20 Minutes**
   All Mini Plyo Hops and Movement Drills (pp. 53–73) All TFW Hip Circuit (pp. 74–83) Upper-Body Band Routine (pp. 84–89)
3. **Metabolic Training, 25 Minutes**
   Category 4 Hurricane Work-to-Rest Method (pp. 137–39)
4. **Core Training, 10 Minutes**
   Swiss Ball Plank Circuit (pp. 317–19)

WEDNESDAY

1. **Prehab 15, 15 Minutes**
   All Prehab 15 Drills (pp. 35-48)
2. **Warrior Warmup, 20 Minutes**
   All Stationary Warmup Drills (pp. 43-48) in *Training for Warriors*) 2 sets of 10 reps All Movement Warmup Drills (pp. 48-50 in *Training for Warriors*) 2 sets of 20 yards All Muscle Activation Exercises (pp. 51-58 in *Training for Warriors*) 1 set of 8 reps (on each side if necessary)
3. **Metabolic Training, 25 Minutes**
   Full-Body Hundred Challenge #1 for 1 set (pp. 269-72) The Gauntlet for 2 sets (pp. 258-63)
4. **Core Training, 10 Minutes**
   Side Plank Circuit (pp. 319-21)

FRIDAY

1. **Prehab 15, 15 Minutes**
   All Prehab 15 Drills (pp. 35-48)
2. **Warrior Warmup, 20 Minutes**
   All Mini Plyo Hops and Movement Drills (pp. 53-73) All TFW Hip Circuit (pp. 74-83) Upper-Body Band Routine (pp. 84-89)
3. **Metabolic Training, 25 Minutes**
   Lower-Body Barbell Complex for 2 sets (pp. 145-47) Four-Way Lunge Circuit for 1 set (pp. 233-35)
4. **Core Training, 10 Minutes**
   Elevated Side Plank Circuit (pp. 322-25)

WEEK 12

The Warrior 7 Performance Evaluation Tests

MONDAY

1. **Prehab 15, 15 Minutes**
   All Prehab 15 Drills (pp. 35-48)
2. **Warrior Warmup, 20 Minutes**
   All Stationary Warmup Drills (pp. 43-48) in *Training for Warriors*) 2 sets of 10 reps All Movement Warmup Drills (pp. 48-50 in *Training for Warriors*) 2 sets of 20 yards All Muscle Activation Exercises (pp. 51-58 in *Training for Warriors*) 1 set of 8 reps (on each side if necessary)
3. **Metabolic Training, 25 Minutes**
   Category 4 Hurricane Best-Time Method (pp. 137-39)
4. **Core Training, 10 Minutes**
   Partner Medicine Ball Circuit (pp. 343-48)

WEDNESDAY

1. **Prehab 15, 15 Minutes**
   All Prehab 15 Drills (pp. 35-48)
2. **Warrior Warmup, 20 Minutes**
   All Mini Plyo Hops and Movement Drills (pp. 53-73) All TFW Hip Circuit (pp. 74-83) Upper-Body Band Routine (pp. 84-89)
3. **Metabolic Training, 25 Minutes**
   Sadiv Set Terrible 275s for 2 sets (p. 252) Dumbbell Shoulder Circuit for 2 sets (pp. 264-67)
4. **Core Training, 10 Minutes**
   Partner Core Drills Circuit (pp. 339-42)

FRIDAY

1. **Prehab 15, 15 Minutes**
   All Prehab 15 Drills (pp. 35-48)
2. **Warrior Warmup, 20 Minutes**
   All Stationary Warmup Drills (pp. 43-48) in *Training for Warriors*) 2 sets of 10 reps All Movement Warmup Drills (pp. 48-50 in *Training for Warriors*) 2 sets of 20 yards All Muscle Activation Exercises (pp. 51-58 in *Training for Warriors*) 1 set of 8 reps (on each side if necessary)
3. **Metabolic Training, 25 Minutes**
   10-Exercise Barbell Complex for 3 sets (pp. 157-66)
4. **Core Training, 10 Minutes**
   Advanced Stabilization Circuit (pp. 326-29)

ACKNOWLEDGMENTS

In life, we are all simply at some level of ignorance about everything. After every event in which my athletes compete, I have developed a habit of not being caught up in the celebration and immediately search for how things could have been even better or what the lessons were to enhance our next performance. I have learned to become as critical of victories as I am of losses, and I believe this helps me to be a better coach and helps our athletes constantly push toward personal improvement. I employed this strategy as I reflected on the success of the first two *Training for Warriors* books, and I received a profound lesson that I believe most people miss in life: "It is not what you know that can hurt you, it is what you don't know you don't know that is truly dangerous!"

This book is my response to that lesson. After going through my previous books, I realized that there was still much I did not cover about the metabolic aspect of the TFW system—partly because I didn't know everything about it! So instead of staying in my comfort zone, I stepped into areas I knew less about. Writing this book reinforced for me that you must focus less on what you know, and start finding out about things that you know you don't know. In order to find out what I didn't know, I had to seek out the people who knew more than I did. I believe that you must surround yourself with people who will expose you to new ideas and push you to explore areas in which you are less knowledgeable. This process is critical for growth and success. The following is a list of the people who have done this for me.

First, I want to thank all the fans of TFW who helped give direction to this book. With the explosion of social media, I was able to poll tens of thousands of people about what they wanted. They showed me again that when it came to what others wanted, I didn't know what I didn't know. This book was my answer to them.

I would like to thank John Berardi. Over the years, John has had a major influence on my own personal dietary philosophy and practice. As one of his biggest fans, I was honored to have him contribute his time and knowledge to this book. He reminded me again that if you don't ask for what you want, you won't get what you want. I also want to thank his team of superwriters, Nate Green and Krista Scott-Dixon, for helping with this aspect of the book. Nate and I have worked on a number of projects together and it was fantastic to do one more.

I would like to thank Dr. Anthony Caterisano. Dr. Caterisano and I first met in a weight room when I was 18 years old, and he has been a great mentor since. To have him on board with the project was special for me, and I think there was no better example of a person who practices what he preaches to use for the science portion of the book.

I would like to thank my editor, Stephanie Meyers, for believing in my ideas and always reminding me that if someone is going to write a great training book, it might as well be me. Now on our third book together, Stephanie is still as upbeat and energetic as she was on the first and has always trusted my concepts as much as I trust her grammar.

Special thanks to the photographer extraordinaire, Lucas Noonan. Lucas has shot all of my TFW books, and I couldn't imagine a better and more patient photographer to work with. He has always gone the extra mile to get the shots we need, and without his photos, the books would all be lifeless and hard to comprehend. Additional thanks to photographers Tom Miles and Petri Litmanen.

The biggest thanks go to my loving and supportive family. First, I must thank my beautiful wife, Amanda. Without her help taking care of all the things I either hate to do or am no good at, I would never have found the time to complete this book. They say behind every great man is an even greater woman. In my case, it is surely true. Also thanks to my three little warrior princesses: Sofia, Kristina, and Keira. I know there were late nights working on this book that caused me to miss time with them, and it is my hope that this book someday affords me the opportunity to get that time back. Thanks to my parents, Martin and Jeanne, and my sister, Kim, for giving me the initial direction and support to have made all of my work possible. Also big thanks to Roger and Michelle Love for holding down the "Rooney Fort" when I traveled for this book and other projects.

Finally, I must thank all the warriors who have helped me develop my system and myself. These are the real people behind TFW:

Ricardo Almeida, Renzo Gracie, Matt Serra, Bill Parisi, Sheikh Tahnoon Bin Zayed Al Nahyan, Barry Friedberg, Fernando Almeida, Rolles Gracie, Igor Gracie, Gregor Gracie, Kyra Gracie, Flavio Almeida, Gordo Correa, Gordinho Correa, Alvaro Romano, Luca Atalla, Nik Fekete, Delson Heleno, Marcio Feitosa, Scott Goodale, Shintaro Higashi, Michal Glogowski, Joe Sampieri, Jamie Crowder, Florina Petcu, Brendan Weafer, Jamal Patterson, Greg Gutman, Shihan Kai Leung, Gene Dunn, Sensei Yoichiro Matsumura, Sean Williams, Rodrigo Gracie, Bruno Fernandez, Oliver Worm, Erik Piispa, Rodrigo Gracie, Sean Alvarez, John Rallo, Rafaello Oliveira, Sabina Skala, Kimberly Root, Max McGarr, Roger Gracie, Braulio Estima, Forrest Griffin, Rich Thurston, Keith Gallas, Dan Payne, Charlie Hoffhine, Scott Altizer, Bill Scarola, Larry Bock, Jim Naugle, John Derent, Jim Miller, Dan Miller, Frankie Edgar, Alan Teo, Sean Santella, Chris Ligouri, Vitor "Shaolin" Riberio, Gianni Grippo, Alberto Marchetti, Mark Leeling, Mark Colangelo, Celita Schutz, Ron Hackaspker, Rich Sadiv, John Annillo, Heather Campanile, Glen Tobias, Rafael "Sapo" Nadal, Daniel Gracie, Peter Lawson, Nieman Gracie, Mike Constantino, Joe Camacho, Richie Mendoza, Neil Wolfson, Todd Hays, Teimoc Johnston-Ono,

Jimmy and Anthony Vennitti, Arthur Canario, Aziz Bendriss, Joe Kenn, Dave Maver, Carl Masaro, Stan Skolfield, Kenny Munson, Vinny Amarino, Pat Hade, Sam Caucci, Diego Baca, Rich Myers, Adam Singer, Fabio Leopoldo, Kazou Misaki, Matt Kreiger, Matt Simms, Dr. Rob Gilbert, Harrison Bernstein, Pat Gray, Kelly Gray, John Annillo, Josh Lehman, Oliver Blanchard, Brian Toal, Henrik Affe, Brian Saxton, Chris Olsen, Chris Poirier, Phil Dozois, Nick Peet, Adam Bornstein, Jim Casey, Nate Green, Bryan Krahn, Charlie Brenneman, Nick Barringer, John Derent, Steven Haase, Joel Snape, Robert Ihlenfeldt, Rannoch Donald, Max Belpulsi, Sean Hyson, Tom Miles, Petri Litmanen, James Jankiewicz, Charles Staley, Sal Alosi, Jerry Palmieri, Antti Nurmi, Tommi Paavola, Lealon Gammel, Colton Brown, Matt Murphy, Keith Mills, Mike Holmgren, and Adam Korn.

ABOUT THE AUTHOR

MARTIN ROONEY, MHS, PT, CSCS

Martin Rooney is an internationally recognized fitness expert and creator of the Training for Warriors system. He holds a Master of Health Science and Bachelor of Physical Therapy from the Medical University of South Carolina and a Bachelor of Arts in Exercise Science from Furman University. Rooney is a former member of the United States Bobsled team, is a four-time All Conference and MVP performer in track and field at Furman, holds a purple belt in Brazilian Jiu Jitsu and a black belt in Kodokan Judo, and currently holds seven WNPF New Jersey State records in Powerlifting.

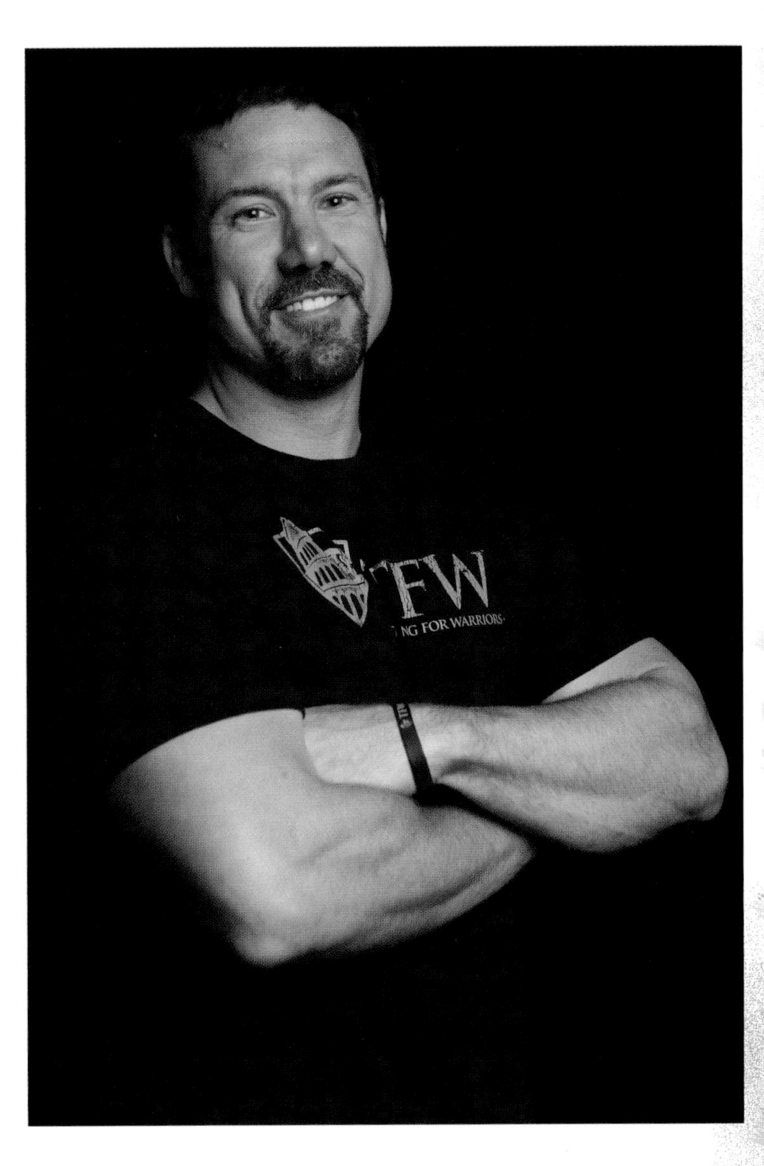

During his career, Rooney has trained thousands of people ranging from UFC champion fighters to Olympic medalists to hundreds of professional and Division I college athletes. Rooney has also served as the martial arts trainer for the New York Jets and the New York Giants and has worked with the physical instructors of the Army Rangers. He regularly lectures and consults around the world for Fortune 500 companies, major universities, professional sports teams, and fitness organizations. Rooney has been on the editorial council for *Gracie Magazine* and is a regular contributor to *Men's Health*, *Men's Fitness*, and *FIGHT!* magazines, as well as websites including Tmuscle.com and LiveStrong.com. His work has also been featured on or in ESPN, Spike TV, Fox Sports Net, HDnet, the NFL Network, and Sirius Satellite Radio, and in the *New York Times*, *USA Today*, *Sporting News*, *Muscle and Fitness*, *Men's Journal*, *Sports Illustrated for Kids*, *Stack Magazine*, and *Fighters Only*.

Currently, Rooney is the Chief Operating Officer of the Parisi Speed School, which has more than seventy-five franchises in twenty-eight states across the country and one in Europe. at the Speed School, Rooney developed one of the top NFL Combine training programs in the country, producing the fastest athlete at the 2001, 2004, 2005, 2006, and 2011 NFL Combine, and 133 athletes Martin trained have been drafted to the NFL.

Rooney is the author of *Train to Win*, *Training for Warriors*, and *Ultimate Warrior Workouts*. He lives in Fair Lawn, New Jersey with his wife, Amanda, and their three daughters, Sofia, Kristina, and Keira.

For more information on the Training for Warriors program, or information on upcoming seminars or Training for Warriors Certification events, please go to www.trainingforwarriors.com, and www.youtube.com/TFWarriors1. You can also follow Martin on Facebook and Twitter at martinrooney1 or check out his bestselling "Push-Up Warrior" app at www.trainingforwarriorsapps.com.

ABOUT THE CONTRIBUTORS

TONY CATERISANO, PHD, FACSM

Dr. Tony Caterisano has spent the last twenty-seven years as a Professor of Exercise Physiology in the Department of Health Sciences at Furman University in Greenville, South Carolina. He coauthored a book on strength and conditioning for football with Virginia Tech Head Strength coach Dr. Mike Gentry (*A Chance to Win: A Complete Guide to Physical Training for Football*, Sports Publishing, Champaign, Ill., 2004).

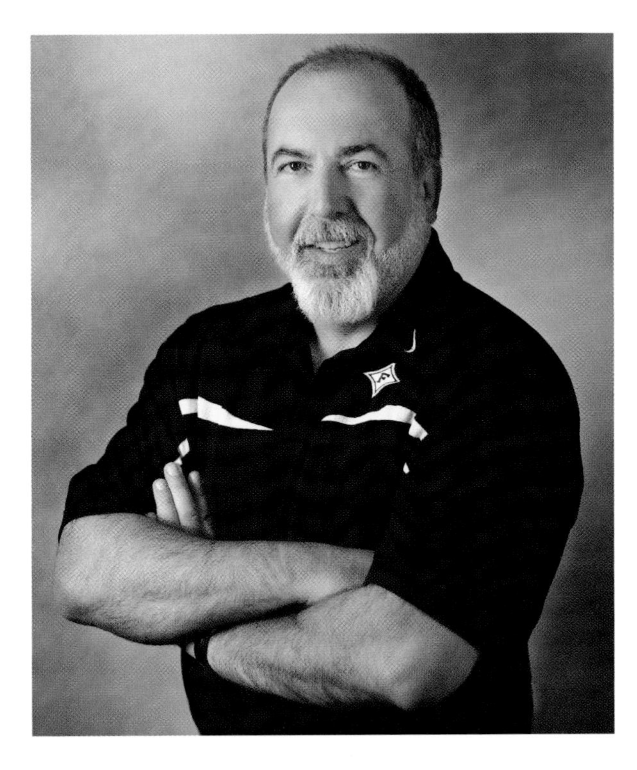

Dr. Caterisano has presented and published dozens of research papers focusing on exercise and resistance training. This includes presentations at the American College of Sports Medicine (ACSM) and National Strength and Conditioning Association (NSCA) national meetings, and publications in such journals as the *Journal of Strength and Conditioning Research*, *American Journal of Sports Medicine*, *Medicine and Science in Sports and Exercise*, and *Journal of Sports Medicine and Physical Fitness*. He has served on the editorial boards of the *Journal of Strength and Conditioning Research* and *Strength and Conditioning Journal* (both of which are official journals of the NSCA). He has also been a reviewer for such journals as *Medicine and Science in Sports and Exercise* and the *British Journal of Sports Medicine*. In addition, he serves on the written examination board of the College Strength and Conditioning Coaches Association (CSCCA). In 2001, Dr. Caterisano was awarded Fellow status in the American College of Sports Medicine.

Dr. Caterisano earned his bachelor's degree from the State University of New York–Brockport in 1974, and his master's degree from the the University of Connecticut in 1979. He spent a year at the University of North Carolina–Chapel Hill in pre-doctoral study in 1980 and completed his doctorate in Exercise Physiology at the University of Connecticut in 1984. He has been certified by the ACSM as an Exercise Test Technologist (ETT), and by the NSCA as a Certified Strength and Conditioning Specialist with Distinction (CSCS*D).

An avid powerlifter, Dr. Caterisano has competed in the World Natural Powerlifting Federation (WNPF) in the Masters 220-pound division, capturing fifteen straight South Carolina state titles as well as national and world titles in 2001, 2002, 2005, 2007, 2008, 2009, and 2010. In 2002 he won a gold medal in the World Championships in the drug-free World Natural Powerlifting Federation with a personal best 370-pound bench press. He has won six more world titles at WNPF World meets. At age 58, he continues to compete in master's-level powerlifting.

Dr. Caterisano also has an impressive résumé as a wrestling coach. He competed in both wrestling and judo at Brockport State in the early 1970s, rising to second-degree black belt in Judo. He has coached college wrestling since 1984, including seven years as an NCAA Division I head coach at Furman. During his tenure as a college wrestling coach, he has produced forty-seven national qualifiers and seven All-Americans. Currently he is coaching his son Mike at Wade Hampton High School in Greenville, South Carolina.

JOHN BERARDI

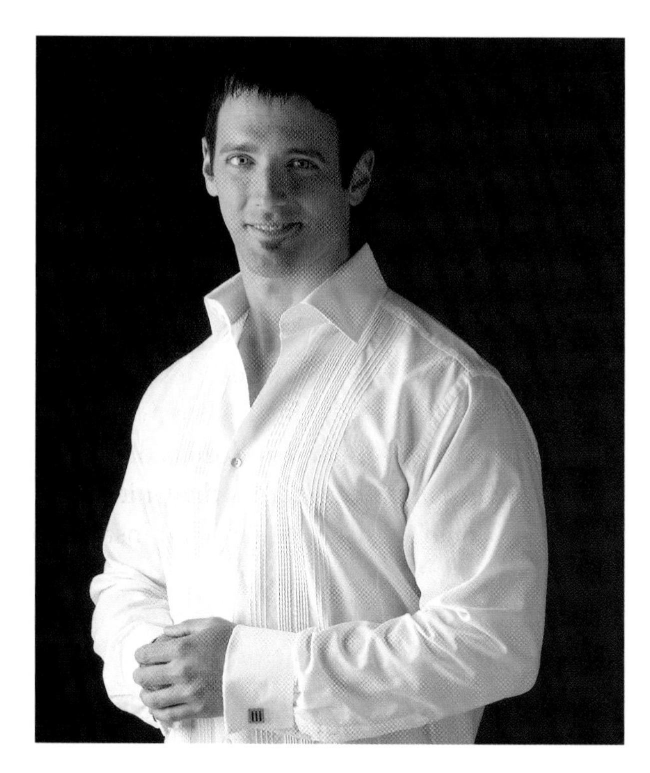

As an elite nutrition coach and exercise physiologist, Dr. Berardi has coached hundreds of elite amateur and professional athletes. In the last two Winter Olympics alone, his athletes collected more than twenty-five medals, twelve of them gold. He is a member of the Nike NFL High-Performance team and and has worked extensively with UFC welterweight champion Georges St. Pierre.

Furthermore, for the last three years, Dr. Berardi has acted as the director of the world's largest body transformation project. This one-of-a-kind fat-loss coaching program has produced more total weight loss than all eleven seasons of *The Biggest Loser* combined. Dr. Berardi received his PhD in Exercise Physiology and Nutrient Biochemistry at the University of Western Ontario, Canada. He is currently an adjunct professor at Eastern Michigan University and the University of Texas.

John Berardi, Nate Green, and Krista Scott-Dixon are all part of the Precision Nutrition team, a group of nutrition and exercise professionals dedicated to helping people look better, feel better, and perform at their highest potential. To learn more about eating for high performance or to participate in one of Dr. Berardi's free 5-day online nutrition courses, visit precisionnutrition.com.

LUCAS NOONAN, PHOTOGRAPHER

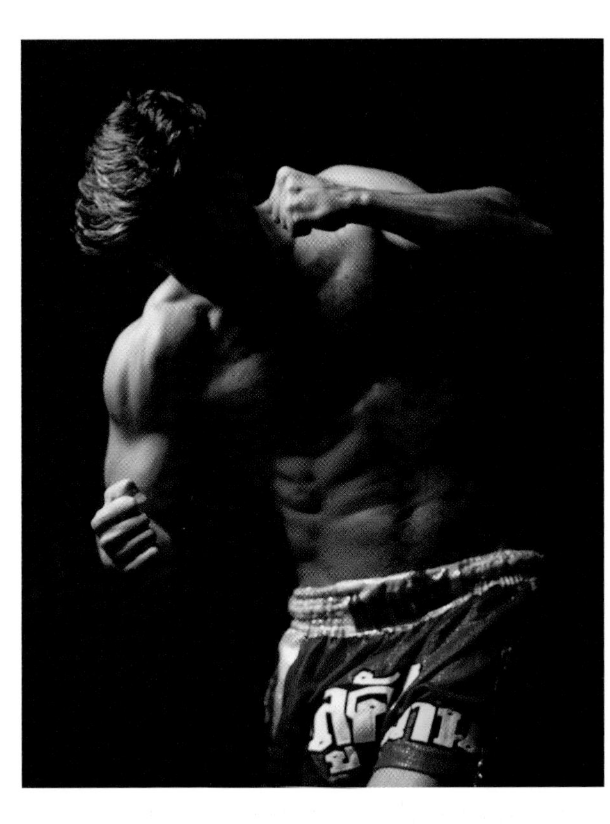

Lucas Noonan is an accomplished sport photographer with work featured in notable sport and fitness magazines including *Men's Health*, *Men's Fitness*, *Gracie Magazine*, *Muscle and Fitness!*, *Train Hard, Fight Easy*, and *Gong Magazine* of Japan. Noonan has shot on location in France, Italy, Ireland, Russia, Scotland, Holland, Brazil, Japan, Sweden, and Spain. He has also shot photos for the International Fight League, for Elite XC, and at dozens of Muay Thai and boxing events across the United States. Noonan is also a Muay Thai instructor at Renzo Gracie and a former Golden Gloves boxing competitor who trained directly under world-renowned trainer Freddie Roach at Wild Card Boxing Club in Hollywood, California.

He lives in New York City, and his work can be seen at lucasnoonan.com.

BOOKS BY MARTIN ROONEY

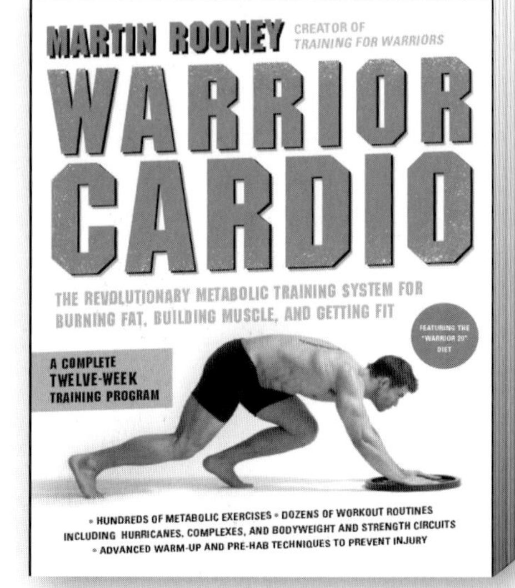

WARRIOR CARDIO

The Revolutionary Metabolic Training System for Burning Fat, Building Muscle, and Getting Fit

ISBN 978-0-06-207428-7 (paperback)

World-renowned fitness expert Martin Rooney delivers a complete, easy-to-follow twelve-week workout and diet plan for anyone looking to shed pounds of fat and increase muscle mass. *Warrior Cardio* is a comprehensive look at cardiovascular training using scientifically proven techniques, paired with a diet plan that delivers.

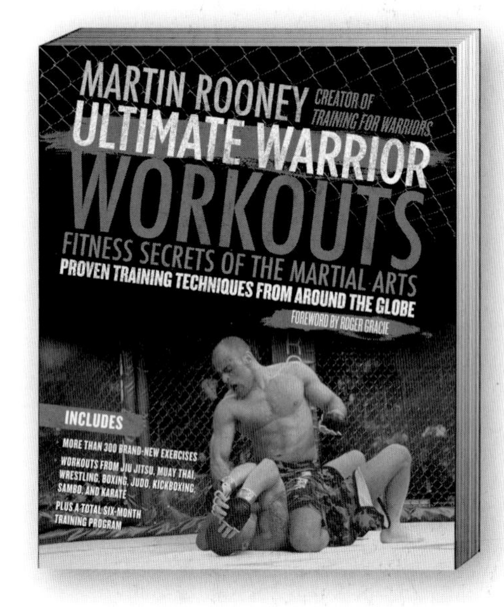

ULTIMATE WARRIOR WORKOUTS

Fitness Secrets of the Martial Arts

ISBN 978-0-06-173522-6 (paperback)

Martin Rooney travels to top-fight destinations around the globe to study and train under the last living masters in the eight core disciplines of Mixed Martial Arts. More than 1,000 full-color photos reveal hundreds of the original training schedules he discovered along the way, from the slopes of Japan's Mt. Fuji and the beaches of Brazil to the streets of Russia.

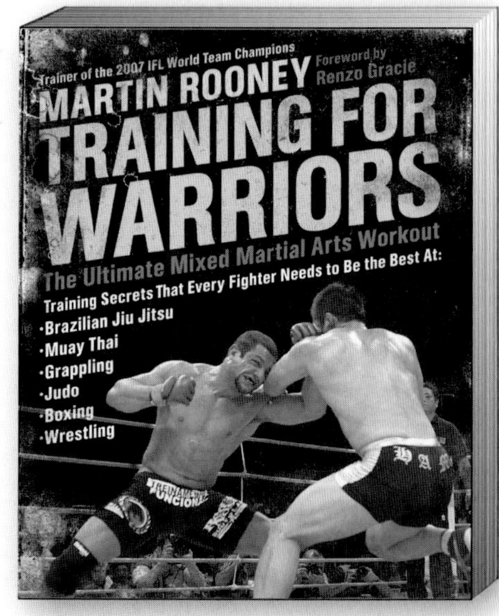

TRAINING FOR WARRIORS

The Ultimate Mixed Martial Arts Workout

ISBN 978-0-06-137433-3 (paperback)

Discover the training secrets that have produced World Champions in MMA, Submission Grappling, Brazilian Jiu Jitsu, and Judo. *Training for Warriors* offers more than 750 color photos that show you how to perform hundreds of exercises designed to specifically target each area of your body and get you fit for whatever battle life throws at you.